CARING FOR LGBTQ2S PEOPLE

A Clinical Guide

Increasing awareness of healthcare disparities and unique health needs of LGBTQ2S people calls for a revitalization of health professional training programs. As new topics become integrated into these programs, there is a great need for a comprehensive resource that aligns with Canadian guidelines and standards of care.

Caring for LGBTQ2S People identifies gaps in care and health care disparities, and provides clinicians with both the knowledge and the tools to continue to improve the health of LGBTQ2S people. Written by expert authors, this fully updated version builds on the critically praised first edition and highlights the significant social, medical, and legal progress that has occurred in Canada since 2003. The book includes general medical information and guidance that is useful for anyone providing care to LGBTQ2S people. Chapters in this edition provide background on the fundamentals of language, cultural competency, and the patient-provider relationship, and include contemporary and expanded discussion on STIs, HIV, substance use, mental health, fertility, and trans health. This clinical guide is written for a general and trainee-level reader in health care and primary care and showcases a comprehensive understanding of LGBTQ2S health while also concluding with unique considerations for those who experience an intersection of diverse identities.

AMY BOURNS is a staff family physician at Sherbourne Health, program director at LGBTQ2S Enhanced Skills Residency Program, and adjunct lecturer in the Department of Family and Community Medicine at the University of Toronto.

EDWARD KUCHARSKI is a family physician at the South East Toronto Family Health Team, chief medical officer at Casey House, and an assistant professor in the Department of Family and Community Medicine at the University of Toronto.

ALLAN PETERKIN is a professor of psychiatry and family medicine at the University of Toronto, where he heads the Program in Health, Arts and Humanities.

CATHY RISDON is a professor and chair in the Department of Family Medicine at McMaster University.

Praise for the First Edition

"With this clinical guide, psychiatrist Allan Peterkin and family physician Cathy Risdon have made an outstanding contribution to the global literature on gay and lesbian health. Anchored solidly in scientific literature and well supported by references, the text is remarkably practical."

CMAJ

"The book is a welcome contribution in a field with few resources, especially for the practitioner who wants to provide the best possible care for the lesbian or gay patient."

JAMA

Caring for LGBTQ2S People

A Clinical Guide

SECOND EDITION

EDITED BY AMY BOURNS
AND EDWARD KUCHARSKI

WITH ALLAN PETERKIN
AND CATHY RISDON

UNIVERSITY OF TORONTO PRESS
Toronto Buffalo London

© University of Toronto Press 2022
Toronto Buffalo London
utorontopress.com

ISBN 978-1-4875-0239-3 (cloth)   ISBN 978-1-4875-1525-6 (EPUB)
ISBN 978-1-4875-2197-4 (paper)   ISBN 978-1-4875-1524-9 (PDF)

Library and Archives Canada Cataloguing in Publication
Title: Caring for LGBTQ2S people : a clinical guide / edited by Amy Bourns and Edward Kucharski with Allan Peterkin and Cathy Risdon.
Names: Bourns, Amy, editor. | Kucharski, Edward, editor. | Peterkin, Allan, editor. | Risdon, Cathy, editor.
Description: Second edition. | Previously published as: Peterkin, Allan. Caring for lesbian and gay people. Toronto; Buffalo: University of Toronto Press, 2003.
Identifiers: Canadiana (print) 20220160023 | Canadiana (ebook) 20220160228 | ISBN 9781487502393 (hardcover) | ISBN 9781487521974 (softcover) | ISBN 9781487515256 (EPUB) | ISBN 9781487515249 (PDF)
Subjects: LCSH: Gays – Medical care. | LCSH: Lesbians – Medical care. | LCSH: Gays – Health and hygiene. | LCSH: Lesbians – Health and hygiene.
Classification: LCC RA564.9.H65 C37 2022 | DDC 362.1086/64 – dc23

We welcome comments and suggestions regarding any aspect of our publications – please feel free to contact us at news@utorontopress.com or visit us at utorontopress.com.

Every effort has been made to contact copyright holders; in the event of an error or omission, please notify the publisher.

We wish to acknowledge the land on which the University of Toronto Press operates. This land is the traditional territory of the Wendat, the Anishnaabeg, the Haudenosaunee, the Métis, and the Mississaugas of the Credit First Nation.

University of Toronto Press acknowledges the financial support of the Government of Canada and the Ontario Arts Council, an agency of the Government of Ontario, for its publishing activities.

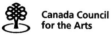

Canada Council   Conseil des Arts
for the Arts   du Canada

ONTARIO ARTS COUNCIL
CONSEIL DES ARTS DE L'ONTARIO
an Ontario government agency
un organisme du gouvernement de l'Ontario

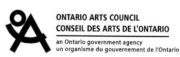

Funded by the   Financé par le
Government   gouvernement
of Canada   du Canada

Canadä

Contents

Figures, Tables, and Boxes

Figures

Tables

Boxes

Foreword

When we published *Caring for Lesbian and Gay People: A Clinical Guide* in 2003, it was the only comprehensive medical textbook of its kind covering the physical and mental health issues faced by sexual minorities. One of its key emphases was how health care providers could improve communication and deepen trust with their queer patients across their entire lifespan, while advocating for better education around the specific needs of these populations. Since then, so much has happened socially, politically, and in health care around human sexuality and gender identity. The editors of this new edition – Amy Bourns and Ed Kucharski – have been at the forefront of many of these changes, creating new international standards of care for trans patients and serving as 2SLGBTQ Leads in the Faculty of Medicine at the University of Toronto (a new and welcome trend in clinical education).

We are happy to pass the editorial torch to Amy and Ed and to the authors they have selected to write new chapters and to provide state-of-the-art clinical updates.

Let's consider some of the key trends, changes, and challenges faced by our patients and their families over the last several years:

- the advance of 2SLGBTQ marriage rights and the emergence of 2SLGBTQ divorce
- advances in trans health care and awareness
- asexuality/asexuals
- ASOs (AIDS service organizations) rebranding as gay men's health units
- awareness of Indigenous health, barriers, and disparities
- the bar culture (the changing landscape in favour of online connections/virtual communities)
- Black Lives Matter/critical race theory

- capital punishment of gay men in certain countries
- co-parenting (new, non-spousal collaborations)
- COVID-19 pandemic
- the criminalization/de-criminalization debates and legal decisions around HIV disclosure/transmission
- crystal meth use with online "Party and Play" communities
- cyberbullying (and ongoing forms of discrimination, harassment, and homophobic/transphobic violence)
- the disappearance of print media in the 2SLGBTQ press
- expansion of areas of prevention (for example, the HPV vaccine)
- Facebook, Twitter, and other social media
- HIV advances in care, undetectable = untransmissable
- improved support and access for transition-related surgeries
- increased awareness of suicide risk, particularly in trans populations
- increased visibility of polyamory
- increasing prevalence of STIs and multi-drug resistance
- location-based social networking and dating platforms such as Grindr, Scruff
- the #MeToo movement
- the opioid crisis
- people coming out earlier (preteen/teen)
- populism as a worldwide political phenomenon, with renewed targeting of sexual and gender minorities
- porn (ubiquitous/free/online) and its impact on sexual behaviour/development/self-esteem
- pre-exposure prophylaxis for HIV
- the Pride movement evolution, as well as criticism and backlash
- pronoun awareness
- surrogacy options in fertility/family planning
- texting/sexting and impacts on privacy and safety
- 2SLGBTQ parenting options/rights (including choices about birth parent registration)
- virtual health care

The chapters that follow will explore many of these themes and how they affect our patients' perceptions of health, identity, community, belonging, and safety. While many 2SLGBTQ civil rights and freedoms have been advanced, we now see the open questioning, devaluing, and devolution of others worldwide. Teaching around culturally appropriate health care standards for sexual and gender minorities remains inconsistent in medical schools and other clinical faculties across North America.

Ready access to attuned, person-centred care and to new treatment protocols remains a problem for many of our patients.

We're reminded of a famous quote: "Eternal vigilance is the price of liberty."

A book like this reminds us that health care is always both personal and political and that ongoing advocacy remains a large part of what caring for our patients requires.

The chapters that follow are authored by experts and champions across professional disciplines and provide a wonderful balance of tips, strategies, protocols, and points of reflection and provocation.

The stories of all the people they have served inform every page and will help to remind us all why we have chosen the work we do and why we care so deeply about it.

Allan Peterkin MD
Cathy Risdon MD

Authors of *Caring for Lesbian and Gay People: A Clinical Guide*
(first edition)

Acknowledgments

We acknowledge that much of this book was written on the sacred land and traditional territories of many Indigenous people and are grateful for the opportunity to think, learn, write, and teach in these communities and territories.

A sincere thank you to our brilliant chapter authors. We are so pleased you embarked on this journey with us! Your expertise and lived experience have added a richness to this text that would not have been possible without you.

We would also like to thank our families for their support: Janet, Mackenzie, and Bryan. There were many weekends, evenings, and summer breaks that were punctuated with this work and we are forever grateful for your patience with us and this project.

Marieclaire White, David McLay, Jen Cutts, Meg Patterson, Leah Connor – without you we would not have been able to move this book forward.

Finally, this book, and our knowledge, are built upon many inspiring people around us and who may have preceded us: Leslie Shanks, Kate Greenaway, Rebecca Hamond, Gail Knudson, Trevor Corneil, Nick Gorton, Maddie Deutsch, Ray Fung, Marcus Law, David McKnight, St. Michael's Hospital Academic Family Health Team, and Sherbourne Health.

Thank you!
Amy and Ed

CARING FOR LGBTQ2S PEOPLE

A Clinical Guide

1 Why a Clinical Guide?

AMY BOURNS AND EDWARD KUCHARSKI

Introduction

When *Caring for Lesbian and Gay People: A Clinical Guide* was first published in 2003, it was the only comprehensive Canadian clinical resource for the 2SLGBTQ (Two-Spirit, lesbian, gay, bisexual, transgender, and queer) community and their health care providers. Since its publication, the text has remained one of only a handful of such resources available globally. While much of the original text remains highly relevant, there have been significant sociocultural and biomedical advances over the past several years pertinent to 2SLGBTQ health, including substantial progression in social acceptance, an evolution of language, changes in legislation, and a slowly growing body of research to support fundamental changes to evidence-based practice. With this update, we aim to provide a current, cohesive, and practical clinical guide to caring for 2SLGBTQ Canadians.

There has been a significant amount of social and political progress in Canada in relation to the rights and freedoms of 2SLGBTQ people. With nationwide marriage equality, inclusion in federal, provincial, and territorial human rights codes, and the growing acceptance of 2SLGBTQ people as part of our diverse landscape, Canada has frequently been referred to as one of the most 2SLGBTQ-friendly countries in the world. It has become the norm for our political leaders to march in Pride celebrations alongside 2SLGBTQ community members. A certain maturity for 2SLGBTQ rights and freedoms is now present in Canada.

At the same time, Canada's post-colonial history of criminalization and psychopathologization of same-sex sexual activity and gender non-conformity continues to leave its mark on the health of our 2SLGBTQ populations. Specifically, the effects of negative societal attitudes, stigma, and discrimination continue to significantly impact health outcomes for 2SLGBTQ people.

Consequently, in 2016 Prime Minister Justin Trudeau announced the appointment of a special advisor on 2SLGBTQ issues to assist in the government's efforts to address these inequities. Following this appointment, the Government of Canada acknowledged discriminatory practices in the federal public service, Canadian Armed Forces, and the Royal Canadian Mounted Police. A formal apology by Prime Minister Justin Trudeau was delivered on 28 November 2017 and outlined

- compensation and expungement of charges for those affected by the government's practices
- access to employment documents and notation in the files of those wrongly dismissed because of historic injustices
- a national monument and travelling exhibits curated by the Canadian Museum of Human Rights to reconcile and memorialize past wrongs[1]

Similarly, Canadian health care–related organizations and systems, including hospitals, are taking an equity approach to the support and inclusion of 2SLGBTQ patients, clients, and staff. Many such organizations have 2SLGBTQ committees, support or offer Pride events, and have developed diversity strategies. However, as in the case of broader society, there remains much work to be done in that many 2SLGBTQ patients continue to feel stigmatized in health care,[2–4] and the transgender community in particular remains one of the most vulnerable and poorly serviced groups of patients.[5] In addition, it is known that 2SLGBTQ people have different health-related concerns and behaviours that can increase their risks for certain conditions.

Programs at universities are increasingly recognizing the unique health needs of the diverse communities they serve. For example, the undergraduate medical school at the University of Toronto has prioritized diversity, appointing a chief diversity officer and faculty leadership in 2SLGBTQ, Black, and Indigenous health, as well as a lead for social justice, anti-oppression, and advocacy. Diversity is now regularly surveyed and expected to be protected and supported in health education by accrediting bodies.[6] Efforts are currently underway at several Canadian medical schools to incorporate curriculum on 2SLGBTQ health at the undergraduate level and during residency training. As 2SLGBTQ-relevant health topics become integrated into these training programs, there is a need for a contemporary resource that aligns with Canadian guidelines and standards of care.

While the original version of the text focused on gay and lesbian individuals, this text includes substantial content on the full spectrum of sexual orientation, gender identity, and gender expression, and explores unique considerations for those who experience an intersectionality of minority identities. Though our intention is to be as inclusive as possible, we have opted not to include discussion of intersex people (i.e., those who experience differences of sexual differentiation or DSDs)* in this expansion. While intersex people often experience the same harmful gender-normalizing social forces as 2SLGBTQ people, there are a number of unique aspects of the experiences and clinical care of intersex people that we feel are best addressed as a separate body of work. We encourage all readers to educate themselves on this topic through existing resources (see, e.g., Accord Alliance, http://www.accordalli ance.org).

For several reasons, which will be explored further in this text, there is a paucity of research specific to 2SLGBTQ health and related health outcomes. Although we will cite Canadian research whenever possible, it is often necessary to rely on studies from other parts of the world, the bulk of which are from the United States. US studies may not, however, accurately reflect the situation in Canada. For example, the lower rates of health care utilization because of the lack of health insurance found in US studies should not be the case in Canada, given the differences in the two countries' health care systems. Societal differences may also impair the application of American findings to the Canadian context.[7]

As is the limitation of all texts, this document does not represent an exhaustive review of the medical literature. We do not present this text as a clinical practice guideline but instead as a resource to help clinicians in their day-to-day practice. Clinicians must use their own expertise and decision-making skills within each clinical encounter. We encourage health care providers to consult other sources of information and seek peer support when needed. Of course, many research articles and guidelines have been reviewed to inform the recommendations in this text; however, some information reflects the opinions and experiences of medical experts and health researchers. We are very fortunate to have chapter contributions from leading experts practising in the diverse fields of 2SLGBTQ medicine and health research across Canada. Since many of the authors are themselves 2SLGBTQ-identified, their perspectives no doubt reflect their experiences as both

---

* Differences in sexual differentiation is used here in place of disorders in sexual differentiation as it is experienced as a less pathologizing term by those affected by DSDs.

providers and 2SLGBTQ community members. We believe this offers a richness to the text that is in keeping with including the voice of patients and families in planning and organizing their care. Readers are also encouraged to turn to collective works such as *The Remedy: Queer and Trans Voices on Health and Health Care*[8] and works that emerged from the arts and community-based Cancer's Margins project[9] to enrich their understanding of 2SLGBTQ communities and health.

Finally, this text was a multiyear project, and in the later stages of production, the COVID-19 pandemic arrived. During this time, many groups have been disproportionately affected by COVID-19, and no doubt this is true for many in the 2SLGBTQ community. We have noted some early information on COVID-19 in the chapters on sexual health and HIV, but we recognize that as this text is being published, research on COVID-19 is nascent. A full understanding of its interplay with 2SLGBTQ communities will be best captured in future editions.

Approach to This Text

Chapters 2 through 5 of this text present foundational knowledge, tools, and recommendations in optimizing an informed approach to care for 2SLGBTQ patients. In the middle, the reader will encounter chapters that are more densely clinical, covering topics including sexually transmitted infections (STIs), human immunodeficiency virus (HIV), substance abuse, reproductive health, and hormone therapy. While providers should be familiar with their content, the level of detail is designed to provide guidance to decision making as situations arise in clinical practice. Last, the final four new chapter topics covering unique considerations for 2SLGBTQ Indigenous people, older adults, disabled people, and newcomer populations by nature lend themselves to a more narrative style such that they are best read from beginning to end.

Language, Terms, and Definitions

The use of language regarding sexual orientation and gender identity is constantly evolving and seldom universally agreed upon. Over the past several years, there has been a proliferation of terms whose meanings may vary over time, and within and between disciplines. Settling with any terminology is bound to be imperfect. Reflecting this diversity of language, our contributing authors may use language and terminology that feels most appropriate to them.

To the extent possible, we have attempted to set out a common understanding of several of the core terms used throughout this text to describe people of varying sexual orientations and gender identities and their experiences. The glossary at the end of this book summarizes the meanings of several of these core terms as they are commonly understood within our current cultural context. As will be discussed in the following chapter, the key when working with patients is to use respectful and affirming language commensurate with a person's self-identification whenever possible.

For the most part throughout this text, we have elected to use the acronym 2SLGBTQ. It is not intended to exclusively represent those who identify as Two-Spirit, lesbian, gay, bisexual, transgender, and queer but to be inclusive of a larger community of sexual and gender minorities. Our intention is to be inclusive but also to have economy of language. We recognize this selection may not sit well with everyone.

The placement of "2S" at the beginning of the acronym is an emerging practice, reflecting the recognition of Two-Spirit Indigenous people as the first sexual and gender minority people in North America.*

Though the existence of sexual and gender minorities is ubiquitous among human populations, each culture has their own way of conceptualizing these characteristics within its social structure. Many cultures, including the traditional cultures of Canada's indigenous people, conceptualize sex and gender minorities differently. The health and well-being of Indigenous Canadians who identify as Two-Spirit or who otherwise differ in their gender identity, gender expression, or sexual orientation will be discussed in chapter 12.

Sex, Gender Identity, and Sexual Orientation

Colloquially, a person's *sex* and their *gender* are often used as interchangeable terms. Distinguishing sex from gender identity and understanding that they are independent of a person's sexual orientation is key to understanding the diversity of sexual and gender minorities.

Sex, in this context, refers specifically to a person's biological makeup and includes their genotypic sex (chromosomal makeup) and their phenotypic sex (primary and secondary sex characteristics). Gender identity, on the other hand, refers to a person's sense of themselves as a girl or woman, boy or man, both, neither, or somewhere in between. The word *gender* is more difficult to define but typically refers to culturally defined norms (behavioral, cultural, or psychological traits) commonly associated with one's sex.

Western society has traditionally conceived of sex and gender identity as a binary system – XX or XY, male or female, man or woman,

* We were unable to use this form of the acronym in the title of the book because of contractual obligations.

masculine or feminine. Sex is assigned to a person based on the appearance of their external genitalia at birth, and their gender identity is presumed to develop in alignment with their sex assigned at birth. When we take a closer look at the variation in human experiences of sex and gender, however, things are not so simple. One framework used to illustrate the diversity in sex, gender identity, and sexual orientation is shown in figure 1.1. Each horizontal line represents a spectrum: while most people fall at one end or the other, some people's experience is of being somewhere in between, spanning both, neither, or in flux.

As we can see, even basic biology thwarts the idea of a simple binary. While most people have sex chromosomes comprising XX or XY, and are born with female or male genitalia respectively, several variations can develop during the process of gametogenesis and fetal development. People with these variations may describe themselves as intersex or as having a DSD.

The conventional thinking also assumes that all females become girls/women and express femininity, while all males become boys/men and express masculinity. Again, this is not always the case. A person's gender identity may not align with the sex they were assigned at birth. *Transgender* (or *trans*) is an umbrella term used to describe people of this experience, while *cisgender* (or *cis*) describes people whose gender identity aligns with the sex they were assigned at birth. Throughout this text, we will use the prefix *cis-* rather than the terms *natal, biological*, or *genetic* to refer to non-trans people as these terms can imply that trans people have a less valid claim to their gender than do cis people.

The term *transgender man* or *trans man* refers to a person who was assigned female at birth but whose sense of self is of being a man. Similarly, the term *transgender woman* or *trans woman* refers to a person who was assigned male at birth but whose sense of self is of being a woman. The terms *transmasculine* and *transfeminine* are often used instead of trans man and trans woman to be inclusive of trans experiences that are less binary. The terms *FTM* (short for *female to male*) and *MTF* (short for *male to female*) have been used to refer to trans men and trans women, respectively, but are considered to be outdated terms in part because they conflate sex with gender identity and reinforce a binary conceptualization of gender. People may feel that their gender identity falls somewhere between the binary notions of man or woman, is both, is neither, or is in flux. Some terms that people may use to describe this experience are *genderqueer, gender fluid, pangender, agender*, or simply as *non-binary*. Of note, one criticism of the framework in figure 1.1 is that while it illustrates spectra, it remains anchored in an underlying binary and does not allow

Figure 1.1. Spectra of Sex, Gender, and Sexual Orientation

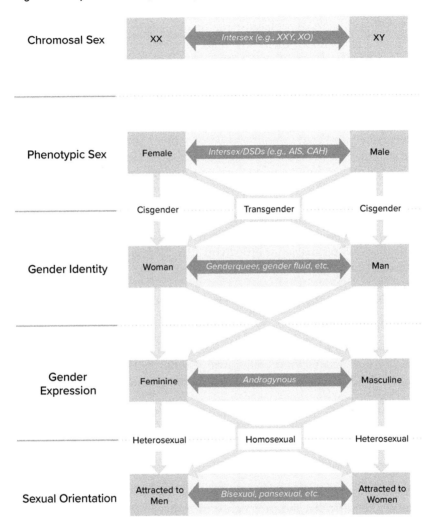

Source: Adapted from R. Hammond. Understanding sex and gender [dissertation]. 2005. Graphic design thanks to Kelly Speck.

a space for those who may present with contrasting masculine and feminine characteristics as part of a genuine expression of gender.

Differing from gender identity, gender expression refers to a person's outward presentation, including their physical appearance, clothing, and communication patterns, which express aspects of their gender identity or role. The terms *masculine, feminine,* and *androgynous* are often used to describe a person's gender expression. Gender expression is often related to but sometimes distinct from a person's gender identity. For example, some cis women or trans women may have a masculine presentation and may identify as *butch* while some cis men or trans men may have a feminine presentation and may identify as *femme*.

The figure can be extended further to illustrate that gender identity and gender expression are distinct from sexual orientation. People who are attracted to members of the opposite sex are considered *heterosexual*, while those attracted to the same sex are considered *homosexual*.* The term *bisexual* refers to those who are attracted to both sexes, while those who experience little to no attraction to anyone often identify as *asexual*.

Who Constitutes the 2SLGBTQ Population?

In his 1940s study, Alfred Kinsey estimated that 10 per cent of the US population was homosexual.[10] However, many researchers now question Kinsey's accuracy and cite lower estimates. The Canadian Community Health Survey completed in 2014 demonstrated the following:

- 1.7 per cent of Canadians ages 18 to 59 reported that they consider themselves to be homosexual (gay or lesbian).
- 1.3 per cent of Canadians ages 18 to 59 reported that they consider themselves to be bisexual.[11]

Unfortunately, this survey did not collect information about gender identity. Historically, the prevalence of transgender people has been thought to have been underestimated as surveys were completed at

---

* Trans PULSE was a multi-year community-based research initiative that used mixed methods to better understand the health of trans communities in Ontario. The core researchers have more recently acquired Canadian Institutes of Health Research (CIHR) funding to conduct a national study – an unparalleled opportunity to gather large-scale, robust data about the health of trans people across Canada. Preliminary findings can be found on the Trans PULSE Canada website: https://transpulsecanada.ca.

specialized gender clinics (precluding those not accessing care in those settings).[12] Contemporary estimates of the prevalence of transgender people in the United States are in the range of 0.5 to 0.6 per cent.[13,14]

There are many reasons why current data may underestimate the 2SLGBTQ population:

- reticence to disclose sensitive information to governments and/or researchers
- internalized trans-, bi-, and/or homophobia
- persons of non-conforming genders and/or orientations may not be given the opportunity to be included or may not be asked appropriately
- questions on surveys often only ask about how one identifies (which differs from attraction and/or behaviour in some individuals)
- mistrust by Indigenous people of governments because of mistreatment

Furthermore, many surveys do not include other demographic information (for example, socioeconomic status, household occupants) that would give a more complete picture of 2SLGBTQ communities.

Although the proportion of the population that is 2SLGBTQ may be smaller than originally thought (or perhaps underestimated), it is likely that physicians and other health care providers continue to underestimate the number of 2SLGBTQ patients they see in their practice.

The Health Needs of 2SLGBTQ People

Two reviews of the international literature previously prepared for Health Canada – *Access to Care*[15] and *Gay Health: Current Knowledge and Future Actions*[16] – demonstrated that gays and lesbians have specific health risks. More recently, two large-scale US reports from the Institute of Medicine and the US Department of Health and Human Services continue to support these findings.[17,18] Groups within the 2SLGBTQ community, are at a higher risk of sexually transmitted infections (including HIV), certain cancers (e.g., anal cancer), obesity, cardiovascular disease, substance misuse disorders, mental health disorders, and victimization by violent crime.

It is important to recognize that many of the health risks experienced by sexual and gender minorities can be attributed to the impact of living with stigma, discrimination, and prejudice, rather than to the inherent state of being 2SLGBTQ. Adapting Meyer's definition of minority stress to the full 2SLGBTQ spectrum, it may be thought of as the chronic psychological strain resulting from stigma and expectations of rejection and discrimination, decisions about disclosure of sexual orientation and/or gender identity, and the internalization of homophobia, biphobia and/or transphobia that 2SLGBTQ people face in a heteronormative, cissexist society.[19] Minority stress may be associated with the adoption of unhealthy behaviours such as smoking and excessive substance use to help cope with heteronormative and cisnormative stressors. Additionally, gender dysphoria may impact a person's relationship with their body and contribute to the development of unhealthy behaviours.[20]

Unfortunately, despite significant social progress, surveys of patient satisfaction with health care received by 2SLGBTQ people report high levels of dissatisfaction across health disciplines.[4,5] It appears that the comprehensive health needs of these populations are not being met. As a result, patients may fear and avoid traditional health care settings and may not be accessing appropriate care. Findings from the Canadian Community Health Survey demonstrate that gay, lesbian, and bisexual Canadians are less likely to have a regular medical doctor (compared to heterosexual peers) and are more likely to feel they needed health care in the past year but did not receive it.[7]

Factors That Affect the Quality of Care for 2SLGBTQ People

Lack of Knowledge and Education

Although 2SLGBTQ people have specific health needs and risks, health care providers across disciplines may be unaware of, or indifferent to, these needs and may have had minimal training in identifying or addressing them. An online questionnaire distributed to 176 medical schools in the United States and Canada demonstrated that medical student respondents

- rated their 2SLGBTQ curriculum as fair or worse 67 per cent of the time
- felt best prepared to care for those with HIV and other STIs
- felt least prepared to discuss hormone therapy and gender affirming surgery

Further focus groups in the same study showed that while medical students felt comfortable working with 2SLGBTQ patients, they did not feel fully prepared and felt the curriculum could be improved.[21]

In a related study, deans of the 150 medical schools in the United States and Canada reported the following:

- The median time dedicated to 2SLGBTQ health was 5 hours, with 9 schools reporting 0 hours.
- The 2SLGBTQ curricular content was rated as "fair" at 44 per cent of schools.[22]

Outside the training environment, a study of clinicians working with 2SLGBTQ youth in British Columbia demonstrated that many lacked cultural competency in caring for these patients, illustrated by both a lack of training and the use of unintentional heteronormative practices.[23] Similarly, a qualitative study involving 13 physicians across Ontario reported that barriers for transgender patients accessing care is multifactorial and called for inclusion of trans health issues in medical education.[24]

Lack of Standards of Care for 2SLGBTQ Patients

The lack of knowledge and training on 2SLGBTQ issues on the part of individual physicians is compounded by a paucity of evidence-based standards of care. McNair et al. found that the existing clinical guidelines for LGB people in primary care did not meet internationally recognized developmental rigour.[25] This is a result of the limited number and poor quality of 2SLGBTQ-specific research studies and the lack of relevant research to guide clinical practice and policymaking.

In 2003, the authors of the original text noted that lesbians and gay men in North America are noticeably absent from much of the reported research in clinical and public health and program evaluation literature, and there is very little research to inform our understanding about health care delivery and access. Unfortunately, this is still true as of 2022. However, we have now seen the inclusion of the LGB communities in the Canadian Community Health Survey, and the emergence of LGB-specific recommendations in mainstream clinical guidelines. For example, cervical cancer screening guidelines include recommendations for screening women who have sex with women and the National Advisory Committee on Immunizations issued a recommendation for all men who have sex with men to receive the human papilloma virus (HPV) vaccine.

A variety of factors affect the 2SLGBTQ health research agenda, including the following:

- Clinical trials, longitudinal cohorts, and population health studies fail to recognize and record sexual orientation as a unit of analysis. In the past, studies in the United States that attempted to do so may have been denied federal funding.
- Fear of stigmatization prevents many people from identifying themselves as 2SLGBTQ when they do access health care. Hidden or "invisible" populations are difficult to access for research purposes.
- Bauer discussed the concept of both informational and institutional erasure of transgender individuals and communities in health care. This erasure can be passive or active. For example, passive erasure might include a lack of identification of trans participants in research studies, whereas active erasure may involve refusal to provide care for trans patients. It is likely that these two forms of erasure compound the invisibility of trans communities.[26]
- Methodological challenges affect the ability to define sexual orientation and gender identity and to recruit and compare study participants. For example, standard definitions of the terms *gay* or *lesbian*, *sex*, and *gender* are not universally applied and may differ significantly between studies.
- There is a lack of coordinating public health infrastructure in Canada to direct and fund 2SLGBTQ health research initiatives.
- Over the last several decades, the bulk of research related to the concerns of gay men has focused on HIV/AIDS to the exclusion of other health concerns.

Negative Social Attitudes: Homophobia, Transphobia, Heterosexism, and Cissexism

The lack of information and standards of care for 2SLGBTQ patients sets the stage for substandard health care, but 2SLGBTQ individuals also face inferior care because of negative social and cultural attitudes on the part of health care providers. All health care is delivered within a general cultural context and reflects prevailing and varied social climates that may be homophobic, biphobic, and transphobic. Bias from health care providers can span from the frequent unintended use of inappropriate language such as failing to use the preferred pronoun of the patient to outright refusal to care for 2SLGBTQ patients. These attitudes and behaviours not only create barriers to care for 2SLGBTQ patients but also likely cause harm.

The American Medical Association in its report, "LGBT Patients: Reluctant and Underserved" stated that 20 per cent of patients delayed care because of negative past experiences.[27] It is likely that trans communities are disproportionately affected. An Ontario study reported both avoidance and poor treatment of trans individuals seeking services in the emergency room.[28]

Negative attitudes and behaviours can be found in the health care professions throughout various levels of training and active practice. In 2000, a qualitative study of gay and lesbian Canadian medical students found that sexual orientation had an effect on their choice to either enter or leave medicine. Further, perceived safety in disclosing sexual orientation often determined residency selection or career path. The author describes the medical school environment for students as follows:

> Considerable energy and emotion are spent by gay and lesbian medical students and residents navigating training programs, which may be, at best, indifferent and, at worst, hostile.[29]

More recent studies demonstrate similar findings. In a 2012 study, medical students across North America reported fear of discrimination as a reason for not disclosing their sexual orientation and/or gender identity. A small number of medical students continued to harbour overtly negative attitudes towards gay men.[30]

More positively, a recent survey of psychiatric residents and psychiatrists reported less negative attitudes towards transgender patients compared to other published data using undergraduate students. The authors point out that a larger study including other specialties would be helpful in determining factors that modify physician attitudes towards trans people. Such information could contribute to the development of educational strategies to improve the experiences of the transgender population in health care.[31]

Conclusion

It is our hope that this text contributes to the positive trajectory of 2SLGBTQ health care that has unfolded since its first edition. Discrimination, barriers to care, and gaps in knowledge continue to face many 2SLGBTQ patients and their providers. We believe that bringing together a pan-Canadian group of authors with a variety of lived experiences will further break down barriers to caring for this population that, while resilient and resourceful, is often poorly served and at risk.

References

1. Government of Canada. LGBTQ2 agreement-in-principle [Internet].
   Ottawa: Government of Canada. 2017. Available from: https://pm.gc.ca
   /en/news/backgrounders/2017/11/28/lgbtq2-agreement-principle.
2. Ng, BE, Moore D, Michelow W, Hogg R, Gustafson R, Robert W, Kanters
   S, Thumath M, McGuire M, Gilbert M. Relationship between disclosure
   of same-sex sexual activity to providers, HIV diagnosis and sexual health
   services for men who have sex with men in Vancouver, Canada. Can J
   Public Health. 2014 Apr;105(3):186–91.
3. Bauer GR, Zong X, Scheim AI, Hammond R, Thind A. Factors impacting
   transgender patients' discomfort with their family physicians: a
   respondent-driven sampling survey. PLoS One. 2015 Dec;10(12):e0145046.
   doi:10.1371/journal.pone.0145046.
4. Steele LS, Daley A, Curling D, Gibson MF, Green DC, Williams CC, Ross
   LE. LGBT Identity, Untreated depression, and unmet need for mental
   health services by sexual minority women and trans-identified people.
   J Women Health (Larchmt). 2017 Feb;26(2):116–27. doi:10.1089
   /jwh.2015.5677.
5. Giblon R, Bauer, GR. Health care availability, quality, and unmet need: a
   comparison of transgender and cisgender residents of Ontario, Canada.
   BMC Health Serv Res. 2017 Apr;17(1):283. doi:10.1186/s12913-017-2226-z.
6. Committee on Accreditation of Canadian Medical Schools. CACMS
   standards and elements, standards for accreditation of medical education.
   June 2015. Available from: https://cacms-cafmc.ca.
7. Tjepkema, M. Health care use among gay, lesbian and bisexual
   Canadians. Health Rep. 2008 Mar; 19(1):53–64.
8. Remedy SZ. The queer and trans voices on health and health care.
   Vancouver: Arsenal Pulp Press; 2017.
9. Cancer's Margins. LGBT cancer [Internet]. Canada. Available from:
   https://www.lgbtcancer.ca/.
10. Kinsey AC, Pomeroy WR, Martin CE. Sexual behavior in the human male.
    Philadelphia (PA): W.B. Saunders; 1948.
11. Statistics Canada. Same-sex couples and sexual orientation … by the
    numbers [Internet]. Statistics Canada; 2015. Available from: http://www
    .statcan.gc.ca/eng/dai/smr08/2015/smr08_203_2015#a3.
12. Spack NP. Management of transgenderism. JAMA. 2013 Feb;309(5):478–
    84. doi:10.1001/jama.2012.165234.
13. Conron KJ, Scott G, Stowell GS, Landers SJ. Transgender health in
    Massachusetts: results from a household probability sample of adults.
    Am J Public Health. 2012 Jan;102(1):118–22. https://doi.org/10.2105
    /AJPH.2011.300315.

14. Flores A, Herman J, Gates G, Brown T. How many adults identify as transgender in the United States? [Internet]. Los Angeles: Williams Institute; 2016 [cited 2019 Feb 4]. Available from: https://williamsinstitute.law.ucla.edu/wp-content/uploads/How-Many-Adults-Identify-as-Transgender-in-the-United-States.pdf.

15. Brotman SL, Ryan B. Access to care: exploring the health and well-being of gay, lesbian, bisexual and Two-Spirit people in Canada. Montreal: McGill Centre for Applied Family Studies, School of Social Work; 2000.

16. Jalbert Y. Gay health: current knowledge and future directions. Ottawa: Health Canada; 1999.

17. Institute of Medicine. The health of lesbian, gay, bisexual, and transgender people: building a foundation for better understanding. Washington (DC): National Academies Press; 2011.

16. U.S. Department of Health and Human Services, Office of Disease Prevention and Health Promotion. Healthy People 2020. Lesbian, gay, bisexual, and transgender health [Internet]. 2014. Available from: http://www.healthypeople.gov/2020/topicsobjectives2020/overview.aspx?topicid=25.

19. Meyer IH. Prejudice, social stress, and mental health in lesbian, gay, and bisexual populations: conceptual issues and research evidence. Psychol Bull. 2003 Sep;129(5):674–97.

20. Bourns A. Guidelines and protocols for hormone therapy and primary care for trans clients. Toronto: Sherbourne Health Centre; 2015.

21. White W, Brenman S, Paradis E, Goldsmith ES, Lunn MR, Obedin-Maliver J, Stewart L, Tran E, Wells M, Chamberlain LJ, Fetterman DM, Garcia G. Lesbian, gay, bisexual, and transgender patient care: medical students' preparedness and comfort. Teach Learn Med. 2015;27(3):254–63.

22. Obedin-Maliver J, Goldsmith ES, Stewart L, White W, Tran E, Brenman S, Wells M, Fetterman DM, Garcia G, Lunn MR. Lesbian, gay, bisexual, and transgender-related content in undergraduate medical education. JAMA. 2011 Sep;306(9):971–7.

23. Knight RE, Shoveller JA, Carson AM, Contreras-Whitney JG. Examining clinicians' experiences providing sexual health services for LGBTQ youth: considering social and structural determinants of health in clinical practice. Health Educ Res. 2014 Aug;29(4):662–70.

24. Snelgrove JW, Jasudavisius AM, Rowe BW, Head EM, Bauer GR. "Completely out-at-sea" with "two-gender medicine": a qualitative analysis of physician-side barriers to providing healthcare for transgender patients. BMC Health Serv Res. 2012 May;12(1):110.

25. McNair RP, Hegarty K. Guidelines for the primary care of lesbian, gay, and bisexual people: a systematic review. Ann Fam Med. 2010 Nov-Dec;8(6):533–41.
26. Bauer GR, Hammond R, Travers R, Kaay M, Hohenadel KM, Boyce M. "I don't think this is theoretical; this is our lives": how erasure impacts health care for transgender people. J Assoc Nurses AIDS Care: JANAC. 2009 Sep-Oct;20(5):348–61. doi:10.1016/j.jana.2009.07.004.
27. American Medical Association. LGBT patients: reluctant and underserved [Internet]. American Medical Association; 2011. Available from: http://www.amednews.com/article/20110905/profession/309059942/4/.
28. Bauer GR, Scheim AI, Deutsch MB, Massarella C. Reported emergency department avoidance, use, and experiences of transgender persons in Ontario, Canada: results from a respondent-driven sampling survey. Ann Emerg Med. 2014 Jun;63(6):713–20.e1.
29. Risdon C, Cook D, Willms D. Gay and lesbian physicians in training: a qualitative study. CMAJ 2000; 162(3):331–4.
30. Matharu K, Kravitz RL, McMahon GT, Wilson MD, Fitzgerald FT. Medical students' attitudes toward gay men. BMC Med Educ. 2012 Aug;12:71.
31. Ali N, Fleisher W, Erickson J. Psychiatrists' and psychiatry residents' attitudes toward transgender people. Acad Psychiatry. 2016 Apr;40(2):268–73.

2 Improving Patient–Provider Relationships and Health Environments for 2SLGBTQ Patients

SYDNEY TAM

Introduction

Most health care professionals will tell you that a good patient–provider relationship is fundamental to providing quality and compassionate care. Most would also agree that this dynamic should be a focus regardless of the patient population. In reality, however, many members of the 2SLGBTQ population feel a deep-seated vulnerability in – if not an abject mistrust and fear of – health care providers and environments.

The history of hetero- and cissexism in medicine is well documented, yet health environments often continue to perpetuate heteronormativity and cisnormativity in an unwitting but systemic fashion. Consider these scenarios:

A lesbian couple brings their daughter to a new pediatrician's office. As they enter, they notice the office is pleasantly decorated. There are pictures and posters on the walls depicting children with both of their parents – moms and dads in happy circumstances. Some are promoting health-focused concepts such as allergy awareness, immunizations, etc. ... The family registers at the front desk and are presented with an intake form that requests the names of both parents, with the headings: "Mother" and "Father." One of the child's moms rolls her eyes at the other, who nods understandingly and sighs, "Just like at the school ..."

A trans woman, who has been on estrogen therapy for over 10 years, arrives at her local hospital for a mammogram. She fills out the medical history form, which asks for a detailed gynecologic history. Some of the questions, however, are only appropriate for cis women; they ask about her last menses, for example, and whether she has any history of hormone replacement therapy (HRT). She answers honestly, stating that she has been on HRT for 10 years, but that she has had neither menses nor a hysterectomy. After handing the questionnaire to the technologist, she explains, rather bravely, that she couldn't answer all of the questions accurately because she is trans. The technologist's expression changes and she abruptly tells the patient, "You people don't need mammograms." The woman leaves embarrassed and confused. Later in the day, she receives two very apologetic calls from the manager and the radiologist ...

These kinds of patient experiences are, unfortunately, not uncommon. For many patients, each such instance can further inflame a sense of victimization and helplessness. No health care provider would want to see their patients face these kinds of barriers. However, without systemic awareness and willingness to facilitate change in the provision of care to marginalized populations, health professionals and organizations will not only contribute to the microaggressions* experienced by 2SLGBTQ people but will also fall short of their ultimate goals.

The Patient Experience of Barriers

Despite societal change and acceptance of 2SLGBTQ people, including a noticeable change of attitude among health care professionals, administrators, and policymakers, there is ongoing evidence of barriers to care. In a 2016 study focused in Nova Scotia, the majority of participants reported that they were uncertain about the level of LGBTQ-friendliness of their primary care provider.[1] Indeed, over half (54.7 per cent) of health care providers surveyed in the same study reported that they had never received training for cultural competence in relation to LGBQ populations, while 60.4 per cent reported never receiving any training regarding trans care.[1]

In a 2017 Ontario study, 47 per cent of younger youth (14–18 years) and 33 per cent of older youth (19–25 years) reported that they had not received needed health care in the past 12 months, with the majority stating this was due to being "afraid of what the doctor would say or do."[2] Supporting this, in a 2015 Canadian survey, only 15 per cent of trans youth asked reported feeling "very comfortable" discussing their trans status and trans-specific health care needs with a family doctor.[3] The survey also found that 47 per cent of 19–25 year olds had not received necessary physical health care in the past year.[3]

---

* *Microaggression* is a term used for brief and commonplace daily verbal, behavioural, or environmental indignities, whether intentional or unintentional, that communicate hostile, derogatory, or negative prejudicial slights and insults towards any group.

To some, it may seem that not much has changed for 2SLGBTQ patients in the decades since the publication of the first edition of this text. However, research illuminating these barriers to care has stimulated nascent changes in some North American health-training programs. Still, the questions remain: What more can be done to disassemble these barriers, and what can be done to continue improving the patient–provider relationship?

An Opportunity for Reflective Practice

Mindfulness of one's own privilege, both earned and unearned, is a key skill for professional and compassionate practice. Most health care providers feel privileged to have the skill and knowledge to contribute toward health and healing for all their patients.

Historically, the provision of health care has followed a hierarchy of power within physician–patient and physician–nurse relationships. This power differential can be offset by approaches that incorporate patient-centred care and shared decision making. However, care providers may not always be mindful of the other forms of privilege that can influence a relationship. Providers may have class privilege, as well as cis and hetero privilege.

Self-awareness of privilege and insight into one's assumptions are important when providing care to any patient, but are particularly important when caring for 2SLGBTQ communities and individuals, given their history of mistreatment in health care.

It is important to note that 2SLGBTQ-identified providers may be perceived (by themselves or others) to be immune from making heteronormative or cisnormative assumptions. Yet they can unintentionally hold on to homophobic or transphobic dogma and pathologization without awareness. For that reason, it is good practice for *all* providers to engage in reflective activities and to create an environment that enables them to receive feedback about their language and care. For example, a provider may advise patients that their organization takes a quality-improvement approach to care and that ensuring culturally competent care is an important part of this work. Thus, if a patient receives care that is not respectful or competent, the patient is encouraged to share their experience.

The use of appropriate and relevant language can build trust and improve care and communication with patients. This includes asking a patient how they prefer to be addressed (i.e., preferred name and pronouns) and how they refer to their body parts (specifically the chest area and genitalia). In addition, asking how someone is sexually active and with what type of partners avoids the pitfall of questions like "are you sexually active?" and "with men, women, or both?" which can imply an expectation of a heteronormative and cisnormative answer. For example, these questions may not prompt a patient to disclose sexual activity with both cis and trans men. Communication during clinical interactions is further discussed in chapter 3.

One framework of cultural competence can be found in the work of Peggy McIntosh, whose landmark 1989 article "White Privilege: Unpacking the Invisible Knapsack"[4] has been adapted and applied to cis and hetero privilege.

Box 2.1. Invisible Knapsack – Sexual Orientation

Sexual Orientation

On a daily basis, as a straight person ...

- I can go for months without being called straight.
- I am not asked to think about why I am straight.
- I am never asked to speak for everyone who is heterosexual.
- People don't ask why I made my choice of sexual orientation.
- Nobody calls me straight as an insult.
- If I pick up a magazine, watch TV, or play music, I can be certain my sexual orientation will be represented.
- I do not have to fear that if my family or friends find out about my sexual orientation there will be economic, emotional, physical, or psychological consequences.
- I can easily find a religious community that will not exclude me for being heterosexual.
- I can count on finding a therapist or doctor willing and able to talk about my sexuality.
- I am guaranteed to find sex education literature for couples with my sexual orientation.
- Because of my sexual orientation, I do not need to worry that people will harass or assault me.
- I am not identified/defined by my sexual orientation.
- I can hold hands or kiss in public with my significant other and not have people double-take or stare.
- I can choose to not think politically about my sexual orientation.

- People can use terms that describe my sexual orientation and mean positive things (e.g., "straight as an arrow," "standing up straight," or "straightened out") instead of demeaning terms (e.g., "eww, that's gay" or being "queer").
- I can be open about my sexual orientation without worrying about my job.

Adapted from McIntosh, "White privilege: Unpacking the invisible knapsack," 1990.[4]

Box 2.2. Invisible Knapsack – Gender Identity

Gender Identity

On a daily basis, as a cisgender person ...

- Strangers don't assume they can ask me what my genitals look like and how I have sex.
- My validity as a man/woman/human is not based upon how much surgery I've had or how well I "pass" as a non-trans person.
- When initiating sex with someone, I do not have to worry that they won't be able to deal with my parts or that having sex with me will cause my partner to question his or her own sexual orientation.
- I am not excluded from events that are either explicitly or de facto* men-born-men or women-born-women only (*basically anything involving nudity).
- I don't have to hear "so have you had THE surgery?" or "oh, so you're REALLY a [incorrect sex or gender]?" each time I come out to someone.
- Strangers do not ask me what my "real name" [birth name] is and then assume that they have a right to call me by that name.
- People do not disrespect me by using incorrect pronouns even after they've been corrected.
- I do not have to worry about whether I will be able to find a bathroom to use or whether I will be safe changing in a locker room.
- I do not have to defend my right to be a part of "Queer," and gays and lesbians will not try to exclude me from OUR movement in order to gain political legitimacy for themselves.

- I do not have to choose between either invisibility ("passing") or being consistently "othered" and/or tokenized based on my gender.
- I do not have to worry that my sexual orientation and gender identity will be conflated.
- If I end up in the emergency room, I do not have to worry that my gender will keep me from receiving appropriate treatment nor will all of my medical issues be seen as a product of my gender. ("Your nose is running and your throat hurts? Must be due to the hormones!")
- My health insurance provider (or public health system) does not specifically exclude me from receiving benefits or treatments available to others because of my gender.
- When I express my internal identities in my daily life, I am not considered "mentally ill" by the medical establishment.
- I am not required to undergo extensive psychological evaluation to receive basic medical care.
- People do not use me as a scapegoat for their own unresolved gender issues.

Adapted from McIntosh, "White privilege: Unpacking the invisible knapsack," 1990.[4]

Despite significant changes to civil rights legislation and attitudes regarding gender and race, people still ubiquitously experience racism and sexism (the two traditional "-isms" in Western society). We have just begun to scratch the surface of addressing homophobia and transphobia from a legal and social perspective. Care providers must therefore consider the layers of bias and discrimination that a person burdened with more than one of the "-isms" faces on a daily basis. When multiple intersections exist, the provider must be aware of the potential complexities and experiences the patient brings to an interaction. It is always advisable to be mindful of one's own biases, to take into account one's own power and privilege as a health care provider, and to always be prepared to recover from missteps in one's assumptions about a patient.[5]

Microaggressions experienced by 2SLGBTQ individuals can easily lead to mistrust and fear of institutions. Providers' positions of privilege can lead to the assumption (and assertion) that an individual provider is not responsible for systemic oppression. However, all providers must be accountable for their positions within systems and acknowledge that by participating in them, we also participate in established systemic bias. The process of building trust, becoming more account-able and participating in, if not leading, systemic change is potentially arduous and challenging – yet it can be professionally and personally rewarding.

Creating a Safer and More Affirming Environment

If you have ever made or agreed with the statements "I'm colour blind" or "Everyone is the same," you have already begun to create an unsafe environment for people with marginalized identities. While equality is ideal, we are living in a time where the historic echoes of oppression continue to impact 2SLGBTQ people.

Appropriate training in cultural competence as an educational tool is a useful and critical step in creating a safer space. Such training is highly recommended for health care providers, as well as health care organizations and their staff – especially front-line staff. Cultural competence training can lead to significant benefits, including an increase in both provider and patient satisfaction.

The creation of a safe and affirming environment can be broad-based, but it does not have to involve radical change – simply being mindful of heterosexism and cissexism, and making changes accordingly in training and practice, can be helpful.

Appropriate resources to further address cultural competence and the creating of affirming environments can be found on the Rainbow Health Ontario (RHO) (https://www.rainbowhealthontario.ca), and Trans Care BC (http://www.phsa.ca/transcarebc/) websites.

The American Medical Association also provides simplified guidelines for creating an 2SLGBTQ friendly practice.[6] The following is adapted from those guidelines:

1. Provide visual cues for 2SLGBTQ patients to identify that your practice is a safe place. Simple ways to create an inclusive office environment include the following:
   - Display brochures and educational materials about 2SLGBTQ health concerns.
   - Display posters from non-profit 2SLGBTQ or HIV/AIDS organizations.
   - Strategically place rainbow stickers or signs stating that your practice or institution is a 2SLGBTQ safe space.
   - Avoid having exclusively heteronormative and cisnormative posters and pictures in waiting areas.
   - Display a privacy policy.

Figure 2.1. An Example of a Non-discrimination Policy from Sherbourne Health

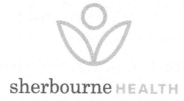

sherbourne HEALTH

We strive to create a safe, respectful and accessible space that affirms the identities, experiences and needs of all service users, staff, providers, students, volunteers and visitors.

Our duties to each other while at Sherbourne:

- Treat everyone with dignity and respect
- Do our part to maintain a safe, clean and pleasant environment
- Be aware of, and follow, Sherbourne's policies and procedures
- Report issues or concerns about Sherbourne's programs and services
- Wear clothes and footwear while in Sherbourne
- Do not use scents and scented products

We will not accept disrespectful comments or discrimination, including homophobia, transphobia, racism, sexism or ableism.

Threats or acts of violence, displaying a weapon, intimidating behavior, or theft may lead to restriction of access to services.

Sherbourne welcomes compliments, complaints and ideas. You can use the feedback form or contact us at feedback@sherbourne.on.ca.

Feedback forms are available in the waiting room and at sherbourne.on.ca.

Sherbourne thanks Client Engagement Forum participants for their input on this statement.
Published August 2018.

Source: Reprinted with permission from Sherbourne Health

2. Customize your patient intake forms and requisitions.
   - Examine the comprehensive Sample New Patient Intake Form found in the appendix to this chapter. Compare it to your current intake form.*
3. Create a clear and enforceable non-discrimination policy and post it in plain view.
   - Include sexual orientation and gender identity.
   - Partner with patients and families to create such policies.
   - See example from Sherbourne Health in figure 2.1.
4. Consider seeking patient feedback and assessing patient needs directly from local 2SLGBTQ communities.
   - For example, when creating a strategic plan, include patient and community advisers.
5. Explicitly use 2SLGBTQ-inclusive language and images on websites and social media.
6. Develop expertise in caring for 2SLGBTQ patients.

Becoming a Better Expert

When seeking to improve one's understanding of issues around 2SLGBTQ health care, it is tempting for a well-intentioned provider to allow the patient to talk about themselves and their experiences. However, this should not be seen as the only opportunity for the provider to educate themselves on the needs of the patient, particularly for populations whose identities intersect so directly with their needs.

Developing expertise around 2SLGBTQ health care is easier than at any other point in medical history. The resources available for professional development are abundant, affordable, and accessible.

Many general primary-care conferences (such as the College of Family Physicians of Canada's annual Family Medicine Forum) now offer at least one session related to 2SLGBTQ health care; additionally, there are specific organizations that offer annual or biannual conferences dedicated to 2SLGBTQ health (examples include RHO and the Canadian Professional Association for Transgender Health). Many organizations offer extensive information on their websites and also offer focused professional training (RHO, Trans Care BC, Fenway Health, and the World Professional Association for Transgender Health).

---

* The two-step method for the collection of gender identity data (i.e., querying both gender identity and sex assigned at birth) has been found to be superior to a single question query and is recommended by several North American medical organizations and the World Professional Association for Transgender Health.[7,8]

It is also important for all health care providers and health service organizations to be aware of any local resources and support groups for 2SLGBTQ individuals, including youth, seniors and others requiring specific support.

The Ongoing Struggle (and Potential)

We are at a time when there is great variation in the ability of health care providers and organizations to deliver culturally competent care for 2SLGBTQ populations. For those with limited experience in this realm of medicine, taking on the task of providing culturally and clinically competent care can feel daunting. However, it may be the best time in history to participate in changing (and challenging) the traditional face of medicine and health care to become accepting, welcoming, and healing to a very diverse and traditionally poorly cared for population of patients. Finally, existing 2SLGBTQ-affirming health care environments and providers should be aware of the ongoing and changing needs of their community and strive to improve their care accordingly.

References

1. Gahagan J, Subirana-Malaret M, Improving pathways to primary health care among LGBTQ populations and health care providers: key findings from Nova Scotia, Canada Int J Equity Health. 2018 Jun;17(1):76.
2. Giblon R, Bauer GR. Health care availability, quality, and unmet need: a comparison of transgender and cisgender residents of Ontario, Canada. BMC Health Serv Res. 2017 Apr;17(1):283.
3. Veale J, Saewyc E, Frohard-Dourlent H, Dobson S, Clark B. Being safe, being me: results of the Canadian trans youth health survey [Internet]. Vancouver (BC): University of British Columbia; 2015. Available from: https://www.saravyc.ubc.ca/2015/04/30/being-safe-being-me-results-of-the-canadian-trans-youth-health-survey/.
4. McIntosh P. White privilege: unpacking the invisible knapsack. Indep Sch. 1990;49(2):31–6.
5. Boogaard K. How successful people recover after making a mistake [Internet]. Inc.com. Inc.; 2016. Available from: https://www.inc.com/kat-boogaard/how-successful-people-recover-after-making-a-mistake.html.
6. Creating an LGBTQ-friendly practice [Internet]. Selecting and using a health information exchange. American Medical Association. Available from: https://www.ama-assn.org/delivering-care/creating-lgbtq-friendly-practice.

7. Tate CC, Ledbetter JN, Youssef CP. A two-question method for assessing gender categories in the social and medical sciences. J Sex Res. 2013;50(8):767–76.
8. Deutsch MB, Green J, Keatley J, Mayer G, Hastings J, Hall AM, et al.; World Professional Association for Transgender Health EMR Working Group. Electronic medical records and the transgender patient: recommendations from the World Professional Association for Transgender Health EMR Working Group. J Am Med Inform Assoc JAMIA. 2013 Jul-Aug;20(4):700–3.

Appendix

sherbourne HEALTH

CLIENT INTAKE FORM FOR HEALTH SERVICES

Date completed:_____

Completing this questionnaire is optional. If you are not comfortable with any of the questions, you do not need to answer them. The information you provide will help us improve the quality of care, and also plan for services and program development. We strive to provide respectful and high quality care to clients with diverse backgrounds and needs.

PERSONAL INFORMATION (aka Who you are and where you're at)

Name (on OHIP or other ID):_____

Preferred Name: _____ Date of Birth: _____/_____/_____
(Day/Month/Year)

☐ OHIP#:_____ Version Code: _____

Expiry Date_____/_____/_____ (Day/Month/Year)   Sex (as per OHIP):   ☐ F   ☐ M

☐ Interim Federal Health Coverage: _____ Expiry Date: _____/_____ (m/y)
☐ NO ONTARIO HEALTH CARD
   Are you in a 3-month waiting period?   ☐ Yes ☐ No   Date you expect to receive your card:_____/_____ (m/y)

Address: _____
          Street Number   Street Name   Apt. Number   City   Postal Code
☐ NO FIXED ADDRESS

Home Phone: (_____)_____-_____ Cell Phone: (_____)_____-_____ Work Phone: (_____)_____-_____

Preferred contact method: ☐ At Home   ☐ On Cell   ☐ At Work
   Can we call you at these numbers?   ☐ At Home   ☐ On Cell   ☐ At Work   ☐ None of these
   Can we leave detailed private messages?   ☐ At Home   ☐ On Cell   ☐ At Work   ☐ None of these
   Can we use your preferred name when calling? ☐ At Home   ☐ On Cell   ☐ At Work   ☐ None of these

Emergency Contact Name:_____ Phone: (_____)_____-_____

If you are under 16 years old please provide the name and phone number of parent or guardian:

   Parent/Guardian Name:_____ Phone: (_____)_____-_____

Do you need an interpreter to communicate in English?   ☐ Yes   ☐ No
What language(s) do you speak?

Gender Identity:
   ☐ Female   ☐ Two Spirit   ☐ Prefer not to answer
   ☐ Male   ☐ Transgender   ☐ Do not know
   ☐ Intersex   ☐ Genderqueer   ☐ Other _____

What sex were you assigned at birth (i.e. on your birth certificate)?
   ☐ Female   ☐ Prefer not to answer   ☐ Other _____
   ☐ Male   ☐ Do not know

What pronouns do you use?_____

1

Reprinted with permission from Sherbourne Health

What is (are) your reason(s) for seeking care with Sherbourne Health Centre?

_____

_____

Please list any health professionals you have seen in the last year (please include nurses, doctors, physiotherapists, chiropractors, naturopaths, counsellors, workers).

_____

_____

Which of the following best describes your racial or ethnic group?

☐ Asian-East (e.g. Chinese, Japanese, Korean)   ☐ Metis

☐ Asian-South (e.g. Indian, Pakistani, Sri Lankan)   ☐ Middle Eastern (e.g. Egyptian, Iranian, Lebanese)

☐ Asian-South East (e.g. Malaysian, Filipino, Vietnamese)   ☐ White-European (e.g. Italian, Portuguese, Russian)

☐ Black-African (e.g. Ghanaian, Kenyan, Somali)   ☐ White-North American (e.g. Canadian, American)

☐ Black-North American (e.g. Canadian, American)   ☐ Mixed heritage (please specify)

☐ Black-Caribbean (e.g. Barbadian, Jamaican)   _____

☐ First Nations

☐ Indian-Caribbean (e.g. Guyanese with origins in India)   ☐ Other (please specify)_____

☐ Indigenous/Aboriginal not included elsewhere   ☐ Prefer not to answer

☐ Inuit   ☐ Do not know

☐ Latin American (e.g. Chilean, Argentinean, Salvadorian)

In what country were you born?

_____   ☐ Prefer not to answer   ☐ Do not know

Are you a Newcomer?   ☐ Yes   ☐ No   Year arrived in Canada: _____

Please list any other countries where you have lived:_____

_____

What type of housing do you live in?

☐ Own/Rent   ☐ Street   ☐ No stable housing

☐ Rooming house   ☐ Supportive housing   ☐ Other_____

☐ Shelter/Hostel   ☐ Family/Friends   ☐ Prefer not to answer

Living arrangements:

☐ Live alone   ☐ With friends   ☐ Other

☐ With partner   ☐ Supportive housing   _____

☐ With children   ☐ With adult family members   ☐ Prefer not to answer

Highest education level completed:

☐ No formal education   ☐ University

☐ Primary school (grade1-8 or equivalent)   ☐ Other _____

☐ High School (grade 9-12 or equivalent)   ☐ Prefer not to answer

☐ College   ☐ Do not know

2

sherbourne HEALTH

Source of income:

- □ No income
- □ Full-time employment
- □ Part-time employment
- □ Student loan

- □ Canadian Pension Plan
- □ Retirement Income
- □ Old Age Security (OAS)
- □ Ontario Works (OW)

- □ Employment Insurance (EI)
- □ Ontario Disability Program (ODSP)
- □ Other_____

Do you have drug coverage?   □ Yes   □ No

What is you total/combined household income?   □ Prefer not to answer   □ Do not know

- □ $0.00-14,999 ($1,249/month [$7.69/hr] or less)
- □ $15,000-19,999 ($1,249-1,667/mo.; $7.69-$10.26/hr)
- □ $20,000-24,999 ($1,667-2,083/mo.; $10.26-$12.82/hr)
- □ $25,000-29,999 ($2,083-2,500/mo.; $12.82-$15.38/hr)

- □ $30,000-34,999 ($2,500-2,916/mo.; $15.38-$17.95/hr)
- □ $35,000-39,999 ($2,916-3,333/mo.; $17.95-$20.51/hr)
- □ $40,000-59,999 ($3,333-4,999/mo.; $20.51-$30.77/hr)
- □ $over $60,000 (over 5,000/mo.; 30.77/hr and up)

How many people are supported by this income? (including parents, children, support payment, etc.)_____   □ Prefer not to answer

Sexual Orientation:

- □ Heterosexual (straight)
- □ Gay
- □ Lesbian
- □ Bisexual

- □ Two-Spirit
- □ Queer
- □ Pansexual
- □ Prefer not to answer

- □ Do not know
- □ Other_____
- □ Not Applicable

Do you have concerns related to your sexual orientation?

- □ Not at all   □ A little   □ Somewhat   □ A lot   □ Prefer not to answer

Are you currently sexually active? ☐   □ Yes ☐   □ No ☐   □ Prefer not to answer
Are you currently in a relationship? ☐   □ Yes ☐   □ No ☐   □ Prefer not to answer
When were you last tested for sexually transmitted infections (STIs)?   _____   □ Never
Is/Are your partner(s):

- □ Female ☐   □ Male ☐   □ Intersex ☐   □ Transgender ☐   □ Two Spirit ☐   □ Other _____

Were your previous partner(s):

- □ Female ☐   □ Male ☐   □ Intersex ☐   □ Transgender ☐   □ Two Spirit ☐   □ Other _____

FAMILY HISTORY

Do any members of your <u>biological family</u> have any health conditions? (mother, father, grandparents, siblings, children)?

- □ Yes (please list below)   □ No   □ Adopted   □ Prefer not to answer   □ Do not know

Relative	Health Conditions
Mother	
Father	
Mother's parents	
Father's parents	
Siblings	
Children	
Other relatives	

sherbourne HEALTH   **LIFESTYLE & OTHER HEALTH-RELATED BEHAVIOURS**

Do you exercise on a regular basis?   □ Yes   □ No   □ Prefer not to answer

If yes, what type of exercise? _____

How many minutes per week do you exercise? _____

Do you have any concerns about your diet/nutrition?   □ Yes   □ No   □ Prefer not to answer

Please describe:_____

_____

Do you smoke cigarettes?   □ Yes   □ Never smoked   □ Used to smoke/quit   □ Prefer not to answer

If yes, for how long? _____ How many cigarettes per day? _____ How many packs per day? _____

If you quit, when did you quit? _____

Do you use any other tobacco or nicotine-containing products?   □ Yes   □ No

If so, please list:_____

Do you drink alcohol?   □ Yes   □ No   □ Prefer not to answer

If yes, how many drinks a week, on average? _____

Do you use any street drugs? □ Yes   □ No   □ Prefer not to answer

If yes, please check:

□ Marijuana   □ Ecstasy/MDMA   □ Hormones or steroids

□ Cocaine   □ Ketamine   □ Other _____

□ Crack   □ GHB

□ Heroin or other opiods   □ Crystal meth

How often do you use them? _____

MEDICAL HISTORY (aka The health stuff)

Do you have any ALLERGIES?   □ Yes (please list below)   □ No   □ Prefer not to answer   □ Do not know

Medicines	
Food	
Environment (eg. grass, pets, dust etc.)	

Do you take any MEDICINES on a regular basis? ⬚ □ Yes   □ No   □ Prefer not to answer

Prescription meds (prescribed by the doctor)	
Non-Prescription (includes lotions/creams, eye drops, etc.)	
Alternative/Herbal	
Vitamins/ Supplements	

Preferred Pharmacy:_____ Phone : (_____)_____-_____ Fax : (_____)_____-_____

4

sherbourne HEALTH

Do you have any current health problems?   □ Yes   □ No   □ Prefer not to answer

If yes, please list and/or describe: _____

_____

_____

Do you have any mental health issues?   □ Yes   □ No   □ Prefer not to answer

If yes, please describe:_____

_____

_____

Do you have any of the following disabilities?

□ No disabilities   □ Physical disability   □ Prefer not to answer
□ Developmental disability   □ Hearing loss   □ Do not know
□ Learning disability   □ Vision loss   □ Other_____

Do you have any accessibility needs or need any accommodations to access care? □ Yes □ No

Please specify:_____

Medeo is our online patient portal for email messaging. Are you interested in signing up?   □ Yes   □ No

Do you have any past health problems (that you have recovered from)?   □ Yes   □ No   □ Prefer not to answer

If yes, please list and/or describe: _____

Please list any previous hospitalizations: □ Prefer not to answer

Reason for hospitalization   Date

_____   _____

_____   _____

Please list any previous surgeries: □ Prefer not to answer

Reason for surgery   Date

_____   _____

_____   _____

When was the last time you had a **vaccine or immunizations**? _____

Please list the dates of any recent **cancer screening test(s)**:   FOBT:_____ PAP:_____ Mammogram:_____

How would you describe your social support network? _____

Is there anything else about your medical history that you think we should know?   □ Yes   □ No
If yes, please explain_____

Is there anything else about you that you feel we should know to provide better care?   □ Yes   □ No
If yes, please describe_____

In general, how would you describe your own health: □ Excellent   □ Very Good   □ Good   □ Fair   □ Poor

3 History and Physical Examination

LAURA STRATTON

Setting the Stage

While the core principles of conducting a history and physical exam in patients who are 2SLGBTQ are no different than with any other patient, there are specific considerations and approaches health care providers should take into account when providing care to members of the 2SLGBTQ community. As discussed in chapter 2, the patient-provider relationship is integral to providing quality health care. This is particularly true in primary care. Many external factors may influence this relationship, including prior interactions with health care providers, systemic hetero- and cisnormative barriers within the health care system, and even societal and media influences at large.[1,2] These factors, to varying degrees, may frame a patient's ideas and expectations leading up to a health care visit, and at times may even prevent patients from accessing care altogether. It is important for providers to be mindful that patients who are 2SLGBTQ face a disproportionate number of barriers before setting foot in the office (or any health care environment). As a result, it is unfortunately common for members of the 2SLGBTQ community to have, for example, decreased rates of cancer screening or to present to care with more advanced stages of disease.[3,4] Recognizing that these barriers exist can help support the practice of remaining non-judgmental when patients present late to care or are guarded, and ideally provide impetus to reduce these barriers.

As outlined in the previous chapter, providers can take many steps to create an inclusive and safe space in the clinic environment to ensure their patients who are 2SLGBTQ feel welcome.

The Significance of Terminology

Terminology is constantly expanding and evolving to capture the diversity within the 2SLGBTQ community. While it is neither possible nor necessary to remain current on *all* terminology to describe sexual orientations and gender identities, it is important to have an understanding of key terminology and concepts, as outlined in chapter 1. Even when health care providers belong to the 2SLGBTQ community, the diversity within the community is vast, it is impossible to fully appreciate and know the experiences of all members. Certain terms may have different meanings to different people, or they may vary based on the context in which they are used, including differences based on geographical location of practice. For example, the term *Two-Spirit* has many definitions but is typically used to describe diversity in gender identity and/or sexual orientation of people who are Indigenous and living on Turtle Island (North America).[5] However, people who identify as Two-Spirit may also choose to identify as LGBTQ or may want to identify by specific terms used within their own Indigenous culture and language. It is always best to ask patients what they mean by certain terms if there is any uncertainty or ambiguity and to never assume that a term used by one patient will have the same meaning for another.

There can also be generational differences with respect to terminology. For example, while the term *queer* has been reclaimed by many members of the 2SLGBTQ community as an inclusive term to describe sexuality, gender, or both, it has historically been used in a derogatory nature, and as such, some people may view it in this light. Reflecting terminology that patients use to describe themselves as opposed to imposing one's own terminology should always be the default. For example, in the case of a ciswoman who describes her sexual orientation as bisexual, avoid referring to her as a lesbian, even if all of her sexual relationships have been with women.

Just as terminology is constantly evolving, so too can an individual's gender identity or sexual orientation. It can be a helpful practice to routinely discuss this with new patients, and give them permission to inform their health care team of any changes that may occur. One might say something such as "gender identity and sexual orientation can change over time, and these are important things for me as your health care provider to know in order to provide the best care for you. Please let me know if anything changes or if we get it wrong." Periodic health reviews can also provide an opportunity to check in with patients if there have been any changes to their identity, orientation, or terminology that they prefer to use.

Despite best intentions and efforts, it is inevitable that health care providers will get it wrong from time to time. When this happens, the advisable course is to apologize, make the correction, and ask for clarification if need be. This can turn the error into an opportunity to build trust in the relationship. Acknowledging the error and making the effort to correct the mistake demonstrates the value providers place on using preferred terminology, pronouns, names, and so on. However, it is also important not to dwell on the error or create an over-the-top apology. This practice serves to shift the focus to the feelings of the person who made the error in an attempt to make them feel better, rather than remaining focused on the patient.

Introductions

When meeting any patient for the first time, introductions are an important part of establishing rapport and trust. This is a patient's first impression of a provider and sets the stage for the remainder of the visit and the ongoing patient–provider relationship. When introducing oneself to patients, including one's pronouns, normalizes the process of exchanging them. For example: "Hi, I am Dr. Doe. My first name is Jane. I use they/them pronouns. What name and pronouns do you use?" Additionally, some providers choose to wear a button to state their pronouns while still providing patients the opportunity to share their pronouns. Including pronouns during introductions helps to facilitate a safe space for patients to comfortably share their pronouns. Routinely doing this helps to avoid potentially harmful and alienating assumptions about a patient's gender presentation and expression, and demonstrates support of trans and gender diverse populations. Often, individuals whose pronoun use matches their gender expression may not feel the need to state their pronouns, whereas for individuals who do not fall into this category, the onus is often placed on them to state their pronouns, which can be an unfair burden. While it may not initially feel comfortable for some providers to ask for and provide their own pronouns, this becomes more natural with practice. Routinely including opportunities for all parties to share their pronouns, whether through intake forms, name tags, introductions, and so on, helps create an environment that promotes diversity and inclusion.

Additionally, taking time at the beginning of an interaction to ask the patient for their preferred or authentic name can avoid future confusion and build trust and respect. This is particularly important for trans or gender diverse patients when their chosen name may not match their given or legal name on their health card. However, providers should keep in mind that not all patients will feel comfortable using the same name in all settings. For example, some trans or gender diverse patients, regardless of stage of transition, may want to use their given name when being called from the waiting room, and use their preferred name only when in private or known safe spaces. Accordingly, it is essential to clarify with patients what they are comfortable with. This is also an opportunity to discuss how providers can help patients with name or gender marker changes on government documentation, should this be something that a patient wants to pursue.

Equally important is ensuring that these preferences are clearly documented in charts and electronic medical records (EMR), and communicated with other members of the health care team so that they too are aware. This is particularly paramount for front desk staff, who are often the first point of contact when patients are checking in. This also avoids situations in which patients are "outed" in waiting rooms. Using a patient's last name to call them from the waiting room is typically a safer choice if there is uncertainty with how a patient wants to be addressed. Then once the patient is in a private setting, clarify their chosen name along with unique identifiers such as date of birth. Making it a routine practice to call all patients by their last name can foster a safe and inclusive environment so as not to single out particular patients.

Consideration should also be given to the referral process for patients who are 2SLGBTQ. Referral letters to specialists or allied health care professionals is a form of indirect introduction and should convey how patients want to be addressed, including preferred name and pronouns. Again, providers should ask patients what they prefer to have included in referrals. For example, some trans or gender diverse patients may not want to include details related to their gender identity, such as previous transition-related surgeries or hormone therapy. Depending on the reason for referral, this may be appropriate to exclude (or have a conversation about why it may be relevant to include). Providers can also create a list of 2SLGBTQ friendly specialists and allied health care professionals. Although the terms *FTM* (female to male) or *MTF* (male to female) typically should be avoided, because of their implied binary notion of gender, it may be helpful to include them in referrals to providers who may not have as much experience providing care to trans and gender diverse patients and associated terminology. Additionally, terminology such as *assigned male at birth* (AMAB) and *assigned female at birth* (AFAB) can be used when communicating with consultants and colleagues. For example, "Thank you for seeing this 25-year-old transman (FTM; assigned female at birth; he/him pronouns) for …"

Taking a History

In primary care, knowing one's patients is essential to providing quality care. This includes having an understanding of patients' values and identities, in addition to detailed and specific clinical information. There are multiple self-imposed and societally driven identities that intersect in any given individual, of which gender identity and sexual orientation comprise a key part. Although simply knowing that someone identifies as 2SLGBTQ does not provide the complete history or knowledge of an individual, it is an important aspect of identity and helps to provide a lens for certain clinical presentations. Prior studies and reports have shown that a lack of disclosure of either sexual orientation or gender identity has been associated with poor health outcomes and psychological well-being.[6,7,8] Regularly including questions regarding gender identity and sexual orientation for all patients allows patients the opportunity to discuss these topics and highlights the importance of these aspects in their overall health. By regularly including opportunities to discuss gender and sexual identity, health care providers can help to alleviate the burden on patients to initiate these discussions, as there are often fears of discrimination (both intentional and unintentional), inadequate care, or poor reactions from health care providers that act as barriers to disclosure.[9] There are also patient-related barriers to disclosure, such as internalized homophobia, and even differences in disclosure among various sexual minorities, with patients who identify as bisexual being less likely to disclose compared to lesbian or gay individuals.[6] Some providers worry that collecting information on sexual orientation or gender identity might offend patients, when in reality this is true for only a small minority of patients.[10] A study involving medical students found that even those who indicated comfort with 2SLGBTQ-identified individuals still rarely routinely asked about sexual orientation.[11] This highlights the importance of making it regular practice to include these topics in periodic health reviews and standard templates. Furthermore, collecting this information enables researchers to serve and guide the care of the 2SLGBTQ community.

Although most patients recognize the importance of gender and sexual identity to their overall health,[10] it may be necessary to frame the questions providers ask to provide context. Simply stating that gender identity and sexual orientation are important for health care providers to know in order to provide appropriate and comprehensive personalized care may be enough to help patients understand why certain questions are being asked. In the context of cancer screening, knowing what body parts are present or surgeries a patient has undergone will help guide which screening tests to recommend. For example, if a patient has been on feminizing hormone therapy, this should prompt providers to discuss breast cancer screening. If they have also had breast augmentation, there may be additional considerations for screening (see chapters

4 and 11 for further discussion on cancer screening). Providing context helps prevent patients from feeling as though questions are being asked simply out of curiosity, which should be avoided. That being said, there are times when such questions are inappropriate and not relevant to the patient encounter. For example, if a patient is presenting with a sprained ankle, it is not an appropriate time to go into a gender history and ask about previous transition-related surgeries, as it is very unlikely to be relevant to the presenting complaint. Unfortunately this does happen, and often can lead to patients feeling "othered."[*,12]

Taking a good social history is imperative. As detailed in other sections of this text, there is a disproportionate degree of housing instability or homelessness, substance misuse, and lack of social or family supports in the 2SLGBTQ community.[13] Enquiring as to where patients are living (and with whom), who makes up their support systems, and if they have any family, both given and/or chosen, helps to provide context to better understand patients, and can help to identify areas requiring additional support. Intimate partner violence (IPV) is frequently overlooked and often not on the radar of providers as something to screen for in 2SLGBTQ relationships.[14] Rates of IPV are just as high or higher than in heterosexual and cisgender populations. A recent US study of young transgender women found a staggering 42 per cent prevalence of IPV in their sample.[15] Similarly, in a 2013 Statistics Canada study, it was reported that "women who self-identified as lesbian or bisexual were significantly more likely than heterosexual women to report violence by a current or previous spouse in the previous five years."[16]

There are clearly inequities faced by many members of the 2SLGBTQ community.[17,18] Having an awareness of these health inequities can be helpful for both patients and providers to engage in appropriate screening and, ideally, to work towards prevention. However, it is equally important to be cognizant of how screening is approached and how messaging around these inequities is presented as providers can inadvertently further stigmatize and marginalize.[19] For example, telling an adolescent who is 2SLGBTQ that they are at higher risk for substance misuse compared to their cisgender or straight peers likely will not prevent this behaviour and may lead to them feeling as though there is something inherently wrong with them. Instead, it may be more fruitful to explore the underlying reasons for the increased risk, such as

---

* To view or treat (a person or group of people) as intrinsically different from and alien to oneself.

stigma and discrimination, and how they may lead to substance use as an unhealthy coping mechanism. Additionally, stating that all patients are asked about alcohol and substance use can help to increase disclosure and minimize patients feeling as though assumptions are being made about them based on their sexual orientation or gender identity.

Gender History

As stated above, there are times when a gender history is clearly inappropriate, but when *is* it indicated? If a patient brings up concerns regarding their gender, this is an appropriate, and necessary, time to discuss a patient's history and experience with gender. Additionally, if a patient is requesting gender-affirming hormone therapy or transition-related surgery, it is important to have a clear gender history in order to help support patients in accessing the appropriate care (see chapter 11, the section "Exploration of Gender Identity and Expression" for sample questions to help guide this conversation). At other times, it may suffice to simply ask how a patient self-identifies and what pronouns they use. If the patient has no specific concerns and no immediate desire for accessing gender-affirming hormone therapy or transition-related surgery, providers can simply state that should anything change, they are available to talk in greater detail. If there are psychosocial concerns, it may also be appropriate to bring up gender identity to inquire if this may be connected to any of the concerns being discussed; in these cases, it is important to allow the patient to decide how in depth to go with respect to gender identity and history. Again, it is important to recognize that gender identity can change over time, and there may be times when providers need to revisit the gender history.

There is much debate and controversy around trans identities and the need for a diagnosis at all, let alone one that is included in the *Diagnostic and Statistical Manual of Mental Disorders* (*DSM-5*). There has been a move towards less pathologizing terminology, such as the change from the previous DSM diagnosis of *gender identity disorder* to the currently used *gender dysphoria*.[20] The latest International Classification of Diseases, ICD-11, has included the use of the term *gender incongruence* and a relocation of the diagnosis from the category of mental health–related conditions to "Conditions Related to Sexual Health or Sexual and Gender Health."[21] On the one hand, having a diagnosis can aid communication between providers and currently may be a necessary requirement for patients to access appropriate interventions. For example, in Ontario patients require the diagnosis of gender dysphoria to obtain government funding for transition-related surgeries. However, labelling individuals who are not cisgender with a diagnosis can be stigmatizing and may cause patients to feel there is something inherently wrong with them. It may therefore be helpful to explain to patients the rationale for having a diagnosis.

When taking a gender history, it is important to appreciate that everyone has their own narrative. When it comes to gender dysphoria or gender incongruence, there are often typical presentations, which can help to guide the types of questions that are asked, but standardized questions should simply act as a guide (see chapter 11). Patients should not feel they need to tell providers a certain narrative to access treatment. This can be done unintentionally based on how questions are framed or asked. Stating that there are no correct answers and that there are many ways in which trans and non-binary identities can emerge over time allows for patients to tell their own story. For example, puberty is often a difficult period of time for trans and gender-diverse patients, but there are also many trans and non-binary people who do not experience significant distress around pubertal changes. Asking open-ended questions about puberty, without implying that it *must* have been difficult, allows for a more honest dialogue.

There are some instances when patients may not feel "trans enough." This can perhaps be thought of more intuitively as applying to individuals who are non-binary, that is, who do not fall within the binary notions of gender, but equally applies to anyone who might feel that their experience does not fit the traditional narrative of being transgender or has not involved as much "dysphoria" as others.[22] One could argue against the very idea of a typical narrative, as everyone's experience of gender identity over time is unique. Providers can support patients by ensuring they do not feel the need to provide certain narratives or answers to questions to gain access to treatment, such as hormones or surgery. Providers can also make every effort to validate patients' experiences.

Sexual History

Taking a sexual history is explored in greater detail in chapter 6; however, there are instances outside of testing for sexually transmitted infections (STIs) in which it may be necessary to ask questions related to sexual orientation and behaviours. For example, having information about a patient's sexual behaviours can help inform whether conversations around potential for pregnancy and options for contraception are needed. When inquiring, remember that sexual orientation and sexual behaviours may not always align. Sexual orientation can be fluid, and as such, there may be a prior history of sexual behaviours that pose a different set of risks compared to current behaviours. There may also be sexual behaviours that are not inherently tied to sexual orientation, such as through sex work.

When asking questions, it is important for providers to think about the reasons behind asking the question and what information is needed to make a clinical decision. For example, when asking about sexual partners, asking if patients are sexually active or have been sexually active with men, women, or both, does not actually provide the information required. Although the question sounds inclusive, it is in fact close-ended and based in heteronormative expectations of what the response should be. This question does not encompass trans or gender diverse partners. For example, if a cismale indicates that they have only been with male partners, providers may inadvertently assume that these partners are all cis men, when in fact the patient may also be with trans masculine partners, in which case a discussion around contraception would be appropriate. Instead, asking patients to describe their sexual partners allows for a more open discussion and does not limit the discussion to binary and cisnormative notions of gender. Some patients, however, may not know how to respond to such an open question (e.g. "Tell me about your sexual partners"), and in these instances it may then be necessary to provide examples to illustrate the rationale behind this line of questioning. For example, if the question is regarding the potential for pregnancy in a ciswoman, providers may want to frame the question as to whether or not she is sexually active with anyone who produces sperm.

Physical Exam

Just as the core principles of conducting a history with 2SLGBTQ community members are no different than in other populations, neither are the core principles of conducting a physical exam. Undergoing a physical exam is a position of vulnerability for most patients and as such, making every effort to create a comfortable environment, such as allowing patients to undress with privacy and having appropriate draping, are key elements in providing a patient-centred physical exam for anyone. This vulnerability can be amplified in those who have experienced adverse childhood events, violence, or abuse, which 2SLGBTQ individuals are at higher risk of having been exposed to.[23] Further, many patients may have had negative past experiences with health care services that can impact their comfort during an exam. Having a trauma-informed approach to care and to conducting physical exams can help build trust and alleviate some of these vulnerabilities.[24] Trauma-informed care is further explored in chapter 9.

Shifting the focus from typically gendered physical exams to ones based on the anatomy and organs present in an individual patient is a helpful first step that allows for a more inclusive exam. Providers should routinely ask questions to determine what anatomy and organs patients have, explaining that to provide appropriate and quality health care it is important to know this information. The World Professional Association for Transgender Health EMR Working Group suggests keeping an inventory of the following organs in EMRs: penis, testes, prostate, breasts, vagina, cervix, uterus, and ovaries.[25] By having an organ inventory for all patients, it makes it clear to all providers involved in a patient's care what anatomy is present, so as to prevent missed diagnoses and to avoid assumptions about a patient's anatomy based on their gender presentation.

Explaining the reason for conducting certain physical exam manoeuvres helps patients understand the relevance of the exam to their care. Historically, transgender bodies have been inappropriately objectified and pathologized.[26,27] Therefore, conducting only physical exams that are medically relevant is essential. In particular, for providers who may not have had much experience providing care to trans patients, it may be viewed as a learning opportunity to have a medically unnecessary physical exam done; however, this is not sufficient justification. Additionally, while having learners present (medical or nursing students, residents, etc.) is an important part of providing care in academic centres, it is equally important to make sure patients do not feel further pathologized by *always* having a learner present or multiple learners at a time. Certain patients may be more than happy to help provide education to others, but providers should be mindful that this is not the patient's role. As with medically unnecessary questions, the frequent involvement of learners can lead to patients' feeling on display and "othered" and in some cases may lead patients to feeling resentful of their health care providers.[12]

When describing physical exams, it is helpful to recognize that in trans and gender diverse populations, certain gendered anatomical terminology may be distressing to a patient. As such, it is important to use terminology that patients also use and are comfortable with. When unsure of a patient's level of comfort with gendered terms, it is always best to ask what terms they are comfortable with – for example, "Are there any words that you use to describe your body parts that you would like me to use?" Or depending on the patient and one's own comfort level, providers can also ask patients to inform them if there are any terms they

Table 3.1. Gendered and Less-Gendered Terms

Gendered Terms	Less-Gendered Terms
Breasts	Chest; upper body; torso
Vulva	External pelvic area
Vagina	Genital opening; frontal pelvic opening; internal canal; front hole
Uterus, ovaries	Internal organs; reproductive organs; estrogen producing tissue
Pap smear	Cancer screening
Bra, panties, boxers, briefs	Underwear
Period, menstruation	(Monthly) bleeding
Testicles	Testosterone-producing tissue; reproductive organs

Adapted from: Bernstein I, Peitzmeier S, Potter J, Reisner S.[28]

are using that the patient feels uncomfortable with. Alternatively, using more neutral terminology until providers are able to determine what the patient prefers is yet another option. A list of examples of gendered and neutral anatomy terms can be found in table 3.1.

Breast and Chest Exams

For patients who are about to start feminizing hormone therapy, a baseline breast/chest exam can be offered. This creates a documented baseline to assess for any changes in breast development with hormone therapy. The Endocrine Society guidelines indicate that the onset of breast development after initiation of feminizing hormone therapy occurs after three to six months, with maximal effects seen after two to three years.[29] Interestingly, a more recent European study found that the majority of breast development occurred within the first six months of hormone therapy.[30] In either instance, breast development is typically modest and variable among individuals, with limited data available to predict breast development outcomes for an individual patient. In certain locations (e.g., Ontario), documentation of amastia (the absence of breast development) following a period of hormone therapy is a criterion to access government funded breast augmentation. Furthermore, for some transfeminine patients, having a breast examination may be an affirming experience.

For patients who have had breast augmentation, consideration should be given to screening and monitoring for implant rupture, which varies based on the type of implant. The majority of saline implant ruptures result in breast asymmetry and notable size changes, and will therefore be evident on clinical exam and/or noticed by patients.[31] In contrast, the majority of silicone implant ruptures are "silent" (i.e., asymptomatic) and not visible on clinical exam.[32] However, for the minority of patients who do present with symptoms or concerns of silicone implant rupture, a physical exam should be conducted to assess for breast asymmetry, palpable nodules or lymph nodes, capsular contracture, or palpable implant shell.[33] Magnetic resonance imaging (MRI) is considered the most widely accepted imaging modality to screen for silicone rupture, but other imaging modalities, such as ultrasound, are often used as well.[33]

Pelvic and Genital Exams

Before starting gender-affirming hormone therapy, it is important to rule out intersex conditions or differences of sex development (DSDs). Historically, this included conducting a genital exam. More recently this recommendation has shifted to simply inquiring whether the patient has a history of ambiguous genitalia and not routinely completing a genital exam unless there are any concerns that arise on history or baseline blood work.

Another instance in which a genital exam may be necessary before hormone therapy is in adolescent populations when considering the use of pubertal suppression agents, or gender-affirming hormone therapy. In this case, clinical assessment to confirm the initiation of puberty through Tanner staging is often recommended.[29,34,35] It can be helpful to inform adolescents before the visit that they will need to have a brief physical exam completed.

For patients who have a cervix and have ever been sexually active, cervical cancer screening should be offered based on local screening guidelines (generally initiating after a certain age, for example 21 or 24). Unfortunately, trans masculine patients are frequently under-screened for a multitude of reasons, including gender dissonance, inaccurate perceptions of risk, discrimination, and lack of provider education.[18,36,37] Further barriers include how screening is tracked. For example, if female sex markers are the only method used to track screening, this will miss patients who have changed their sex marker to male. Again, this highlights the importance of moving away from a gendered division of care to one that is based on present anatomy/organs and risk. Additionally, women who have sex with women encompass another group who are frequently underscreened for cervical cancer.[38]

When completing a Papinicoulau (Pap) test there are some strategies to help make the process more comfortable and inclusive for 2SLGBTQ patients. It can be helpful to explain the steps involved beforehand so that patients know what to expect and can ask questions before being undressed and in a vulnerable position. Some patients may feel more comfortable being able to see and handle the speculum beforehand, whereas others may not want to see the speculum at all. If this is the first time that a patient is having a Pap test and they have not had receptive (frontal) intercourse, it may be helpful for patients to try inserting a speculum at home themselves or with a trusted partner. It is also worthwhile to have smaller speculum sizes and/or pediatric-sized speculums available. When conducting or describing a Pap test, it is best to use terminology that the patient is comfortable with to refer to their anatomy. As with anyone, providers should explain what is being done at each stage of the exam, but more time between steps may be required for patients who are 2SLGBTQ. Some patients may also feel more comfortable having a support person in the room or to hold their hand or may prefer to listen to music as a distraction technique. If a patient is on testosterone, there is often vaginal atrophy and fewer secretions, and therefore using lubrication can help ensure the exam is less painful. If the exam is particularly painful, topical lidocaine jelly can be applied several minutes before the exam if there are no contraindications. In some circumstances, intravaginal estrogen can be used for the week before the exam. Patients may also prefer to have the option to insert the speculum themselves. Once the exam is complete, it is important to indicate if a patient is on testosterone on the lab requisition, as it can impact the interpretation of the results.[39]

In other instances where pelvic exams may be necessary, such as STI screening, it may be a reasonable option to consider having patients do their own self-swabs. There is growing evidence that self-swabbing for human papillomavirus (HPV) testing or certain infections, such as candida or bacterial vaginosis, are just as effective, if not more, than provider-collected swabs.[40,41]

For patients who have had vaginoplasty, it is recommended that yearly neovaginal exams be done. This can be done with either a speculum or an anoscope, and is approached similarly to that of cis women or trans masculine patients, as described above. For patients who are assigned male at birth and have undergone vaginoplasty, the prostate will remain in situ anterior to the neovagina. Examination of the prostate can be done either rectally or via the neovagina. It is expected that the prostate will decrease in size with feminizing hormone use.

Box 3.1. Key Points

- Include the pronouns you use when introducing yourself. For example, "Hi, I'm Dr. Doe. My first name is Jane. I use they/them pronouns. What name and pronouns do you use? Please let me know if this changes."
- Ask open-ended questions whenever possible, using inclusive language.
- Never make any assumptions about a person's sexual orientation or gender identity, regardless of their presentation.
- Sexual orientation and gender identity are fluid and can change over time. Always check in with patients if there have been any changes.
- Use terminology that patients use to describe their identity and anatomy. Ask if you are unsure.
- Mistakes are inevitable – apologize, correct yourself, and move on.
- Physical exams are a position of vulnerability for patients. Make every effort to ensure patients understand the reasoning for a specific exam and that a comfortable and safe environment is created.

References

1. Paterson JL, Brown R, Walters MA. The short and longer term impacts of hate crimes experienced directly, indirectly, and through the media. Pers Soc Psychol Bull. 2019 Jul;45(7):994–1010.
2. Card KG, Hawkins BW, Mortazavi L, Gregory A, Ng KH, Lachowsky NJ. Stigma, the media, and pre-exposure prophylaxis for HIV prevention: observations for enhancing knowledge translation and resisting stigma in the Canadian context. AIDS Behav. 2019 Jul;23(7):1877–87.
3. Bristowe K, Hodson M, Wee B, Almack K, Johnson K, Daveson BA, Koffman J, McEnhill L, Harding R. Recommendations to reduce inequalities for LGBT people facing advanced illness: ACCESSCare national qualitative interview study. Palliat Med. 2018 Jan;32(1):23–35.
4. Gonzales G, Zinone R. Cancer diagnoses among lesbian, gay, and bisexual adults: results from the 2013–2016 National Health Interview Survey. Cancer Causes Control. 2018 Sep;29(9):845–54.
5. Robinson M. Two-Spirit and bisexual people: different umbrella, same rain. J Bisex. 2017 Jan;17(1):7–29.
6. Durso LE, Meyer IH. Patterns and predictors of disclosure of sexual orientation to healthcare providers among lesbians, gay men, and bisexuals. Sex Res Soc Policy. 2013 Mar;10(1):35–42.

7. Quinn GP, Schabath MB, Sanchez JA, Sutton SK, Green BL. The importance of disclosure: lesbian, gay, bisexual, transgender/transsexual, queer/questioning, and intersex individuals and the cancer continuum. Cancer. 2015 Apr;121(8):1160–3.

8. Aleshire ME, Ashforord K, Fallin-Bennett A, Hatcher J. Primary care providers' attitudes related to LGBTQ people: a narrative literature review. Health Promot Pract. 2019 Mar;20(2):173–87. doi:10.1177/1524839918778835.

9. Brooks H, Llewellyn CD, Nadarzynski T, Pelloso FC, De Souza Guilherme F, Pollard A, Jones CJ. Sexual orientation disclosure in health care: a systematic review. Br J Gen Pract. 2018 Mar;68(668):e187–96.

10. Maragh-Bass AC, Torain M, Adler R, Schneider E, Ranjit A, Kodadek LM, Shields R, German D, Snyder C, Peterson S, Schuur J, Lau B, Haider AH. Risks, benefits, and importance of collecting sexual orientation and gender identity data in healthcare settings: a multi-method analysis of patient and provider perspectives. LGBT Health. 2017 Apr;4(2):141–52.

11. Stott DB. The training needs of general practitioners in the exploration of sexual health matters and providing sexual healthcare to lesbian, gay and bisexual patients. Med Teach 2013 Sep;35(9):752–9.

12. McPhail D, Rountree-James M, Whetter I. Addressing gaps in physician knowledge regarding transgender health and healthcare through medical education. Can Med Educ J. 2016 Oct;7(2):e70–8.

13. Hadland SE, Yehia BR, Makadon HJ. Caring for lesbian, gay, bisexual, transgender, and questioning youth in inclusive and affirmative environments. Pediatr Clin North Am. 2016 Dec;63(6):955–69.

14. Ard KL, Makadon HJ. Addressing intimate partner violence in lesbian, gay, bisexual, and transgender patients. J Gen Intern Med. 2011 Aug;26(8):930–3.

15. Garthe RC, Hidalgo MA, Hereth J, Garofalo R, Reisner SL, Mimiaga MJ, et al. Prevalence and risk correlates of intimate partner violence among a multisite cohort of young transgender women. LGBT Health. 2018 Aug/Sep;5(6):333–40.

16. Sinha M. Measuring violence against women: statistical trends. Ottawa: Canadian Centre for Justice Statistics, Statistics Canada; 2013.

17. Hafeez H, Zeshan M, Tahir MA, Jahan N, Naveed S. Health care disparities among lesbian, gay, bisexual, and transgender youth: a literature review. Cureus. 2017 Apr;9(4):e1184.

18. James SE, Herman JL, Rankin S, Keisling M, Mottet L, Anafi M. The report of the 2015 U.S. Transgender Survey [Internet]. Washington (DC): National Center for Transgender Equality. 2016 [cited 2019 Aug 8] Available from: https://www.transequality.org/sites/default/files/docs/USTS-Full-Report-FINAL.PDF.

19. Mendez IM, Averett PE, Lee JG. Messaging lesbian, gay, bisexual, and transgender health inequities: a qualitative exploration. Health Promot Pract. 2019 Jan;20(1):18–21.
20. Byne W, Karasic DH, Coleman E, Eyler AE, Kidd JD, Meyer-Bahlburg HF, Pleak RR, Pula J. Gender dysphoria in adults: an overview and primer for psychiatrists. Transgend Health. 2018 May;3(1):57–70.
21. Reed GM, Drescher J, Krueger RB, Atalla E, Cochran SD, First MB, Cohen-Kettenis PT, Arango-de Montis I, Parish SJ, Cottler S, Briken P, Saxena S. Disorders related to sexuality and gender identity in the ICD-11: revising the ICD-10 classification based on current scientific evidence, best clinical practices, and human rights considerations. World Psychiatry. 2016 Oct;15(3):205–21.
22. Garrison S. On the limits of "trans enough": authenticating trans identity narratives. Gend Soc. 2018 Jun;32(5):613–37.
23. McKay T, Lindquist CH, Misra S. Understanding (and acting on) 20 years of research on violence and LGBTQ+ communities. Trauma Violence Abuse. 2019 Dec;20(5):665–78. doi:10.1177/1524838017728708.
24. Purkey E, Patel R, Phillips SP. Trauma-informed care: better care for everyone. Can Fam Physician. 2018 Mar;64(3):170–2.
25. Deutsch MB, Green J, Keatley J, Mayer G, Hastings J, Hall AM, et al.; World Professional Association for Transgender Health EMR Working Group. Electronic medical records and the transgender patient: recommendations from the World Professional Association for Transgender Health EMR Working Group. J Am Med Inform Assoc. 2013 Jul-Aug;20(4):700–3.
26. Winter S, De Cuypere G, Green J, Kane R, Knudson G. The proposed ICD-11 Gender Incongruence of Childhood diagnosis: a World Professional Association for Transgender Health membership survey. Arch Sex Behav. 2016 Oct;45(7):1605–14.
27. Davy Z. The DSM-5 and the politics of diagnosing transpeople. Arch Sex Behav. 2015 Jul;44(5):1165–76.
28. Bernstein I, Peitzmeier S, Potter J, Reisner S. If you have it, check it: overcoming barriers to cervical cancer screening with patients on the female-to-male transgender spectrum. Baltimore (MD): National LGBT Health Education Center; 2014.
29. Hembree WC, Cohen-Kettenis PT, Gooren L, Hannema SE, Meyer WJ, Murad MH, Rosenthal SM, Safer JD, Tangpricha V, T'Sjoen GG. Endocrine treatment of gender-dysphoric/gender-incongruent persons: an Endocrine Society clinical practice guideline. J Clin Endocrinol Metab. 2017 Nov 1;102(11):3869–903.
30. de Blok CJM, Klaver M, Wiepjes CM, Nota NM, Heijboer AC, Fisher AD, Schreiner T, T'Sjoen G, den Heijer M. Breast development in transwomen

after 1 year of cross-sex hormone therapy: results of a prospective multicenter study. J Clin Endocrinol Metab. 2018 Feb;103(2):532–8.

31. Baek WY, Lew DH, Lee DW. A retrospective analysis of ruptured breast implants. Arch Plast Surg. 2014 Nov;41(6):734–9.

32. Handel N, Garcia ME, Wixtrom R. Breast implant rupture: causes, incidence, clinical impact, and management. Plast Reconstr Surg. 2013 Nov;132(5):1128–37.

33. Hillard C, Fowler JD, Barta R, Cunningham B. Silicone breast implant rupture: a review. Gland Surg. 2017 Apr;6(2):163–8.

34. Bonifacio HJ, Rosenthal SM. Gender variance and dysphoria in children and adolescents. Pediatr Clin North Am. 2015 Aug;62(4):1001–16.

35. Conard LAE, Corathers SD, Trotman G. Caring for transgender and gender-nonconforming youth. Curr Pediatr Rep. 2018;6(2):139–46.

36. Seay J, Ranck A, Weiss R, Salgado C, Fein L, Kobetz E. Understanding transgender men's experience with and preferences for cervical cancer screening: a rapid assessment survey. LGBT Health. 2017 Aug;4(4):304–9.

37. Gatos KC. A literature review of cervical cancer screening in transgender men. Nurs Womens Health. 2018 Feb;22(1):52–62.

38. Peitzmeier S. Promoting cervical cancer screening among lesbians and bisexual women [Internet]. Baltimore (MD): Fenway Institute; 2013 [cited 2019 Aug 8]. Available from: https://www.lgbthealtheducation.org /wp-content/uploads/Promoting_Cervical_Cancer_Screening _LBWomen.pdf.

39. Potter J, Peitzmeier SM, Bernstein I, Reisner SL, Alizaga NM, Agénor M, Pardee DJ. Cervical cancer screening for patients on the female-to-male spectrum: a narrative review and guide for clinicians. J Gen Intern Med. 2015 Dec;30(12):1857–64.

40. McDowell M, Pardee DJ, Peitzmeier S, Reisner SL, Agénor M, Alizaga N, Bernstein I, Potter J. Cervical cancer screening preferences among trans-masculine individuals: patient-collected human papillomavirus vaginal swabs versus provider-administered Pap tests. LGBT Health. 2017 Aug;4(4):252–9.

41. Gaydos CA, Beqaj S, Schwebke JR, Lebed J, Smith B, Davis TE, Fife KH, Nyirjesy P, Spurrell T, Furgerson D, Coleman J, Paradis S, Cooper CK. Clinical validation of a test for the diagnosis of vaginitis. Obstet Gynecol. 2017 Jul;130(1):181–9.

4 Prevention and Screening for 2SLGBQ People

ALEXANDRE COUTIN, EDWARD KUCHARSKI,
AMY BOURNS, AND LISA SMITH*

Central tenants for primary care and community medicine include prevention and screening, and in many respects they are the same for 2SLGBTQ people as they would be for any individual or population. For example, the broad lifestyle recommendations of not smoking (or smoking cessation), consuming very little or no alcohol, eating four to five servings of fruits and vegetables daily (potatoes don't count), and exercising and maintaining a healthy body weight to prevent cancer and chronic disease[1] are gender identity and/or sexual orientation agnostic.

What may be different is the milieu in which patients experience these areas of risk and health care – from cigarette companies targeting the 2SLGBTQ community to challenges accessing culturally competent primary care and outright discrimination in the health care setting.[2] There are some behaviours in the 2SLGBTQ community that are more pronounced or different, and thus can confer a higher (and sometimes lower) risk of disease. This chapter reviews prevention and screening for members of sexual minority (2SLGBQ) populations, and recommendations for trans and non-binary (TNB) populations are covered in chapter 11, as hormonal and surgical interventions impart additional unique considerations. Areas of prevention and screening that will not be explicitly highlighted here are those that are applicable to any clinical scenario (for example, hypertension) for anyone, not just those who are 2SLGBQ. Regularly reviewing *Choosing Wisely* and *Canadian Task Force on Preventive Health Care* recommendations will help inform providers to deliver appropriate, evidence-based care. This practice, and familiarity with the contents of this chapter, in addition to providing a welcoming, culturally competent care environment will enable providers to successfully implement prevention and screening care with their 2SLGBQ patients.

---

* literature review

Last, given there is a greater burden of sexually transmitted infections, mental health issues, and substance use disorders within sexual minority communities (along with TNB communities), these are explored more broadly in their own dedicated chapters (6, 8, and 9, respectively).

Women who have sex with women (WSW) and men who have sex with men (MSM) – a large proportion of whom identify as Two-Spirit, lesbian, gay, bisexual, or queer (2SLGBQ) – are no doubt present in many if not all Canadian providers' practices.* For many providers, their 2SLGBQ patients' sexual orientation is either unknown to them, suspected, not discussed, or thought to be of no significant importance to their care. Indeed, many providers may want to treat all of their patients similarly in an effort to minimize bias and discrimination. However, such an approach is ill-advised as the 2SLGBQ population (and the 2SLGBTQ population more broadly) is one that is at increased risk for certain health conditions and one for which routine primary care is often suboptimal.[3-12] Most patients are willing to discuss their identity if asked,[4,13,14] and this chapter will outline why it is imporant to inform prevention and screening for 2SLGBQ patients.

Accurately determining the prevalence of those who identify as sexual minorities is challenging. Previous studies[15-18] have yielded a range of results depending on methodology, definitions used, and geographical range. Overall, findings suggest that approximately 3 to 8 per cent of the North American population identifies as 2SLGBQ. This proportion is increasing with a concurrent change in social landscape, and previous inquiries have likely underestimated true prevalence.

When considering the health care needs of 2SLGBQ patients, clinicians may be unaware of the patient's sexual orientation and/or practices, as well as harbour heteronormative assumptions that can interfere with the effectiveness of the patient–physician relationship. Such assumptions may also lead the provider to miss crucial data during a clinical encounter (see chapters 2 and 3).

At times, the provider's knowledge of a patient's 2SLGBQ identity can lead to other assumptions that may impede care via missed

---

* We have divided this chapter broadly into cis-WSW and cis-MSM and use a broader acronym of 2SLGBQ to describe both of these populations. This terminology is intended to improve the ease of reading and not meant to exclude any particular identity. Readers are encouraged to approach each patient as an individual, rather than making assumptions based on oversimplified categories. Furthermore, categories used in research are often inconsistent. Accordingly, the reader is encouraged to seek out a specific reference for clarity when needed.

prevention and screening opportunities and lack of anticipatory care. To most effectively counter erroneous assumptions, clinicians should remember two key factors:

1. Sexual identity is fluid and may change over time.
2. Sexual identity and behaviours are different and may or may not overlap.

In general, behaviours take precedence over identity in situations where an ongoing relationship between clinician and patient is unlikely (i.e., emergency departments, clinics for sexually transmitted infections [STIs]). These clinical encounters tend to focus on an acute problem. For example, knowing when a cis woman last had vaginal intercourse with someone who can make sperm is of high importance when ruling out an ectopic pregnancy in the emergent clinical presentation of abdominal pain. However, primary care providers must explore both identity and behaviours to understand their patients' nuanced experiences, especially when there is an ongoing relationship.

Women Who Have Sex with Women (WSW)

Use of Health Care Services

Lifetime prevalence of same-sex behaviour is estimated to be 7.1 to 11.2 per cent among women,[19] while approximately 4.4 to 6.7 per cent of women identify as LGBQ.[20] Despite positive shifts in societal attitudes, WSW continue to face various barriers to optimal health. Further, negative interactions in clinical settings lead them to delay or avoid health care.[10,21] Such interactions may include heteronormative assumptions of the gender of partners, the need for contraception, and desires for fertility or outright exclusion of partners, as well as erroneously recommending against cervical cancer screening (see Cervical Cancer Screening below).

Lesbian-identified women have in the past avoided periodic health reviews and postponed seeking necessary treatments longer than their heterosexual counterparts.[22,23] Practice websites and brochures often feature only heterosexual couples and families, intake forms lack inclusive options, and clinic spaces have an overwhelming paucity of visuals indicating queer-positivity.[10,20,24-27] Practitioners likely contribute to these unwelcoming spaces because of lack of knowledge regarding WSW health needs and hesitancy to broach topics pertaining to patients' sexual identity.[4,10,12,13,28,29]

Primary and Preventive Care Needs

The majority of primary care concerns for WSW are similar to those of any general practice population; however, some risks and needs pertain more specifically to WSW.[8] That said, researchers have historically and erroneously regarded the health needs of WSW as synonymous with the collective sexual minority population. Therefore, focused evidence-based guidelines pertaining to the health needs of WSW are lacking, especially those considering the intersections of ethnic identity, racialized identity, socioeconomic status, and geography.[8]

Cardiovascular Disease and Diabetes

Cardiovascular disease (CVD) has been a longstanding leading cause of mortality for all populations in North America and for a number of reasons, is a particular health concern for sexual minority women.[30–33] WSW exhibit a greater prevalence of CVD risk factors, including stress, tobacco use, alcohol consumption, substance use, mental health disparities, lower socioeconomic status, and higher body mass index.[34–36]

Additionally, WSW who identify as non-heterosexual have an even greater disparity of CVD risk compared to WSW who identify as heterosexual, suggesting that non-heterosexual identity is the primary driver of CVD risk rather than same-sex sexual activity. This finding may be explained using Meyer's theory of minority stress: such stress may result in biological processes that confer increased CVD risk, or it may precipitate negative coping behaviours that increase these risks.[34,37]

LGB adults are more likely to experience adverse cardiovascular outcomes,[34,36] and WSW seem to have greater odds of heart disease, diabetes, obesity, and hypercholesterolemia.[24,38,39] Though sexual minority women may be at increased risk for diabetes, no studies concretely show a significant difference in prevalence of diabetes by sexual orientation.[34]

CVD risk factors should be addressed in preventive health visits with WSW patients, particularly those with a family history of CVD, cerebrovascular disease, or diabetes. Future study is required to better understand CVD in 2SLGBQ women and overcome barriers that have thus far hindered its understanding.[40]

Cervical Cancer Screening

Compared to the general population, WSW have decreased rates of cervical cancer screening and tend to initiate this screening late. A 2010 report on a survey of 225 lesbian women from a mid-size

American city found as many as 25 per cent reported delaying Pap testing out of a fear of discrimination.[41] Other research has estimated that screening rates are 5 to 18 per cent lower for WSW, with a greater time interval between Pap tests, particularly in those having had only female partners, because of the perceived lack of exposure risk (see Risk Factors for Cervical Cancer, below).[42-53] In fact, studies have suggested sexual minority women believe themselves to be at lower risk for STIs, that human papillomavirus (HPV) is not spread between females, and that they don't need to engage in sexual risk reduction behaviours.[34,43,54,55] Though previous studies have suggested a lower rate of STIs between lesbians, more recent evidence indicates that HPV is common in lesbians and is transmitted through sexual contact.[20,56]

The following are risk factors for cervical cancer:[57]

- HPV (human papillomavirus) infection
- smoking
- multiparity (because of increased hormone exposure)
- sex before age 18 (because of cervical vulnerability during this period)
- multiple partners (because of increased exposure to HPV)
- inadequate Papanicolaou (Pap) testing
- oral contraceptive use
- STI infection (HIV, chlamydia, syphilis)

WSW may contract HPV via any sexual activity (for example, genital-genital, oral-genital, or digital-genital contact). Sharing toys can also transmit the virus.[43] Those who are sexually active and have not had receptive penetrative vaginal or anal sex are still at risk for HPV infection and cervical cancer.[42]

Lesbians report higher rates of sexual intercourse before the age of 18 and more sexual partners overall, compared with heterosexual women.[43] Lesbian women more often have high body mass index (BMI) scores and increased alcohol consumption, both of which have been linked to gynecological cancers.[42,43] However, sexual minority women are more likely to be nulliparous and have lower rates of oral contraceptive use than the general public.[58,59] Finally, lesbians, and particularly bisexual women, may be at increased risk of cervical cancer because of higher rates of smoking.[41,42,58,60,61]

Despite a higher prevalence of some risk factors, a 2014 US study found the risk of abnormal Pap and HPV testing to be modestly lower in WSW.[62] However, both cervical cytology abnormalities and HPV infection are more common in HIV seropositive women regardless of sexual partners.

Health care and WSW communities must be made aware that regular Pap and HPV testing is as important for WSW as it is in the general population.[34,42,43,55,62,63] Evidence strongly supports physician recommendation as a determinant of regular screening behaviour.[42,64]

Unfortunately, many providers continue to neglect offering cervical cancer screening because of an outdated belief that WSW are at lower or no risk of cervical cancer. This misconception has led to the explicit statements in various guidelines to include WSW in cervical cancer screening and for those at average risk to be screened in a manner similar to heterosexual women.

Breast Cancer

Risk factors for breast cancer that have been identified among the general population include the following:[65]

- family history, particularly genetic mutations (for example, BRCA1, BRCA2)
- Ashkenazi Jewish ancestry
- increased breast tissue density
- early menarche
- late menopause
- late pregnancy
- nulliparity
- exposure to ionizing radiation (for example, radiotherapy for cancer treatment)
- hormone replacement therapy
- hormonal contraception use
- alcohol use
- increased BMI
- sedentary lifestyle
- higher socioeconomic status
- smoking (likely)

WSW have been shown to have a higher prevalence of a number of these risk factors, namely, higher rates of nulliparity, older age at first live birth, fewer pregnancies, fewer total months pregnant, fewer total months breastfeeding, higher BMIs, greater alcohol consumption, and less exercise.[42,66–72]

Conversely, some research indicates that sexual minority women have a lower prevalence of ever having used oral contraception compared to heterosexual women (61 versus 84 per cent) and shorter mean duration of birth control use (2.57 versus 5.99 years).[72] Also, breast cancer rates are higher in more affluent women, yet income levels in lesbian and bisexual women are comparatively low.[42]

Participation in breast cancer screening is also an important determinant of morbidity and mortality from breast cancer. Findings with respect to sexual minority women's participation in mammography screening have been inconsistent. Some studies suggest WSW are less likely to have had a recent mammogram,[46,50] whereas others have reported no difference or a higher likelihood of mammography.[42,52,66,73] A tailored risk counselling approach has been shown to be successful in increasing lesbian patients' mammography screening.[64]

A tailored risk assessment for cis women can be created at mycanceriq .ca. This is an online risk assessment portal from Ontario Health (Cancer Care Ontario), that identifies a cis woman's risk of breast (and several other cancers) as being low, average, or increased. The tool then provides suggested behaviours to reduce risk (for example, reducing alcohol consumption, engaging in screening). A randomized control trial demonstrated this approach reduces perceived risk of breast cancer, reduces anxieties and fears about breast cancer, and increases screening rates.[74]

Despite these risk factors and screening disparities, it remains unclear whether breast cancer is truly more prevalent in WSW.[42] Lesbian women have been estimated to have a greater disease-specific mortality age-adjusted relative risk (RR) for breast cancer but did not differ in their overall risk for all-cause mortality.[42] Women in same-sex relationships also had greater age-adjusted RR for fatal breast cancer but did not differ in their overall risk for all-cause mortality.[75]

The few published prevalence estimates in the WSW population are unreliable because of small sample sizes and poor study design. Large cohort studies pooled from sexual orientation data collection in routine statistics and cancer registries are needed.[71] Further inquiry is required to determine if known risks translate into increased mortality and to uncover culturally appropriate ways to modify these risks among sexual minority women.[69]

Bacterial Vaginosis (BV)

BV is a common cause of vulvovaginal symptoms in cis women and is characterized by a shift in vaginal flora from the dominant *Lactobacillus* to a polymicrobial flora.[76] It is associated with preterm birth, increased susceptibility to pelvic inflammatory disease, and certain STIs such as herpes simplex virus (HSV)-2 and HIV.[56,76]

BV has been associated with smoking,[77,78] receptive oral sex,[79,80] a higher number of female partners or a partner with BV,[81,82] and use of vaginal lubrication or sharing vaginal sex toys.[61,79] A number of these risk factors have a higher prevalence among WSW.

Though investigation of BV as a sexually transmitted entity is limited by the absence of a clear microbiological etiology, the epidemiological profile of BV is similar to that of established STIs.[82] Particularly in WSW, BV should be clinically regarded as sexually transmitted.[78,80,81] In fact, some data demonstrate AFAB partners can share strain-specific genital bacteria and that specific bacterial species are associated with treatment failure in BV.[56]

Although BV is common among all cis women, and likely even more so among WSW, routine screening for BV is currently not recommended, nor is the treatment of asymptomatic partners of women with BV.[42,56,78,81] Currently, providers should encourage awareness of signs and symptoms of BV in WSW and promote healthy sexual practices such as cleaning shared sex toys between uses.[56] For more information on STIs and screening, please see chapter 6.

Vaccinations

Unlike for MSM, there are no unique guidelines or recommendations for vaccinations for WSW outside of the routinely recommended immunizations for all adults. However, a tailored approach should be taken to assess for other risks in WSW to consider additional immunizations (for example, vaccinating for hepatitis A and B in the context of liver disease).

Further Health Considerations for WSW

There are other health care disparities seen in the WSW population that despite their importance are not explored in detail in this chapter. At the very least, being aware that WSW may also struggle with higher rates of disability, polycystic ovary syndrome (PCOS), asthma, and chronic lung disease (undoubtedly from higher rates of smoking) will be helpful in clinical care.[83,84]

Fortunately, there is strong evidence for both colorectal and lung cancer screening, and this will be discussed in the later section on gender-agnostic screening for any member of the 2SLGBTQ community.

There are few evidence-based guidelines (if any) supportive of screening for several other forms of cancer (for example, ovarian, endometrial), despite a strong desire from both patients and providers to be able to intervene and detect cancer at early stages, when treatments are often more effective and less toxic.

Fortunately, it is estimated that people can reduce the risk of cancer (and other chronic diseases) by 40 to 50 per cent by engaging in healthy lifestyle behaviours, as outlined at the start of this chapter. Further, directing patients to online risk-assessment tools (for example, mycanceriq.ca) can empower engagement in health behaviours that reduce risks for several types of cancer and chronic diseases.

Men Who Have Sex with Men (MSM)

Historically, MSM have been vulnerable to certain cancers, CVD, STIs, mental illness, substance use disorders, smoking, trauma, and HIV/AIDS (and their related health impacts). In the late 1990s before the advent of effective HIV treatments, the life expectancy of gay men in a large Canadian city was estimated to be 8 to 20 years less than for all men.[85-87]

Thankfully, much progress has been made in offsetting the health inequities of sexual minority men. That said, sexual minority stress and its deleterious health effects continue to affect this population.[25]

2SGBQ Men's Use of Health Care Services

Gay men's access to health care services varies. A large British survey reported that gay men, but not bisexual men, were more likely than heterosexual men to have seen a family practitioner in the past three months.[88] In a US survey, there was no significant difference between gay men and straight men in having a usual source of care when sick.[89]

In Canada, gay men are more likely to consult a medical specialist compared with heterosexual men (29 versus 19 per cent), but are not different in their likelihood of consulting a family doctor (75 versus 69 per cent). Likewise, more gay men than heterosexual men consult psychologists (8 versus 3 per cent) and social workers or counsellors (about 7 versus 4 per cent). Bisexual men do not differ from heterosexual men in their consultations with doctors, though they do have more frequent contact with social workers or counsellors.[89]

At the same time, gay men may face several barriers when accessing care, including trouble finding a provider and lacking trust and confidence in a doctor, as well as problems communicating with a doctor or nurse.[90,91] These issues can lead to a decrease in overall satisfaction in care received, as well as to postponing care.[91,92] Some of these barriers are easily overcome with simple interventions, such as offering 2SLGBQ-affirmative publications in waiting rooms, while some no doubt will require more resources.

Interestingly, a Dutch study reported no difference between gay and bisexual men versus heterosexual men in their levels of confidence in different aspects of the healthcare system.[93] The authors hypothesize this may be due to the more accepting social attitudes towards sexual minorities in the Netherlands.

Disclosure of sexual orientation to health care providers improves care. More than 80 per cent of youth reported a positive or neutral impact on their care.[92] And young gay men in New York City were more likely to have at least one health visit in the past year if they had disclosed their sexual orientation to their primary care provider.[94]

Coronary Artery Disease (CAD) and Diabetes

There is no conclusive evidence that MSM are at higher risk of CAD and diabetes than the general population. However, certain risk behaviours like smoking and/or stimulant use, for example, likely increase the risk of CAD. It is recommended that screening and treatment of dyslipidemia, diabetes, and hypertension be undertaken according to guidelines used and accepted in general primary care for all patients. In addition, HIV infection and its treatment can have an impact on the cardiovascular system (see chapter 7 for a full discussion).

Vaccinations

MSM are at higher risk of some vaccine-preventable infectious diseases. In addition to routine vaccinations, MSM should receive vaccination for hepatitis A and B (see chapter 6). The National Advisory Committee on Immunization states that despite a lack of evidence for vaccinating MSM above the age of 27, strong consideration should be given to HPV vaccination for MSM of all ages.[95] In particular, MSM with HIV are at higher risk for anal cancer when infected with HPV.[96]

There have been several outbreaks of meningococcal meningitis in MSM communities in cities across North America and Europe in recent decades.[97] Some experts recommend vaccination in the context of an outbreak for those with close contacts.[98] Currently, there are no evidence-based recommendations to routinely vaccinate MSM for meningococcal disease, except in the setting of HIV infection (see chapter 7 for more information on vaccines for people living with HIV).

Prostate Cancer Screening

The Canadian Task Force on Preventive Health Care (CTFPHC) has recommendations for prostate cancer screening. These screening recommendations are no different for MSM than for other men. While very limited evidence suggests that gay men may have lower risk and prevalence of prostate cancer, screening recommendations should be applied consistently for all men, regardless of orientation.[42]
Broadly, the task force recommends not routinely offering prostate cancer screening, in particular, given the harms of many false-positive results. However, it does recommend a conversation with patients about screening, and for some who place a high value on testing, it might be considered.[99] An excellent video was created by Dr. Mike Evans describing both the European and the American large randomized controlled trials for screening and help in decision making for patients. The video is widely available online and accessible using any search platform with the terms "Mike Evans" and "prostate screening."

Anal Cancer

We know that the risk of HPV-related anal cancer is higher in MSM than in the general population.[100] This is true for both HIV-negative and -positive men with the latter being at highest risk.[97] The incidence of anal cancer among MSM has been estimated at 37 cases per 100,000 person-years, while the rate among MSM living with HIV is reported as 131 cases per 100,000 person-years.[100,97]
The idea for anal cytological screening (anal Pap test) rests on the similarities between anal dysplasia and cervical dysplasia and the success of cervical Pap screening programs. In Canada, anal Pap testing for gay men (regardless of HIV status) is not considered standard of care at this time; however, it is being performed in some health care centres.[101] No published randomized controlled trials that demonstrate a benefit of anal cancer screening have been published; however, one such study is underway.
Some experts recommend a digital anorectal exam (DARE) and/or anal cytology every one to two years for screening of people at high risk of anal cancer (see boxes 4.1 and 4.2 below, respectively).[102] DARE may also be completed in any patient who reports a symptomatic complaint of anal pain, discomfort, or bleeding. Generally for concerning symptoms,

endoscopy and/or referral to a gastroenterologist is recommended (this should be differentiated from screening, as screening is undertaken in an asymptomatic patient). Note that if one is completing anal cytology, performing a DARE following the collection of cells is likely a better approach to avoid getting lubricant in the cytology sample. Because of the lack of clear evidence and guidelines on anal cancer screening, the preferable approach likely involves an ongoing conversation between clinician and patient and shared decision making.

Box 4.1. Performing a DARE (Digital Anorectal Exam)

- Inspect the perianal skin for any nodules, erosions, or fissures.
- Complete a quadrant-by-quadrant sweep of the anal canal (with plenty of lubricant, or with lidocaine jelly).
- Palpate thoroughly the mucosa, feeling for induration, nodules, or tenderness
- Intra-anal warts can be identified by their verrucous texture and lack of pain or tenderness on examination.
- The presence of painful warty nodules may indicate an underlying cancer.
- Exquisite generalized tenderness may indicate an anorectal infection, such as lymphogranuloma venereum; obtain swabs for chlamydia and gonorrhea.

Source: Adapted from Weiss, Anal cancer: information to get you out of the dark!, 2019.[102]

Box 4.2. Performing an Anal Cytology Swab

- Patients should insert nothing into their anus, including an enema or a douche, for 24 hours before the exam.
- Lubricants should be avoided before sampling because they may affect processing and interpretation of the sample.
- Patients are typically asked to lie on their left side, but other positions are also possible.
- Retract the buttocks to expose the anal opening; insert a Dacron or polyester tipped swab moistened with tap water into the anus as far

as it will go, typically to a depth of 5 to 7.5 centimetres (2 to 3 inches); the swab can be felt to pass through the internal sphincter so the sample is obtained from the junction of the anus and rectum, which is where most HPV-related lesions are found.

- Rotate the swab through full circles in both directions with firm lateral pressure applied to the swab (this pressure ensures that the mucosal surface, rather than rectal contents, are sampled); then slowly withdraw from the anus, continuously rotating the swab in both directions and taking 15 to 30 seconds to withdraw completely.
- Smear the swab directly onto a glass slide and fix as a conventional cytology smear by placing it into alcohol, or place the swab in a preservative vial and agitate vigorously to disperse the cells for liquid-based cytology.
- Fix the sample quickly if using a glass slide, within 15 seconds, to avoid drying artefact

Source: Adapted from University of California, Obtaining a specimen for anal cytology.[103]

Gender-Agnostic Screening Recommendations

Cancer Screening

Since the first edition of this text, there have been many advances in cancer screening and updated evidence-based guidelines. Further, new recommendations have been published about both prostate (see above) and lung cancer screening. Unfortunately, there is still wide debate and variable practice in screening for cancers that undoubtedly confuse both patients and providers.

The CTFPHC publishes screening guidelines for several cancers and can be found online at www.canadiantaskforce.ca.

Lung Cancer Screening

As mentioned, since many 2SLGBTQ people smoke at a higher rate than the general population, they are likely to be at higher risk of lung cancer. The CTFPHC recommends lung cancer screening according to the criteria of the National Lung Cancer Screening Trial (smokers ages 55 to

74, with at least a 30-pack/year history who currently smoke or quit less than 15 years ago) with low-dose CT at a centre that has experience with screening. Ontario has also started a lung cancer screening program in several centres using a more sensitive risk calculator to select persons at higher risk of lung cancer and most likely to benefit from screening.

Colorectal Cancer Screening

There are now many organized screening programs for colorectal cancer screening, and general screening recommendations should be applied for all patients, regardless of sexual orientation or gender identity. There is no clear evidence that members of the 2SLGBTQ population are at higher risk of colorectal cancer. Age and family history are generally the most common risk factors. However, other factors (for example alcohol use, sedentary lifestyle, higher BMI), may increase risk and be over-represented in some 2SLGBTQ groups.

Conclusion

Many providers select primary care as an area of focus since prevention and screening are logical interventions to reduce morbidity and mortality and often reduce the burden of disease on patients, their families, communities, and the broader health system. This remains true for the 2SLGBTQ community. While some areas often require some added attention in various members of these communities, the vast majority of prevention and screening remains the same in stewarding their health. Providers and leaders should continue to advocate for prevention and screening for cancer and chronic disease at patient, organization, and government levels as it is believed that upwards of 40 per cent of many diseases can be prevented through these early and often accessible lifestyle changes and health care manoeuvres.

References

1. Cancer Care Ontario [Internet]. Toronto: Cancer Care Ontario. Feb 2019 [cited 2020 Jan 8]. Cancer fact: updated cancer prevention guidelines incorporate a holistic view of nutrition. Available from: https://www.cancercareontario.ca/Cancerfacts.
2. Washington HA. Burning Love: big tobacco takes aim at LGBT youths. Am J Public Health. 2002;92(7):1086–95. doi:10.2105/AJPH.92.7.1086.
3. Bostwick WB, Hughes TL, Everett B. Health behavior, status, and outcomes among a community-based sample of lesbian and bisexual women. LGBT Health. 2015 Jun;2(2):121–6. doi:10.1089/lgbt.2014.0074.

4. Law M, Mathai A, Veinot P, Webster F, Mylopoulos M. Exploring lesbian, gay, bisexual, and queer (LGBQ) people's experiences with disclosure of sexual identity to primary care physicians: a qualitative study. BMC Fam Pract. 2015 Dec;16(1):175. doi:10.1186 /s12875-015-0389-4.

5. Wilkin T. Primary care for men who have sex with men. N Engl J Med. 2015 Aug;373(9):854–62. doi:10.1056/NEJMcp1401303.

6. Torke AM, Carnahan JL. Optimizing the clinical care of lesbian, gay, bisexual, and transgender older adults. JAMA Intern Med. 2017 Dec;177(12):1715–16. doi:10.1001/jamainternmed.2017.5324.

7. Coutin A, Wright S, Li C, Fung R. Missed opportunities: are residents prepared to care for transgender patients? A study of family medicine, psychiatry, endocrinology, and urology residents. Can Med Educ J. 2018 Jul;9(3):e41–55. doi:10.36834/cmej.42906.

8. Mayer KH, Bekker LG, Stall R, Grulich AE, Colfax G, Lama JR. Comprehensive clinical care for men who have sex with men: an integrated approach. Lancet. 2012 Jul;380(9839):378–87. doi:10.1016 /S0140-6736(12)60835-6.

9. Duarte MT, de Freitas AP, Andrade J, Ignacio MA. P5.19 Health needs of women who have sex with women and access to health services. Sex Transm Infect. 2017;93 Suppl 2:A242.

10. Knight DA, Jarrett D. Preventive health care for women who have sex with women. Am Fam Physician. 2017 Mar;95(5):314–21.

11. Knight DA, Jarrett D. Preventive health care for men who have sex with men. Am Fam Physician. 2015 Jun;91(12):844–51.

12. Sharma M, Pinto AD, Kumagai AK. Teaching the social determinants of health: A path to equity or a road to nowhere? Acad Med. 2018 Jan;93(1):25–30.

13. Scheck A. Special Report: LGBT patients in the ED (do ask, do tell). Emerg Med News. 2015 Jul;37(7):16–17.

14. Maragh-Bass AC, Torain M, Adler R, Ranjit A, Schneider E, Shields RY, et al. Is It Okay To Ask: transgender patient perspectives on sexual orientation and gender identity collection in healthcare. Acad Emerg Med. 2017 Jun;24(6):655–67.

15. Heilman B, Barker G, Harrison A. The man box: A study on being a young man in the US, UK, and Mexico: key findings. Washington (DC): Promundo US and Unilever; 2017.

16. Kraus K, Moizo M [Internet]. Paris, France: IFOP; 2017 Jan [cited 2018 Sep 25]. To bi or not to bi ? Enquête sur l'attirance sexuelle entre femmes. Available from: https://www.ifop.com/publication/ to-bi-or-not-to-bi-enquete-sur-lattirance-sexuelle-entre-femmes/.

17. Gates GJ [Internet]. Los Angeles: The Williams Institute, UCLA Scool of Law; [2011 Apr]. How many people are lesbian, gay, bisexual, and

transgender? Available from https://williamsinstitute.law.ucla.edu
/publications/how-many-people-lgbt/.

18. Statistic Canada [Internet]. Ottawa: Government of Canada; 2015 [cited 2018 Sep 25]. Same-sex couples and sexual orientation … by the numbers. Available from: https://www.statcan.gc.ca/eng/dai/smr08/2015/smr08_203_2015.

19. Everett BG. Sexual orientation disparities in sexually transmitted infections: examining the intersection between sexual identity and sexual behavior. Arch Sex Behav. 2013 Feb;42(2):225–36.

20. Marrazzo JM, Gorgos LM. Emerging sexual health issues among women who have sex with women. Curr Infect Dis Rep. 2012 Feb;14(2):204–11.

21. Khalili J, Leung LB, Diamant AL. Finding the perfect doctor: identifying lesbian, gay, bisexual, and transgender-competent physicians. Am J Public Health. 2015 Jun;105(6):1114–19.

22. Harrison AE, Silenzio VM. Comprehensive care of lesbian and gay patients and families. Prim Care. 1996 Mar;23(1):31–46.

23. Carroll NM. Optimal gynecologic and obstetric care for lesbians. Obstet Gynecol. 1999 Apr;93(4):611–13.

24. ACOG Committee on Health Care for Underserved Women. ACOG Committee Opinion No. 525: health care for lesbians and bisexual women. Obstet Gynecol. 2012 May;119(5):1077–80.

25. Frost DM, Lehavot K, Meyer IH. Minority stress and physical health among sexual minority individuals. J Behav Med. 2015 Feb;38(1):1–8.

26. McNair RP, Hegarty K. Guidelines for the primary care of lesbian, gay, and bisexual people: a systematic review. Ann Fam Med. 2010;8(6):533–41.

27. Tang H, Tang G, Coutin A, Nyhof-Young J, Biro L. Taking pride in a novel LGBTQ health infographic for first year medical students. Poster session presented at: The Canadian Condernce on Medical Education; 2017 Apr 29–May 2; Winnipeg, MB.

28. Bidell MP. The Lesbian, Gay, Bisexual, and Transgender Development of Clinical Skills Scale (LGBT-DOCSS): establishing a new interdisciplinary self-assessment for health providers. J Homosex. 2017;64(10):1432–60.

29. Obedin-Maliver J, Goldsmith ES, Stewart L, White W, Tran E, Brenman S, Wells M, Fetterman DM, Garcia G, Lunn MR. Lesbian, gay, bisexual and transgender-related content in undergraduate medical education. JAMA. 2011 Sept;306(9):971–7.

30. Ulstad VK. Coronary health issues for lesbians. J Gay Lesbian Med Assoc. 1999;3(2):59–66.

31. Nair C, Colburn H, McLean D, Petrasovits A. Cardiovascular disease in Canada. Health Rep. 1989;1(1):1–22.

32. Institute for Health Metrics and Evaluation [Internet]. Seattle (WA): University of Washington; 2018 [cited 2019 Dec 4]. Canada profile. Available from http://www.healthdata.org/Canada.

33. Institute for Health Metrics and Evaluation [Internet]. Seattle (WA): University of Washington; 2018 [cited 2019 Dec 4]. United States profile. Available from http://www.healthdata.org/united-states.

34. Makadon HJ, Mayer KH, Potter J, Goldhammer H, American College of Physicians, R2 Digital Library, editors. The Fenway guide to lesbian, gay, bisexual, and transgender health. 2nd ed. Philadelphia: American College of Physicians; 2015.

35. Caceres BA, Brody A, Luscombe RE, Primiano JE, Marusca P, Sitts EM, et al. A systematic review of cardiovascular disease in sexual minorities. Am J Public Health. 2017;107(4):e13–e21.

36. Hatzenbuehler ML, McLaughlin KA, Slopen N. Sexual orientation disparities in cardiovascular biomarkers among young adults. Am J Prev Med. 2013;44(6):612–21.

37. Farmer GW, Jabson JM, Bucholz KK, Bowen DJ. A population-based study of cardiovascular disease risk in sexual-minority women. Am J Public Health. 2013;103(10):1845–50.

38. Blosnich JR, Hanmer J, Yu L, Matthews DD, Kavalieratos D. Health care use, health behaviors, and medical conditions among individuals in same-sex and opposite-sex partnerships: A cross-sectional observational analysis of the Medical Expenditures Panel Survey (MEPS), 2003–2011. Med Care. 2016;54(6):547–54.

39. Diamant AL, Wold C. Sexual orientation and variation in physical and mental health status among women. J Womens Health (Larchmt). 2003;12(1):41–9.

40. Caceres BA, Brody A, Chyun D. Recommendations for cardiovascular disease research with lesbian, gay and bisexual adults. J Clin Nurs. 2016;25(23–4):3728–42.

41. Tracy JK, Lydecker AD, Ireland L. Barriers to cervical cancer screening among lesbians. J Womens Health (Larchmt). 2010;19(2):229–37.

42. Quinn GP, Sanchez JA, Sutton SK, Vadaparampil ST, Nguyen GT, Green BL, et al. Cancer and lesbian, gay, bisexual, transgender/transsexual, and queer/questioning (LGBTQ) populations. CA Cancer J Clin. 2015 Sep-Oct;65(5):384–400.

43. Waterman L, Voss J. HPV, cervical cancer risks, and barriers to care for lesbian women. Nurse Pract. 2015;40(1):46–53.

44. Curmi C, Peters K, Salamonson Y. Barriers to cervical cancer screening experienced by lesbian women: a qualitative study. J Clin Nurs. 2016;25(23–4):3643–51.

45. Curmi C, Peters K, Salamonson Y. Lesbians' attitudes and practices of cervical cancer screening: a qualitative study. BMC Womens Health. 2014;14(1):153.
46. Kerker BD, Mostashari F, Thorpe L. Health care access and utilization among women who have sex with women: sexual behavior and identity. J Urban Health. 2006;83(5):970–9.
47. Marrazzo JM, Koutsky LA, Kiviat NB, Kuypers JM, Stine K. Papanicolaou test screening and prevalence of genital human papillomavirus among women who have sex with women. Am J Public Health. 2001;91(6):947.
48. Cochran SD, Mays VM, Bowen D, Gage S, Bybee D, Roberts SJ, et al. Cancer-related risk indicators and preventive screening behaviors among lesbians and bisexual women. Am J Public Health. 2001;91(4):591.
49. Diamant AL, Wold C, Spritzer K, Gelberg L. Health behaviors, health status, and access to and use of health care: a population-based study of lesbian, bisexual, and heterosexual women. Arch Fam Med. 2000;9(10):1043–51.
50. Buchmueller T, Carpenter CS. Disparities in health insurance coverage, access, and outcomes for individuals in same-sex versus different-sex relationships, 2000-2007. Am J Public Health. 2010;100(3):489–95.
51. Cahill S, Makadon H. Sexual orientation and gender identity data collection in clinical settings and in electronic health records: A key to ending LGBT health disparities. LGBT Health. 2014;1(1):34–41.
52. McElroy JA, Wintemberg JJ, Williams A. Comparison of lesbian and bisexual women to heterosexual women's screening prevalence for breast, cervical, and colorectal cancer in Missouri. LGBT Health. 2015;2(2):188–92.
53. Matthews AK, Brandenburg DL, Johnson TP, Hughes TL. Correlates of underutilization of gynecological cancer screening among lesbian and heterosexual women. Prev Med. 2004;38(1):105–13.
54. Henderson AW, Lehavot K, Simoni JM. Ecological models of sexual satisfaction among lesbian/bisexual and heterosexual women. Arch Sex Behav. 2009;38(1):50–65.
55. Marrazzo JM, Coffey P, Bingham A. Sexual practices, risk perception and knowledge of sexually transmitted disease risk among lesbian and bisexual women. Perspect Sex Reprod Health. 2005;37(1):6–12.
56. Gorgos LM, Marrazzo JM. Sexually transmitted infections among women who have sex with women. Clinical Infectious Diseases. 2011;53(suppl_3):S84–S91.
57. Canadian Cancer Society [Internet]. Toronto: Canadian Cancer Society; [cited 2018 Dec 7]. Risk factors for cervical cancer. Available from: http://www.cancer.ca/en/cancer-information/cancer-type/cervical/risks/.

58. Case P, Austin SB, Hunter DJ, Manson JE, Malspeis S, Willett WC, et al. Sexual orientation, health risk factors, and physical functioning in the Nurses' Health Study II. J Womens Health (Larchmt). 2004;13(9):1033–47.
59. Stoffel C, Carpenter E, Everett B, Higgins J, Haider S. Family planning for sexual minority women. Semin Reprod Med. 2017;35(5):460–8.
60. Bryant LO, Bowman L. Tobacco use among sexual minorities. New Dir Adult Contin Educ. 2014;2014(142):63–72.
61. Roberts SJ. Primary care of women who have sex with women: recommendations from the research. Nurse Pract. 2015;40(12):24–32.
62. Massad LS, Xie X, Minkoff H, Darragh TM, D'Souza G, Sanchez-Keeland L, et al. Abnormal Pap tests and human papillomavirus infections among HIV-infected and uninfected women who have sex with women. J Low Genit Tract Dis. 2014;18(1):50–6.
63. Henderson HJ. Why lesbians should be encouraged to have regular cervical screening. J Fam Plann Reprod Health Care. 2009;35(1):49–52.
64. Brown JP, Tracy JK. Lesbians and cancer: an overlooked health disparity. Cancer Causes Control. 2008;19(10):1009–20.
65. Canadian Cancer Society [Internet]. Toronto: Canadian Cancer Society; [cited 2018 Dec 8]. Risk factors for breast cancer. Available from: http://www.cancer.ca/en/cancer-information/cancer-type/breast/risks/.
66. Clavelle K, King D, Bazzi AR, Fein-Zachary V, Potter J. Breast cancer risk in sexual minority women during routine screening at an urban LGBT health center. Womens Health Issues. 2015;25(4):341–8.
67. Austin SB, Pazaris MJ, Rosner B, Bowen D, Rich-Edwards J, Spiegelman D. Application of the Rosner-Colditz risk prediction model to estimate sexual orientation group disparities in breast cancer risk in a U.S. cohort of premenopausal women. Cancer Epidemiol Biomarkers Prev. 2012;21(12):2201–8.
68. Boehmer U, Miao X, Maxwell NI, Ozonoff A. Sexual minority population density and incidence of lung, colorectal and female breast cancer in California. BMJ Open. 2014;4(3):e004461.
69. Zaritsky E, Dibble SL. Risk factors for reproductive and breast cancers among older lesbians. J Womens Health (Larchmt). 2010;19(1):125–31.
70. Brandenburg DL, Matthews AK, Johnson TP, Hughes TL. Breast cancer risk and screening: a comparison of lesbian and heterosexual women. Women Health. 2007;45(4):109–30.
71. Meads C, Moore D. Breast cancer in lesbians and bisexual women: systematic review of incidence, prevalence and risk studies. BMC Public Health. 2013;13(1):1127.
72. Dibble SL, Roberts SA, Nussey B. Comparing breast cancer risk between lesbians and their heterosexual sisters. Womens Health Issues. 2004;14(2):60–8.

73. Grindel CG, McGehee LA, Patsdaughter CA, Roberts SJ. Cancer prevention and screening behaviors in lesbians. Women Health. 2006;44(2):15–39.

74. Bowen DJ, Powers D, Greenlee H. Effects of breast cancer risk counseling for sexual minority women. Health Care Women Int. 2006;27(1):59–74.

75. Cochran SD, Mays VM. Risk of breast cancer mortality among women cohabiting with same sex partners: findings from the National Health Interview Survey, 1997–2003. J Womens Health (Larchmt). 2012;21(5):528–33.

76. Onderdonk AB, Delaney ML, Fichorova RN. The human microbiome during bacterial vaginosis. Clin Microbiol Rev. 2016;29(2):223–38.

77. Bradshaw CS, Walker SM, Vodstrcil LA, Bilardi JE, Law M, Hocking JS, et al. The influence of behaviors and relationships on the vaginal microbiota of women and their female partners: the WOW Health Study. J Infect Dis. 2014;209(10):1562–72.

78. Bailey JV, Farquhar C, Owen C. Bacterial vaginosis in lesbians and bisexual women. Sex Transm Dis. 2004;31(11):691–4.

79. Marrazzo JM, Thomas KK, Agnew K, Ringwood K. Prevalence and risks for bacterial vaginosis in women who have sex with women. Sex Transm Dis. 2010;37(5):335–9.

80. Vodstrcil LA, Walker SM, Hocking JS, Law M, Forcey DS, Fehler G, et al. Incident bacterial vaginosis (BV) in women who have sex with women is associated with behaviors that suggest sexual transmission of BV. Clin Infect Dis. 2015;60(7):1042–53.

81. Forcey DS, Vodstrcil LA, Hocking JS, Fairley CK, Law M, McNair RP, et al. Factors associated with bacterial vaginosis among women who have sex with women: a systematic review. PloS One. 2015;10(12):e0141905.

82. Fethers KA, Fairley CK, Hocking JS, Gurrin LC, Bradshaw CS. Sexual risk factors and bacterial vaginosis: a systematic review and meta-analysis. Clin Infect Dis. 2008;47(11):1426–35.

83. Fredriksen-Goldsen KI, Kim HJ, Barkan SE. Disability among lesbian, gay, and bisexual adults: disparities in prevalence and risk. Am J Public Health. 2012;102(1):e16–21.

84. Agrawal R, Sharma S, Bekir J, Conway G, Bailey J, Balen AH, et al. Prevalence of polycystic ovaries and polycystic ovary syndrome in lesbian women compared with heterosexual women. Fertil Steril. 2004;82(5):1352–7.

85. Peterkin A, Risdon C. Caring for lesbian and gay people: A clinical guide. Toronto: University of Toronto Press; 2003.

86. Jalbert Y. Gay health: Current knowledge and future directions. Ottawa: Health Canada; 1999.

87. Cochran SD, Björkenstam C, Mays VM. sexual orientation and all-cause mortality among US adults aged 18 to 59 Years, 2001–2011. Am J Public Health. 2016;106(5):918–20.

88. Urwin S, Whittaker W. Inequalities in family practitioner use by sexual orientation: evidence from the English General Practice Patient Survey. BMJ Open. 2016;6(5):e011633.

89. Tjepkema M. Health care use among gay, lesbian and bisexual Canadians. Health Rep. 2008;19(1):53–64.

90. Dahlhamer JM, Galinsky AM, Joestl SS, Ward BW. Barriers to health care among adults identifying as sexual minorities: A US National Study. Am J Public Health. 2016;106(6):1116–22.

91. Elliott MN, Kanouse DE, Burkhart Q, Abel GA, Lyratzopoulos G, Beckett MK, et al. Sexual minorities in England have poorer health and worse health care experiences: a national survey. J Gen Intern Med. 2015;30(1):9–16.

92. Macapagal K, Bhatia R, Greene GJ. Differences in healthcare access, use, and experiences within a community sample of racially diverse lesbian, gay, bisexual, transgender, and questioning emerging adults. LGBT Health. 2016;3(6):434–42.

93. Bakker FC, Sandfort TG, Vanwesenbeeck I, van Lindert H, Westert GP. Do homosexual persons use health care services more frequently than heterosexual persons: findings from a Dutch population survey. Soc Sci Med. 2006;63(8):2022–30.

94. Griffin-Tomas M, Cahill S, Kapadia F, Halkitis PN. Access to health services among young adult gay men in New York City. Am J Men Health. 2019;13(1):1557988318818683.

95. Public Health Agency of Canada [Internet]. Ottawa: Government of Caanda; 2020 [cited 2020 Jan 8]. Canadian immunization guide: part 4 – active vaccines. Available from: https://www.canada.ca/en/public-health/services/canadian-immunization-guide.html.

96. Silverberg MJ, Lau B, Justice AC, Engels E, Gill MJ, Goedert JJ, et al.; North American AIDS Cohort Collaboration on Research and Design (NA-ACCORD) of IeDEA. Risk of anal cancer in HIV-infected and HIV-uninfected individuals in North America. Clin Infect Dis. 2012;54(7):1026–34.

97. Centers for Disease Control and Prevention. Notes from the field: serogroup C invasive meningococcal disease among men who have sex with men – New York City, 2010–2012. MMWR Morb Mortal Wkly Rep. 2013 Jan;61(51–2):1048.

98. Dhanireddy S [Internet]. Waltham, MA: UpToDate; 2019 [cited 2019 Nov 29]. Primary care of gay men and men who have sex with men.

Available from: https://www.uptodate.com/contents/primary
-care-of-gay-men-and-men-who-have-sex-with-men/.

99. Bell N, Connor Gorber S, Shane A, Joffres M, Singh H, Dickinson J, et al.;
Canadian TaskFOrce on Preventive Health Care. Recommendations
on screening for prostate cancer with the prostate-specific antigen test.
CMAJ 2014;186(16):1225–34.

100. Daling JR, Weiss NS, Hislop TG, Maden C, Coates RJ, Sherman KJ, et
al. Sexual practices, sexually transmitted diseases, and the incidence of
anal cancer. N Engl J Med. 1987;317(16):973–7.

101. BC Centre for Excellence in HIV/AIDS [Internet]. Vancouver: BC Center
for Excellence in HIV/AIDS; 2015 Aug [cited 08 Jan 2020]. Primary
care guidelines for the management of HIV/AIDS in British Columbia.
Available from: http://cfenet.ubc.ca/therapeutic-guidelines
/primary-care-guidelines.

102. Weiss E [Internet]. Vancouver: UBC; 2017 Apr 17 [cited 2020 Jan 08]. Anal
cancer: information to get you out of the dark! Available from: https://
thischangedmypractice.com/anal-cancer-info-dare/.

103. University of San Francisco [Internet]. San Francisco: University of San
Francisco; [cited 13 Jan 2020]. Obtaining a specimen for anal cytology.
Available from: https://analcancerinfo.ucsf.edu/obtaining
-specimen-anal-cytology.

5 2SLGBTQ Children and Youth

CATHERINE MASER AND ASHLEY VANDERMORRIS

Introduction

Childhood and adolescence are dynamic life stages during which key facets of an individual's physical, emotional, cognitive, and interpersonal self are emerging and evolving. The most recent Canadian census found that between 4 and 10 per cent of Canadian youth identify as homosexual or bisexual.[1] In population health surveys, approximately 1 per cent of youth state they are transgender,[2] while several more recent studies suggest that 1.2 per cent to 4.1 per cent of adolescents report a gender identity that differs from the gender assigned at birth.[3]

Working with 2SLGBTQ children, youth, and their families provides an opportunity to positively engage individuals in health care in a collaborative, respectful, and affirming manner that can have implications that reverberate throughout the life course. To effectively address the needs of 2SLGBTQ children, youth and their families, practitioners must adopt a developmentally informed stance so that interactions and interventions are appropriately tailored to meet the child or youth where they are while also supporting them in moving forward along a healthy developmental trajectory.

In this chapter, we will begin by presenting frameworks that inform current understandings of development across childhood and adolescence. We will then explore the emergence of gender and sexual identities within the context of these developmental stages. Finally, we will apply a developmental lens to outline key considerations in crafting an affirming patient encounter and will present the HEEADSSS framework as a valuable tool in addressing the critical domains that can influence 2SLGBTQ adolescents both in illness and in health.

Developmental Considerations

Erik Erikson was a psychologist who proposed a psychosocial development theory that is still widely used to understand how social interactions and relationships influence the development of personality in humans. He describes a series of stages that occur sequentially and are based upon a specific area of conflict or crisis between the needs of the individual and the needs of society. He suggests that we must accomplish or be successful in each stage to develop competence in motives, behaviours, and actions that would enable us to then move on to the next. The theory consists of eight stages, five of which are in childhood, further emphasizing the vast amount of personality development that is established prior to adulthood (see table 5.1). Alternative theories of development exist and some experts have a preference based on their areas of interest and expertise. For example a task-based approach to development is presented in this book in chapter 8 on mental health.

Adolescence can be further subdivided into three stages as delineated in table 5.2. Within each stage, intra- and interpersonal development across a number of domains contributes to the adolescent's emerging sense of self. Healthy and supported navigation of these stages culminates in accomplishment of the fundamental developmental tasks of adolescence – achieving independence from parents; adopting peer codes and lifestyles; assigning importance to and accepting one's body image; and establishing sexual, ego, vocational, and moral identities.[5] Features of this progression that are particularly salient to 2SLGBTQ youth may include a shift from a desire to align with dominant gender and sexual identities during early adolescence to a more sophisticated appreciation of and comfort with diversity and a recognition of societal prejudices in late adolescence.[6]

Adolescent Neurodevelopment

Adolescence is a time of marked neurodevelopment, which manifests as profound physical, cognitive, and socioemotional change.[7-11] Early adolescence is heralded by a second surge of neuronal proliferation, which then is followed by a lengthy process of myelination and synaptic pruning that spans the teenage years and continues, in certain areas of the cortex, well into an individual's twenties.[9-11] Myelination serves to optimize efficiency of meaningful connections within the brain, while dendritic pruning eliminates unused synapses.[9] These processes underpin the remarkable neuroplasticity of adolescence and highlight

Table 5.1. Erikson's Stages

Stage/Age	Psychosocial Crisis	Basic Virtue
Infancy 0 to 1 year	Trust vs mistrust	Hope and optimism
Toddler (1–3 years)	Autonomy vs shame and doubt	Self-control and willpower
Preschool/primary grades (3–6 years)	Initiative vs guilt	Direction and purpose
School age (6–12 years)	Industry vs inferiority	Competence
Adolescence (12–18 years)	Identity vs role confusion	Fidelity and devotion (to others and ideas)

Source: Adapted from Perry, Hockenberry, Lowdermilk, and Wilson, Maternal child nursing care. 2010.[4]

Table 5.2. Stages of Adolescence

	Early Adolescence (10–13 Years)	Middle Adolescence (14–16 Years)	Late Adolescence (17–19 Years)
Cognitive and Moral	Concrete Inability to perceive long-term outcome of current decision-making	Emergence of abstract thought Questioning of mores	Future-oriented with sense of perspective Idealism Ability to think things through independently
Self-Concept/ Identity Formation	Preoccupation with changing body Self-consciousness about appearance and attractiveness	Concern with attractiveness "Stereotypical adolescent"	More stable body image Attractiveness may still be a concern Firmer identity
Family	Increased need for privacy	Conflicts over control and independence Struggle for acceptance or greater autonomy	Emotional and physical separation from family Increased autonomy
Peers	Seeking of same-sex peer affiliation to counter instability	Intense peer group involvement Preoccupation with peer culture Peers provide behavioural example	Peer group and values recede in importance Intimacy/possible commitment takes precedence

(Continued)

Table 5.2. (Continued)

	Early Adolescence (10–13 Years)	Middle Adolescence (14–16 Years)	Late Adolescence (17–19 Years)
Sexual	Increased interest in sexual anatomy Anxieties and questions about genital changes, size Limited dating and intimacy	Testing of ability to attract partner Initiation of relationships and sexual activity Questions of sexual orientation	Consolidation of sexual identity Focus on intimacy and formation of stable relationships

Adapted from Kliegman, R.M., Stanton, B.M., St. Geme, J., Schor, N.F., and Behrman, R.E. Nelson Textbook of Pediatrics. 2011.[5]

the significant potential influence of experience and environment on final adult cognitive architecture and associated function.

MRI studies have revealed that the dynamic process of neurodevelopment is completed in the most primitive areas of the brain first and then progresses "back to front," culminating with refinement of the most evolutionarily "new" systems last.[8,9,12] Thus, areas such as the limbic system, which played a role in early species survival because of its central role in emotion, reward pathways, impulse and instinct, motivation, and selective memory retrieval, reaches full maturity relatively early in adolescence. In contrast, the prefrontal cortex, which confers executive functions such as abstract thought, judgment, emotional modulation, impulse control, and complex problem solving, continues to mature well into an individual's mid-twenties.[9,12–14]

This dyssynchrony between full maturation of different regions of the brain, and in particular between the earlier-maturing limbic system and later-maturing prefrontal cortex, is then further compounded by changes in the brain's response to neurotransmitters during adolescence. Two key neurotransmitters implicated in adolescent behaviour are dopamine and serotonin.[9] Basal levels of dopamine, which plays a prominent role in reward pathways and emotional responses, decrease during adolescence, and the dynamics of dopamine release during this developmental stage are altered. This can result in difficulties with emotional regulation, as well as unique responses to rewarding stimuli.[9,15] Levels of serotonin, which is critical to mood modulation and impulse control, are similarly decreased during adolescence.[9,16]

Figure 5.1. Adolescent Health: Pubertal Transitions in Health

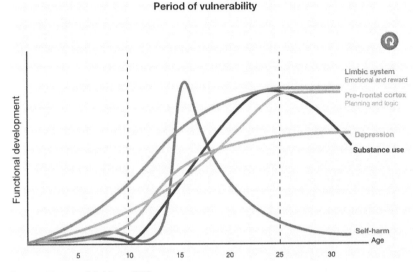

Period of vulnerability

Source: Patton, GC, Viner, R.[17]

The above factors all converge to introduce into adolescence a period that has been referred to as a "window of vulnerability."[17] During this period adolescents are uniquely susceptible to social influence and emotionally driven responses, and may have the capacity to understand information but not to integrate that information into their decision making.[9,18] This is thought to be the basis for the risk-taking behaviour that can characterize adolescence. This period is also a window of opportunity during which respectful, responsive, and reinforcing interpersonal interactions can have significant positive impact.[19] As a health care provider, understanding adolescent neurodevelopment can help to identify not only potential susceptibilities but also the unique strengths of adolescents, which can be leveraged to support the development of healthy habits and behaviours (see figure 5.1).

Development of Gender Identity and Sexual Orientation

It is thus critical to consider how the formation of gender identity and sexual orientation fit within the complex and dynamic developmental system of each child and adolescent.

Gender Identity Formation

Gender identity formation first arises in early childhood and evolves as children and then adolescents come to have an increasingly sophisticated sense of themselves in relation to others. Key stages of gender identity formation include the following:[20]

Two to three years:

- Children become conscious of the physical differences between boys and girls.
- Before their third birthday, most are easily able to label themselves as either a boy or a girl.

Four to five years:

- Most children have a stable sense of their gender identity. Their identity is not yet "fixed," but they know which gender they identify with.
- During this same time, children learn gender role behavior. They become aware of "things that boys do" or "things that girls do" and can identify toys "typically used by boys or by girls."
- They begin to play with children with similar genders.

Six to seven years:

- Children may feel more comfortable with their identity and reduce outward expressions of gender.
- Children who feel their gender identity is different from the sex assigned to them at birth may experience increased social anxiety as they feel different from their peers or that they don't fit in.

Eight years old and up:

- Some stereotypic gender behaviours may appear.
- As puberty approaches some realize their identity is different from that assigned at birth.
- Pubertal changes can be very distressing.

Emergence of Sexual Orientation

A discussion of the factors influencing an individual's sexual orientation is beyond the scope of this chapter. However, relevant to work with 2SLGBTQ children and youth is a consideration of the experiences that may be encompassed by the process of *identifying with* one's sexual orientation.

Historical approaches to understanding this process tended to favour a "stage" conceptualization of sexual orientation identity formation. Troiden in 1989 synthesized features of existing proposed models of non-heterosexual identity formation into a four-stage model:[21]

Stage 1: Sensitization

- Sense of being different but this is not identified as being related to sexuality
- May begin to have awareness of non-heterosexual feelings/behaviours
- Typically occurs before onset of puberty

Stage 2: Identity confusion

- Begin to identify non-heterosexual feelings/behaviours
- May have anxiety arising from conflict between feelings and emerging sense of self
- May have sense of isolation

Stage 3: Identity assumption

- Identity is adopted and shared with some others
- May continue to struggle with internalized homophobia
- Positive social connections with other sexual minority individuals may help to provide coping skills or to enhance comfort with identity

Stage 4: Commitment

- Satisfaction with identity, self-acceptance, unwillingness to alter identity
- Comfort with sharing sexual identity with broader social network

Of note, Troiden framed these stages as overlapping and clarified that identity formation is rarely linear; rather, he likened the process to a "horizontal spiral,"[21] with individuals often moving back and forth between stages at different times.

More recently, the limitations of a stage model of identity formation inadequately capturing the unique and diverse experiences of sexual minority youth has been acknowledged.[22–24] Debates exist regarding the sequence of key milestones such as identity disclosure (particularly to parents) and self-acceptance, though these milestones are commonly agreed upon to be central to the identity formation process.[24] Factors that may influence the temporality of experiences that contribute to identity formation may include geography, ethnoracial background, culture, individual sexual experiences, and gender.[24]

More contemporary studies of youth who identify as non-hetero-sexual propose a diverse range of developmental trajectories. Work by Savin-Williams and Cohen suggests that many adolescents may not experience "identity confusion" but rather may assume a non-heterosexual identity without any notable distress.[22] Reasons for this may include both methodological limitations of earlier studies, which may not have been able to access representative samples, as well as evolving societal responses to homosexuality,[22] which may enable youth to be less distressed by an emerging awareness of non-heterosexuality.

Finally, it is important to note that the sexual orientation identity that an adolescent assumes may not conform to traditional categories such as "homosexual" or "bisexual."[25–27] Younger generations may describe themselves using what Watson et al. refer to as "self-generated" or "emerging" identity labels that are neither bound by binary conceptu-alizations of gender nor by historically assumed associations between sexual attraction, sexual activity, and sexual orientation.[25] Furthermore, identity is not static; it is important not to presume that a young per-son who has articulated a particular sexual orientation has completed a finite process of "identity formation." Rather, as a health care pro-vider one must engage in an ongoing dialogue that offers the adoles-cent patient the opportunity to explore their lived experiences and to articulate their own interpretations of how these experiences relate to their current sense of identity.

Framing the Visit

How then does a care provider set the stage for an affirming medical encounter in which safe and meaningful dialogue can occur? We will outline five considerations for cultivating an inclusive and affirming care environment for children and youth.

1. *Create physically affirming space.* Adolescents are neurodevelopmen-tally primed to respond emotionally to environmental cues.[18] Being thoughtful and deliberate in how a care environment is designed

can immediately signal to a teen that the providers working in that space are safe and welcoming.[28] Considerations that can achieve this include the following:[3,27-31]

- Display a clinic mission statement that articulates the clinic's commitment to providing inclusive and affirming care.
- Have posters that depict youth in same-sex and opposite sex couples, as well as youth with diverse gender expression.
- Hang notices on the wall about support group meetings for sexual minority and gender diverse youth.
- Create intake forms and questionnaires that are inclusive and allow for diverse responses to demographic questions.
- Avoid displaying brochures that assume heterosexuality or binary gender identities.
- Display stickers or symbols that indicate that your office is a "safe space,"
- Ensure the clinic has single-occupancy, gender-non-specific bathrooms.
- Have providers wear pins or lanyards indicating their "affirming" stance.
- Ensure all office staff are welcoming and non-judgmental.

Actions such as these promote a safe and positive clinical space not only for 2SLGBTQ youth but for all youth accessing care.[27,28]

2. *Ensure confidentiality.* Confidentiality is critical to developing open, trusting, and sustained care relationships with 2SLG-BTQ adolescents.[28,32] Confidentiality must be emphasized by all members of the care team and staff, not only by the direct health care provider.[30] To ensure that adolescents are not put in the position of having to advocate for their privacy to parents/caregivers, policies around confidentiality should be clearly articulated to parents/caregivers and youth jointly, and should be reviewed at every encounter. This allows for any questions to be addressed transparently and promotes clear expectations and boundaries.[30,33]

A portion of every encounter should involve the health care provider meeting with the adolescent one on one.[27,34] This not only is important for developing a trusting provider-patient relationship but has been shown to increase the willingness of the adolescent to disclose information and enhances the accuracy of the information that is shared.[28,34,35] Should issues arise that require mandatory disclosure (for example, acute suicidality), only the minimum amount of information necessary to ensure safety should be disclosed.[27,28]

3. *Employ inclusive language.* The use of open and non-judgmental language by health care providers can promote a safe and trusting clinical environment. Patients report that visiting health care settings in which diversity is acknowledged through language, even on standard forms, promotes a sense of inclusivity.[29] The use of a transgender adolescent's chosen name in multiple contexts has been found to mitigate mental health risks.[36] In the clinical setting, providing adolescents with the opportunity to articulate the terminology that best resonates with their individual experiences and identities, and then using these terms, can cultivate a sense of respect and collaboration that sets an affirming tone for the entire encounter.[27]

When obtaining a history, phrase questions in gender-neutral and non-binary terms. Encounters are most likely to be inclusive and affirming if the language used avoids labels and instead focuses on experiences.[27,30] Identity should be discussed independently of activity as the two are not synonymous. Examples of questions relevant to providing adolescent care that can be presented in a neutral manner include the following:

- "Who makes up your family?" (rather than "Do you live with your mother and father?")
- "Are you in a romantic relationship?" (rather than "Do you have a boyfriend/girlfriend?")
- "Have you had any sexual contact with anyone?" (rather than "Are you sexually active?")
- "Is there a way you typically describe your sexual orientation?" (rather than "Are you attracted to males or females?")
- "Is there a way you would like me to refer to your gender?" (rather than "What's your gender identity?")
- "What pronouns do you prefer that I use?" (rather than "Do you use male or female pronouns?")

When in doubt, ask. The language used by youth may be fluid and may change from encounter to encounter as their identity and sense of self continues to develop and evolve. Inviting an adolescent to explain the terminology they use and what it means to them can be a therapeutically valuable undertaking as it provides the adolescent with a sense of control and expertise while affording the provider insight into the perspectives and conceptualizations of the young person.

4. *Adopt a collaborative stance.* Developing a strong rapport with an adolescent is foundational to engaging that young person in care. Adolescents tend to respond more positively if they feel that their perspective and voice are respected and valued as paramount within the health care encounter.[3,37] Principles of motivational interviewing and a collaborative conversational approach to exploring and promoting an individual's motivation underpin the key features of an adolescent-oriented interviewing style:[37]

   - Start from a strengths-based position.
   - Ask open-ended questions.
   - Respond with reflections rather than directives.
   - Employ techniques of restatement and summation to encourage additional comments from the adolescent.
   - Engage in conversational clarification to help crystallize the presenting issue.
   - Explore the adolescent's insight – for example, "When are you the happiest?" or "If you had one wish, what would it be?"
   - Express support and offer validation.
   - Strive for collaborative decision making.

   A respectful, collaborative approach to working with adolescents can foster self-efficacy and autonomy by indicating that the health care provider trusts in the adolescent's capacities and understanding of their own experiences and needs. An affirming approach should never be directive, but rather should facilitate the adolescent identifying and moving along the trajectory that best aligns with their individual goals for health and wellness.[3]

5. *Enhance accessibility.* The World Health Organization (WHO) has developed a set of standards for the health care of all adolescents. Within these standards, accessibility encompasses aspects of health care delivery that optimize the likelihood of adolescents reaching and receiving the care they need.[33,38] In one study of transgender youth, 84 per cent reported not receiving the health care they felt they needed in the preceding year.[39] As 2SLGBTQ adolescents are over-represented among homeless youth, this population may be more likely than other young people to be navigating the health care system independently, making accessibility particularly

relevant.[27,40] Accessibility of care for all adolescents can be enhanced by the following:[27,38,41,42]

- expanded working hours (i.e., outside school hours)
- flexible appointment procedures (e.g., drop-in rather than previously scheduled)
- accommodating late arrivals
- adaptable care plans that account for constraints adolescents may face (e.g., single-dose rather than multi-day treatments when possible; multiple interventions during a single encounter when appropriate)

The HEEADSSS Assessment

The HEADS (home, education, activities, drug use, and sexual behaviour) acronym was first developed in 1974 by Dr. Harry S. Berman as a teaching tool in the Mount Sinai School of Medicine in New York City. The addition of another S for suicidality and depression expanded the tool for use in interviewing high-risk youth and has been used in all encounters since 1982 at Children's Hospital Los Angeles in its high-risk youth programs.[43] It has subsequently been updated to reflect changes in social context for youth, including eating and body image (E); accessing the Internet, cell phones, and social media/safety (S); and spirituality (S).[44]

The HEEADSSS psychosocial interview tool prompts practitioners to ask questions they may not otherwise consider and promotes a conversation that elicits valuable information when assessing youth in all settings. It enables providers to gain insight into how a young person is engaged in the world and provides context for many health risks and concerns. See table 5.3 for some examples of questions drawn from the HEEADSSS framework adapted to working with 2SLGBTQ youth.

Contextualizing the HEEADSSS Assessment

H – HOME
Children and adolescents are best able to meet developmental milestones and learn to navigate the complexities of the world when they have a stable, supportive home environment. It may be challenging for 2SLGBTQ youth to disclose their identities or orientation to family for fear of punishment, harassment, or rejection, or risk of losing their housing. Recent studies indicate that they are over-represented

Table 5.3. HEEADSSS Assessment with 2SLGBTQ Lens

Home	Do the people who live with you know that you are 2SLGBTQ? (Who?)
	How did they find out, and how did they react?
	Do you feel you can be yourself at home?
	Do you talk to your family about medical options for transition?
	Does your family help you financially to purchase gender-affirming devices/clothing/makeup?
Education	Do people at school know that you are 2SLGBTQ? (Who?)
	How did they find out and how did they react?
	Are you able to express your gender and orientation safely at school?
	Do teachers (and classmates?) use your preferred name and pronouns?
	Do you have access to a bathroom that fits with your gender identity?
	Have you ever been harassed or attacked at school/work?
	Do you skip or miss classes? How often? What do you do instead?
	Do you ever worry about your academic/work future as a 2SLGBTQ person?
Eating/Body Image	What do you like and not like about the way you look?
	Do you wish you could look different? (How?)
	What is your ideal image?
	Do you eat more/less when you are under stress or to obtain this image of yourself?
	(Consider those who may restrict nutritional intake to achieve pubertal suppression.)
Activities	Do any of your friends know that you are 2SLGBTQ?
	How did they find out, and how did they react?
	Do you know any other 2SLGBTQ people? How did you meet them?
	Do you attend any groups/drop ins for 2SLGBTQ youth?
	How much time do you spend on the Internet each week?
Drugs	Do you ever use drugs/alcohol to cope with stress?
	What do you think is a safe limit for drug and alcohol use? Have you ever crossed that limit? (How often?)
	Have you ever done things when you were drunk or high that you regretted afterwards?
	Have you experienced black outs or memory loss after using drugs/alcohol?
	Review the CRAFFT screening tool (see table 5.4).
Sexuality and Gender	How would you describe your sexual orientation?
	Have any of the people you've dated known that you are 2SLGBTQ? How did they find out, and how did they react?
	Is being trans a part of your sex life? (How?)
	Are there parts of your body that are off-limits sexually?
	Do you use dating apps? Do you ever meet up with people you meet online?

(Continued)

Table 5.3. (Continued)

Suicide/Mental Health	Do you worry about people finding out you are 2SLGBTQ? Do you ever wish you weren't 2SLGBTQ? Does thinking about trans/orientation issues ever make you feel stressed, sad, lonely? Do you ever feel that your situation is hopeless? Do you have thoughts of suicide or self-harm? (Do further investigation if SI or SH is present.)
Safety	Has anyone ever threatened to "out" you as 2SLGBTQ? Do you worry about this happening? Have you ever been threatened or attacked because you are 2SLGBTQ, or for other reasons? Do you worry about this happening? How safe do you feel in your neighbourhood or the places where you hang out? Has anyone offered you money, clothes, alcohol, or drugs in exchange for sex? Has anyone tried to get you involved in the sex trade?
Spirituality	Do you consider yourself religious or spiritual? Does that impact your identity or your relationship with family?

in the child welfare system and in unstable or insecure housing and lack access to the resources that would support transition out of homelessness.[40,45]

Homeless 2SLGBTQ youth or those in foster care experience increased school absenteeism, report higher amounts of substance use, and have poorer mental health outcomes when compared to their non-2SLGBTQ peers in unstable housing.[27,40] It is essential then, to get a sense of the home environment and to establish the level of support and safety provided by caregivers and family members.

Parent and caregiver responses to a young person coming out as 2SLGBTQ can vary widely and their support is essential to the health and wellness of sexual minority and gender diverse youth. A supportive relationship with an adult has been shown to enhance the architecture of the developing brain and helps to promote resilience through adolescence and into adulthood.[46] Supportive families can mitigate the negative effects of high-risk behaviours, poor mental health, and suicidality, and they too may need support from primary health care providers and community resources.[30,47] Useful online resources for families include Families in Transition (https://familyservicetoronto .org/our-services/programs-and-services/families-in-transition) and the Family Acceptance Project (https://familyproject.sfsu.edu).

E – EDUCATION

Educational engagement can serve as an important protective factor in the lives of children and youth. High school graduation is associated with improved long-term health outcomes, employment opportunities, and living conditions.[48] Interestingly, high school attendance is a better indicator of an adolescent's likelihood of dropping out of school than is academic achievement, highlighting the importance of keeping children and adolescents engaged in school.[49] Key factors that influence educational engagement include mental health, physical health, a sense of safety, and social connectedness.[48] All of these domains must be explored and supported when working with 2SLGBTQ children and adolescents.

Having a sense of school safety has been shown to reduce the risk of depression and suicidal ideation among 2SLGBTQ students.[50,51] Unfortunately, over half of 2SLGBTQ adolescents report experiencing some form of harassment while at school, and almost 60 per cent report feeling unsafe at school.[31,52] Racialized 2SLGBTQ youth are even more likely to have experienced harassment of some form.[53] Transgender youth who report a sense of school connectedness are twice as likely to report good mental health; however, most transgender youth do not report having the experience of strong connectedness to school.[39,54]

Working with patients and their communities to address opportunities to enhance the learning environment for 2SLGBTQ students has the potential to improve outcomes not only for 2SLGBTQ adolescents but for all students. An improved school climate has been associated with higher school-wide standardized test scores.[55] School environments in which gender and sexual orientation-related harassment is not tolerated have been found to have significantly less bullying, aggression, and victimization among all students.[56] Gay-straight alliances, sometimes referred to as gender and sexuality alliances, have been found to reduce gender and sexuality-based discrimination and can promote a school environment that all students describe as safer and more accepting.[57]

E – EATING/BODY IMAGE

Adolescents often develop unhealthy eating habits, and many are at risk for obesity related to poor nutrition and lack of exercise. This is a time of heightened body image awareness, and many adolescents may worry that social acceptance is connected to body weight, shape, and size. For gender diverse youth, puberty and a changing body can contribute to increased dysphoria, leading to poorer mental health outcomes, which often include disordered eating.[58]

Youth assigned female at birth may restrict intake to minimize chest tissue growth or to cause delayed onset or cessation of menses. A large cohort study of college students found that transgender and sexual minority young adults reported higher use of laxatives, diet pills, and vomiting when compared to heterosexual cisgender women.[59] The National Eating Disorders Association and the Trevor Project[60] surveyed over 1000 LGBTQ youth and found that the majority had been diagnosed with an eating disorder and that greater than 75 per cent suspected they had an eating disorder. Even more concerning is the finding that 58 per cent of youth who had been diagnosed had considered suicide.

Proper nutrition has vast implications for healthy growth and development and the ability to participate in daily activities, to concentrate, and to be successful academically. Eating patterns and associated behaviours, as well as a youth's perception of their body, should be discussed at every encounter.

A – ACTIVITIES

Adolescence is a time of social receptiveness and openness to exploring new experiences. Positive interpersonal encounters can promote prosocial behaviours and decisions among adolescents.[19] Involvement in extracurricular activities has been identified as a facilitator of positive youth development.[61] Social connectedness is a critical protective factor that bolsters resilience among 2SLGBTQ youth.[62]

A significant proportion of 2SLGBTQ students, however, report barriers to engagement in extracurricular activities.[52] These barriers range from non-affirming policies in relation to gender identity and gendered sporting activities (e.g., team membership, locker room use) to outright discouragement from participation in extracurricular opportunities. In the clinical context, health care providers should work to support their 2SLGBTQ patients in identifying opportunities for positive social engagement, such as formal peer networks or affirming organizations, while also leveraging their clinical roles to advocate against barriers to extracurricular involvement for 2SLGBTQ adolescents.

One domain of engagement that is of particular relevance to 2SLGBTQ adolescents may be Internet and social media use. Use of online spaces and resources is more prevalent among 2SLGBTQ adolescents as compared to non-2SLGBTQ youth.[63] 2SLGBTQ youth are more likely to access health information online, to use online spaces to develop supportive social networks, and to characterize the Internet as a platform for positive civic engagement.[63] Internet-based technologies have been found to provide 2SLGBTQ youth with strategies to overcome experiences of marginalization to promote a sense of well-being.[64] However, 2SLGBTQ adolescents are also nearly three times as likely to be bullied or harassed online, and safety regarding an adolescent's online presence must be assessed. Therefore, exploring how the Internet and social media factor into a 2SLGBTQ adolescent's day-to-day life should be a part of the clinical encounter.

D – DRUGS

Minority stress refers to the notion that "minorities experience distinct, chronic stressors related to their stigmatized identities, including victimization, prejudice, and discrimination."[6] 2SLGBTQ youth experience minority stress as a matter of course in society and as such may be prone to considering the use of substances as a means of managing or coping with the stressors of homophobia, transphobia, or heterosexism.[30,65,66]

When compared to their heterosexual peers, sexual minority youth report an increased incidence of driving after using alcohol or cannabis, current or frequent use of cigarettes, and a higher incidence of drinking alcohol before age 13.[67] Similarly, in a sampling of high school students reporting high risk behaviours, gender minority youth have increased incidence of using alcohol, cannabis, and other illicit substances.[65]

The CRAFFT has been validated as an effective screening tool to assess substance use in adolescents[44,68] and can be easily administered in the

Table 5.4. CRAFFT Screening Tool

CRAFFT	Question
Car	Have you ever ridden in a car driven by someone (including you) who had been using drugs or alcohol?
Relax	Do you use alcohol or drugs to relax, feel better about yourself, or fit in?
Alone	Do you ever use alcohol or drugs by yourself?
Forget	Do you ever forget things you did while using drugs or alcohol?
Friends	Do friends or family members ever tell you that you should cut down on your drinking or drug use?
Trouble	Have you ever gotten into trouble while you were using alcohol or drugs?

Scoring:
A "no" response = 0 points
A "yes" response = 1 point
0–1 = negative screen
2–6 = positive screen
Consider a safety contract for "yes" to the "car" question regardless of overall score.

Source: Adapted from Robert E Rakel, ed. Textbook of Family Medicine, 2011.[69]

context of the HEEADSSS interview. A positive screen indicates the need for a more in-depth assessment of potentially problematic substance use.

2SLGBTQ youth face barriers to obtaining supportive health care[30,70] and as such may not be able to access medications such as hormones by prescription. A discussion of substance use should therefore also include assessment for potential use of hormones or steroids obtained without a prescription.

S – SEXUALITY AND GENDER

2SLGBTQ youth are more likely than non-2SLGBTQ youth to be sexually active, to report early sexual debut, to have not used a condom at the most recent sexual contact, and to have multiple sexual partners.[30,67,71] Structural issues such as stigmatization and isolation that can act as barriers to care, combined with unique physiologic vulnerability associated with age and sexual practices, make 2SLGBTQ youth more likely than their peers to have poor sexual health outcomes.[71-73] Racialized and gender diverse youth experience even greater disparities.[30,71] It is imperative, therefore, that 2SLGBTQ youth are provided with comprehensive sexual health care delivered in a confidential, nonjudgmental, and patient-centred manner.

Starting the Conversation.   The same principles that set the stage for any successful adolescent health care encounter are critical to creating a safe and respectful environment in which a 2SLGBTQ adolescent's sexual health needs can be effectively identified and addressed. Important considerations when working with 2SLGBTQ youth within the context of sexual health care provision include the following:[30,71]

- Use inclusive and respectful language.
- Avoid making assumptions – identity, attraction, expression, and activity are each independent facets of an adolescent's sexuality.
- Start with open-ended questions, then clarify through close-ended, specific questions when needed (for example, ask concretely about specific symptoms of sexually transmitted infections [STIs]).
- Make decisions collaboratively – offer options when feasible (for example, urine versus self-swab-based screening).
- Follow the patient's lead regarding comfort level (for example, avoid unnecessary physical exams or offer alternatives for physical exam procedures).
- Provide adequate information for patients to understand and prepare for next steps.
- Promote adolescent self-efficacy by discussing potential preventive strategies rather than lecturing on possible negative outcomes.

Promoting Positive Sexuality. Providers working with 2SLGBTQ older children and adolescents must seek out opportunities to discuss and facilitate healthy sexuality among this population. In addition to universal hepatitis B vaccination, many jurisdictions also recommend hepatitis A vaccination as an intervention to mitigate risk of hepatitis-associated morbidity. Adolescence is an opportune time to review and address hepatitis vaccination status.[74-76] Vaccination with the nonavalent (9-valent) human papillomavirus (HPV) vaccine is recommended for children and adolescents of all genders, ideally between the ages of 9 and 13, to prevent high-risk HPV. A discussion about HPV vaccination can be framed to both children and parents as an opportunity for health promotion independent of sexual activity status.[77,78]

For those engaged in sexual activity known to be associated with high risk of human immunodeficiency virus (HIV) transmission, education around HIV pre-exposure prophylaxis (PrEP) is a critical component of care. HIV PrEP is discussed in detail in chapter 7. Relevant to caring for adolescents is the 2018 FDA approval of PrEP for adolescents at risk of HIV and endorsement of its use by the Society for Adolescent Health and Medicine and the WHO.[79-81] Optimal adherence to PrEP among adolescents is supported by monthly physician visits, with adherence declining when visits are reduced to a quarterly regimen.[82]

Another facet of healthy sexuality is knowledge of and access to methods for contraception. This is a topic relevant to all adolescents regardless of activity, orientation, or identity; adolescent assigned females who have been sexually active with assigned females have been shown to be at higher risk of pregnancy than peers who have sex exclusively with assigned males,[73,83] and adolescent assigned females who report being "unsure" of their sexuality report markedly lower rates of contraceptive use than their heterosexual peers.[30] Current guidelines recommend long-acting reversible contraceptives (i.e., intrauterine contraceptives) as the first-line option for adolescents.[84-86] Information on types of emergency contraception should also be reviewed.[30] The importance of ongoing use of a barrier form of STI protection (condom or dental dam) regardless of use of another type of contraceptive should be emphasized.[30]

Addressing Sexual Health Conditions. When addressing sexual health concerns, it is important to tailor recommendations, diagnostics, and interventions to adolescents' sexual practices and anatomy rather than their sexual orientation, and to be cognizant of the unique implications of age and specific behaviours for risk profiles.[87] For example, there are physiologic features of the rectal mucosa that render those engaging in receptive anal intercourse at higher risk of STI acquisition, while the columnar cells that compose the adolescent cervical epithelium are more susceptible to infection than the squamous cells of the more mature cervical epithelium.[88]

Adolescents as a broad demographic are over-represented in population-level STI prevalence. STI screening intervals for 2SLGBTQ adolescents should be aligned with up-to-date jurisdiction-specific guidelines. Guidelines should be interpreted with the recognition that sexual activity under age 25 is considered an independent risk factor for STI acquisition and that additional risk factors may emerge or recede over the course of adolescence, necessitating an iterative approach to determination of screening frequency.[89-91] STI screening as frequently as every three months may be indicated for some youth.[89] The American Academy of Pediatrics has recommended screening all youth for STIs by the age of 16 to 18, independent of reported sexual activity, because evidence suggests significant underreporting of sexual activity among adolescents.[92]

The diagnosis and treatment of specific STIs in 2SLGBTQ adolescents should be consistent with existing jurisdictional guidelines. These are typically congruent with management recommendations for adults; details of the management of specific infections are outlined in chapter 6 of this book. Management protocols that minimize the requirement for sustained adherence on the part of the adolescent may be preferable for some youth (for example, selecting a single-dose over a multi-day treatment if effectiveness of the two regimens is largely equivalent).[87]

Providing Gender-Related Care.   This chapter reviews approaches to promoting affirming care for 2SLGBTQ children and youth. A discussion of potential interventions to support gender diverse children and youth is beyond the scope of this chapter. For more information on this topic please refer to the UCSF Center of Excellence for Transgender Health at prevention.ucsf.edu/transhealth. Of note, training sessions for primary care and other providers wanting to extend care to children and youth (including puberty suppression) are currently available through Rainbow Health Ontario. The Gender Creative Kids website (https://gendercreativekids.ca) is also an important resource for families and communities wishing to support gender diverse children.

S – SUICIDE/MENTAL HEALTH

Half of all mental health conditions have their onset by age 14.[93] An emerging body of literature posits that in addition to the heightened susceptibility to mental health conditions associated with adolescence, minority stress (defined above) is a key social determinant of mental health among 2SLGBTQ youth.[6,94] Minority stress can be influenced by structural factors (e.g., institutionalized discrimination), interpersonal experiences (positive or negative), and intrapersonal processes (e.g., internalized homophobia, emotional regulation, coping)[6]; the interplay of these factors is unique to each individual and may contribute to increased vulnerability to mental health conditions in some adolescents while promoting enhanced resilience among others.

2SLGBTQ youth are more likely than their non-2SLGBTQ counterparts to experience depression, suicidal ideation, social anxiety, substance use disorders, post-traumatic stress disorder, and other mental health conditions.[30] 2SLGBTQ adolescents experiencing mental health symptoms may benefit from being referred to a skilled and affirming mental health practitioner. If such a referral is made, it should be emphasized to the adolescent that the referral is not because of their sexual orientation or gender identity, but rather to connect them to resources that may support them in leading healthy and fulfilling lives as the person they are. "Conversion" or "reparative" therapies should never be offered or endorsed.[30,58,73]

Almost half (42.8 per cent) of lesbian, gay, and bisexual adolescents report having seriously considered suicide.[95] Studies of transgender youth have reported rates of past year serious contemplation of suicide as high as 69 per cent.[2,39] All 2SLGBTQ adolescents should be routinely screened for suicidality with a validated suicide risk screening tool;[96] one example, the National Institute of Mental Health's "Ask suicide-screening questions" or ASQ, is included here (see figure 5.2) and others can be found at the links listed below. If an adolescent endorses suicidal ideation, the nature of this ideation should be explored and the adolescent should be asked if they have a suicide plan. A thorough safety assessment by an experienced and skilled provider may be indicated. While non-suicidal self-injury (NSSI), often referred to as *self-harm*, should not be misinterpreted as a suicide attempt, such behaviours are an independent risk factor for suicidality and disclosure of NSSI necessitates further assessment.[97,98] NSSI is more common among early as compared to late adolescents, and has been found to be particularly common among 2SLGBTQ adolescents.[39]

In addition to directly targeting interventions to children and adolescents experiencing mental health concerns, providers should explore potential opportunities to enhance external protective factors such as family connectedness and positive school environments.[6,96] Parental acceptance has been identified as a key mitigator of mental health vulnerability among 2SLGBTQ youth.[49,99] Transgender children who are socially transitioned and supported in their gender identity have rates

Figure 5.2. ASQ Screening Tool

NIMH TOOLKIT

asQ — Suicide Risk **Screening Tool**

Ask Suicide-Screening Questions

Ask the patient:

1. In the past few weeks, have you wished you were dead?   ○ Yes   ○ No

2. In the past few weeks, have you felt that you or your family would be better off if you were dead?   ○ Yes   ○ No

3. In the past week, have you been having thoughts about killing yourself?   ○ Yes   ○ No

4. Have you ever tried to kill yourself?   ○ Yes   ○ No

   If yes, how? _____

   _____

   When? _____

   _____

If the patient answers Yes to any of the above, ask the following acuity question:

5. Are you having thoughts of killing yourself right now?   ○ Yes   ○ No

   If yes, please describe: _____

Next steps:

- If patient answers "No" to all questions 1 through 4, screening is complete (not necessary to ask question #5). No intervention is necessary (*Note: Clinical judgment can always override a negative screen*).

- If patient answers "Yes" to any of questions 1 through 4, or refuses to answer, they are considered a positive screen. Ask question #5 to assess acuity:

   ☐ "Yes" to question #5 = acute positive screen (imminent risk identified)
   - Patient requires a STAT safety/full mental health evaluation.
   - Patient cannot leave until evaluated for safety.
   - Keep patient in sight. Remove all dangerous objects from room. Alert physician or clinician responsible for patient's care.

   ☐ "No" to question #5 = non-acute positive screen (potential risk identified)
   - Patient requires a brief suicide safety assessment to determine if a full mental health evaluation is needed. Patient cannot leave until evaluated for safety.
   - Alert physician or clinician responsible for patient's care.

Provide resources to all patients

- 24/7 National Suicide Prevention Lifeline 1-800-273-TALK (8255) En Español: 1-888-628-9454
- 24/7 Crisis Text Line: Text "HOME" to 741-741

asQ Suicide Risk Screening Toolkit | NATIONAL INSTITUTE OF MENTAL HEALTH (NIMH) NIH 6/13/2017

Source: National Institute of Mental Health. Suicide Risk Screening Tool. 2017.[101]

of mental health conditions comparable to their cisgender peers.[100] Engaging and educating parents and family to nurture affirming intra-familial relationships may therefore offer an additional crucial platform for intervention.

- Suicide Behaviors Questionnaire – Revised – http://youth suicideprevention.nebraska.edu/wp-content/uploads/2019/09 /SBQ-R.pdf
- Columbia Suicide Severity Rating Scale – https://cssrs.columbia .edu/wp-content/uploads/C-SSRS_Pediatric-SLC_11.14.16.pdf
- Patient Health Questionnaire (PHQ-9) – https://www.ncbi.nlm.nih .gov/pmc/articles/PMC1495268/#app1title

S – SAFETY

2SLGBTQ youth are consistently over-represented in assessment of safety and high-risk behaviours. We have previously addressed the importance of assessing for safe home and school environments for 2SLGBTQ youth and of being cognizant of the increased risk for sub-stance misuse and for suicidal ideation and attempts when compared to their peers.

Large scale surveys also report that sexual minority youth disclosed higher rates of carrying a weapon, carrying a weapon on school prop-erty, being threatened or injured by a weapon on school property, and being in a physical fight. Other high-risk behaviours with higher incidence include seldom or never wearing a seatbelt, riding with a driver who has been drinking alcohol, and driving after consuming alcohol.[67]

Most youth are increasingly connecting with peers online, via social media, and by texting. 2SLGBTQ youth find connection, social support and community in online environments and often have fewer friends in person than online.[102] This mode of communication also makes them more vulnerable to harassment and bullying.[103] Youth and their care-givers should be aware of Internet safety and the risks of using dating apps, providing personal information, or meeting in person with indi-viduals they meet online.[104]

S – SPIRITUALITY

Adolescence is a time of self-reflection and discovery. Youth are tasked with establishing their identities in a multitude of contexts: gender identity, sexual orientation, vocational goals, social connection, moral-ity, and spirituality. As providers we often overlook the positive effects of spirituality as a means to develop resilience and manage the many stressors and barriers we have previously discussed in this chapter. See specific considerations for those who identify as Two-Spirit in chapter 13 of this book.

Kim and Esquivel[105] further suggest that spirituality not only acts as a protective factor in moderating adversity but also acts to positively enhance mental health, psychological well-being, and academic learning. Recognizing that many 2SLGBTQ youth face challenges at home, in school, and in the community, it is optimal to inquire about their spiritual beliefs and sources of hope and practices, and to work with youth to include and optimize this domain in their lives.

Conclusion

Childhood and adolescence are times of incredible opportunity and potential. Health care providers are optimally positioned to support children and adolescents as they navigate the complex processes encompassed by growth and development. Engaging 2SLGBTQ children and youth in a respectful, collaborative, and responsive manner can have a transformative impact on the health and health care experiences of this population. This can have implications that resonate throughout the life course of the individual and more broadly throughout society as these happy and healthy children and adolescents grow into confident, capable, and contributory adults.

References

1. Statistics Canada [Internet]. Ottawa: Government of Canada; 2018. A portrait of Canadian youth. Available from: https://www150.statcan.gc.ca/n1/pub/11-631-x/11-631-x2018001-eng.htm.
2. Veale JF, Watson RJ, Peter T, Saewyc EM. Mental health disparities among Canadian transgender youth. J Adolesc Health. 2017;60:44–9. doi:10.1016/j.jadohealth.2016.09.014 PMID:28007056.
3. Bonifacio JH, Maser C, Stadelman K, Palmert M. Management of gender dysphoria in adolescents in primary care. CMAJ. 2019;191(3):E69–75. doi:10.1503/cmaj.180672.
4. Perry S, Hockenberry M, Lowdermilk D, Wilson D, editors. Maternal child nursing care. 4th ed. Missouri: Elsevier; 2010.
5. Kliegman RM, Stanton BM, St. Geme J, Schor NF, Behrman RE. Nelson textbook of pediatrics. 19th ed. Philadelphia (PA): Elsevier Health Sciences; 2011.
6. Russell ST, Fish JN. Mental health in lesbian, gay, bisexual, and transgender (LGBT) youth. Annu Rev Clin Psych.ol 2016;12(1):465–87.

7. Vijayakumar N, Op de Macks Z, Shirtcliff EA, Pfeifer JH. Puberty and the human brain: insights into adolescent development. Neurosci Biobehav Rev. 2018 Sep;92:417–36.

8. Gogtay N, Giedd JN, Lusk L, Hayashi KM, Greenstein D, Vaituzis AC, et al. Dynamic mapping of human cortical development during childhood through early adulthood. Proc Natl Acad Sci USA. 2004;101(21):8174–9. doi:10.1073/pnas.0402680101.

9. Arain M, Haque M, Johal L, Mathur P, Nel W, Rais A, et al. Maturation of the adolescent brain. Neurophsychiatr Dis Treat. 2013;9:449–61. doi:10.2147/NDT.S39776.

10. Giedd JN. The teen brain: insights from neuroimaging. J Adolesc Health. 2008;42(4):335–43. doi:10.1016/j.jadohealth.2008.01.007.

11. Gerber AJ, Peterson BS, Giedd JN, Lalonde FM, Celano MJ, White SL, Wallace GL, Lee NR, Lenroot RK. Anatomical brain magnetic resonance imaging of typically developing children and adolescents. J Am Acad Child Adolesc Psychiatry. 2009 May;48(5):465–70. doi:10.1097/CHI.0b013e31819f2715.

12. Fine JG, Sung, C. Neuroscience of child and adolescent health development. J Couns Psychol. 2014;61(4):521–7.

13. Lenroot RK, Giedd JN. Brain development in children and adolescents: insights from anatomical magnetic resonance imaging. Neurosci Biobehav Rev. 2006;30:718–29. doi:10.1016/j.neubiorev.2006.06.001.

14. Casey BJ, Jones RM, Hare TA. The adolescent brain. Ann N Y Acad Sci. 2008;1124:111–26.

15. Wahlstrom D, White T, Luciana M. Neurobehavioral evidence for changes in dopamine system activity during adolescence. Neusci Biobehav Rev. 2010;34(5):631–48. doi:10.1016/j.neubiorev.2009.12.007.

16. Glick, AR. The role of serotonin in impulsive aggression, suicide, and homicide in adolescents and adults: a literature review. Int J Adolesc Med Health. 2015;27(2):143–50. doi:10.1515/ijamh-2015-5005.

17. Patton, GC, Viner, R. Commission findings. Paper presented at: Our future: a Lancet Commission on adolescent health and wellbeing;2016 Jun 9; Washington, DC.

18. Schriber RA, Guyer AE. Adolescent neurobiological susceptibility to social context. Dev Cogn Neurosci. 2016;19:1–18.

19. Van Hoorn J, Van Dijk E, Güroğlu B, Crone EA. Neural correlates of prosocial peer influence on public goods game donations during adolescence. Soc Cogn Affect Neurosci. 2016;11(6):923–33. doi:10.1093/scan/nsw013.

20. Caring for Kids [Internet]. Ottawa: Canadian Paediatric Society; [updated May 2018]. Gender identity. Available from: https://www.caringforkids.cps.ca/handouts/gender-identity.

21. Troiden R. The formation of homosexual identities. J Homosex. 1989;17(1–2):43–73. doi:10.1300/J082v17n01_02.
22. Savin-Williams RC, Cohen KM. Developmental trajectories and milestones of lesbian, gay, and bisexual young people. Int Rev Psychiatry. 2015;27(5):357–66. doi:10.3109/09540261.2015.1093465.
23. Rosario M, Schrimshaw EW, Hunter J. Different patterns of sexual identity development over time: implications for the psychological adjustment of lesbian, gay, and bisexual youths. J Sex Res. 2011;48(1):3–15.
24. Maguen S, Floyd FJ, Bakeman R, Armistead L. Developmental milestones and disclosure of sexual orientation among gay, lesbian, and bisexual youths. J Appl Dev Psychol. 2002;23(2):219–33. doi:10.1016/s0193-3973(02)00105-3.
25. Watson RJ, Wheldon CW, Puhl RM. Evidence of Diverse Identities in a Large National Sample of Sexual and Gender Minority Adolescents. J Res Adolesc. 2020 Feb;30 Suppl 2:431–42. doi: 10.1111/jora.12488. Epub 2019 Feb 13.
26. White AE, Moeller J, Ivcevic Z, Brackett MA. Gender identity and sexual identity labels used by U.S. high school students: a co-occurrence network analysis. Psychol Sex Orientat Gend Divers. 2018;5(2):243–52. doi:10.1037/sgd0000266.
27. Hadland SE, Yehia BR, Makadon HJ. Caring for lesbian, gay, bisexual, transgender, and questioning youth in inclusive and affirmative environments. Pediatr Clin North Am. 2016;63(6):955–69. doi:10.1016/j.pcl.2016.07.001.
28. Kaufman M; Canadian Paediatric Society; Adolescent Health Committee. Adolescent sexual orientation. Paediatr Child Health. 2008;13(7):619–30. doi:10.1093/pch/13.7.619.
29. Pinto AD, Aratangy T, Abramovich A, Devotta K, Nisenbaum R, Wang R, Kiran T. Routine collection of sexual orientation and gender identity data: a mixed-methods study. CMAJ. 2019;191(3):E63–8.
30. Levine D; Committee on Adolescence. Office-based care for lesbian, gay, bisexual, transgender, and questioning youth. Pediatrics. 2013;132(1):e297–313. doi:10.1542/peds.2013-1283.
31. Rafferty J; Committee on Psychosocial Aspects of Child and Family Health; Committee on Adolescence; Section on Lesbian, Gay, Bisexual, and Transgender Health and Wellness. Ensuring comprehensive care and support for transgender and gender-diverse children and adolescents. Pediatrics. 2018;142(4):e20182162. doi: 10.1542/peds.2018-2162.
32. Allen LB, Glicken AD, Beach RK, Naylor KE. Adolescent health care experience of gay, lesbian, and bisexual young adults. J Adolesc Health. 1998;23(4):212–20.

33. Tylee A, Haller DM, Graham T, Churchill R, Sanci LA. Youth-friendly primary-care services: how are we doing and what more needs to be done? Lancet. 2007;369(9572):1565–73. doi:10.1016/S0140-6736(07)60371-7.

34. Ford C, English A, Sigman G. Confidential health care for adolescents: position paper for the Society for Adolescent Medicine. J Adolesc Heal. 2004;35(2):160–7. doi:10.1016/j.jadohealth.2004.03.002.

35. Ford CA, Millstein SG, Halpern-Felsher BL, Irwin CE. Influence of physician confidentiality assurances on adolescents' willingness to disclose information and seek future health care: a randomized controlled trial. JAMA. 1997;278(12):1029–34. doi:10.1001/jama.1997.03550120089044.

36. Russell ST, Pollitt AM, Li G, Grossman AH. Chosen name use is linked to reduced depressive symptoms, suicidal ideation, and suicidal behavior among transgender youth. J Adolesc Health. 2018;63(4):503–5. doi:10.1016/j.jadohealth.2018.02.003.

37. Woods ER, Neinstein LS. Office visit, interview techniques, and recommendations to parents. In: Neinstein LS, Gordon CM, Katzman DK, Rosen D, Woods ER, editors. Adolescent health care: A practical guide. 5th ed. Philadelphia: Woltser Kluwer; 2008; pp. 32–43.

38. World Health Organization. Global standards for quality health-care services for adolescents: a guide to implement a standards-driven approach to improve the quality of services for adolescents. Volume 1: standards and criteria [Internet]; 2015. Available from: http://apps.who.int/iris/bitstream/handle/10665/183935/9789241549332_vol1_eng.pdf.

39. Saewyc E, Pyne J, Frohard-Dourlent H, Travers R, et al. Being safe, being me in Ontario: regional results of the canadian trans youth health survey. Vancouver (BC): Stigma and Resilience Among Vulnerable Youth Centre, School of Nursing, University of British Columbia; 2017.

40. Baams L, Wilson BD, Russell ST. LGBTQ youth in unstable housing and foster care. Pediatrics. 2019;143(3):e20174211. doi:10.1542/peds.2017-4211.

41. Ambresin AE, Bennett K, Patton GC, Sanci LA, Sawyer SM. Assessment of youth-friendly health care: a systematic review of indicators drawn from young people's perspectives. J Adolesc Health. 2013;52(6):670–81. doi:10.1016/j.jadohealth.2012.12.014.

42. Elliott AS; Canadian Paediatric Society, Asolescent Health Committee. Meeting the health care needs of street-involved youth. Paediatr Child Health. 2013;18(6):317–26. doi:10.1093/pch/18.6.317.

43. Cohen E, Mackenzie RG, Yates GL. HEADSS, a psychosocial risk assessment instrument: implications for designing effective intervention programs for runaway youth. J Adolesc Health. 1991;12(7):539–44.

44. Klein DA, Goldenring JM, Adelman WP. HEEADSSS 3.0: the psychosocial interview for adolescents updated for a new century fueled by media. Contemp Pediatr. 2014;1:1–16.
45. Abramovich A, Shelton J. Where am I going to go?: Intersectional approaches to ending LGBTQ2S homelessness in Canada & the US. Toronto: Canadian Observatory on Homelessness Press; 2017.
46. Center on the Developing Child [Internet]. Cambridge (MA): Harvard University; 2017. Three principles to improve outcomes for children and families. Available from: https://developingchild.harvard.edu/resources /three-early-childhood-development-principles-improve-child-family -outcomes/.
47. Travers R, Bauer G, Pyne J, Bradley K, for the Trans PULSE Project; Gale L, Papadimitriou M. Impacts of strong parental support for trans youth: a report prepared for Children's Aid Society of Toronto and Delisle Youth Services [Internet]. London (ON): Western University; 2012. Available from: https://transpulseproject.ca/wp-content/uploads/2012/10 /Impacts-of-Strong-Parental-Support-for-Trans-Youth-vFINAL.pdf.
48. Robert Wood Johnson Foundation [Internet]. New Jersey: Robert Wood Johnson Foundation; 2016. The relationship between school attendance and health. Available from: https://www.rwjf.org/en/library/research/2016/09 /the-relationship-between-school-attendance-and-health.html.
49. Anglin TM, Grant LM. Addressing chronic absenteeism among adolescent students. Poster session presented at: Cultivating connections: 2017 Annual Meeting of the Society for Adolescent Health aand Medicine; 2017 Mar 8–11; New Orleans, LA.
50. Eisenberg ME, Resnick MD. Suicidality among gay, lesbian and bisexual youth: the role of protective factors. J Adolesc Health. 2006;39(5):662–8. doi:10.1016/j.jadohealth.2006.04.024.
51. Birkett M, Espelage DL, Koenig B. LGB and questioning students in schools: the moderating effects of homophobic bullying and school climate on negative outcomes. J Youth Adolesc. 2009;38(7):989–1000. doi:10.1007/s10964-008-9389-1.
52. Kosciw JG, Greytak EA, Zongrone AD, Clark CM, Truong, NL. The 2017 National School Climate Survey: The experiences of lesbian, gay, bisexual, transgender, and queer youth in our nation's schools. New York: GLSE; 2018.
53. Taylor C, Peter T, McMinn TL, Elliott T, et al. Every class in every school: The first national climate survey on homophobia, biphobia, and transphobia in Canadian schools. Final report. Toronto: Egale Canada Human Rights Trust; 2011.
54. Gower AL, Saewyc EM, Corliss HL, Kne L, Erickson DJ, Eisenberg ME. The LGBTQ supportive environments inventory: methods for quantifying

supportive environments for LGBTQ youth. J Gay Lesbian Soc Serv. 2019;31(3):314–31.

55. Cornell D, Huang F, Datta P, Malone M et al. Technical Report of the Virginia Secondary School Climate Survey: 2016 Results for 9th–12th Grade Students and School Staff. Charlottesville, VA: Curry School of Education, University of Virginia; 2016.

56. Espelage DL. Ecological Theory: preventing youth bullying, aggression, and victimization. Theory Prac. 2014;53(4):257–64. doi:10.1080/00405841.20 14.947216.

57. Li G, Wu AD, Marshall SK, Watson RJ, Adjei JK, Park M, Saewyc EM. Investigating site-level longitudinal effects of population health interventions: Gay-Straight Alliances and school safety. SSM Popul Health. 2019 Jan;7:100350. doi:10.1016/j.ssmph.2019.

58. Bonifacio HJ, Rosenthal SM. Gender variance and dysphoria in children and adolescents. Pediatr Clin North Am. 2015;62(4):1001–16. doi:10.1016/j.pcl.2015.04.013.

59. Diemer EW, Grant JD, Munn-Chernoff MA, Patterson DA, Duncan AE. Gender identity, sexual orientation, and eating-related pathology in a national sample of college students. J Adolesc Health. 2015;57(2):144–9. doi:10.1016/j.jadohealth.2015.03.003.

60. The Trevor Project; National Association of Eating Disorders. Eating disorders among LGBTQ youth. A 2018 national assessment [Internet]. West Hollywood (CA): Trevor Project; 2018. Available from: https://www.thetrevorproject.org/wp-content/uploads/2018/03/Suicidality-and-Eating-Disorders-Among-LGBTQ-Youth-2018-2.pdf.

61. Hallingberg BE, Van Goozen SH, Moore SC. Characteristics associated with risk taking behaviours predict young people's participation in organised activities. J Adolesc. 2016;53:189–94. doi:10.1016/j.adolescence.2016.10.008.

62. DiFulvio GT. Sexual minority youth, social connection and resilience: from personal struggle to collective identity. Soc Sci Med. 2011;72(10):1611–17. doi:10.1016/j.socscimed.2011.02.045.

63. Gay, Lesbian & Straight Education Network; Center for Innovative Public Health Research; Crimes against Children Researh Centre. Out online: The experiences of lesbian, gay, bisexual and transgender youth on the Internet [Internet]. New York: GLSEN; 2013. https://www.glsen.org/sites/default/files/Out%20Online%20FINAL.pdf.

64. Palmer NA. LGBT youth online and in person: Identity development, social support, and extracurricular and civic participation in a positive youth development framework. Nashville: Vanderbilt University; 2013.

65. Reisner SL, Greytak EA, Parsons JT, Ybarra ML. Gender minority social stress in adolescence: disparities in adolescent bullying and substance use

by gender identity. J Sex Res. 2015;52(3):243–56. doi:10.1080/00224499 .2014.886321.

66. Rainbow Health Ontario [Internet]. Toronto: Rainbow Health Ontario; 2015. Fact sheet: LGBTQ people, drug use & harm reduction. Available from: https://www.rainbowhealthontario.ca/resources/rho-fact -sheet-lgbt2sq-people-drug-use-harm-reduction/.

67. Kann L, McManus T, Harris WA, Shanklin SL, Flint KH, Queen B, et al. Youth risk behavior surveillance: United States, 2017. MMWR Surveill Summ. 2018;67(No. SS-8):1–114. doi:doi:10.15585/mmwr.ss6708a1.

68. Knight JR, Sherritt L, Shrier LA, Harris SK, Change, G. Validity of the CRAFFT substance abuse screening test among adolescent clinic patients. Arch Pediatr Adolesc Med. 2002;156:607–14.

69. Rakl RE, editor. Textbook of family medicine. 8th ed. Philadelphia: Saunders; 2011.

70. Gridley SJ, Crouch JM, Evans Y, Eng W, Antoon E, Lyapustina M, et al. Youth and caregiver perspectives on barriers to gender-affirming health care for transgender youth. J Adolesc Health. 2016;59(3):254–61. doi:10.1016/j.jadohealth.2016.03.017.

71. Wood SM, Salas-Humara C, Dowshen, NL. Human immunodeficiency virus, other sexually transmitted infections, and sexual and reproductive health in lesbian, gay, bisexual, transgender youth. Pediatr Clin North Am. 2016;63(6):1027–55.

72. Mustanski B, Van Wagenen A, Birkett M, Eyster S, Corliss HL. Identifying sexual orientation health disparities in adolescents: analysis of pooled data from the Youth Risk Behavior Survey, 2005 and 2007. Am J Public Health. 2014;104(2):211–17. doi:10.2105/AJPH.2013.301748.

73. Institute of Medicine, Committee on Lesbian, Gay, Bisexual, and Transgender Health Issues and Research Gaps and Opportunities. The health of lesbian, gay, bisexual, and transgender people: Building a foundation for better Understanding. Washington (DC): National Academies Press; 2011.

74. Public Health Agency of Canada [Internet]. Ottawa: Government of Canada; 2016. Canadian immunization guide. Available from: https:// www.canada.ca/en/public-health/services/publications/healthy-living /canadian-immunization-guide-part-4-active-vaccines.html.

75. Schillie S, Vellozzi C, Reingold A, et al. Prevention of hepatitis B virus infection in the United States: Recommendations of the Advisory Committee on Immunization Practices. MMWR Recomm Rep 2018;67(No. RR-1):1–31. doi:10.15585/mmwr.rr6701a1external icon.

76. Fiore AE, Wasley, A, Bell, BP. Prevention of hepatits A through active or passive immunization. MMWR Recomm Rep. 2006;55(RR07):1–23. Available from: https://www.cdc.gov/mmwr/preview/mmwrhtml/rr5507a1.htm.

77. Salvadori MI. Human papillomavirus vaccine for children and adolescents. Paediatr Child Health. 2018;23(4):262–5. Available: https://www.cps.ca /en/documents/position/HPV.

78. Petrosky E, Bocchini JA Jr, Hariri S, Chesson H, Curtis CR, Saraiya M, et al.; Centers for Disease Control and Prevention. Use of 9-valent human papillomavirus (HPV) vaccine: updated HPV vaccination recommendations of the advisory committee on immunization practices. MMWR Morb Mortal Wkly Rep. 2015;64(11):300–4.

79. Centers for Disease Control and Prevention. Preexposure prophylaxis for the prevention of HIV infection in the United States 2017 Update: a clinical practice guideline [Internet]. Atlanta (GA): CDC; 2018. Available from: https://www.cdc.gov/hiv/pdf/risk/prep/cdc-hiv-prep -guidelines-2017.pdf.

80. Society for Adolescent Health and Medicine. HIV pre-exposure prophylaxis medication for adolescents: a position paper of the Society for Adolescent Health and Medicine. J Adolesc Health. 2018;63(4):513–16. doi:10.1016/j.jadohealth.2018.07.021.

81. World Health Organization [Internet]. Geneva, Switzerland; 2017. Implementation tool for pre-exposure prophylaxis (PrEP) of HIV infection. Available from: https://www.who.int/hiv/pub/prep/prep -implementation-tool-policy/en/.

82. Hosek SG, Landovitz RJ, Kapogiannis B, Siberry GK, Rudy B, Rutledge B, et al. Safety and feasibility of antiretroviral preexposure prophylaxis for adolescent men who have sex with men aged 15 to 17 years in the United States. JAMA Pediatr. 2017;171(11):1063–71. doi:10.1001/ jamapediatrics.2017.2007.

83. Lindley LL, Walsemann KM. Sexual orientation and risk of pregnancy among New York City high-school students. Am J Public Health. 2015;105(7):1379–86. doi:10.2105/AJPH.2015.302553.

84. Di Meglio G, Crowther C, Simms J. Contraceptive care for Canadian youth. Paediatr Child Health. 2018;23(4):271–7. Available from: https:// www.cps.ca/en/documents/position/contraceptive-care.

85. Black A, Guilbert E, Costescu D, Dunn S, Fisher W, Kives S, et al. Canadian contraception consensus (part 3 of 4):Chapter 7-Intrauterine contraception. J Obstet Gynaecol Can. 2016;38(2):182–222. doi:10.1016/j. jogc.2015.12.002.

86. Ott MA, Sucato GS; Committee on Adolescence. Contraception for adolescents. Pediatrics. 2014;134(4):e1257–81. doi:10.1542/peds.2014-2300.

87. Centers for Disease Control and Prevention [Internet]. Atlanta (GA): CDC; 2015. Sexually transmitted diseases treatment guidelines. Available from: https://www.cdc.gov/std/tg2015/chlamydia.htm.

88. Neinstein LS, Gordon CM, Katzman DK, Rosen D, Woods ER, editors. Adolescent health care: A practical guide. 5th ed. Philadelphia: Woltser Kluwer; 2008.
89. Public Health Agency of Canada [Internet]. Ottawa: Government of Canada; 2013. Canadian guidelines on sexually transmitted infections: primary care and sexually transmitted infections. Available from: https://www.canada.ca/en/public-health/services/infectious-diseases /sexual-health-sexually-transmitted-infections/canadian-guidelines /sexually-transmitted-infections/canadian-guidelines-sexually-transmitted-infections-17.html#a6.
90. Public Health Agency of Canada. Canadian communicable disease report. CCDR. 2018;44(2). Available from: https://www.canada.ca/content /dam/phac-aspc/documents/services/reports-publications/canada -communicable-disease-report-ccdr/monthly-issue/2018-44/issue-2 -february-1–2018/issue-2-eng.pdf.
91. Centers for Disease Control and Prevention. Sexually transmitted sisease surveillance, 2013. Atlanta (GA): CDC; 2014.
92. Emmanuel PJ, Martinez J; Committee on Pediatric AIDS. Adolescents and HIV infection: the pediatrician's role in promoting routine testing. Pediatrics. 2011;128(5):1023–9. doi:10.1542/peds.2011-1761.
93. Substance Abuse & Mental Health Services Administration. Key substance use and mental health indicators in the United States: Results from the 2016 National Survey on Drug Use and Health [Internet]. Washington (DC): U.S. Department of Health and Human Services; 2017. Available from: https://www.samhsa.gov/data/sites /default/files/NSDUH-FFR1-2016/NSDUH-FFR1-2016.pdf.
94. Hatzenbueler ML, Pachankis JE. Stigma and minority stress as social determinants of health among lesbian, gay, bisexual, and transgender youth: research evidence and clinical implications. Pediatr Clin North Am. 2016;63(6):985–97. doi:10.1016/j.pcl.2016.07.003.
95. Kann L, Olsen EO, McManus T, Harris WA, Shanklin SL, Flint KH, et al. Sexual identity, sex of sexual contacts, and health-related behaviors among students in grades 9–12. United States and selected sites, 2015. MMWR Surveill Summ. 2016;65(9):1–202.
96. Guss C, Shumer D, Katz-Wise SL. Transgender and gender nonconforming adolescent care: psychosocial and medical considerations. Curr Opin Pediatr. 2015 Aug;27(4):421–6.
97. Grandclerc S, De Labrouhe D, Spodenkiewicz M, Lachal J, Moro MR. Relations between nonsuicidal self-injury and suicidal behavior in adolescence: a systematic review. PLoS One. 2016;11(4):e0153760.
98. Whitlock J, Minton R, Babingto, P, Ernhout C. The relationship between non-suicidal self-injury and suicide. Ithaca (NY): Cornell University Press; 2015.

99.   Katz-Wise SL, Rosario M, Tsappis M. Lesbian, gay, bisexual, and transgender youth and family acceptance. Pediatr Clin North Am. 2016;63(6):1011–25.
100. Olson KR, Durwood L, DeMeules M, McLaughlin KA. Mental health of transgender children who are supported in their identities. Pediatrics 2016;137(3):e20153223.
101. National Institute of Mental Health. asQ Suicide Risk Screening Tool [Internet]. Bethesda (MD): National Institutes of Health; 2017. Available from: https://www.nimh.nih.gov/labs-at-nimh/asq-toolkit-materials /asq-tool/screening-tool_155867.pdf.
102. Ybarra ML, Mitchell KJ, Palmer NA, Reisner SL. Online social support as a buffer against online and offline peer and sexual victimization among U.S. LGBT and non-LGBT youth. Child Abuse Negl. 2015;39:123–36. doi:10.1016/j.chiabu.2014.08.006.
103. Mitchell KJ, Ybarra ML, Korchmaros JD. Sexual harassment among adolescents of different sexual orientations and gender identities. Child Abuse Negl. 2014;38(2):280–95. doi:10.1016/j.chiabu.2013.09.008.
104. Norris ML. HEADSS up: adolescents and the internet. Paediatr Child Health. 2007;12(3):211–16.
105. Kim S, Esquivel GB. Adolescent spirituality and resilience: Theory, research, and educational practices. Psychol Sch. 2011;48(7):755–65. doi:10.1002/pits.20582.

6 Sexual Health

IAN ARMSTRONG AND JORDAN GOODRIDGE

Introduction

> Sexual health is a state of physical, mental and social well-being in relation
> to sexuality. It requires a positive and respectful approach to sexuality and
> sexual relationships, as well as the possibility of having pleasurable and
> safe sexual experiences, free of coercion, discrimination, and violence.[1]

For many patients, sexual health is an important dimension of their overall well-being; if neglected, this can negatively impact self-image, relationships, and risk-associated behaviours. Sexually transmitted infections
(STIs), if unrecognized or untreated, lead to additional morbidity such
as susceptibility to other STIs, infertility, and chronic pain, and to interpersonal effects of population spread and congenital disease. This chapter aims to inform clinicians on how to facilitate sexual health for their
patients. This includes information on history taking, sexual function,
specific STIs, undifferentiated syndromes, laboratory investigations, and
preventive strategies. Of note, HIV is discussed separately in chapter 7,
including transmission, risk, testing, management, and prevention.

History Taking

Sexual History

The sexual history should identify opportunities to enhance quality of
life, presence or absence of symptoms, and history of exposures and
risk factors for current and future STIs. A sexual history sensitive to
diverse genders and sexual practices can also build a patient's sense of
safety with a provider, by recognizing non-normative sexual practices,
and validating experiences of trauma, shame, and judgment that may

be associated with these topics. The US Centers for Disease Control and Prevention suggest the five *P*'s mnemonic for sexual history taking,[2] elaborated in box 6.1:

- partner(s)
- practices
- protection from STIs
- past history of STIs
- pregnancy prevention

Some clinicians also include a sixth *P*, performance, for satisfaction with sexual function.

Box 6.1. Sample Sexual History Questions

PARTNER(S)	PRACTICES	PROTECTION
Have you had any sexual partners? How many in the last 12 months? What gender or genders have they been? Are they casual or regular partners?	What types of sexual activity do you have? Oral, vaginal, anal? If anal sex, insertive (top) and/or receptive (bottom)? Any use of sex toys or hands? Have you combined drugs with sex?	What do you think about using condoms? Do you use condoms some, most, or all the time? Have you had any slips or breaks?
PAST HISTORY	PREGNANCY	PERFORMANCE
Have you ever been diagnosed with or treated for an STI? When were you last tested?	Is there any possibility that you (or your partner) could become pregnant? Why do you say that?	Do you have any concerns about sexual desire, or how your body works during sex?

Screening for a history of sexual violence is also recommended as this could complicate the examination and testing. Trauma-informed care specialist Dr. L. Elizabeth Lincoln suggests including questions such as "Is there anything in your history that makes having a physical examination difficult?" and "Is there anything I can do to make your visit and exam easier?" Explaining the rationale for sensitive questions and examinations, and respecting patient autonomy if they decline examination or testing, are other elements of trauma-informed care.[3]

Sexual history taking and risk reduction counselling for transgender individuals necessitates additional considerations.[4] Many trans individuals experience dysphoria related to gendered connotations of anatomic terms, and may feel more comfortable if the clinician clarifies or mirrors the words they use for their genitals. It may be helpful to take an inventory of the patient's anatomy (any surgical changes to internal and external genitals), as well as use of hormones, to better understand their health needs.

There is limited literature on how hormone therapy or genital surgeries change susceptibility of trans individuals to STIs; thus, best practices include screening/testing individuals based on their behaviour, partner risk factors, and current anatomy.[5,6]

Symptoms

Patients should be asked about symptoms that may indicate an underlying STI. Based on site of exposure, patients may have symptoms consistent with urethritis, epididymitis, prostatitis, genital ulcers, genital warts, proctitis, vaginitis, and/or pelvic inflammatory disease. These symptoms include penile/vaginal discharge, dysuria, and vaginal bleeding after sex; scrotal/testicular swelling, pain, and tenderness; rectal pain, discharge, and bleeding; and abnormal lesions in the genito-anal region including vesicles, ulcers, buboes, and warts. See the section on undifferentiated syndromes and the individual sections on common STIs for more information regarding their common presentations.

Risk Factors

Although identity categories such as gay, lesbian, bisexual, heterosexual, and asexual tend to carry importance in a person's understanding of themselves, sexual orientation does not always correlate with behaviours and past partner selection. For this reason, epidemiologic categories such as men who have sex with men (MSM) and women who have sex with women (WSW) are preferred in some contexts.

Because of higher STI prevalence among certain subpopulations, it is important to identify behavioural risks of infections. These include MSM and their partners, those who combine sex with drugs (particularly intravenous drugs), sex workers or those who engage in survival sex and their partners, and those with multiple sexual partners.[7] A 2SLGBTQ identity is not in itself a risk factor for STIs.

Sexual Health and Function

Asexuality

Asexuality is a heterogeneous self-identification that is best understood as a unique sexual orientation.[8] This may be thought of as a spectrum, including asexuality (typically never having experienced sexual attraction), grey-asexuality (occasionally experiencing sexual attraction), and demi-sexuality (only experiencing sexual attraction after an established emotional bond). Individuals identifying as asexual may still experience romantic attraction without sexual attraction,[9] non-partner-oriented sexual desire,[10,11] and variable appreciation, indifference, or aversion to sexual organs and sexual behaviour.[12] Asexual-spectrum individuals may have received or internalized messages that this represents a deficiency or pathology and may choose not to disclose to health professionals for fear of being pathologized.[8] However, many self-identified asexuals embrace this identity with a sense of pride and positivity.[13] Clinicians should take an open-minded approach when individuals describe an absence of sexual desire and only pursue workup if it is prioritized by the patient, if it causes distress for the patient, or if there are associated symptoms warranting investigation.

Asexuality appears to be more common among trans individuals, with up to 74 per cent of trans women and 30 per cent of trans men reporting they have never or rarely felt sexual desire.[14] Autism spectrum disorder also appears to be overrepresented among asexuals,[15] and, incidentally, in trans individuals.[16] Asexuality does not appear to be a risk factor for depression but is associated with social withdrawal.[10]

Sexual Dysfunction

Sexual dysfunction refers to concerns around desire, arousal, and orgasm. Each of these may relate to medical causes (see table 6.1), psychiatric causes (including depression, anxiety, and posttraumatic stress disorder [PTSD]), or stressors (including fatigue, partner factors, relationship factors, body image, cultural or religious factors, and response to traumatic events). Regardless of the presumed etiology, exploration of the psychological and relational context of sexual dysfunction by a physician or by a sex therapist may be helpful.[17]

Table 6.1. Common Organic Conditions Associated with Types of Sexual Dysfunction

	Low Libido/ Low Sexual Desire	Vaginal Dryness	Premature Ejaculation	Delayed Ejaculation	Orgasmic Disorder
Diabetes mellitus[18,19]	✓	✓	✓		✓
Hypothyroidism[20,21]	✓			✓	
Hyperthyroidism[21,22]	✓		✓		
Hypogonadism*	✓	✓			
Hyperprolactinemia	✓			✓	
Oral contraceptives[23]	✓				
Psychotropics[24]	✓			✓	✓
Antihypertensive[25,26]	✓	✓		✓	✓
Antiepileptics[27]	✓		✓	✓	
Multiple sclerosis[27]	✓			✓	✓
Parkinsonism[27]			✓		
Acquired brain injury[27]		✓	✓	✓	

* Hypogonadism may be primary or secondary to chronic use of alcohol[28] or opioids.[29]

Erectile dysfunction, or ED, is caused by a disruption of the balance of blood into and out of the penis. ED may have psychogenic causes, organic causes (see table 6.2), or an interplay between the two; some experts argue that all ED has a psychological component.[17] To differentiate psychogenic contributions to ED, a sexual history should focus on the specific onset, the absence/presence of nocturnal or spontaneous erections, and erectile function during masturbation.[30] ED also has important predictive value as an early manifestation of atherosclerosis: new onset erectile dysfunction in an individual with vascular risk factors is a strong predictor of developing cardiovascular disease, and in patients with known cardiovascular disease, it is a predictor of all-cause mortality.[31–33]

Among cis MSM, surveys of self-reported ED show rates that are comparable[35,36] or lower[37,38] than the general cis male population. Among gay and bisexual men, negative feelings about body image predict erectile dysfunction.[39] A subset of MSM experience ED associated specifically with condom use;[40,41] it is unclear whether ED pharmacotherapy would motivate condom use in these individuals.

Table 6.2. Organic Causes of Erectile Dysfunction

Vascular	Neurologic
• atherosclerosis	• multiple sclerosis, Parkinson's disease, spinal cord injury
Endocrine	
• diabetes mellitus, hypogonadism, hyperprolactinemia, hyperthyroidism or hypothyroidism	**Substance-related**
	• alcohol, nicotine
Anatomic	**Iatrogenic**
• venous leak	• medications (antihypertensives, antidepressants, antipsychotics, corticosteroids, opioids)
• abnormalities causing penile pain (phimosis, lichen sclerosus, Peyronie's disease, corporal fibrosis secondary to priapism)	• radical pelvic surgery
	• radiotherapy for prostate cancer

Source: Adapted from Jenkins L, Albersen M, Corona G, Isidori AM, Goldfarb S, et al. 2017.[34]

Feminizing hormone therapy has a variable effect on sexual desire and erectile function, with the most frequent outcome being reduced erectile function.[14] However, this decrease does not bear a linear correlation with suppression of testosterone levels:[42] in one case series of transfeminine individuals, suppressed testosterone levels predicted fewer spontaneous erections but not fewer sexually induced erections.[43] Transfeminine individuals who want to retain erectile function may be supported by reducing their dose of feminizing hormones or using low-dose testosterone or oral PDE5 inhibitors.[44]

In transmasculine individuals, arousal is associated with physiologic engorgement of the clitoris or post-metoidioplasty penis, and this response can be augmented by PDE5 inhibitors.[45] More than 90 per cent of individuals reported complete satisfaction with erectile function after metoidioplasty, although the majority had insufficient length for vaginal penetration.[46] After phalloplasty, prostheses can enable non-arousal-dependent erections, which are associated with better realization of expectations but more pain with intercourse than phalloplasty without prosthesis.[47,48] For more information on transition-related surgeries, see Rainbow Health Ontario resources at https://www.rainbowhealthontario.ca.

Treatment of ED may be targeted to the cause, such as lifestyle modification, smoking cessation, treatment of co-morbidities,[49,50] and psychosocial interventions.[51,52] Mechanism-independent approaches, such as oral PDE5 inhibitors, vacuum devices, intracavernosal/intraurethral prostaglandins, and penile prosthesis surgery, may also be indicated.

Sexual Satisfaction – Women Who Have Sex with Women

Studies of sexual satisfaction among WSW tend to be descriptive surveys, and often do not include trans WSW. Sexual satisfaction is similar between married heterosexual women and WSW in monogamous committed relationships greater than one year, and is tied closely to relationship satisfaction; other parameters linked to higher sexual satisfaction included socio-economic status, sexual function, and sexual frequency.[53] Another study of WSW found that overactive bladder symptoms were linked to sexual dissatisfaction and sexual dysfunction; however, there was no link with depressive or anxious symptoms.[54] Compared to heterosexual women, lesbians reported higher orgasm frequency and less vaginal discomfort with sexual activity, and bisexual women reported higher sexual interest and higher vulvar discomfort with sexual activity; no difference was reported in orgasm pleasure or satisfaction with sex life across these three groups.[36]

Sexual Satisfaction – Men Who Have Sex with Men

Some studies have suggested that gay and bisexual identified men report lower satisfaction with sex life and orgasm pleasure than heterosexual men, despite equivalent erectile and orgasmic function.[36] A study of young MSM ages 16–29 found that orgasmic satisfaction and global sexual satisfaction were correlated with perceived acceptance within their neighbourhood and inversely correlated with participant's internalized stigma.[38] Among MSM, 42 per cent reported their feelings about their body had negative effects on the quality of their sex life.[55] Additionally, a survey of MSM on HIV PrEP found that this population experienced greater sexual satisfaction after PrEP initiation.[56]

There is mixed literature on the link between circumcision status and sexual satisfaction. Studies of adult circumcision report decreased sexual enjoyment after adult circumcision,[57] no difference in sexual satisfaction and function,[58] or improved erectile function and overall satisfaction.[59] A convenience sample of cisgender men with diverse orientations (48.2 per cent with homosexual or bisexual identity) found that happiness with one's circumcision status, and not circumcision status itself, was associated with better sexual functioning.[60]

Some MSM use substances to augment sexual performance or satisfaction and relieve anxiety around sex. This is referred to as "party and play," "PnP," or "chemsex" and may include a broad range of substances including methamphetamine, GHB, cocaine, ketamine, mephedrone, ecstasy, PDE5 inhibitors, or "poppers."[61] Practitioners should provide a non-judgmental and supportive environment so that their patients can safely express how substance use facilitates their sexual fulfillment. This way, practitioners can tailor counselling on harm reduction or abstinence to the needs and readiness of the patient.[62] For more information about substance use, see chapter 9.

Alkyl nitrites (including amyl nitrite and isobutyl nitrite), or "poppers," are volatile inhaled substances causing a brief "rush," vasodilation, and smooth muscle relaxation. They are used by MSM almost exclusively in sexual contexts, as they facilitate receptive anal intercourse by relaxing the internal anal sphincter. In many countries, including Canada, poppers are illegal because of risk of methemoglobinemia following accidental oral ingestion[63] and rarely following inhalation.[64] Poppers can cause a contact dermatitis presenting as ulceration.[65,66] Chronic inhalation is also associated with maculopathy.[67] Additionally, poppers and sildenafil were found as part of a cocktail on overdose autopsy, with a hypothesized synergy causing drastic vasodilation.[68] This led to product labelling for PDE5 inhibitors warning against co-administration with alkyl nitrites.[69]

Sexual Satisfaction – Transfeminine Individuals

Historically, gatekeeping policies restricted access to gender-affirming care for trans and non-binary individuals whose gender history did not fit a stereotyped script. As a result, some trans and non-binary patients may still feel inhibited when speaking with providers about their sexuality.[44]

The majority of the literature on sexual satisfaction among transfeminine individuals relates to post-surgical outcomes. Following orchiectomy, transfeminine individuals may produce ejaculate, which is thought to arise from the prostate.[47] Systematic reviews of surgical literature have reported that following vaginoplasty, 64 to 98 per cent of transfeminine individuals were satisfied with general sexual outcomes.[70] Eighty-nine per cent maintained erogenous sensation,[71] and 80 per cent could achieve orgasm (in studies specifying type of orgasm, 36 per cent experienced vaginal orgasm and 83 per cent experienced clitoral orgasm).[70] Fifty-six to 100 per cent were satisfied with neovaginal dimensions and intercourse.[72] Penile inversion vaginoplasty may be associated with unsatisfactory physiologic lubrication during intercourse.[70-75] Some 19.7 per cent of individuals experienced dyspareunia, which may be ameliorated with physical therapy or extra lubricant.[70] Following colovaginoplasty, transfeminine individuals typically experience adequate lubrication for receptive intercourse[76] and, in rare cases, excessive discharge in the early post-operative period.[77]

Prospective survey data has shown that breast augmentation[78] and feminizing hormone therapy[79] also improved sexual satisfaction. Although hypogonadism in cis men can cause low libido, one study found no correlation between testosterone levels and libido in transfeminine individuals.[80]

Although only a minority of transfeminine individuals undergo gender affirming surgery, transfeminine individuals who do not undergo gender-affirming surgeries are an understudied population. A Canadian survey studying sexual inactivity among sexually experienced transfeminine individuals found that 43 per cent reported no sexual activity in the past year, and sexual activity was 3.7 times more prevalent among those with a history of genital surgery. Hormone use and living in their felt gender were not predictive of sexual inactivity.[81]

Sexual Satisfaction – Transmasculine Individuals

Similar to the case for transfeminine individuals, there is a paucity of literature on sexual satisfaction among transmasculine individuals outside surgical outcomes. Rates of orgasmic ability among transmasculine individuals after bottom surgery (i.e., metoidioplasty or phalloplasty) range from 25 to 100 per cent.[44] Rates of phalloplasty sensation and orgasm are typically high; with radial forearm flap phalloplasty, one centre reported at 23 months' follow-up that 15 out of 20 subjects could achieve orgasm, which increased at 54 months' follow-up to 20 out of 20.[81] Masculinizing chest surgery[82] and masculinizing hormone therapy[83] also improved sexual satisfaction. Additionally, no correlation was found between serum testosterone levels and desire in transmasculine individuals.[83]

BDSM

In some circumstances, patients may seek advice from clinicians around practices of bondage, discipline, domination, submission, and sadomasochism (BDSM). This may be relevant if patients request advice on minimizing risks of harm, if they have a medical condition that may require them to modify or limit participation in certain activities, and when BDSM practices pose a risk of injury or infection. For instance, conditions that can cause loss of consciousness (including seizure disorders, vasovagal events, hypoglycemia) may preclude some types of immobilization or physical impact. Patients may also benefit from advice around preventing bondage-related nerve injury or joint strain and aseptic techniques to use when skin is intentionally broken.[84]

Studies of those who engage in BDSM have found no link with psychopathology or psychiatric symptoms of depression, anxiety, obsessive compulsive disorder (OCD), or PTSD.[85]

Some practices that eroticize pain may produce lesions that clinically resemble trauma, infection, or dermatologic pathology. Providers should also be able to distinguish BDSM from abuse. BDSM scenes take place within a context of negotiations and knowledgeable consent, and either party can stop what is happening with a mechanism such as a "safeword."[84] However, abuse can take place in the context of a relationship that involves BDSM. Clinicians are advised to ask questions in a non-judgmental manner, and to seek clarification if they believe it serves the patient's interests.

Vaginal Douching

Vaginal douching is highly prevalent in high-resource countries, with 32 per cent of US women reporting douching in the last 12 months and higher rates observed in non-Hispanic Black women and women with lower levels of education.[86] This is often associated with misconceptions that douching can prevent STIs, prevent pregnancy, hide evidence of infidelity, and tighten the vagina.[87] However, vaginal douching can alter vaginal pH (normally 3.8 to 4.5 for premenopausal adults), predisposing towards bacterial vaginosis.[88] Additionally, chemical additives in commercial douching products may cause irritation. Douching has been associated with STIs, pelvic inflammatory disease (PID), and ectopic pregnancy;[89] however, this may in part be confounded by symptomatic individuals attempting to self-treat with douching. Because of these associated harms, and a lack of physiologic benefit, douching is discouraged.[87] Effects of douching in relation to HIV have also been investigated. Vaginal douching is associated with an elevated risk of HIV acquisition, particularly if soap is used.[90]

Neovaginal Douching

In contrast, neovaginal douching for transfeminine individuals is necessary, especially in the early recovery period to facilitate clearance of dead skin and clots, typically by using normal saline multiple times daily.

After the immediate post-operative period, douching with tap water is safe to continue (frequency per surgeon's recommendations). Since the tissue lining after penile inversion vaginoplasty is not a mucosa, lifelong douching is necessary to clear sebum and dead skin.[5,91] Following colovaginoplasty, douching is not mandatory after the initial recovery period; however, 80 per cent of transfeminine individuals who had undergone this procedure continued to douche at six-year follow-up.[92]

Rectal Douching

Pre-coital rectal douching is frequently practiced by MSM, although concerns about health implications have been raised. Observational data shows douching is associated with a higher odds of lymphogranuloma venereum (LGV),[93,94] hepatitis C,[95] HIV,[96] hepatitis B,[97] and HPV;[98] however, it is unclear whether this represents increased susceptibility caused by douching or association with higher-risk behaviours.[99,100] Some research has found that rectal douching more than once weekly increased the risk of rectal gonorrhea or chlamydia even when controlling for episodes of unprotected receptive anal intercourse, number of male partners, and substance use,[101] but other studies have found no association with rectal STIs.[102]

There has been insufficient published research on safety and harms of rectal douching to guide clinical recommendations. Research on frequent large-volume enemas has shown potential for rectal surface epithelium loss (especially with use of soapsuds[103]) and hyponatremia.[104] Bowel preparation for colonoscopy is known to cause significant and persistent changes in bowel microflora load and composition.[105,106] In the absence of high-quality evidence, experts recommend douching no more than two to three times per week, using tap water for infrequent douching or normal saline for frequent douching, and avoiding soap or other chemicals that can cause irritation.[107]

Fisting

Fisting refers to the insertion of a hand or fist into the rectum or vagina. There is a paucity of literature to guide clinicians on counselling patients around these practices. Among WSW, vaginal fisting is thought to increase the risk of HIV;[108] use of gloves may reduce the risk of STIs.[109] Among MSM, receptive anal fisting is associated with increased risk of hepatitis C[110,111] and HIV.[112] Clinicians should screen for concomitant chemsex and fisting, as there are rare reports of intestinal perforation.[113]

Vulvar Pathology

A variety of dermatologic conditions affecting the vulva may impact the sexual well-being of individuals assigned female at birth. Medical treatments are summarized in table 6.3.

Table 6.3. Treatments for Non-infectious Vulvar Conditions

Atrophic vaginitis	Over-the-counter: water-based lubricants Conjugated estrogen cream 0.25mg/g, 0.5 g PV daily for 2 weeks, then twice weekly Estradiol 17β 10 mcg tab PV daily for 2 weeks, then twice weekly
Lichen simplex chronicus[120]	Clobetasol 0.05% cream or ointment once daily for 3–4 weeks, then transition to lower potency steroid or taper over 3–6 months Hydroxyzine 25 mg TID-QID PRN Lidocaine 2% viscous or pramoxine cream 1%–2.5% applied TID-QID PRN
Lichen sclerosus[120,127]	Clobetasol 0.05% BID for 1 week, then once daily for 5 weeks or until symptom resolution, then taper to 1–3 times a week for indefinite maintenance therapy
Lichen planus[120]	Clobetasol 0.05% daily for 2–3 months, then taper to 1–3 times weekly for indefinite maintenance therapy

Atrophic vaginitis refers to symptomatic changes in the vaginal epithelium due to a hypoestrogenic state. It arises with menopause and primary ovarian insufficiency, as well as with testosterone therapy in transmasculine people.[114] Symptoms can include vulvovaginal dryness, burning, pruritus, dysuria, and dyspareunia. Affected individuals may also have a heightened risk for urinary tract infections,[115] vulvovaginal *Candida*, and bacterial vaginosis.[116] Treatments can include vaginal moisturizers, lubricants, and topical estrogen therapy (cream or suppository). Of note, vaginal suppository[117] and intravaginal cream[118] result in elevated serum levels of estradiol and estrone. This is unlikely to cause clinical feminization with ongoing testosterone therapy, but transmasculine individuals may nonetheless opt to pursue non-hormonal methods, which are equally effective.[119]

Lichen simplex chronicus is a thickening of the vulvar skin associated with pruritus and burning pain. It arises from a chronic 'itch-scratch' cycle; the preceding dermatitis can involve atopic dermatitis, allergic or irritant contact dermatitis, or vulvovaginal infection with *Candida*.[120] In lichen simplex chronicus, the thickened vulva appears erythematous and may develop papillae or edema; patients experience pruritus and burning pain. Investigations can include patch testing and biopsy. Lichen simplex chronicus is managed with avoidance of behavioural or irritant causes, and symptomatic medical therapy to eliminate scratching. This can include topical steroids, oral antihistamines, and topical anaesthetics.[120]

Lichen sclerosus is a chronic inflammatory dermatologic condition of unknown etiology that usually affects the anogenital region.

It primarily affects cis women, with the highest prevalence in prepubertal and postmenopausal age groups.[121] Lichen sclerosus has been documented in a transgender woman eight years after penile inversion vaginoplasty,[122] although there are no reported cases affecting transmasculine individuals. Lichen sclerosus presents as thinning and white plaques associated with pruritus, pain, dyspareunia, and dysuria; it can progress to fissuring, atrophy, and midline fusion of the vulva starting from the clitoral hood.[123] Lichen sclerosus typically spares the vaginal mucosa.[120] It is usually a clinical diagnosis though it can be confirmed by biopsy.[123] Treatment is aimed at managing symptoms and reducing the risk of malignant transformation, which occurs in 2 to 5 per cent of individuals.[120] This involves patient education about the course of disease and the importance of avoiding irritants and scratching, and medical therapy with topical high-potency corticosteroids or topical calcineurin inhibitors.[123]

Lichen planus is an inflammatory mucocutaneous condition that can affect multiple sites including oral and genital mucosa, skin, hair, and nails. The etiology is unknown, but it is thought to involve T-cell mediated autoimmunity. It produces glazed erythematous erosions, violaceous papules, or rough hypertrophic lesions of the vulva.[120] Associated symptoms include burning pain, pruritus, and vaginal discharge.[124] Diagnosis is confirmed by biopsy. Lichen planus is treated with topical high-potency steroids or calcineurin inhibitors, with indefinite maintenance therapy to prevent relapse.[125] Severe cases may also benefit from a four- to six-week course of systemic corticosteroids. In the event of adhesions and vaginal stenosis, dilators or surgical dilation may also be indicated.[120,126]

Dyspareunia, or pain with receptive vulvovaginal intercourse, has a broad differential diagnosis. The majority of clinical literature on dyspareunia is focused on the act of penile-vaginal penetration; however, vulvovaginal pain may arise from a variety of sexual acts between sexual minority women.[128] Clinicians should take a detailed history including timeline, associated symptoms, and location of pain. Superficial pain raises suspicion for vulvar pathology, infections such as *Candida* or vulvodynia; deep pain during insertive vaginal sex suggests pathology such as endometriosis, interstitial cystitis, PID, or musculoskeletal (MSK) dysfunction.

Vulvodynia is a poorly understood chronic pain condition of the vulva that can have significant impacts on sexual function. It is estimated to affect 16 per cent of cis women.[129] It can be localized, usually to the vaginal vestibule, or generalized. It may be provoked (by contact including postcoital worsening) or unprovoked; clinically, it is replicated by light touch of a cotton swab to the posterior fourchette

("Q-tip test"). Research has suggested that these syndromes may be related to vaginismus, previously defined as painful vaginal spasm that prevents penetrative intercourse; however, muscle spasm may be a defensive *response* to vulvar pain, rather than the primary cause of pain.[130,131] Beyond affecting sexual functioning, vulvodynia complicates pelvic examination and may lead to avoidance of Pap screening. Initial treatment involves elimination of irritants, physical therapy, topical anaesthetics, and tricyclic antidepressants; in resistant cases, a vestibulectomy may be offered.[132]

There is little research on the experience and prevalence of vulvodynia among cisgender WSW, perhaps because of a phallocentric concept of female sexual function. However, survey data shows that vulvodynia among cis WSW affects sexual functioning, though not relationship satisfaction, and that vulvar pain in self-identified bisexual women can reduce interest in pursuing sexual experiences with cis men.[128] In another survey, bisexual cis women in relationships with cis men were more likely to report pain than heterosexual women in relationships with cis men, with lesbian women and bisexual women in same-sex relationships being least likely to report pain.[133] However, vulvodynia in lesbian cis women had less effect on sexual aspects of the relationship, compared to bisexual and heterosexual cis women.[133]

Pain with intercourse is reported by 9 to 45 per cent of transfeminine individuals after vaginoplasty.[71,73,75] This may be related to inadequate lubrication, STIs,[134] neovulvar pathology,[122] post-operative neuropathic pain, or dimensions of the neovagina (related to surgical technique or neovaginal stenosis).[44]

Perianal Health

A variety of non-infectious conditions can affect the perianal skin such as hemorrhoids, fissures, and fistulas, which may impact sexual wellbeing. There is limited to no evidence investigating prevalence of these complaints among MSM or comparing incidence with the general population. Treatment recommendations are generally the same as for the general population, but patients should be advised that topical medications may include components (such as mineral oil) that can weaken latex condoms.

Hemorrhoids, varicose veins from the rectal venous plexus, cause a variety of anal symptoms. The prevalence of hemorrhoids in the general population, based on incidental diagnosis on colonoscopies for colorectal cancer screening (ages 20 to 85), is estimated to be 39 per cent.[135] Their pathophysiology is poorly understood, although studies

Table 6.4. Hemorrhoid Grading, Symptoms, and Treatment

	Grade I Internal	Grade II Internal	Grade III Internal	Grade IV Internal	Mixed or External
Definition[141]	No protrusion past dentate line (visible only on anoscopy)	Prolapse out of the canal with straining, but reduce spontaneously	Prolapse out of the canal with straining, require manual reduction	Irreducible prolapse	Arise distal to dentate line
Symptoms	Painless bleeding	Painless bleeding, pruritus	Painless bleeding, pruritus, swelling, fecal incontinence	Pain, bleeding, swelling, fecal incontinence	Pruritus/ swelling, painful thrombosis
Treatment[132]	Conservative management, banding	Conservative management, banding	Conservative management, banding, or surgery	Conservative management or surgery	Conservative management or surgery

of asymptomatic patients on screening colonoscopy have shown a correlation between hemorrhoids and constipation[136] and diarrhea;[137] there is conflicting evidence for a link with obesity or sedentary behaviour.[135,136] They are also more common during and after pregnancy.[138] There have been no studies evaluating a possible link between receptive anal intercourse and perianal conditions such as hemorrhoids.

Hemorrhoids can be classified as internal, which originate above the dentate line and are covered with insensate mucosa, or external, from below the dentate line and covered with highly sensitive anoderm.[138] Internal hemorrhoids can present with painless bleeding, or prolapse (graded I to IV based on degree of prolapse: see table 6.4). External hemorrhoids can present with perianal pruritus, prolapse, or thrombosis (associated with excruciating pain and swelling). Hemorrhoids are diagnosed clinically on examination with digital anorectal exam or anoscopy.[139] Despite their prevalence, it is dangerous to assume rectal bleeding is related to hemorrhoids without additional investigations if indicated; the differential diagnosis includes gastrointestinal malignancies, STIs, and anal fissures. Initial conservative management of any hemorrhoids involves sitz baths and fibre supplementation, with topical low-potency corticosteroids or analgesics as needed.[138] Internal hemorrhoids may be managed in the office with band ligation, sclerotherapy, or infrared coagulation; or surgically with hemorrhoidectomy.[139] External hemorrhoids that are severe or refractory require surgery to resolve. Thrombosed external hemorrhoids may also be excised for immediate symptom relief, if they present within 72 hours of onset.[140]

Anal fissures are superficial ulcers or tears distal to the dentate line, which cause sharp pain associated with bowel movements and sometimes bleeding. They are typically caused by local trauma, including anal sex, constipation, or diarrhea. They may also occur secondary to STIs (chlamydia, primary or secondary syphilis, HIV), granulomatous diseases, and inflammatory bowel disease.[142,143] Traumatic anal fissures usually occur on the midline; those outside the midline should be investigated for secondary causes. If present less than three months, anal fissures can be treated conservatively with sitz baths and fibre supplementation, or medical therapy including topical anaesthetics and topical smooth muscle relaxants.[142] Chronic anal fissures are those present more than a few weeks and may develop induration and an associated skin tag. These are more likely to require invasive therapy such as botulinum toxin or surgery.[144]

Perianal fistulas are tracts extending from the anal canal to the perianal skin; they can result from anorectal abscess, Crohn's disease, obstetric trauma, or local irradiation.[139,145] Fistulas may present with discharge, pain, swelling, or bleeding, and examination may show granulation tissue, a palpable cord, or expressible discharge.[146] Visualization and characterization of the fistula system may also require examination under anaesthesia or magnetic resonance imaging. Abscesses and fistulas are not typically attributed to sexual activity unless they result from LGV proctitis.[147] Conservative treatment includes fibre supplementation, analgesics, and sitz baths. Failure of conservative management, or complex risk factors, should be referred for surgery.[139]

Pruritus ani is a presenting complaint with a broad differential diagnosis. Among MSM, care should be taken to exclude rectal chlamydia, condylomata, or herpes simplex viruses (HSV), as well as non-STIs including Candida intertrigo or pinworm. Non-infectious causes include local irritation secondary to moisture, chemical irritants, or excoriation; dermatologic conditions such as atopic dermatitis, psoriasis, or lichen sclerosus; and premalignant or malignant conditions.[148] If the cause is not apparent on history and examination, investigations such as STI swabs, fungal scrapings, and punch biopsy can be considered. Initial treatment should be targeted at an underlying cause, if identified. The approach to idiopathic anal pruritus involves patient education

Table 6.5. Treatments for Perianal Conditions

External hemorrhoids	Over-the-counter: zinc oxide, bulk-forming laxatives, hydrocortisone 1% cream Pramoxine 1% foam or ointment, up to 5 times daily PRN Nitroglycerin 0.2%–0.5% ointment BID PRN
Anal fissures	Nifedipine 0.2%–0.3% cream/ointment BID-QID for 4 weeks Nitroglycerin 0.2%–0.5% ointment BID for up to 3 weeks Lidocaine 2% viscous applied TID-QID PRN
Pruritus ani	Over-the-counter: hydrocortisone 1% cream BID-QID for 2–4 weeks Hydroxyzine 25 mg PO TID-QID PRN Capsaicin 0.006% cream TID for 14 days

Source: Adapted from Fargo MV, Latimer KM[139]

(avoiding scratching or scrubbing the area, avoiding soaps and scented wipes, avoiding dietary triggers), conservative measures (such as barrier creams, baby powder, fibre supplementation), and consideration of topical steroids or calcineurin inhibitors.[139,148]

Treatment recommendations for perianal conditions are summarized in table 6.5.

Rectal prolapse refers to protrusion of all layers of the rectum; this is distinguished from mucosal prolapse secondary to hemorrhoids.[19] There is no evidence linking sexual practices such as receptive anal intercourse with rectal prolapse; identified risk factors include obstetric trauma, chronic constipation, and advanced age.[149,150]

Despite widespread concerns about harms associated with anal intercourse in the lay press, there is little published literature on the topic. A history of receptive anal intercourse is associated with a lower resting anal canal tone in MSM.[151] A large cross-sectional study ($n = 4170$) found increased rates of fecal incontinence among individuals with a history of receptive anal intercourse versus no history of receptive anal intercourse (11.6 per cent versus 5.3 per cent for men, and 9.9 per cent versus 7.4 per cent for women).[152] Another study of cis women ($n = 1003$) found that risk of fecal incontinence was not higher with any history of anal intercourse, but was higher with anal intercourse in the last month.[153]

Anal Dyspareunia

Anal intercourse is not inevitably painful, but can cause pain without sufficient relaxation, lubrication, and digito-anal foreplay,[154] and/or in the presence of pathology described above. Distinct from this, anodyspareunia is a term proposed to describe persistent and severe pain associated with receptive anal intercourse. In one survey of cis MSM,[155] 14 per cent of respondents reported frequent and severe pain with receptive anal intercourse. This pain was lifelong in 60 per cent, acquired in 2 per cent, situational in 21 per cent, or "other" in 15 per cent. Frequent, severe pain was associated with behavioural and mechanical factors (not feeling relaxed, large insertive penis, and insufficient foreplay) and reduced relationship satisfaction; it was not correlated with internalized homonegativity scores or with being "out of the closet." Further research is necessary to characterize anodyspareunia as a distinct clinical phenomenon.

Specific Infections

Chlamydia

Chlamydia trachomatis (CT) is a bacterium spread by contact with infected bodily fluids. It can live in the vagina, cervix, rectum, urethra, pharynx, and eyes. In Canada, young individuals (ages 15 to 29) are most affected by chlamydia.[156]

Studies in MSM have observed more anorectal than urethral or pharyngeal infections of chlamydia.[157-161] Although transmission between cis WSW is less studied, more recent data suggests transmission of chlamydia is possible. Screening should be considered at least annually in all sexually active individuals and more frequently in populations with a high burden of infection, such as MSM.[162]

Screening of asymptomatic individuals preferably includes a urine sample, cervical swab, or vaginal self-swab[163] for nucleic acid amplification testing (NAAT), because of the greater sensitivity and specificity of NAAT compared to cultures.[156] Recommendations for the use of rectal and/or pharyngeal NAAT swabs for chlamydia detection vary by province and territory. For instance, in Ontario, these swabs are only recommended if *unprotected* oral or anal sex is reported by MSM (we would extend this recommendation to transfeminine patients who have sex with men), sex workers of any gender and their contacts, and known contacts of an individual infected with gonorrhea or chlamydia.[164] Testing at these sites for chlamydia can be considered in other individuals who have sex with men (e.g., average risk cis women, transmasculine individuals), but cost–benefit analyses are lacking in these groups, who have comparatively lower risks of isolated extragenital infections (in which chlamydia would be missed from routine urine screening alone).[165,166] Rectal swabs can be collected through an anoscope or blindly, the latter of which can be done by the provider or by the patient. The use of an anoscope, which minimizes fecal contamination, is preferred for symptomatic individuals. Blind swabs should be inserted two to three centimetres into the rectal canal, with lateral pressure to avoid fecal contamination.

In transfeminine individuals who have had vaginoplasty, the role of neovaginal specimens to detect chlamydia – as opposed to urine testing only – is unknown.[167] At this time, neovaginal NAAT swabs may be considered in addition to urine NAAT testing as it is possible that it may increase chlamydia detection rates. There are no published reports of urethral STIs affecting transmasculine individuals post-phalloplasty, but routine testing for chlamydia using urine NAAT should be recommended when the neophallus is involved in sexual activities.

Long-term asymptomatic carriage of chlamydia is possible.[168] Although infection with chlamydia is typically asymptomatic, a patient may develop vaginal/cervical symptoms (e.g., discharge, abnormal vaginal bleeding, lower abdominal pain, deep dyspareunia), urethral symptoms (dysuria, discharge, itch), scrotal/testicular symptoms (testicular pain and/or swelling), or rectal symptoms (pain and discharge with proctitis) depending on the site of infection. The typical incubation period before symptom onset is two to three weeks.[156]

Chlamydia can be treated with either azithromycin 1 g by mouth single dose, or doxycycline 100 mg by mouth twice a day for seven days. However, for anorectal chlamydia, doxycycline has a superior cure rate over azithromycin.[169] See table 6.9 at the end of this section for more information regarding management and counselling of suspected or confirmed cases of chlamydia. Repeat screening for new infection is recommended after three months.[156,162]

LGV

LGV – caused by *Chlamydia trachomatis* serovars L1, L2, L2b and L3 – has expanded past parts of Africa, Asia, South America, and the Caribbean region, where it is endemic, to cause primarily rectal infection in MSM in many urban locations in North America and Europe.[169-178]

LGV typically causes a painless papule that may ulcerate at the site of inoculation within a month of infection. Subsequently, systemic symptoms typically develop along with unilateral lymphadenopathy (inguinal, femoral) or hemorrhagic proctitis.[156,178] If there is clinical suspicion of LGV chlamydia, LGV-specific testing should be performed on samples taken for chlamydia testing (i.e., culture or NAAT). In recent years, male rectal specimens positive for chlamydia are automatically sent for LGV testing in certain regions, such as Ontario.[179,180] Treatment of LGV requires a prolonged course of antibiotics, such as doxycycline 100 mg by mouth twice a day for three weeks.[156,179] While Canadian guidelines recommend a test of cure after treatment of LGV, the US Centers for Disease Control and Prevention does not unless an alternative treatment regimen is used or the treated patient is pregnant.[162] Consider local guidelines when determining appropriate follow-up. See table 6.9 at the end of this section for more information regarding management and counselling of suspected or confirmed LGV.

Gonorrhea

Neisseria gonorrhoeae is an intracellular bacterium spread by contact with infected bodily fluids. Much like chlamydia, *N. gonorrhoeae* can live in the vagina, cervix, rectum, urethra, pharynx, and eyes. In Canada, the majority of reported gonorrhea cases occur in young men and women (ages 15 to 29), with an increasing number of cases in MSM.[156] More recently, throat-to-throat transmission (through kissing), throat-to-anus transmission, and anus-to-throat transmission (through oro-anal sex) have been proposed as modes of gonorrhea transmission in MSM.[181] These theories are supported by the higher incidence for anal gonorrhea in those receiving oro-anal sex,[182] the higher incidence for pharyngeal gonorrhea in those performing insertive oro-anal sex (or anilingus),[183] and the frequent detection of gonorrhea in the saliva of men with pharyngeal infection.[184,185]

Asymptomatic screening should always include a urine sample, vaginal swab, or cervical swab,[186] for NAAT. For gonorrhea, Canadian guidelines recommend pharyngeal testing for all individuals with a history of performing oral sex and rectal testing for individuals with a history of receptive anal intercourse, *irrespective* of whether condoms were used.[156] This differs from more recent provincial and territorial recommendations, such as Ontario's public health guidelines recommending screening for extragenital gonorrhea and chlamydia only after *unprotected* oral or anal sex in MSM (and presumably transfeminine individuals who have sex with men), sex workers and their contacts, and known contacts of an individual infected with gonorrhea or chlamydia.[187] Similar to the case for chlamydia, cost–benefit analyses are lacking in lower-risk populations where isolated extragenital gonorrhea infection is less common.[165,166]

Gonorrhea infection has been documented in transfeminine individuals post-vaginoplasty with penile inversion[188,189] and colovaginoplasty,[190] and may be symptomatic[189,190] or asymptomatic.[188] As with chlamydia, it may be prudent to supplement urine NAAT with neovaginal swab NAAT to optimize detection of gonorrhea in asymptomatic individuals.[167] Additionally, transmasculine individuals post-phalloplasty should have routine testing for gonorrhea using urine NAAT when the neophallus is used in sexual activities.

Symptomatic individuals suspected of having gonorrhea should have a culture taken to determine antimicrobial sensitivities; this is particularly important for symptomatic MSM, in whom antimicrobial resistance is more common.[156]

Long-term asymptomatic carriage of pharyngeal or rectal gonorrhea is possible,[191] but the majority of urethral and cervical infections are symptomatic. Infection with gonorrhea mimics that of chlamydia, with the potential for vaginal/cervical symptoms (i.e., mucopurulent discharge, abnormal vaginal bleeding, lower abdominal pain, deep dyspareunia), urethral symptoms (dysuria, mucopurulent discharge, itch), scrotal/testicular symptoms (testicular pain and/or swelling), or rectal symptoms (pain and discharge with proctitis). Incubation period is typically two to seven days.[156]

First-line treatment for suspected or confirmed gonorrhea varies by guideline. Traditionally, dual therapy was widely recommended with ceftriaxone 250 mg intramuscular injection [IM] once, with azithromycin 1 g orally once,[156] for synergistic effect to prevent resistance. The 2020 CDC guideline updated its recommendation to ceftriaxone 500 mg IM once (if the patient weighs less than 150 kg).[192] This change responds to an increasing prevalence of azithromycin-resistant *N. gonorrhoeae*, which is, in fact, higher in Canada (7.6 per cent in 2018)[193] than in the United States (4.6 per cent in 2018).[192] The WHO recommends discontinuing the use of a particular empiric antibiotic once 5 per cent of locally acquired isolates of *N. gonorrhoae* demonstrate resistance to that antibiotic.[194] More information regarding management and counselling of suspected or confirmed cases of gonorrhea can be found in table 6.9 at the end of this section.

Since the discovery of penicillin and its application for treating STIs, gonorrhea strains resistant to multiple classes of antibiotics have emerged. At this time, gonorrhea resistant to ceftriaxone has been reported in Canada,[195] and strains resistant to ceftriaxone and azithromycin have been reported in the United Kingdom.[196] Therefore, it is prudent to refer to regional public health treatment guidelines for up-to-date empiric regimens and to consider gonorrhea culture and sensitivities in the event of suspected or confirmed treatment failure.

Canadian guidelines recommend a test of cure using either gonorrhea cultures three to seven days after the completion of therapy or NAAT two to three weeks after the completion of treatment, *particularly* in specific cases (see box 6.2).[156] Repeat screening for new infection is recommended after three months.[156,162]

Box 6.2. Situations in Which Follow-Up Gonorrhea Cultures for Test of Cure Are Particularly Recommended

- All pharyngeal infections
- Persistent symptoms or signs post-treatment
- Case treated with a non-first-line regimen
- Culture from case (or a linked case) demonstrates antimicrobial resistance to the administered treatment
- A linked case has had treatment failure with the same antibiotic
- Treatment failure for gonorrhea has occurred previously in the case
- Compliance is uncertain
- Case is re-exposed to an untreated partner
- Infection during pregnancy
- Disseminated gonococcal infection
- Case is a child
- Cases with PID (and positive gonorrhea testing)
- Women undergoing therapeutic abortion (because of an increased risk of developing PID)

Source: Canadian Guidelines on Sexually Transmitted Infections[156]

Syphilis

Syphilis is caused by infection with the bacterium *Treponema pallidum subsp. pallidum*, which is most readily transmitted through oral, anal, and vaginal sex. While direct contact with lesions pose the highest risk of transmission, lesions are often not apparent (especially when internal). Rarely, transmission has been reported through kissing and through blood-borne routes.[156]

Rates of syphilis in Canada increased dramatically between 2009 and 2018. In 2018, incidence in men was over three times that in women, with the majority of infections occurring in the MSM population.[197,198] Syphilis transmission between WSW is unlikely but still possible,[199,200] and so screening should be considered in all individuals whose practices include oral-genital, anal-genital, and genital-genital sex.

Symptoms of syphilis infection are outlined in table 6.6. Though often subtle, untreated infection typically proceeds in a step-wise manner from one or more primary chancre sore(s), to secondary systemic spread with a diffuse rash and condyloma lata lesions, to tertiary syphilis, with asymptomatic periods in between. These asymptomatic

Table 6.6. Typical Manifestations of Syphilis in Its Various Stages

Stage of Syphilis	Typical Manifestations	Typical Incubation Period: Time to Onset (Range)
Early Stage (Infectious)		
Primary	Chancre (usually a painless, single indurated ulcer with a clean base and rolled borders; often multiple ulcers in HIV-infected patients), regional lymphadenopathy	3 weeks (3–90 days)
Secondary	Rash (typically maculopapular or papulosquamous) on palms, soles, trunk, extremities; fever, malaise, generalized lymphadenopathy; mucus lesions; condyloma lata; alopecia	2–12 weeks (2 weeks–6 months)
Hepatitis	Elevated liver enzymes (ALP > AST/ALT), normal bilirubin (Much more common in HIV-infected patients, up to 30% prevalence)	2–12 weeks (2 weeks–6 months)
Neurosyphilis		
Asymptomatic	None	Unknown, likely within days
Acute meningitis	Headache, meningismus, confusion	<2 years
Ocular	Uveitis, keratitis, optical neuritis	<2 years
Early latent	None	<1 year
Late Stage (Non-infectious)		
Late latent	None	>1 year
Tertiary (Rare)		
Neurosyphilis	Often asymptomatic; Early symptoms: headaches, vertigo, personality changes; Late symptoms: dementia, ataxia, presence of Argyll Robertson pupil (small pupil that lacks light reflex but demonstrates preserved constriction during accommodation and convergence for near objects)	<2–20 years

(Continued)

Table 6.6. (Continued)

Stage of Syphilis	Typical Manifestations	Typical Incubation Period: Time to Onset (Range)
Cardiovascular	Aortic aneurysm, aortic insufficiency, coronary ostial stenosis	10–30 years
Gumma	Tissue destructive, immune-mediated soft granulomas occurring in any organ, usually skin or bone	15 years (1–46 years)

ALP = alkaline phosphatase; AST = aspartate aminotransferase; ALT = alanine aminotransferase

Source: Adapted from Canadian Guidelines on Sexually Transmitted Infections[156] and Lewis J, Seña AC[201]

periods are termed *early latent* syphilis when under one year, and *late latent* syphilis when more than one year from infection.[156]

Syphilis testing is complicated by the fact that *T. pallidum* cannot be cultured, and infection can be latent. Laboratory diagnosis involves treponemal and non-treponemal tests. Treponemal tests detect antibodies to *T. pallidum* and include EIA (enzyme immunoassay), CMIA (chemiluminescent microparticle immunoassay), CLIA (chemiluminescent immunoassay), MFI (multiplex flow immunoassay), TP-PA (*T. pallidum* particle agglutination), and FTA-ABS (fluorescent treponemal antibody-absorbed). Non-treponemal tests detect specific antigens released by host cells damaged by *T. pallidum*, such as cardiolipin or lecithin, or antigens released by *T. pallidum*, such as lipoprotein-like material.[202] Non-treponemal tests are reported as a titre, which typically reflects disease activity but may plateau after treatment instead of returning to an undetectable level. Serologic syphilis testing algorithms vary across Canada, with the typical initial screen involving either a treponemal immunoassay or a non-treponemal test. Confirmation may be done using TP-PA or FTA-ABS, which are the most sensitive treponemal tests. Because treponemal tests remain positive for life, the non-treponemal rapid plasma reagin (RPR) titre is particularly important for those who have previously been treated for syphilis, as a four-fold increase in RPR indicates a new infection. RPR may be initially negative, in which case serology should be repeated in two to four weeks if clinical suspicion of early syphilis infection is high. Interpretation of syphilis serologic testing is summarized in table 6.7, and table 6.8 summarizes the possible causes of false-positive results.

Table 6.7. Interpretation of Syphilis Serology Results

Tests			
Treponemal (e.g., EIA, CMIA, CLIA, MFI)	Non-treponemal (RPR, VDRL)	Confirmatory Treponemal (TP-PA)	Interpretation
NR	NR	Test not done	Negative
R	R	R/I	Recent or prior infection*
R	NR	R	Recent or prior infection*
R	R	NR	Inconclusive†
R	NR	I	Inconclusive†
R	NR	NR	False positive

Source: Adapted from Toronto Public Health[203]

CLIA = chemiluminescent immunoassay; CMIA = chemiluminescent microparticle immunoassay; EIA = enzyme immunoassay; FTA-ABS = fluorescent treponemal antibody-absorbed; I = indeterminate; MFI = multiplex flow immunoassay; NR = non-reactive; R = reactive; RPR = rapid plasma regain; TP-PA = Treponema pallidum particle agglutination; VDRL = Venereal Disease Research Laboratory

* May indicate infectious syphilis, latent syphilis (unknown duration), old treated syphilis, or cross-reactivity from other treponemal infections. Repeat in 2–4 weeks for change in titre.

† May indicate incubating primary syphilis, old syphilis (treated or untreated), or a false positive.

Table 6.8. Possible Causes of False-Positive Syphilis Serology

False-Positive Treponemal Tests	False-Positive Non-treponemal Tests
Infectious: malaria, infectious mononucleosis, LGV, varicella, tuberculosis, viral hepatitis, bacterial endocarditis, chancroid, pneumonia (mycoplasma, pneumococcus, viral), other treponemal infections (yaws, pinta, bejel) **Non-infectious:** chronic liver disease, immunizations, IV drug use, advanced age, pregnancy, connective tissue disease, multiple myeloma, malignancy, ulcerative colitis	**Infectious:** malaria, infectious mononucleosis, genital herpes, other treponemal infections (yaws, pinta, bejel) **Non-infectious:** chronic liver disease, advanced age, systemic lupus erythematosus, thyroiditis

Source: Adapted from Toronto Public Health. 2018.[203]

Additionally, chancre(s) consistent with syphilis can be tested directly and may yield a positive result before serology. Testing varies by region; in Ontario, the direct fluorescence antibody test is done on specimens collected by applying a slide directly onto the lesion.[204] See Public Health Agency of Canada (PHAC) 2010 guidelines for more information regarding laboratory testing for syphilis.[156]

Syphilis infection can progress to involve the central nervous system (CNS) in any stage;[162] this progression occurs more commonly in HIV-positive individuals.[205] If undetected, T. pallidum can form a reservoir in the CNS, and fail to respond to treatment for early disease or late latent disease.[156,162] Cerebrospinal fluid (CSF) examination should be considered if neurologic symptoms or signs are present or in certain individuals who are being treated for syphilis but have a suboptimal decline in VDRL/RPR titre – that is, less than a four-fold decrease in titre within 6 to 12 months of treatment for early syphilis, or within 12 to 24 months of treatment for late latent syphilis.[162,206] Other indications for CSF examination when the neurological examination is normal are controversial because they have not been associated with improved outcomes.[206] These indications include VDRL/RPR ≥ 1:32 dilutions – which has been associated with CNS/CSF abnormalities in some but not all studies[204–206] – as well as HIV-positive individuals with a CD4 ≤ 350 to 500 cells/μL.[207–209]

Syphilis treatment depends on the stage of infection (see table 6.9 at the end of this section). Primary syphilis, secondary syphilis, and early latent syphilis are treated with penicillin G 2.4 million units IM single dose. Because of a theoretical concern that T. pallidum in late stage disease may divide more slowly,[162] late latent syphilis is treated with penicillin G 2.4 million units IM once a week for three weeks. Neurosyphilis is treated with penicillin G 3–4 million units IV every four hours for 10 to 14 days. See table 6.9 at the end of this section for more information regarding management and follow-up of suspected or confirmed cases of syphilis.

A Jarisch-Herxheimer reaction has been well documented in 30 to 50 per cent of patients treated for syphilis. Patients should be counselled that this reaction – a response to the breakdown of spirochetes characterized by flu-like symptoms – is not harmful, represents neither a drug reaction nor an allergy, resolves within 24 hours, and can be managed with over-the-counter antipyretics and hydration.[210]

Mycoplasma and Ureaplasma

Mycoplasma genitalium is one of the smallest known organisms capable of independent growth. It can be isolated from the urogenital tract of approximately 1 per cent of adults,[211] and it may be more common among men who have sex with women than MSM.[212] *M. genitalium* has demonstrated sexual transmission.[213] However, its pathogenicity has been a subject of debate. A recent meta-analysis showed *M. genitalium* was significantly associated with increased risk of clinical cervicitis and PID, and a trend towards risk of infertility.[214] A causal link between PID and *M. genitalium* is also supported by its isolation from endometrial biopsies in many cases of nongonococcal non-chlamydial PID.[215] *M. genitalium* is also consistently associated with nongonococcal urethritis among individuals with penises.[212,216] It has been shown to colonize the rectum but has not been linked to symptomatic proctitis.[217]

M. genitalium can be detected with NAAT, if regionally available. Current guidelines recommend testing only in the event of clinical cervicitis, recurrent urethritis, or PID.[218]

Of the empiric treatments for cervicitis or urethritis, a single dose of azithromycin 1 g by mouth is more effective at eradicating *M. genitalium* than doxycycline 100 mg twice a day for seven days.[219] However, this approach may select for macrolide resistance, and therefore the recommended treatment regimen for confirmed *M. genitalium* is azithromycin 500 mg orally on day one, followed by 250 mg orally on days two to five.[218] Azithromycin treatment failure may necessitate second-line treatment with moxifloxacin 400 mg daily for seven days.[218] There is insufficient evidence to justify routine contact tracing, but expert opinion supports treatment of current partners to prevent reinfection.[218]

Mycoplasma hominis is part of the vaginal microflora that is sometimes isolated in women with PID or bacterial vaginosis, but its significance is unclear.[220]

Ureaplasma spp. are ubiquitous bacteria that colonize 30 to 40 per cent of asymptomatic sexually active men. Despite conflicting data on association with urethritis, epidemiologic[221] and experimental[222,223] data suggest *U. urealyticum* is a cause of nongonococcal urethritis, while *U. parvum* is a commensal organism. There is inconsistent evidence for an association between *U. urealyticum* and symptomatic cervicitis, conflicting data on an association with preterm delivery, and no association with PID or infertility.[224]

HPV-Associated Disease

Over 40 strains of human papillomavirus (HPV) are known to infect the anogenital tract, oral cavity, and oropharynx, and are separate from strains linked to warts of the skin.[156] HPV strains are typically divided into low-risk strains (those associated with anogenital warts and low or no cancer risk) and high-risk or oncogenic strains (those associated with high-risk dysplasia, including high-grade squamous intraepithelial lesion [HSIL], and cancer).[156] HPV transmission occurs through penetrative sex (vaginal, anal and oral), and non-penetrative sex (digital-vaginal sex, sharing sex toys, and skin-to-skin contact).[156,225]

Infection with HPV is very common, with an estimated 70 per cent of Canadians acquiring at least one genital HPV infection over their lifetime.[226] Populations at highest risk for infection include adolescents and young sexually active adults, although prevalence in males is high at all ages.[156]

Prevention strategies have focused on encouraging the use of barrier methods during sex, which are largely but not completely protective,[162] and immunization efforts against various strains of HPV. See the section on prevention for more information. With the relatively recent implementation of national HPV vaccination programs – first in 2006 in many jurisdictions – HPV incidence is likely to decrease with increased uptake. However, vaccine introduction is still lacking in many countries, particularly those of lower income.[227]

Anogenital warts are caused in 90 per cent of cases by low-risk HPV types 6 and 11.[228] These are protected against by HPV4 and HPV9 vaccines.

While incidence of genital HPV infection and genital warts is similar in sexually active men regardless of the sex of their partners,[229,230] anal HPV infection is significantly more common in MSM.[231,232] Cases of internal genital warts among transfeminine individuals who have undergone vaginoplasty have been reported,[233,234] but there are no published reports of genital or urethral warts affecting transmasculine individuals who have undergone phalloplasty or metoidioplasty.

Anogenital warts typically appear as multiple, asymmetrical, polymorphic growths that are papular, leaf-like, or cauliflower-like. While usually asymptomatic, they can occasionally cause itching, local discharge, and bleeding. They are diagnosed by visual inspection; laboratory tests are generally unnecessary.[156] Warts of significant size should be analysed by pathology, as one study found that anal warts requiring surgical excision were positive for intraepithelial neoplasia or squamous cell carcinomas in 26 per cent of HIV-negative MSM and 47 per cent of HIV-positive MSM.[235]

Screening for internal genital warts in individuals with a cervix can be performed visually during routine Pap tests.[156] Recommendations regarding screening for anal warts in asymptomatic individuals are lacking. However, because external perianal warts are often accompanied by internal anal warts, especially in individuals with HIV,[156] these individuals could benefit from inspection of the anal canal through digital examination or anoscopy.[162]

Left untreated, most anogenital warts will spontaneously clear by six months.[156] External warts can be treated at home by the individual with imiquimod 3.75% or 5% cream, podophyllotoxin/podofilox 0.5% solution, or sinecatechins 10% ointment. External or internal warts can be treated by clinicians using cryotherapy, trichloroacetic acid (TCA) 50%–90% solution in 70% alcohol, or ablative or surgical treatments. Patients with intra-urethral warts should be referred to a urologist.[156] Neovulvar warts can safely and effectively be treated with imiquimod[236] or CO_2 laser.[237] Of note, treatment does not prevent transmission or recurrence, both of which are common.

HPV-related anogenital dysplasia and cancers are associated, in 64 to 87 per cent of cases, with high-risk HPV strains 16 and 18.[238] Because HPV can be transmitted by non-penetrative sexual contact, digital intercourse, and fomites, all sexually active individuals with a cervix are at risk for cervical cancer. High-risk HPV DNA[239] and cervical neoplasia[240,241] have been documented in cis women with no history of a partner with a penis. As such, screening recommendations are the same for all sexually active individuals with a cervix. A careful surgical history is important as a transmasculine individual may have a total hysterectomy (removal of uterus and cervix), subtotal hysterectomy (uterus removed but cervix left in place), with or without colpoclesis/vaginectomy (removal of vaginal mucosa). Although most vaginoplasty techniques do not involve creation of a cervix, transfeminine patients may nonetheless be susceptible to HPV-related cancers of the neovagina.[242] Several experts recommend annual visual inspection of the neovagina for hair growth, warts, and other lesions, which may also include a vaginal Pap smear to detect occult dysplastic changes. For more information on recognition of HPV-associated dysplasia and cancer, see chapter 4.

Molluscum

Molluscum contagiosum is a poxvirus that spreads by auto-inoculation and skin contact. It is estimated to affect 2 to 10 per cent of the population.[243,244] The most common routes of spread are physical contact and fomites;[245] it can also be associated with contact sports, tattoos,[246] electrolysis,[247] and school swimming pools.[248]

Molluscum presents as flesh-coloured, umbilicated papules, which occur in clusters. Typical distribution involves the face, trunk, groin, and inner thighs; larger and more profuse lesions occur in the context of immunosuppression. Diagnosis is usually clinical but can be confirmed by curettage and smearing or biopsy to reveal a characteristic histology.

Lesions appear after an incubation period of 14 days to 6 months.[249] If untreated, they can be present for years. It is critical to educate patients to avoid scratching, which can lead to reinfection and auto-inoculation. Treatment options include cryotherapy (blanching lesions every 10 to 14 days until resolved), vesicants (0.7 per cent cantharidin every 14 days until resolved), irritants (iodine applied by toothpick), or curettage (can cause scarring).[249]

HSV

Genital herpes is the predominant cause of genital ulcer disease in North America and worldwide.[156,162,250] While most cases are caused by HSV-2, the proportion of cases caused by HSV-1 is increasing, especially among young women and MSM.[162] Women are more affected than men.[156]

Most individuals with genital HSV are unaware that they are infected, and individuals may have long periods without symptoms, in which anogenital subclinical shedding occurs. Consequently, despite increased infectivity during symptomatic periods, most anogenital herpes infections are actually transmitted during asymptomatic periods.[251] Unlike other STIs, HSV-2 is often transmitted within long-term couples rather than high-risk core groups. Longitudinal studies of HSV-2-serodiscordant couples demonstrate annual seroconversion rates of 3 to 12 per cent among negative partners,[252–254] suggesting that prevention efforts (such as the use of barriers during intercourse) should target these couples. Transmission occurs through anogenital-anogenital contact and, to a lesser extent, oro-genital contact. While the risk of infection of neovaginal tissue is largely unknown, neolabial infection has been described.[255] HSV should be considered in any individual where suggestive symptoms develop.[167]

The presentation of HSV-1 and HSV-2 are similar. First episodes present with genital or perianal vesicles that typically ulcerate, though less commonly may lack lesions and manifest as genital pain or urethritis, cervicitis, proctitis, or aseptic meningitis.[156] First episodes are often accompanied by bilateral inguinal, with or without femoral, lymphadenopathy. Chronic infection then develops in many patients, with varying frequency of recurrent episodes. Overall, genital infections caused by HSV-2 compared to HSV-1 tend to have more frequent symptomatic recurrences[256-260] and higher rates of subclinical shedding.[259] In both cases, recurrence rates typically decrease over time, with a faster rate of decrease observed for HSV-1.[260]

HSV is not routinely tested for in asymptomatic individuals. When lesions are present, they should be unroofed and fluid should be swabbed and sent for HSV culture (the most common method of testing in Canadian laboratories) or HSV NAAT via PCR (more sensitive and specific, but less widely available).[156] Type-specific HSV IgG serology (for HSV-1 antibodies and HSV-2 antibodies) can be considered. However, because serology does not differentiate between acute and chronic infection, its main utility is in patients with (1) recurrent genital symptoms or atypical symptoms with negative HSV culture or PCR, (2) initial genital HSV identified during pregnancy, to determine whether the infection is new or recurrent (absence or presence of antibodies, respectively), or (3) no symptoms but whose partner has genital herpes, to counsel on the risk of transmission if HSV-serodiscordant.[156,162] While HSV-2 antibodies are relatively helpful, HSV-1 antibodies do not differentiate between orolabial infection and anogenital infection. Orolabial infection ("cold sores") is extremely common – even without symptoms – and often acquired in childhood. An additional shortcoming of this test is its relatively long window period; by 12 weeks after infection, it is estimated that greater than 70 per cent of individuals will be HSV-antibody positive.[156]

Treatment of HSV involves antivirals such as acyclovir, valacyclovir, famciclovir, or foscarnet. Dose and duration depend on the site of infection, HIV status, and number of episodes per year. See table 6.10 at the end of this section for information on the management of genital HSV among HIV-negative individuals; consult local guidelines for treatment of HIV-positive individuals or individuals seeking treatment for orolabial infection.

Prevention of HSV can involve condom use, which may reduce transmission by about 50 per cent,[253] and/or suppressive therapy with antiviral medication. A study in HIV-negative, heterosexual individuals demonstrated a 50 per cent reduction in HSV transmission to sexual partners when the person with HSV took daily suppressive valacyclovir 500 mg.[252] This should be routinely considered in individuals who have one or more HSV-negative partners. Unfortunately, studies have not found a reduction in either HSV transmission or HIV transmission when co-infected individuals were treated with acyclovir.[261,262]

Chancroid

Chancroid, which is caused by *Haemophilus ducreyi*, appears to have declined worldwide as a cause of genital ulcer disease, although infection might still occur in certain regions in Africa and the Caribbean.[162] Infections in Canada and the United States are very rare and usually tied to sporadic outbreaks.[156,162] Chancroid is transmitted via genital-genital sex *only* when ulcerations are present, the usual reservoir being vulnerable individuals (e.g., sex workers with limited access to care) with multiple sexual partners.[156]

The ulcer(s) associated with chancroid are typically painful, ragged, and dirty-based, with non-indurated borders. Unilateral lymphadenopathy may develop, suppurate, and spontaneously rupture.[156]

In Canada, the diagnosis of chancroid is made preferably by using material from the base of an ulcer or an aspirate of buboe(s) if present, which can be sent for culture for *H. ducreyi*.[263] Consult with your local laboratory for more information on the specialized culture or transport medium required. Other causes of genital ulcer disease – including syphilis and HSV – should be ruled out with appropriate testing. Patients in whom chancroid is suspected should have routine STI screening done concurrently, and HIV serology repeated in 1.5 to 3 months if initial serology is negative, as co-infection rates are high.[156,162,264] STI prevention strategies, including barrier methods, HIV PrEP, and vaccination, should be discussed as indicated.

Treatment of chancroid should be considered if the clinical suspicion is high, particularly if testing for syphilis and HSV is negative. In Canada and the United States, once dose of azithromycin 1 g orally has shown excellent cure rates with the advantage of single-dose therapy.[156,162] See local guidelines for treatment options and requirements regarding contact tracing and follow-up recommendations.

Hepatitis A

Hepatitis A (HAV) infection is caused by an RNA virus. Approximately half of reported cases in Canada are linked to travel.[265] It is generally transmitted via fecal-oral routes, such as through contaminated food or water, or through sexual activities such as anilingus (oro-anal contact), anal-finger contact, penile-anal contact, and indirectly if objects that have come into contact with an infected individual's anus then enter another person's mouth.[266] Transmission through infected blood has also been reported.[265] Populations at highest risk include MSM, people who inject drugs, and individuals with chronic liver disease; national immunization recommendations target these groups.[265,266] See the section on prevention for information on hepatitis A vaccination.

Infection with the hepatitis A virus is typically symptomatic, with an incubation period varying from 2 weeks to 1.5 months.[265,266] Prodromal symptoms, such as poor appetite, nausea, fatigue, and a low-grade fever, may occur. Jaundice is more common in adults than children.[265] Abdominal pain may also be a presenting feature, and light-coloured stool and dark urine are also very common signs.[266] Anti-HAV IgM can be ordered to assess for acute or recent HAV infection. By symptomatic presentation, approximately 90 per cent of infected individuals will have anti-HAV IgM antibodies; levels should be subsequently repeated if initially negative.[267] See table 6.11 for more information regarding management of hepatitis A.

Hepatitis B

Hepatitis B, considerably more infectious than HIV or HCV, is a DNA virus transmitted through exposure to an infected person's blood or body fluids. This includes breaks in mucosal surfaces during insertive/receptive penile, vaginal, oral, and anal intercourse.[268]

As with hepatitis A, hepatitis B transmission can be prevented through vaccination. Numerous countries have implemented universal immunization programs – see the section on prevention for more information. In HIV-infected individuals, anti–hepatitis B antibody titres should be ordered at the time of HIV diagnosis, as well as one to two months[162,269] or one to six months[270] after completion of the vaccine series, and can be considered periodically afterwards depending on level of immunocompromise and risk for hepatitis B infection.[162,268–270]

Infection with hepatitis B can be acute and self-limited or chronic (which occurs in 5 per cent of individuals infected in adulthood versus 90 per cent of infants infected at birth).[268] About half of hepatitis B infections are symptomatic, presenting similarly to acute hepatitis A infection but with a longer incubation period of about one to six months.[270] Those who go on to develop chronic infection are at risk for cirrhosis, end-stage liver disease, and/or hepatocellular carcinoma. See table 6.11 for more information regarding management of hepatitis B.

Hepatitis C

Hepatitis C (HCV) is an RNA virus typically transmitted through exposure to an infected individual's blood through breaks in the skin or in the lining of the nose and mouth.[271] Like the hepatitis B virus, it can survive outside of the body for days. Common means of transmission include shared needles, transfusion of contaminated blood products, and unsafe medical practices. Sexual transmission of hepatitis C is rare in the general population but has become increasingly recognized in certain groups of MSM,[272-275] including those co-infected with HIV and other STIs, those engaging in sexual behaviours that tend to induce mucosal trauma (e.g., receptive fisting and vigorous use of sex toys, group sex),[95,276] and those using drugs in relation to sex (e.g., methamphetamines, cocaine, gamma hydroxy butyrate [GHB]).[95,276-278] See the section "Screening" later in the chapter for more information.

Most individuals infected with HCV are asymptomatic. Acute symptoms, when present, resemble those of hepatitis A and hepatitis B infection, with a typical incubation period between two weeks and six months.[279] While some individuals spontaneously clear the virus, it progresses to chronic infection in most individuals. See table 6.11 for more information regarding management of chronic hepatitis C.

Trichomonas Vaginalis

Trichomoniasis – infection with the parasitic protozoan *Trichomonas vaginalis* – can be transmitted sexually and via fomite. Transmission between cis women and partners of any gender is well documented.[156,280,281] In patients with a penis, *T. vaginalis* has been occasionally reported among MSM in association with urethritis and proctitis in regions with high prevalence,[282] but it is rare among cis MSM in high-resource countries.[283,284] No neovaginal or neophallic trichomonas infections have been described in the literature. There are limited data on the prevalence and burden of extragenital *T. vaginalis*, and at this time rectal and oral testing for *T. vaginalis* are not recommended.[162]

Most infections with trichomonas are asymptomatic, especially in patients with a penis. If symptoms develop, they usually include yellow-green vaginal discharge, pruritus, and dysuria; or urethritis, epididymitis, and/or prostatitis.[156,162] Untreated asymptomatic vaginal/cervical infections might persist for months to years without symptoms,[285-288] while penile infections have high rates of spontaneous resolution and generally last less than 10 days.[289-291] Screening asymptomatic individuals is not routinely recommended, though it might be considered in individuals at high risk for infection (e.g., multiple sexual partners, illicit drug use, history of prior STI); data are lacking on whether this practice is beneficial.[162] In contrast, individuals who are immunocompromised or living with HIV and have a uterus should have routine screening because of increased risk of PID[162,269,292] and because treatment reduces vaginal HIV shedding.[293,294] See table 6.14 for more information regarding screening.

Trichomonas is treated either with a single dose of metronidazole 2 g orally, or a seven-day course of metronidazole 500 mg orally twice a day. The seven-day course has a higher cure rate for vaginal infection in HIV-positive[294] and HIV-negative[295,296] individuals, but the single dose may be preferred for convenience or unpredictable adherence.

See tables 6.14 and 6.15 later in the chapter for more information regarding testing for trichomonas, and see table 6.9 at the end of this section for more information regarding management of suspected or confirmed cases of trichomonas. Of note, sexual partners of individuals with trichomonas should be treated empirically; testing is not necessary in contacts.[156]

Shigella

Shigella is a genus of bacteria causing dysentery with fecal-oral transmission. It is a common cause of diarrhea in resource-limited settings through contaminated food or water but also occurs in outbreaks among MSM as a result of direct or indirect anal-oral contact.[297] After an incubation period of one to seven days, patients may present with fever, abdominal pain, mucoid or bloody diarrhea, and vomiting.[297] It is diagnosed by stool culture or molecular testing; culture would be preferred if resistance is regionally prevalent. The illness is generally self-limiting and resolves in an average seven days among immunocompetent hosts, with fecal shedding up to six weeks;[298] however, HIV-positive individuals are at increased risk of complications such as bacteremia.[299] Other rare complications include hemolytic-uremic syndrome and reactive arthritis. Antibiotics can be used to shorten duration of symptoms and shedding[300] or to prevent complications in immunocompromised states. Because of documented resistance to multiple antibiotic classes observed among MSM, treatment guided by culture may be warranted.[301–303]

Giardia

Giardia lamblia is a protozoan that can cause diarrheal illness. Parasitic cysts are shed in stool and can survive externally for prolonged periods; following ingestion, the trophozoite form is released in the small bowel. It is spread by the fecal-oral route and may come from contaminated food or water, or direct sexual contact.[304] Adult infection with giardia is mainly asymptomatic but may cause a spectrum of disease, from mild self-limiting symptoms to chronic malabsorptive illness. Symptoms include diarrhea, abdominal cramps, anorexia, flatulence, weight loss, fever, and urticaria,[305] and appear within 4 to 10 days.[306] In contrast to other gastrointestinal pathogens, HIV and immunosuppression do not cause more severe giardial illness.[304] Giardia infection is diagnosed by stool examination or molecular testing. Mild symptoms generally resolve spontaneously within 10 days or within 72 hours of antibiotics.[305] In asymptomatic or untreated individuals, cyst shedding can persist up to 14 months.[305,307] Giardia can be treated with metronidazole 500 mg orally twice a day for five to seven days;[308] other antimicrobials such as paromomycin and albendazole may also be used if available.[304] See table 6.9 for information on management of patients with giardia.

Entamoeba Histolytica

Entamoeba histolytica is an enteric pathogen that can cause intestinal and extraintestinal disease. Infectious cysts are spread by contaminated water/food or fecal-oral contact.[309] Cysts remain viable in the environment for weeks to months and ingestion of a single cyst can lead to infection. Cysts transform into active trophozoites in the small intestine, which either shed asymptomatically in stools or invade the colon lining to cause bloody diarrhea. Particularly virulent strains can cause extraintestinal disease such as liver abscess. Although invasive strains are rare, they have been observed to spread in MSM,[310] WSW,[311] and heterosexual networks,[312] as well as within households.[313] Rare cases of cutaneous amoebiasis, from insertive anal intercourse, have also been described.[314,315]

Its diagnosis is complicated by its microscopically identical appearance to *E. dispar*, a non-pathogenic organism. Therefore, initial diagnosis by stool ova + parasites (at least three samples from separate days are recommended to increase sensitivity)[316] would be confirmed with stool antigen testing, *E. histolytica* serology, or PCR.

While *E. dispar* infection does not warrant treatment, all confirmed *E. histolytica* infections should be treated, whether symptomatic or not, to minimize risk of invasion and spread.[317] Treatment consists of systemic therapy with oral metronidazole 750 mg orally three times a day for 7 to 10 days, followed by paromomycin 25 to 35 mg/kg/day divided three times a day for 7 days.[317]

Quick Reference: Management of Common STIs

Table 6.9. Management of Common Bacterial STIs in Canada
Refer to the sections "Screening" and "Undifferentiated Syndromes" for screening/testing indications for each STI.

STI	Treatment of Uncomplicated Infections (Recommended First-Line Regimens)[162,206,318]	Usual Time to Symptom Resolution after Treatment	Contact Trace-Back Period[162]	Minimum Time of Abstinence after Treatment*,[162]	Follow-Up after Treatment[162]
Chlamydia trachomatis	Azithromycin 1g PO x1 for most cases, Doxycycline 100 mg PO BID x1 week PO x1 week preferred for anorectal chlamydia	Improvement within days, complete resolution within 2–4 weeks[319]	60 days	1 week	Repeat screening (for new infection) after 3–6 months
LGV (C. trachomatis serovars L1, L2, L2b, and L3)	Doxycycline 100 mg PO BID x3 weeks	Not well documented in the literature; symptoms should improve with treatment, and patients should be followed to symptom resolution[156,162]	60 days	Abstinence until completion of treatment	TOC (e.g., NAAT > 3 weeks after treatment completion) Consider HCV testing if suspected to be acquired in Canada, as there is a high rate of LGV-HCV co-infection

(Continued)

Table 6.9. (Continued)

STI	Treatment of Uncomplicated Infections (Recommended First-Line Regimens)[162,206,318]	Usual Time to Symptom Resolution after Treatment	Contact Trace-Back Period[162]	Minimum Time of Abstinence after Treatment*,[162]	Follow-Up after Treatment[162]
Neisseria gonorrhea	Currently, Canadian guidelines recommend ceftriaxone 250 mg IM once + azithromycin 1 g PO once; consider instead ceftriaxone 500 mg IM once, or 1 g IM once if weight > 150 kg[192]	Resolution within 3–5 days[162]	60 days	1 week	TOC with culture 3–7 days or NAAT 2–3 weeks after treatment completion; repeat screening in 3–6 months
Syphilis	Early disease (primary, secondary, and latent up to 1 year of duration): Penicillin G 2.4 million units IM x1 Late latent syphilis (>1 year): Penicillin G 2.4 million units IM q1week x3 doses Neurosyphilis: Penicillin G 3–4 million units IV q4h x10–14 days	Primary syphilis: lesions begin to resolve within a few days[206] Less well defined in the literature for other stages.	Primary: 3 months Secondary: 6 months Early latent: 1 year Late latent: Variable	1 week	Early disease: 3, 6, 12 months after treatment[†] Late syphilis (except neurosyphilis): 12, 24 months after treatment[†] Neurosyphilis: 6, 12, and 24 months after treatment[†] If living with HIV (any stage): serology 3, 6, 9, 12, 24 months[†]

Organism	Treatment	Time to improvement	Partner/contact management	Time to follow-up	Follow-up recommendations
Mycoplasma genitalium	If not empirically treated with azithromycin‡: azithromycin 500 g PO on day 1, 250 mg PO on days 2–5. If azithromycin treatment failure: moxifloxacin 400 mg daily x7 days	Not well defined	Not routine; consider treating current partners	Not defined in guidelines	No follow-up necessary unless symptoms recur
Trichomonas vaginalis	Metronidazole 2 g PO in a single dose OR metronidazole 500 mg PO BID x1 week	Improvement usually noticed within 1 week of single dose treatment (in 92%)[320]	Treat current partners	1 week[321] vs symptom resolution[162,322]	Guideline recommendations vary: e.g., no follow-up necessary unless symptoms recur[156] vs in <3 months if initial infection is vaginal§,[162]
Shigella	Treat according to stool culture and sensitivity	Usually 48–72 h, may depend on antibiotic choice[300]	Recommend testing sexual and household contacts, no defined trace back period	1 week if treated; 4–6 weeks if untreated	Monitoring until symptom resolution

(Continued)

Table 6.9. (Continued)

STI	Treatment of Uncomplicated Infections (Recommended First-Line Regimens)[162,206,318]	Usual Time to Symptom Resolution after Treatment	Contact Trace-Back Period[162]	Minimum Time of Abstinence after Treatment*,[162]	Follow-Up after Treatment[162]
Giardia lamblia	Metronidazole 500 mg PO BID x5–7 days[308]	Within 72 h	Recommend testing sexual and household contacts, no defined trace back period	Up to 14 months if untreated	No follow-up necessary unless symptoms persist
Entamoeba histolytica	Metronidazole 750 mg PO TID x7–10 days, THEN paromomycin 25–35 mg/kg/day divided TID x7 days[317]	Not well defined	Recommend testing sexual and household contacts, no defined trace back period	Not well defined	Monitoring until complete symptom resolution

LGV = lymphogranuloma venereum; TOC = test of cure

* Patients should be informed to abstain until minimum time of abstinence listed and until symptom resolution.

† For early syphilis, expect a four-fold decline in RPR/VDRL titres by 12 months. [162,323] For late syphilis, expect a four-fold decline in RPR/VDRL by 2 years, regardless of HIV status. [162,323] For neurosyphilis, CSF parameters may normalize at different times, but an initial high CSF-VDRL titre should decline four-fold within a year. [156]

‡ PHAC guidelines recommend a five-day course of azithromycin as the first-line treatment for M. genitalium and moxifloxacin as second-line. However, symptomatic cases should have already received empiric urethritis treatment (azithromycin single dose or doxycycline) by the time M. genitalium is confirmed. Therefore, a five-day course of azithromycin would only be prescribed is if doxycycline were used empirically, or for partner treatment.

§ There is insufficient data to support retesting penile trichomonas infections. [162]

Table 6.10. Management of Common Viral STIs in Canada

Refer to sections "Screening" and "Undifferentiated Syndromes" for screening/testing indications for each STI.

STI	Treatment of Uncomplicated Infections (Recommended Regimens)[150,197]	Usual Time to Symptom Resolution after Treatment	Contact Trace-Back Period[156]	Minimum Time of Abstinence after Treatment*,[156]	Follow-Up after Treatment
Genital HSV[156]	First clinical episode (within 3 days of onset): valacyclovir 1 g PO BID x10 days, or acyclovir 200 mg PO five times daily x5–10 days Recurrent episodes (within 12 h of symptoms): valacyclovir 500 mg PO BID x3 days, or acyclovir 200 mg PO five times daily x5 days Suppression of frequent recurrences (≥6/year): valacyclovir 500–1000 mg PO daily, or acyclovir 400 mg PO BID Suppression to prevent transmission: valacyclovir 500 mg PO daily	Initial symptomatic episode: ~9 days with treatment[324] • Without treatment: ~2–3.5 weeks Recurrent episode: ~4–5 days[325-327] • Without treatment: ~6–10 days in most[325,326,328]	N/A, although patients are encouraged to inform current and future partners	From prodromal symptoms until complete healing of lesions (highest risk of transmission)	N/A

(Continued)

Table 6.10. (Continued)

STI	Treatment of Uncomplicated Infections (Recommended Regimens)[150,197]	Usual Time to Symptom Resolution after Treatment	Contact Trace-Back Period[156]	Minimum Time of Abstinence after Treatment*,[156]	Follow-Up after Treatment
HPV (warts)	Optimal treatment depends on lesion characteristics, e.g., external vs internal. See the HPV-Associated Disease section for more information.	Variable, depending on treatment	N/A	N/A; infectivity remains after treatment of lesions	If external perianal warts are present, follow-up with anoscopy after treatment is recommended because of high likelihood of internal anal warts

* Patients should be informed to abstain until minimum time of abstinence listed *and* until symptom resolution.

Table 6.11. Management of Viral Hepatitis in Canada
Refer to the section "Screening" for screening indications.

STI	Treatment of Uncomplicated Infections (Recommended Regimens)	Follow-Up after Treatment/ Immunization
Hepatitis A	Symptomatic treatment[266]	Acute infection: HAV IgM antibodies (may persist for 3–6 months)[265] Post-immunization: consider anti-HAV total or IgG 1–2 months after last dose for those with HIV[269]
Hepatitis B	Acute hepatitis B: no available treatment Chronic hepatitis B*: nucleos(t)ide analogues with a high barrier to resistance, such as tenofovir or entecavir, are preferred.[329,268] Post-exposure prophylaxis (if patient anti-HBs negative): HBIg and immunization with HB vaccine within 1 week of blood exposure, or within 2 weeks of sexual exposure[330]	Acute infection: HBsAg and anti-HBc IgM Chronic infection: HBsAg persistence for >6 months[268] Post-immunization: recommended anti-HBs in 1–2 months for certain high-risk groups (e.g., individuals living with HIV, IVDU)[162,268,269]
Hepatitis C	Treatment recommendations depend on HCV genotype, treatment history, presence or absence of cirrhosis, and other co-morbidities including HIV infection[331,332]	HCV RNA (as anti-HCV Ab remains detectable after clearance of the virus)

* HIV PrEP with tenofovir/emtricitabine simultaneously provides adequate treatment for chronic hepatitis B. Individuals on tenofovir/emtricitabine should not discontinue treatment without switching to another antiviral active against hepatitis B, or without close clinical follow-up, because of the risk of chronic hepatitis B flare.[333] Individuals co-infected with HIV must be treated with *two* drugs active against HBV, preferably with tenofovir and lamivudine or emtricitabine.[334]

Undifferentiated Syndromes

Urethritis

Urethritis, or inflammation of the urethra, is a common presentation that can occur in all individuals regardless of assigned sex at birth. Symptoms range from itching to dysuria and discharge, which may be mucoid, mucopurulent, or purulent. It is important to consider gonorrheal and chlamydial infections; other possible causes are bacterial (*Mycoplasma genitalium, Ureaplasma urealyticum*), viral (HSV), and parasitic (*Trichomonas vaginalis*, which is more common in individuals performing insertive vaginal sex). These infections are described elsewhere in this chapter. Less common considerations include adenovirus and *Candida albicans*. Despite exhaustive testing, a specific pathogen cannot be identified in 25 to 40 per cent of cases of urethritis.[335]

Differential diagnosis includes urinary tract infection (often manifesting as dysuria with frequency, urgency; hematuria; fever, chills) and prostatitis (which may also present with irritative and obstructive urinary tract symptoms, including nocturia, hesitancy, weak stream, and incomplete voiding).

On physical examination of individuals with a penis, spontaneous discharge may be present; if not, discharge may be expressed by having the patient or provider compress the urethra from the base of the penis to the glans penis. Examination of the testes and epididymis is important to distinguish a complicated infection, such as orchitis or epididymitis. Inguinal and/or femoral lymphadenopathy may also be present.

First-catch urine NAAT remains the most sensitive test for chlamydia and gonorrhea, although an additional endourethral swab (inserted two centimetres into the urethra and rotated) for gonorrhea culture is recommended for antimicrobial resistance testing. If available, a point-of-care Gram stain of discharge or endourethral specimen for polymorphonuclear leukocytes (PMNs; suggestive of urethritis) and Gram-negative diplococci (specific for gonorrhea) can be done. Testing for *Trichomonas vaginalis* could be considered in individuals performing insertive vaginal sex.

Individuals assigned female at birth should also be evaluated with a urinalysis and culture to rule out a urinary tract infection. Consider testing for syphilis, HIV, and hepatitis as part of a comprehensive STI screening as indicated.

Individuals suspected of having urethritis can be empirically treated if follow-up cannot be assured.[150] Unless a Gram stain is available at the point of care to rule out gonorrheal infection, therapy should cover both gonorrhea and chlamydia (e.g., azithromycin 1 g orally single dose, plus either ceftriaxone 250 mg IM single dose, per Canadian guidelines,[156] or ceftriaxone 500 mg IM single dose, per CDC 2021 guidelines[162]), regardless of the characteristics of the discharge. Abstinence is recommended for at least one week following initiation of treatment.

Symptom resolution may take up to seven days post-treatment completion.[156] Persistent symptoms and documented inflammation (e.g., PMNs on microscopy as described above), despite adequate treatment and after excluding reinfection, is concerning for persistent urethritis. The subsequent antimicrobial regimen should cover for resistant strains of *Mycoplasma genitalium* (e.g., moxifloxacin 400 mg orally daily for seven days), as well as for *T. vaginalis* for individuals engaging in insertive vaginal intercourse (e.g., metronidazole 2 g orally once).[162]

Alternative initial treatment regimens are discussed in their relevant sections, and contact tracing and other management recommendations are discussed for each organism elsewhere in this chapter.

Vaginal Discharge

In people assigned female at birth, the three most common causes of vaginal discharge are bacterial vaginosis, vaginal candidiasis, and trichomoniasis.[336] These are summarized in table 6.12. Other less common causes include normal physiologic variation, contact irritation, STI, or retained foreign body.

Clinical assessment of patients with vaginal discharge should include history, examination with visualization of the cervix, and assessment of discharge. Workup may include a saline wet mount, KOH preparation, litmus testing, Gram stain, molecular testing, and cultures (for trichomonas vaginalis and *Candida*).[336]

Bacterial vaginosis (BV) is a disruption of the normal vaginal microflora, in which lactobacilli fail to maintain an acidic pH, resulting in overgrowth of other commensal bacteria. This presents with vaginal discharge (classically grey and watery), vulvar pruritus or irritation, and vaginal odour (classically "fishy" smelling). BV may result from hormonal changes (such as menopause or testosterone therapy[337]), sexual transmission of anaerobic bacteria among WSW[338,339] and WSM,[340] and hygiene practices such as douching. Prevalence of BV is higher among WSW (45.2 per cent) than women with no history of cis female partners,[341] particularly with higher number of recent and lifetime female partners, and confirmed BV in one's partner.[342-344] However, no specific sexual practices among WSW have been found to be associated with BV.[343]

Treatment options include metronidazole (oral or intravaginal) and intravaginal clindamycin.[162] *Lactobacillus* probiotics are under investigation but at this time have not demonstrated efficacy.[345] Treatment of partners with penises has been shown not to improve outcomes;[346] there is no evidence on co-treatment of partners with vaginas or neovaginas, but it may be considered.[336]

Table 6.12. Common Causes of Vaginal Discharge

	Bacterial Vaginosis	Vulvovaginal Candidiasis	Trichomoniasis
Risk factors	Vaginal douching Sexual activity	Antibiotic use Immunocompromise Diabetes	Multiple sexual partners
Symptoms	Discharge, "fishy" odour	Discharge, pruritus	Discharge, pruritus
Signs	White or grey discharge	White clumpy discharge, vaginal erythema	"Frothy" discharge, "strawberry cervix"
Treatment	Metronidazole 500 mg PO BID x7 days, OR Metronidazole 0.75% 5 g PV qhs x10 days, OR Clindamycin 2% 5 g PV qhs x7 days	Clotrimazole 1% 5 g PV qhs x7–14 days, OR Fluconazole 150 mg PO x1, OR Miconazole 2% 5 g PV qhs x3 days	Metronidazole 2 g PO x1, OR Metronidazole 500 mg PO BID x7 days, AND Partner treatment

Source: Adapted from Canadian Guidelines on Sexually Transmitted Infections[156]

BV can recur within 12 months of successful treatment in approximately 58 per cent of cases.[342] In one study of BV treated with intravaginal metronidazole, BV persistence (defined by Gram stain) was not related to any specific sexual activity, including cis male or cis female partners, use of sex toys, use of condoms, receptive oral/anal sex, or genital-genital contact.[347] Use of gloves for digital-vaginal sex following treatment with intravaginal metronidazole did not decrease recurrence.[348]

Candida albicans exists as part of the normal flora of the skin and GI tract and can be isolated intermittently from the vaginal microbiome in 70 per cent of cis women followed for 12 months.[349] However, overgrowth and yeast germination results in vulvovaginal candidiasis. Symptoms include discharge (classically described as "cottage cheese–like"), acute pruritus, burning, ranging to edema, fissuring, and skin breakdown in severe cases. Although uncomplicated vulvovaginal candidiasis is estimated to affect 70–75 per cent of cis women in their lifetime, frequent or severe candidiasis have been associated with both host and behavioural practices. Antibiotics frequently trigger symptomatic vulvovaginal candidiasis among cis women who are already colonized. Both *Candida* colonization and symptomatic vulvovaginal candidiasis are more frequent among cis women with uncontrolled diabetes but not controlled diabetes.[350] Vulvovaginal candidiasis occurs more frequently among cis women with HIV, with the highest prevalence in those with lower CD4 counts.[351] Small and low-quality studies have also suggested association with oral and barrier contraceptives, but this has not been borne out in larger studies.[352] The possibility of sexual transmission has also been investigated. Oral and anal intercourse have been associated with incident *Candida* vulvovaginitis.[353] In one study where 13 pairs of cis WSW partners were both colonized with *Candida*, the strains were genetically different within each pair, suggesting a lack of transmission between partners with vaginas.[354]

Treatment of asymptomatic vaginal colonization is not recommended. For treatment of symptomatic vulvovaginal candidiasis, treatment options include a variety of intravaginal antifungal creams or suppositories for one to seven days, or a single dose of oral fluconazole 150 mg. For severe vulvovaginal candidiasis (skin breakdown, fissuring, edema), 7 to 10 days intravaginal azole or two doses of oral fluconazole may be prescribed.[336] In the event of recurrent vulvovaginal candidiasis (four or more episodes within one year), a longer initial azole antifungal course can be given orally (e.g., three doses fluconazole 200 mg orally, one every 72 hours) or topically (10 to 14 days), followed by a three- to six-month maintenance regimen of oral (e.g., fluconazole 200 mg orally every week for six months).[336] Vaginal culture and expert consultation may also be considered if there is concern about resistance. There is no benefit to treating asymptomatic partners with penises;[355,356] treatment of asymptomatic partners with vaginas has not been studied.

Trichomonas vaginalis is discussed separately above.

Neovaginal Discharge

The qualities and microflora of a neovagina differ from the vagina of a cis female, so an assessment of neovaginal discharge requires special consideration. A penile inversion neovagina typically has a pH of 5.0 to 7.0[357] and has a microflora similar to skin flora, with lactobacilli present 75 per cent of the time.[358] In contrast, the pH of a sigmoid neovagina is 7 to 9, with a microflora of predominantly facultative anaerobes (at lower counts than in the rectum).[359]

The differential diagnosis for neovaginal discharge following penile inversion includes microflora overgrowth, accumulation of sebum or dead skin cells, STIs, candidiasis, and hypergranulation tissue.[337,360] In this context, malodorous discharge does not correlate with vaginal pH or with leukocytes on Gram stain.[357] Evaluation should include examination for granulation tissue and swabs for *Candida*. Conservative treatment with increased douching frequency or douching with vinegar solution or povidone iodine may resolve bacterial overgrowth; otherwise, a five-day course of vaginal metronidazole can be trialled.[337]

In addition to the above, neovaginas of sigmoid origin may develop diversion neovaginitis, an inflammatory syndrome of pain and malodorous discharge, which can present years after colovaginoplasty. After confirmation by inspection and biopsy, initial treatment is topical 5-ASA derivatives or short-chain fatty acids, with reanastomosis in severe cases.[361] For an individual with sigmoid vaginoplasty, inflammatory bowel disease should also be considered: Crohn's disease[362] or ulcerative colitis[363] can flare with sigmoid neovaginal involvement years after surgery. However, observations of neovaginal sparing during ulcerative colitis flares may suggest it is less susceptible to flares than other colonic tissue.[364]

Cervicitis

Cervicitis refers broadly to inflammation of the cervix. While it is most commonly caused by *C. trachomatis* or *N. gonorrhea*;[365] it has also been associated with *T. vaginalis*,[366] *M. genitalium*,[211] HSV,[367] and BV.[368] Uncommonly, cervicitis can be attributed to *M. tuberculosis*[369] or cytomegalovirus (CMV) in immunocompetent individuals.[367,370]

Cervicitis is often asymptomatic but can cause symptoms of mucopurulent vaginal discharge, intermenstrual or postcoital bleeding, dyspareunia, and dysuria.[365] Pelvic examination shows pathognomonic purulent discharge from the cervical os and cervical erythema; *T. vaginalis* is also associated with cervical petechiae ("strawberry cervix"), while there may be vesicular or ulcerative lesions with HSV. Features of cervical motion tenderness, uterine tenderness, or adnexal tenderness suggest an alternative diagnosis of PID. Cervicitis workup includes testing for GC/CT, BV, TV, and possibly *M. genitalium* if NAAT is available. Non-infectious differential diagnosis includes cervico-vaginal dermatoses and contact dermatitis.

Uncomplicated cervicitis can be treated presumptively if there is high suspicion of bacterial STI (age under 25, new sexual partner, multiple sexual partners) with azithromycin 1 g single dose or doxycycline 100 mg twice a day for seven days.[268] If there is low suspicion of sexually transmitted infection, it is also appropriate to wait until diagnostic tests are reported.[371] The goals of treatment are to relieve symptoms, prevent progression to PID, and halt transmission to partners. Because cervicitis increases HIV viral shedding by HIV-positive cis women,[372] treatment may also reduce HIV transmission.

Pelvic Inflammatory Disease

The endocervical canal forms a barrier between the vaginal flora and the aseptic upper genital tract. PID results when cervicitis compromises this barrier function and allows ascending infection. As a result, PID is considered a polymicrobial infection. PID causes a wide range of clinical presentations, from asymptomatic upper genital tract inflammation (detected later as tubal scarring during a fertility workup) to subtle acute lower abdominal/pelvic pain to tubo-ovarian abscess or sepsis.[373]

The approach to treatment for WSW and transmasculine people does not differ from non-2SLGBTQ patients: empiric antibiotic treatment with polymicrobial coverage (outpatient or inpatient depending on severity) and workup to exclude other possible diagnoses. For transmasculine individuals on testosterone therapy, atrophic changes reduce but do not eliminate susceptibility to PID,[374] as in postmenopausal cisgender women.[375]

Proctitis

Proctitis describes inflammation of the rectal mucosa, and the term proctocolitis is used when the sigmoid colon is also involved. Proctitis presents with anorectal pain, bleeding, purulent discharge, and tenesmus; diarrhea, abdominal pain, and bloating may also be present in the case of proctocolitis. Common causes of proctitis to evaluate for include gonorrhea, chlamydia (especially LGV serotypes), and HSV;[162] uncommon causes include CMV, and syphilis.[376,377] Although proctitis associated with HSV-1, HSV-2, and CMV can affect immunocompetent individuals, they are more prevalent in MSM with HIV.[378-380] HIV also increases the risk of proctitis from group A *Streptococcus*;[381] CD4-dependent opportunistic infections such as microsporidium, cryptosporidium, and Mycobacterium avium complex (MAC); as well as proctitis where no pathogen is identified.[377,378] The non-infectious differential for proctitis includes inflammatory bowel disease,[382] anal cancer, radiation changes, and chronic rectal ischemia.[383] Acute anal pain without bleeding or discharge should raise suspicion of anal gland abscesses, malignancy, thrombosed hemorrhoid, anal fissures, and proctalgia fugax.

Examination includes assessment for perianal ulceration, inguinal lymphadenopathy, and anoscopy. Investigations may include anal swabs (GC, CT, HSV), serology for syphilis and HIV, or CD4 count if known or suspected HIV.

Empiric therapy is indicated for MSM with clinical proctitis. This involves coverage for gonorrhea and chlamydia using ceftriaxone IM as a single dose and doxycycline 100 mg twice a day for seven days.[162] If ulcers or bleeding are present, or if LGV is confirmed by testing, then doxycycline should be extended to 100 mg twice a day for 21 days, although there is some evidence that a 7- to 14-day course of doxycycline may be effective for cure.[384] If ulcers are observed on examination, presumptive treatment should cover HSV, such as acyclovir 400 mg three times a day for 7 to 10 days or valacyclovir 1 g twice a day for 7 to 10 days.[162] CMV proctitis may be self-limiting,[378] but treatment with IV ganciclovir and monitoring for peritoneal signs are indicated with immunosuppression or severe symptoms.[377]

Balanitis

Balanitis refers to inflammation of the glans penis; the term *balanoposthitis* can be used to describe inflammation of the glans and foreskin. The lifetime prevalence is 3 to 11 per cent of individuals with a penis. Balanitis and balanoposthitis present with pruritus, pain, erythema, edema, and discharge from under the foreskin.[385]

Balanitis has a broad differential diagnosis, which includes incomplete personal hygiene, infectious causes, chemical irritants, trauma, dermatologic conditions, and neoplastic conditions. The most common cause is incomplete hygiene and accumulation of smegma in uncircumcised individuals.[385,386] Infectious etiologies include *Candida*, HSV,[387] low-risk and high-risk HPV subtypes,[388] primary syphilis,[389,390] *E. histolytica*,[391] *T. vaginalis*,[392] anaerobic bacteria,[393] and group A *Streptococcus pyogenes*.[394-396] See table 6.13 for a summary of causes of balanitis.

The normal penile microflora includes *Candida* in 16 per cent of individuals; higher rates of colonization are observed in uncircumcised individuals and those with diabetes.[397,398] However, colonization can progress to candidal balanitis in conditions which promote yeast growth, such as insufficient hygiene, diabetes mellitus, and phimosis.[385,397] Diagnosis can be confirmed with *Candida* culture, and other investigations should include screening for diabetes and HIV.[386] Candidal balanitis is treated with one to three weeks of topical antifungals, and testing and treatment of partners with a vagina if applicable. If untreated, chronic or recurrent balanitis in diabetes can result in fibrosis of the foreskin and acquired phimosis.[398]

Table 6.13. Common Causes and Characteristics of Balanitis

	Candida	HSV	T. vaginalis	Anaerobes	S. pyogenes
Symptoms	Pain, discharge, pruritus	Pain, ulcers	Pruritus, discharge	Pain, discharge	Pain, discharge
Signs	White sub-preputial discharge, erythema, erosions	Vesicles, ulcers, erosions	Urethral discharge	Foul-smelling sub-preputial discharge, inguinal lymphadenopathy	Purulent discharge, inflammation
Diagnosis	Culture	Viral culture	Gram stain, NAAT	Gram stain, culture	Gram stain, culture
Treatment	Clotrimazole 1% BID x1–3 weeks[385]	See table 6.10 for treatment options	Metronidazole 2 g PO x1[156]	Metronidazole 200–400 mg PO TID-QID x5 days[393]	Cephalexin 500 mg PO QID x7 days

Balanitis resulting from aerobic skin flora, such as virulent strains of *S. pyogenes* and *S. aureus*, has been shown to be transmitted by oral intercourse.[396]

Circinate balanitis, a phenomenon associated with reactive arthritis, causes shallow ulcers to the glans penis. It is often painless, and resolves spontaneously, but may be treated with topical glucocorticoids if symptomatic.[399]

Balanitis xerotica obliterans is the term used when the penis is affected by lichen sclerosus, a progressive inflammatory dermatosis. It presents with white or purple plaques and induration involving the foreskin, frenulum, or urethral meatus. In chronic cases, it can progress to phimosis, pain with erections, urethral stenosis, or atrophy of the glans.[400] Mild disease may respond to high-potency topical steroids, but surgeries such as circumcision or urethroplasty are indicated for more advanced disease.[401] Patients with balanitis xerotica obliterans should be monitored for development of squamous cell carcinoma.[400] Other rare dermatoses of the glans penis include Zoon balanitis, penile lichen planus, and psoriasis.[402]

Investigations, based on history, can include STI screening and swabs for fungal and bacterial cultures, with or without Gram stain microscopy. Empiric therapy with topical antifungals is indicated for most patients, along with conservative measures such as education on cleaning, saline baths, and talcum powders to reduce moisture. If cellulitis is present, a first-generation cephalosporin may be added.[385] If there is no response, clinicians should consider anaerobic infection, dermatologic pathology, or malignancy. If phimosis is present, this can be managed with stretching exercises with or without mid-potency steroids[403] or consideration of elective circumcision (emergent circumcision if paraphimosis occurs).

Epididymitis

Epididymitis refers to inflammation of the epididymis; progression to involve the testes would be considered epididymo-orchitis. In both syndromes, the differential diagnosis includes infectious, inflammatory, and traumatic causes, with infectious causes typically presenting acutely.[162] Common mechanisms of infection are ascent of organisms causing urethritis (*C. trachomatis, N. gonorrhea, M. genitalium, Ureaplasma spp.*); descent of organisms causing cystitis, particularly in the context of benign prostatic hyperplasia, prostate biopsy, or urinary tract instrumentation (*E. coli*, other enteric microbes, *Pseudomonas spp.*); and coliforms transferred via insertive anal intercourse.[156,394] In the context of immunosuppression, rarer pathogens should be considered such as CMV, salmonella, toxoplasmosis, *Corynebacterium* species, and *Mima polymorpha*.[156] Non-infectious causes of epididymitis to consider include reflux of sterile urine into the epididymis secondary to urinary retention, and adverse reactions to medications such as amiodarone.[404] The history, physical exam, and investigations should also exclude other causes of acute scrotal pain, including testicular torsion, Fournier's gangrene, trauma, and inguinal hernia,[405,406] whereas chronic scrotal pain suggests traumatic, neoplastic, autoimmune, granulomatous, and idiopathic causes.[162]

Investigations for acute epididymitis include urethral Gram stain, urinalysis, first-void urine NAAT for GC and CT, and mid-stream urine culture, as well as scrotal ultrasound. Doppler ultrasound and C-reactive protein can also be used to exclude testicular torsion.[404]

Empiric therapy when infectious epididymitis is suspected is indicated to prevent infertility and chronic scrotal pain. In cases where there is high suspicion of chlamydia or gonorrhea, treatment involves ceftriaxone 250 mg IM single dose with doxycycline 100 mg twice a day for 10 days. In individuals who practise insertive anal sex, the preferred empiric regimen is ceftriaxone 250 mg IM single dose and levofloxacin 500 mg daily for 10 days. Finally, if suspicion is limited to enteric organisms, empiric treatment is levofloxacin 500 mg daily for 10 days. Providers should be vigilant for rarer causes if symptoms do not resolve within 72 hours.[162]

Screening

Who Should Be Screened?[156,162]

Clinicians should not provide STI testing only to those who request it but should also offer screening opportunistically to patients presenting for other concerns or periodic health reviews. This recommendation is of particular importance for those with risk factors for STIs, such as the following:

- Demographic-related risks/considerations
  - sexually active <25 years of age
  - men who have sex with men (MSM) and transfeminine individuals who have sex with men
  - street-involved or homeless individuals
  - pregnant individuals (at least at the first prenatal visit, more frequently as indicated)
- Activity-related risks
  - known contact with any STI
  - new or multiple sexual partner(s)
  - sex without use of barrier methods – oral, anal, or vaginal
  - shared sex toys
  - substance use, particularly if associated with sexual activity
  - sex workers, their clients, and those engaging in survival sex (exchanging sex for money, drugs, shelter, or food)
- Victims of sexual assault/abuse
- People with previous STIs

Which STIs?

Patients should be told what they are being tested for and informed that we do not and cannot routinely test for all STIs – for instance, HPV and HSV infections.[156] Patients should be educated about their risks of acquiring these STIs, even when they and their partners test negative on routine screening. They should be encouraged to obtain testing and treatment if and when suggestive symptoms arise.

Routine STI screening *commonly* includes:

- chlamydia (CT) – consider urine and swabs as appropriate
- gonorrhea (*Neisseria gonorrhoeae*, NG) – consider urine and swabs as appropriate
- HIV (see chapter 7 for more information on HIV testing)
- syphilis

Consider the following, based on risk factors:

- HPV-related dysplasia (e.g., cervical cancer screening, anal cancer screening), particularly for those with HIV
- hepatitis B (if unvaccinated and at risk); also consider periodic anti-HBs testing of at-risk individuals in certain groups, such as those with HIV or other immunocompromised patients, even when previously immunized[270]
- hepatitis C in certain high-risk groups, such as IV drug users,[407] and MSM with risk factors such as HIV,[408,409] use of HIV PrEP,[333] high-risk behaviours such as receptive fisting and group sex,[95,276] substance use during sex,[95,111,276,278] and hepatitis C contacts. It can also be considered for individuals born between 1945 and 1975.[331,410]

How and When?[156]

Asymptomatic screening should be recommended every three months to one year in most sexually active individuals, depending on sexual activities (see table 6.14).

If a physical examination is required for someone with a neovagina, an anoscope may be more ergonomic than a speculum since the neovagina lacks fornices and may have reduced elasticity (depending on tissue origin).[337]

Diagnostic Testing

In addition to the screening tests described in table 6.14, symptomatic individuals should be offered testing based on clinical presentation and organisms of concern (see table 6.15).

Prevention

Advice on STI risk reduction should be tailored to the patient's values and practices. This may include behavioural strategies, physical barriers, vaccination, and chemoprophylaxis.

Table 6.14. STI Testing Recommendations for Asymptomatic Individuals

STI	Site of Screening	Specimen Type	Lab Testing (Preferred)[156,162]	Window for Testing after Exposure
Chlamydia, gonorrhea	Genital (urethra, vagina, cervix)	Urine* OR Vaginal swab† OR Cervical swab	NAAT NAAT‡	NAAT, culture: Inadequately studied; proposed to be 1 day (24 hours) for gonorrhea and 2–7 days for chlamydia[411]
	Pharynx§	Swab	NAAT	
	Rectum‖	Swab	NAAT	
Trichomonas (only screen certain populations)	Vagina#	Swab	NAAT	Inadequately reported in the literature
Syphilis	All sites	Blood	Syphilis serology	>3–6 weeks**
HIV	Blood borne	Blood	HIV serology	1.5 months (4th generation test) to 3 months[264]
Hepatitis A (if unvaccinated)	Screening asymptomatic individuals not typically advised			
Hepatitis B (if unvaccinated and at risk)	Blood borne	Blood	Anti-HBs (immunity) HBsAg, anti-HBc (current/prior infection)[412]	HBsAg detected by 9 weeks; resolves by 15 weeks after symptom onset if no chronic infection[412]
Hepatitis C (for high-risk groups)	Blood borne	Blood	Anti-HCV (HCV RNA if anti-HCV+)	Anti-HCV detected in >97% after 6 months[413]

Note: These investigations should be considered in addition to those outlined in table 6.15 when evaluating symptomatic individuals, as guidelines recommend routine screening in patients presenting with symptoms of a specific STI.

(Continued)

Table 6.14. (Continued)

*10–20 mL, preferably >2 hours since last void.

† Vaginal swab for NAAT is the preferred method for detection of gonorrhea/chlamydia in asymptomatic individuals with a vagina because of NAAT's excellent sensitivity.[163]

‡ Chlamydia and gonorrhea cultures are required for sexual assault cases.

§ For all individuals performing oral sex (per Canadian guidelines).[156]

‖ For receptive anal sex, irrespective of condom use (per Canadian guidelines).[156] Swab can be collected through an anoscope or blindly, and either by the provider or by the patient. The use of an anoscope, which minimizes fecal contamination, is preferred for symptomatic individuals. Blind swabs should be inserted 2–3 cm into the rectal canal, with lateral pressure to avoid fecal contamination.

Trichomonas screening is recommended in asymptomatic individuals living with HIV who have a uterus because of their increased risk of pelvic inflammatory disease[162,269,292] and because treatment reduces vaginal HIV shedding.[293,294]

** Treponemal IgM (which can be detected using CMIA) can usually be detected by 3–6 weeks after exposure. Note that a minority of patients will not have detectable IgM antibodies in the early infection.[414] Tests such as CMIA also pick up IgG antibodies later in infection, so repeat serology is warranted with high clinical suspicion.

Table 6.15. Additional STI Testing Recommended for Symptomatic Patients[156]
Consider empiric treatment if high clinical suspicion of sexually transmitted infection and/or concerns regarding a patient's ability to follow up.

Presentation	Common STIs of Concern	Typical Incubation Period before Symptoms[156,415,416]	Specimen Type and Lab Testing
Urethritis, cervicitis:§ penile/vaginal discharge +/– dysuria +/– vaginal bleeding after sex	Gonorrhea	<1 week*	*In addition* to NAAT, consider urethral/cervical swab for NG *culture* to determine antimicrobial sensitivity†
	Chlamydia	2–3 weeks	CT NAAT is sufficient for diagnosis; if LGV suspected, order LGV testing on NAAT
	Trichomonas vaginalis	Within 4 weeks[417]	If persistent AND initial tests are negative for GC/CT, consider vaginal/cervical/urethral swab, OR urine, for *T. vaginalis* NAAT‡
	Mycoplasma genitalum	Unknown, likely >2–8 weeks[418]	If persistent AND initial tests are negative for GC/CT, consider vaginal/cervical/urethral swab, OR urine,[218] for *M. genitalum* NAAT
Epididymitis (scrotal/testicular swelling, pain, and tenderness)	Gonorrhea, chlamydia, enteric pathogens	Not well documented in the literature	Additional testing depends on other symptoms. Consider a mid-stream urine if enteric pathogens are suspected (e.g., individuals performing insertive anal sex, older non-sexually active individuals)

(Continued)

Table 6.15. (Continued)

Presentation	Common STIs of Concern	Typical Incubation Period before Symptoms[156,415,416]	Specimen Type and Lab Testing
Proctitis[||] (e.g., rectal pain, discharge, bleeding)	Chlamydia esp LGV	LGV: 3–30 days	Rectal swab for chlamydia and LGV testing[||,#] (NAAT)[156]
	Gonorrhea	<1 week*	*In addition* to NAAT, consider *adding* rectal swab for GC *culture*[†]
	HSV	1 week	Swab (unroof vesicles if present for fluid collection), for HSV NAAT (if available) or culture
Vesicles	HSV		
Ulcer(s):Painful erosions	HSV		
Painless single ulcer (sometimes multiple) with a clean base	Primary Syphilis (see section on *Syphilis*)	Primary: 3 weeks (3 days to 3 months)	Dark-field microscopy, direct fluorescence antibody test, or NAAT. Contact your local laboratory for availability of syphilis tests and collection instructions
One or multiple painful ulcer(s) with dirty base(s)	Chancroid (*H. ducreyi*)	5–14 days	Chancroid (*H. ducreyi*) culture (requires specialized culture or transport media, with variable regional availability)
Small painless papule or ulcer	LGV	3–30 days	Swab for LGV NAAT or culture
Buboes		Within 6 weeks of initial lesion (see above)	Aspirate for LGV NAAT or culture
Anogenital warts	HPV	3 weeks to 8 months	N/A – diagnosed by visual inspection

* Better characterized for urethral and cervical infections.

[†] Cultures and sensitivities allow for monitoring local antimicrobial susceptibility trends. As with NAAT testing, urethral cultures for chlamydia and gonorrhea are more sensitive >2 hours since last void.

[‡] NAAT testing for *T. vaginalis* in men is becoming increasingly available in Canada. Check with your local laboratory for more information about testing requirements.

§ Also consider other causes of vaginal discharge (see "Vaginal Discharge" section). Consider acute PID if abnormal vaginal discharge is accompanied by lower abdominal pain, intermenstrual bleeding, and/or dyspareunia. Chronic PID may or may not present with cervicitis. Pelvic examination may demonstrate cervical motion, uterine, and/or adnexal tenderness.

|| Proctitis: provider-collected rectal swab via anoscopy is preferred for symptomatic individuals over blind swab. Assess for rectal erythema, purulent discharge, erosions, or ulcers.

Some local laboratories automatically arrange for LGV testing on rectal specimens positive for chlamydia. Otherwise, LGV testing should specifically be requested in those cases where clinical suspicion is high.

Table 6.16. Hepatitis A, B, and C: Typical Incubation Periods. See sections on Hepatitis A, B, and C for more information.

	Incubation Period
Hepatitis A[265,266]	2 weeks to 1.5 months
Hepatitis B* (acute)[270]	~1–6 months
Hepatitis C* (asymptomatic in most patients)[279,415,416]	2 weeks to 6 months

* Symptomatic patients who initially tested seronegative should be retested in three months.

Behavioural Approaches

Behavioural approaches include reducing the number of sexual partners, avoiding substance use around intercourse, or participating in sexual activities that carry a lower risk of infections. These can include manual genital stimulation, frottage ("body grinding"), intercrural sex (thrusting the penis between the partner's thighs), and not sharing sex toys. An increased frequency of testing may also reduce STI risk since having an asymptomatic STI increases susceptibility to other STIs.

Barrier Methods

Barrier methods reduce the risk of many STIs by preventing the exchange of body fluids. External condoms (also referred to as "male condoms") are used to cover a penis or sex toy during oral or insertive intercourse. Individuals should be counselled on proper application to prevent breakage or exposure to pre-ejaculate. Internal condoms (also referred to as *female condoms*) are designed to remain in the vagina, but can be used for receptive anal intercourse if the inner ring is removed. Dental dams can be used for cunnilingus or anilingus. Gloves can be used for digital or manual penetration, to protect against vaginal or rectal mucus, to protect small cuts on the hands, and to cover fingernails. A glove can also be cut into an impromptu dental dam, or into a condom for a post-metoidioplasty neophallus. Patients should be advised that barrier methods are less effective at preventing STIs that rely on skin-skin contact, such as parasites, HPV, or HSV,[419,420] than they are at preventing bacterial STIs[421] or HIV.[422] Barriers are commonly made of latex, polyurethane, polyisoprene, or nitrile. Latex and polyisoprene are weakened by oil-based lubricants;[423] polyurethane can endure oil-based lubricants but is more prone to breakage and slippage than latex.[424] Animal membrane condoms are intended for contraception, but are not recommended for STI prevention because of porosity.[423]

Vaccination

Various immunizations reduce the transmission of STIs. Vaccines for HPV, hepatitis A, and hepatitis B are currently available.

HUMAN PAPILLOMAVIRUS VACCINATION
There are currently three vaccines available to prevent HPV infection, with coverage of different HPV strains. HPV2 protects against high-risk strains HPV 16 and 18; HPV4 covers HPV 6, 11, 16, and 18; and HPV9 covers HPV 6, 11, 16, 18, 31, 33, 45, 52, and 58.

HPV 6 and 11 account for 90 per cent of genital warts.[228] Most HPV-related cancers are associated with HPV 16 and 18, which is included in all current HPV vaccinations; further protection is added with HPV9. Most cases of cervical, vaginal, and anal cancer are related to HPV, and a significant proportion of vulvar, penile, and oropharyngeal cancers are also related to HPV infection.

Currently, individuals assigned female at birth may receive any of the above vaccines, while only HPV4 or HPV9 are indicated for individuals assigned male at birth. Using the same vaccine for the entire series is preferred but not mandatory.[425]

Routine HPV vaccination should be initiated at 11 to 12 years of age. Catch-up immunization up to age 26 is recommended for cis females, MSM, transgender people, and individuals with immunocompromising conditions including HIV.[162,426] HPV4 and HPV9 may be offered over age 26, although potential benefit may be reduced.[426]

Hepatitis A Vaccination

Populations at highest risk of acquiring hepatitis A include travellers to HAV-endemic countries (including many parts of Asia, Africa, and

Latin America), MSM (via oral-anal contact), and people who inject drugs.[265] Those at risk for severe infection with hepatitis A include individuals with pre-existing chronic liver disease, including hepatitis B and C. National immunization recommendations target these groups.[265,266] Primary immunization typically involves two doses of monovalent hepatitis A vaccine (6–36 months apart) or three doses of combined hepatitis A and hepatitis B vaccines.

Nearly 100 per cent of hepatitis A vaccine recipients develop seroprotective concentrations of antibody after receiving two doses of vaccine.[265] Protective anti-HAV antibody generally persists for over 20 years. Furthermore, demonstrated immune memory (the anamnestic response) likely indicates protection even without detectable antibody levels.[265] Canadian guidelines therefore recommend *against* routine serologic testing post–hepatitis A vaccination.[265]

Individuals living with HIV, however, should have anti-HAV IgG or total serology done at the time of HIV diagnosis, regardless of immunization history.[269,334] Guidelines differ on whether to routinely check serologic response in HIV-positive individuals one to two months after hepatitis A vaccination;[265,269,334] therefore, clinical judgment should guide this decision.

Hepatitis B Vaccination

Numerous countries have implemented universal two-dose or three-dose hepatitis B immunization programs, including the United States in 1991 and Canada in the mid-1990s. Groups at elevated risk of infection, to whom hepatitis B immunization should routinely be offered *if not already received*, include persons with multiple sexual partners, MSM, and injection drug users.[270] If unsure about vaccination history, anti-HBs antibody titres and HBsAg can be ordered to assess for immunity and rule out asymptomatic chronic infection in these and other high-risk groups.

Vaccination with a higher than standard dose (40 μg) of HBV vaccine is recommended by some guidelines for individuals with conditions such as HIV or chronic renal disease.[269,270]

Seroprotective levels for anti–hepatitis B (>10 mIU/mL) typically develop in greater than 95 per cent of individuals following a three-dose vaccine series,[427,428] though a recent review of studies looking at a combined hepatitis A and B vaccine found the seroprotection rate for anti–hepatitis B ranged from 82 per cent to 100 per cent of individuals one month after vaccine series completion.[429] Risk factors for poor response to vaccination include HIV or other immunosuppressive conditions/medications, chronic renal disease, and diabetes mellitus.[427-429]

Antibody levels may decline over time, as evidenced by studies in which seroprotective anti–hepatitis B levels were found in approximately 60 to 85 per cent of individuals at 10 years and 30 to 40 per cent of individuals at 15 years after primary immunization in infancy.[318] However, this does *not* account for the presence of T- and B-cell memory. Studies on the anamnestic response estimate that protection against HB infection is actually likely 95 to 100 per cent at 10 years and 85 to 100 per cent at 15 years after HB immunization in infancy.

As a result of the above data, Canadian guidelines do *not* recommend routine serologic testing or booster doses of hepatitis B vaccine for most healthy individuals (including certain high-risk groups such as MSM) who have completed a recommended hepatitis B immunization schedule.[270,330] Post-immunization anti–hepatitis B titres (one to six months after completion of the series) are recommended only in certain circumstances, such as immunocompromise (HIV, solid organ transplant recipients), potential percutaneous or mucosal exposure (sexual or household contacts of confirmed acute cases of chronic carriers of hepatitis B), and health care workers.[270] Similarly, annual anti–hepatitis B monitoring is only indicated with immunocompromise and dialysis.[270,430–432]

Circumcision

Circumcision has been shown to reduce heterosexual transmission of HIV in endemic countries, and is recommended as a prevention strategy in these areas.[433] However, a meta-analysis found circumcision did *not* reduce odds of acquiring HIV for MSM in high-income countries,[434] so it is not recommended for HIV prevention in these areas. Circumcision may reduce odds of HSV, HPV, and trichomonas,[435–438] but does not alter risk of chlamydia, gonorrhea, non-specific urethritis, or syphilis.[434,439,440]

Microbicides

Microbicides are an area of active research for STI prevention, including HIV PrEP,[441] but none are commercially available at the time of this publication.

Chemoprophylaxis (PrEP and PEP, Antivirals)

HIV pre-exposure prophylaxis (PrEP) and post-exposure prophylaxis (PEP) are evidence-based interventions to reduce the spread of HIV. The impact of PrEP on rates of other STIs remains unclear, with mixed findings around the impact of risk compensation,[442,443] and regular screening for high-risk groups. See chapter 7 for more details on HIV PrEP and PEP.

As discussed in the HSV section above, individuals with HSV who are in long-term sexual relationships with HSV-negative individuals may reduce transmission risk by taking suppressive antiviral medications. Risk of HSV transmission is reduced by approximately 50 per cent through the use of suppressive therapy with antiviral medication.[250] Unfortunately, the same results have not been replicated in studies of HIV-positive individuals with HSV.

Box 6.3. The COVID-19 Pandemic and 2SLGBTQ Sexual Health

- The SARS-CoV2 pandemic reshaped many dimensions of people's lives, including their sexual lives. With recommendations around physical distancing, many MSM reduced their number of sexual partners,[448-453] stopped taking PrEP,[452,454-456] and shifted to monogamy.[457] For some individuals, these changes were associated with reduced quality of their sex life,[450,458] while some couples experienced greater relationship satisfaction.[12] This population-level shift in behaviour, as well as public health's necessary focus on preventing COVID-19, led to a drastic reduction in testing for HIV and other STIs.[456,460,461] A subset of MSM did not reduce their sexual activity.[448,462,463] In some settings, this correlated with lower income,[448] lower level of education,[448,462] drug and alcohol use,[448,462,464-466] and high impact on daily life from sheltering in place.[463,467,469] Many reported a sense of shame or guilt for not adhering to physical distancing recommendations.[463,468] Some centres observed an increase in presentations for HIV PEP[469] and sexually transmitted infections,[470,471] suggesting an increase in sexual risk-taking among a subset of the population. This macro-level behavioural heterogeneity provides a window into the complex dynamics and risk factors for individual sexual decision making during experiences of uncertainty, unpredictability, and isolation.

- The pandemic necessitated precautions to reduce exposure of health care workers and accordingly saw an uptake of self-testing for HIV (approved in Canada in November 2020),[472] pharyngeal and rectal swabs for chlamydia and gonorrhea (approved but not in widespread use),[473,474] and virtual care.[460] These innovations have the potential mitigate geographic barriers to testing and care beyond the pandemic.

There have also been small studies on the efficacy of PrEP and PEP for bacterial STIs. These generally use doxycycline, which is indicated in STI treatment, acne treatment, and malaria prophylaxis. Randomized trials have investigated doxycycline among high-risk MSM as PEP, as well as PrEP. PEP reduced new diagnoses of chlamydia and syphilis but not gonorrhea,[444] while PrEP reduced overall STI incidence.[445] However, national guidelines in the United Kingdom[446] have recommended against these approaches to prevent antibiotic resistance among chlamydia[447] and other community acquired pathogens.

References

1. World Health Organization. Defining sexual health [Internet]. Geneva: WHO; 2006 [cited 2019 May 24]. Available from: https://www.who.int /reproductivehealth/publications/sexual_health/defining_sexual _health.pdf.
2. Centers for Disease Control and Prevention. A guide to taking a sexual history [Internet]. Atlanta (GA): US Department of Health and Human Services; 2011 [cited 2019 May 20]. Available from: https://www.cdc.gov /std/treatment/sexualhistory.pdf.
3. Tello M. Trauma informed care: what it is, and why it's important. 2018 Oct 16 [cited 2019 Jun 12]. In Harvard Health Blog [Internet]. Cambridge (MA): The President and Fellows of Harvard College. Available from: https://www.health.harvard.edu/blog/trauma-informed-care-what -it-is-and-why-its-important-2018101613562.
4. Centers for Disease Control and Prevention. Taking a sexual history from transgender people [Internet]. Atlanta (GA): US Department of Health and Human Services; 2017 [cited 2019 May 20]. Available from: https:// www.cdc.gov/actagainstaids/campaigns/transforminghealth /healthcareproviders/sexual-history.html.
5. Deutsch, MB [Internet]. San Francisco: University of California San Francisco Medical Centre; 2016 [cited 2019 Jun 18]. Guidelines for the primary and gender-affirming care of transgender and gender nonbinary people. Available from: http://transhealth.ucsf.edu/protocols.
6. Workowski KA, Bolan GA; Centers for Disease Control and Prevention. Sexually transmitted diseases treatment guidelines, 2015. MMWR Recomm Rep. 2015 Jun;64 RR-03:1–137.
7. Hegazi A, Lee MJ, Whittaker W, Green S, Simms R, Cutts R, et al. Chemsex and the city: sexualised substance use in gay, bisexual and other men who have sex with men attending sexual health clinics. Int J STD AIDS. 2017;28(4):362–6. doi:10.1177/0956462416651229.
8. Brotto LA, Yule M. Asexuality: sexual orientation, paraphilia, sexual dysfunction, or none of the above? Arch Sex Behav. 2017;46:619–27. doi:10.1007/s10508-016-0802-7.

9. Scherrer KS. Coming to an asexual identity: negotiating identity, negotiating desire. Sexualities. 2008;11(5):621–41. doi:10.1177/1363460708094269.
10. Brotto LA, Knudson G, Inskip J, Rhodes K, Erskine Y. Asexuality: a mixed-methods approach. Arch Sex Behav. 2010;39(3):599–618. doi:10.1007/s10508-008-9434-x.
11. Prause N, Graham CA. Asexuality: classification and characterization. Arch Sex Behav. 2007;36(3):341–56. doi:10.1007/s10508-006-9142-3.
12. Van Houdenhove E, Gijs L, T'Sjoen G, Enzlin P. Asexuality: a multidimensional approach. J Sex Res. 2015;52(6):669–78. doi:10.1080/0022 4499.2014.898015.
13. Jones C, Hayter M, Jomeen J. Understanding asexual identity as a means to facilitate culturally competent care: a systematic literature review. J Clin Nurs. 2017;26:3811–31. doi:10.1111/jocn.13862.
14. Wierckx K, Elaut E, Van Hoorde B, Heylens G, De Cuypere G, Monstrey S, et al. Sexual desire in trans persons: associations with sex reassignment treatment. J Sex Med. 2014;11:107–18. doi:10.1111/jsm.12365.
15. George R, Stokes MA. Sexual orientation in autism spectrum disorder. Autism Res. 2018;11(1):133–41. doi:10.1002/aur.1892.
16. Strang JF, Janssen A, Tishelman A, Leibowitz SF, Kenworthy L, McGuire JK, et al. Revisiting the link: evidence of the rates of autism in studies of gender diverse individuals. J Am Acad Child Adolesc Psychiatry. 2018;57(11):885–7.
17. Jannini EA, McCabe MP, Salonia A, Montorsi F, Sachs BD. Organic vs. psychogenic? The Manichean diagnosis in sexual medicine. J Sex Med. 2010;7:1726–33. doi:10.1111/j.1743-6109.2010.01824.x.
18. Erol B, Tefekli A, Ozbey I, Salman F, Dincag N, Kadioglu A, et al. Sexual dysfunction in type II diabetic females: a comparative study. J Sex Marital Ther. 2002;28(2 Suppl 1):55–62. doi:10.1080/00926230252851195.
19. Bellastella G, Maiorino MI, Olita L, Della Volpe E, Giugliano D, Esposito K. Premature ejaculation is associated glycemic control in type 1 diabetes. J Sex Med. 2015;12:93–9.10.1111/jsm.12755.
20. Carani C, Isidori AM, Granata A, Carosa E, Maggi M, Lenzi A, et al. Multicenter study on the prevalence of sexual symptoms in male hypo- and hyperthyroid patients. J Clin Endocrinol Metab. 2005;90:6472–9. doi:10.1210/jc.2005-1135.
21. Gabrielson AT, Sartor RA, Hellstrom WJ. The impact of thyroid disease on sexual dysfunction in men and women. Sex Med Rev. 2019;7:57–70. doi:10.1016/j.sxmr.2018.05.002.
22. Cihan A, Demir O, Demir T, Aslan G, Comlekci A, Esen A. The relationship between premature ejaculation and hyperthyroidism. J Urol. 2009;181:1273–80. doi:10.1016/j.juro.2008.10.150.

23. Boozalis A, Tutlam NT, Chrisman Robbins C, Peipert JF. Sexual desire and hormonal contraception. Obstet Gynecol. 2016;127(3):563–72. doi:10.1097/AOG.0000000000001286.
24. Montejo AL, Montejo L, Navarro-Cremades F. Sexual side effects of antidepressant and antipsychotic drugs. Curr Opin Psychiatry. 2015;28:418–23. doi:10.1097/YCO.0000000000000198.
25. Latif RA, Muhamad R, Ann AY, Sidi H, Nik Jaafar NR, Midin M, et al. Duration of hypertension and antihypertensive agents in correlation with the phases of female sexual response cycle. Compr Psychiatry. 2014 Jan;55 Suppl 1:S7–12. doi:10.1016/j.comppsych.2012.10.008.
26. Al Khaja KAJ, Sequeira RP, Alkhaja AK, Damanhori AHH. Antihypertensive drugs and male sexual dysfunction: a review of adult hypertension guideline recommendations. J Cardiovasc Pharmacol Ther. 206;21(3):233–44. doi:10.1177/1074248415598321.
27. Rees PM, Fowler CJ, Maas CP. Sexual function in men and women with neurological disorders. Lancet. 2007;369:512–25. doi:10.1016/S0140-6736(07)60238-4.
28. van Thiel DH, Gavaler JS, Eagon PK, Chiao YB, Cobb CF, Lester R. Alcohol and sexual function. Pharmacol Bioch Behav. 1980;13 Suppl 1:125–9. doi:10.1016/s0091-3057(80)80020-7.
29. Gudin JA, Laitman A, Nalamachu S. Opioid related endocrinopathy. Pain Med. 2015;16:S9–15.
30. Muneer A, Kalsi J, Nazareth I, Arya M. Erectile dysfunction. BMJ. 2014;348:g129. doi:10.1136/bmj.g129.
31. Araujo AB, Hall SA, Ganz P, Chiu GR, Rosen RC, Kupelian V, et al. Does erectile dysfunction contribute to cardiovascular disease risk prediction beyond the Framingham risk score? J Am Coll Cardiol. 2010;55(4):350–6. doi:10.1016/j.jacc.2009.08.058.
32. Vlachopoulos CV, Terentes-Printzios DG, Ioakeimidis NK, Aznaouridis KA, Stefanadis CI. Prediction of cardiovascular events and all-cause mortality with erectile dysfunction: a systematic review and meta-analysis of cohort studies. Circ Cardiovasc Qual Outcomes. 2013;6(1):99–109. doi:10.1161/CIRCOUTCOMES.112.966903.
33. Raheem OA, Su JJ, Wilson JR, Hsieh TC. The association of erectile dysfunction and cardiovascular disease: a systematic critical review. Am J Men's Health. 2017;11(3):522–63. doi:10.1177/1557988316630305.
34. Yafi FA, Jenkins L, Albersen M, Corona G, Isidori AM, Goldfarb S, et al. Erectile dysfunction. Nat Rev Dis Primers. 2016;2:16003. doi:10.1038/nrdp.2016.3.
35. Shindel AW, Rowen TS, Lin TC, Li CS, Robertson PA, Breyer BN. An internet survey of demographic and health factors associated with risk of sexual dysfunction in women who have sex with women. J Sex Med. 2012;9(5):1261–71. doi:10.1111/j.1743-6109.2012.02659.x.

36. Flynn KE, Lin L, Weinfurt KP. Sexual function and satisfaction among heterosexual and sexual minority US adults: a cross-sectional survey. PLoS One. 2017;12(4):e1074981. doi:10.1371/journal.pone.0174981.

37. Vansintejan J, Vandevoorde J, Devroey D. The Gay Men Sex Studies: erectile dysfunction among Belgian gay men. Int J Gen Med. 2013;6:527–34. doi:10.2147/IJGM.S45783.

38. Li DH, Remble TA, Macapagal K, Mustanski B. Stigma on the streets, dissatisfaction in the sheets: Is minority stress associated with decreased sexual functioning among young men who have sex with men? J Sex Med. 2019;16(2):267–77. doi:10.1016/j.jsxm.2018.12.010.

39. Levitan J, Quinn-Nilas C, Milhausen R, Breuer R. The relationship between body image and sexual functioning among gay and bisexual men. J Homosex. 2019;66(13):1856–81. doi:10.1080/00918369.2018.1519301.

40. Cove J, Petrak J. Factors associated with sexual problems in HIV-positive gay men. Int J STD AIDS. 2004;15:732–6.

41. Adam BD, Husbands W, Murray J, Maxwell J. AIDS optimism, condom fatigue, or self-esteem? Explaining unsafe sex among gay and bisexual men. J Sex Res. 2005;42(3):238–48. doi:10.1080/00224490509552278.

42. Elaut E, De Cuypere G, De Sutter P, Gijs L, Van Trotsenburg M, Heylens G, et al. Hypoactive sexual desire in transsexual women: prevalence and association with testosterone levels. Eur J Endocrinol. 2008;158:393–9. doi:10.1530/EJE-07-0511.

43. Bettocchi C, Palumbo F, Cormio L, Ditonno P, Battaglia M, Selvaggi FP. The effects of androgen depletion on human erectile function: a prospective study in male-to-female transsexuals. Int J Impot Res. 2004;16:544–6. doi:10.1038/sj.ijir.3901216.

44. Holmberg M, Arver S, Dhejne C. Supporting sexuality and improving sexual function in transgender persons. Nat Rev Urol. 2019;16:121–39. doi:10.1038/s41585-018-0108-8.

45. Cohanzad S. Extensive metoidioplasty as a technique capable of creating a compatible analogue to a natural penis in female transsexuals. Aesthetic Plast Surg. 2016;40:130–8. doi:10.1007/s00266-015-0607-4.

46. Vukadinovic V, Stojanovic B, Majstorovic M, Milosevic A. The role of clitoral anatomy in female to male sex reassignment surgery. ScientificWorldJournal. 2014;2014:437378. doi:10.1155/2014/437378.

47. De Cuypere G, T'Sjoen G, Beerten R, Selvaggi G, De Sutter P, Hoebeke P, et al. Sexual and physical health after sex reassignment surgery. Arch Sex Behav. 2005;34(6):679–90. doi:10.1007/s10508-005-7926-5.

48. Wierckx K, Van Caenegem E, Elaut E, Dedecker D, Van de Peer F, Toye K, et al. Quality of life and sexual health after sex

reassignment surgery in transsexual men. J Sex Med. 2011;8:3379–88. doi:10.1111/j.1743-6109.2011.02348.x.

49. Glina S, Sharlip ID, Hellstrom WJ. Modifying risk factors to prevent and treat erectile dysfunction. J Sex Med. 2013;10:115–19. doi:10.1111/j.1743-6109.2012.02816.x.

50. Rew KT, Heidelbaugh JJ. Erectile dysfunction. Am Fam Physician. 2016;94(10):820–7.

51. McCabe MP, Price E, Piterman L, Lording D. Evaluation of an internet-based psychological intervention for the treatment of erectile dysfunction. Int J Impot Res. 2008;20:324–30. doi:10.1038/ijir.2008.3.

52. Melnik T, Soares BG, Nasselo AG. Psychosocial interventions for erectile dysfunction. Cochrane Database Syst Rev. 2007 Jul;3(3):CD004825. doi:10.1002/14651858.CD004825.pub2.

53. Henderson AW, Lehavot K, Simoni JM. Ecological models of sexual satisfaction among lesbian/bisexual and heterosexual women. Arch Sex Behav. 2009;38(1):50–65. doi:10.1007/s10508-008-9384-3.

54. Shindel AW, Rowen TS, Lin TC, Li CS, Robertson PA, Breyer BN. An Internet survey of demographic and health factors associated with risk of sexual dysfunction in women who have sex with women. J Sex Med. 2012;9(5):1261–71. doi:10.1111/j.1743-6109.2012.02659.x.

55. Peplau LA, Frederick DA, Yee C, Maisel N, Lever J, Ghavami N. Body image satisfaction in heterosexual, gay, and lesbian adults. Arch Sex Behav. 2009;38:713–25. doi:10.1007/s10508-008-9378-1.

56. Montgomery MC, Ellison J, Chan PA, Harrison L, van den Berg JJ. Sexual satisfaction with daily oral HIV pre-exposure prophylaxis (PrEP) among gay and bisexual men at two urban PrEP clinics in the United States: an observational study. Sex Health. 2021;18(4):319–26. doi:10.1071/SH20207.

57. Kim D, Pang MG. The effect of male circumcision on sexuality. BJU Int. 2007;99:619–22.

58. Kigozi G, Watya S, Polis CB, Buwembo D, Kiggundu V, Wawer MJ, Serwadda D, Nalugoda F, Kiwanuka N, Bacon MC, Ssempijja V, Makumbi F, Gray RH. The effect of male circumcision on sexual satisfaction and function, results from a randomized trial of male circumcision for human immunodeficiency virus prevention, Rakai, Uganda. BJU Int. 2008 Jan;101(1):65–70.

59. Senel FM, Demirelli M, Misirlioglu F, Sezgin T. Adult male circumcision performed with plastic clamp technique in Turkey: results and long-term effects on sexual function. Urol J. 2012;9(4):700–5.

60. Bossio JA, Pukall CF. Attitude toward one's circumcision status is more important than actual circumcision status for men's body image and sexual functioning. Arch Sex Behav. 2018;47:771–81. doi:10.1007/s10508-017-1064-8.

61. Giorgetti R, Tagliabracci A, Schifano F, Zaami S, Marinelli E, Busardò FP. When "chems" meet sex: a rising phenomenon called "chemsex." Curr Neuropharmacol. 2017;15:762–70. doi:10.2174/1570159X15666161117151148.

62. Frankis J, Clutterbuck D. What does the latest research evidence mean for practitioners who work with gay and bisexual men engaging in chemsex? Sex Transm Infect. 2017;93(3):153–4. doi:10.1136/sextrans-2016-052695.

63. Al-Lawati A, Murch N. Acquired methemoglobinemia. Sultan Qaboos Univ Med J. 2012;12(2):237–41.

64. Bradberry SA, Whittington RM, Parry DA, Vale JA. Fatal methemoglobinaemia due to inhalation of isobutyl nitrite. J Toxicol Clin Toxicol. 1994;32(2):179–84. doi:10.3109/15563659409000448.

65. Latini A, Lora V, Zaccarelli M, Cristaudo A, Cota C. Unusual presentation of poppers dermatitis. JAMA Dermatol. 2017;153(2):233–4. doi:10.1001/jamadermatol.2016.4262.

66. Schauber J, Herzinger T. 'Poppers' dermatitis. Clin Experimental Dermatol. 2012;37:587–8.

67. Van Bol LB, Kurt RA, Keane PA, Pal B, Sivaprasad S. Clinical phenotypes of poppers maculopathy and their links to visual and anatomic recovery. Ophthalmology. 2017;124(9):1425–7.

68. Zamora JH. Viagra a killer when combined with "poppers." San Francisco Star [Internet]. 1998 July 28 [cited 2019 May 20]. Available from: https://www.sfgate.com/news/article/Viagra-a-killer-when-combined-with-poppers-3077700.php.

69. Pfizer Canada Inc. Viagra: consumer information [monograph on the Internet]. Kirkland, QC: Pfizer Inc; 2018 Sept 18 [cited 2019 May 20]. Available from: https://www.pfizer.ca/pi/en/Viagra.pdf.

70. Kloer C, Parker A, Blasdel G, Kaplan S, Zhao L, Bluebond-Langner R. Sexual health after vaginoplasty: a systematic review. Andrology. 2021 Apr 21. doi:10.1111/andr.13022. Epub ahead of print.

71. Dunford C, Bell K, Rashid T. Genital reconstructive surgery in male to female transgender patients: A systematic review of primary surgical techniques, complication profiles, and functional outcomes from 1950 to present day. Eur Urol Focus. 2021;7(2):464–71. doi:10.1016/j.euf.2020.01.004.

72. Hess J, Rossi Neto R, Panic L, Rübben H, Senf W. Satisfaction with male-to-female gender reassignment surgery. Dtsch Arztebl Int. 2014;111(47):795–801. doi:10.3238/arztebl.2014.0795.

73. Lawrence AA. Patient-reported complications and functional outcomes of male-to-female sex reassignment surgery. Arch Sex Behav. 2006;35:717–27. doi:10.1007/s10508-006-9104-9.

74. Weyers S, Elaut E, De Sutter P, Gerris J, T'Sjoen G, Heylens G, et al. Long-term assessment of the physical, mental, and sexual health among transsexual women. J Sex Med. 2009;6:752–60. doi:10.1111/j.1743-6109.2008.01082.x.

75. Imbimbo C, Verze P, Palmieri A, Longo N, Fusco F, Arcaniolo D, et al. A report from a single institute's 14-year experience in treatment of male-to-female transsexuals. J Sex Med. 2009;6:2736–45. doi:10.1111/j.1743-6109.2009.01379.x.

76. Georgas K, Belgrano V, Andreasson M, Elander A, Selvaggi G. Bowel vaginoplasty: a systematic review. J Plast Surg Hand Surg. 2018;52(5):265–73. doi:10.1080/2000656X.2018.1482220.

77. Manrique OJ, Sabbagh MD, Ciudad P, Martinez-Jorge J, Kiranantawat K, Sitpahul N, et al. Gender-confirmation surgery using the pedicle transverse colon flap for vaginal reconstruction: a clinical outcome and sexual function evaluation study. Plast Reconstr Surg. 2018;141(3):767–71. doi:10.1097/PRS.0000000000004122.

78. Weigert R, Frison E, Sessiecq Q, Al Mutairi K, Casoli V. Patient satisfaction with breasts and psychosocial, sexual, and physical well-being after breast augmentation in male-to-female transsexuals. Plast Reconstr Surg. 2013;132:1421–9. doi:10.1097/01.prs.0000434415.70711.49.

79. Manieri C, Castellano E, Crespi C, Di Bisceglie C, Dell'Aquila C, Gualerzi A, Molo M. Medical treatment of subjects with gender identity disorder: the experience in an Italian public health center. Int J Transgenderism. 2014;15(2):53–65.

80. Elaut E, De Cuypere G, De Sutter P, Gijs L, Van Trotsenburg M, Heylens G, et al. Hypoactive sexual desire in transsexual women: prevalence and association with testosterone levels. Eur J Endocrinol. 2008;158:393–9. doi:10.1530/EJE-07-0511.

81. Scheim AI, Bauer GR. Sexual inactivity among transfeminine persons: A Canadian respondent-driven sampling survey. J Sex Res. 2019:56(2):264–71. doi:10.1080/00224499.2017.1399334.

82. Agarwal CA, Scheefer MF, Wright LN, Walzer NK, Rivera A. Quality of life improvement after chest wall masculinization in female-to-male transgender patients: A prospective study using the BREAST-Q and Body Uneasiness Test. J Plast Reconstr Aesthet Surg. 2018;71:651–7. doi:10.1016/j.bjps.2018.01.003.

83. Costantino A, Cerpolini S, Alvisi S, Morselli PG, Venturoli S, Meriggiola MC. A prospective study on sexual function and mood in female-to-male transsexuals during testosterone administration and after sex reassignment surgery. J Sex Marital Ther. 2013;39:321–25. doi:10.1080/0092 623X.2012.736920.

84. Thorp S. [Internet]. Washington (DC): American Medical Students Association; April 2010 [cited 2019 Mar 16]. Beyond whips & chains: what medical students need to know about BDSM. Available from: https://www.amsa.org/members/career/scholars-programs/sexual-health -leadership-course/projects/more-sexual-health-topics/.

85. Connolly PH. Psychological functioning of bondage/domination/sado-masochism (BDSM) practitioners. J Psychol Human Sex. 2006;18(1): 79–120. doi:10.1300/J056v18n01_05.

86. Chandra A, Martinez GM, Mosher WD, Abma JC, Jones J. Fertility, family planning, and reproductive health of U.S. women: data from the 2002 National Survey of Family Growth. National Center for Health Statistics. Vital Health Stat 23(25). 2005.

87. Cottrell BH. An updated review of evidence to discourage douching. MCN Am J Matern Child Nurs. 2010;35(2):102–7. doi:10.1097/NMC.0b013e3181cae9da.

88. Beigi RH, Wiesenfeld HC, Hillier SL, Straw T, Krohn MA. Factors associated with absence of H_2O_2-producing Lactobacillus among women with bacterial vaginosis. J Infect Dis. 2005;191:924–9.

89. Martino JL, Vermund SH. Vaginal douching: evidence for risks or benefits to women's health. Epidemiol Rev. 2002;24(2):109–24.

90. McClelland RS, Lavreys L, Hassan WM, Mandaliya K, Ndinya-Achola JO, Baeten JM. Vaginal washing and increased risk of HIV-1 acquisition among African women: a 10-year prospective study. AIDS. 2006;20:269–73.

91. GrS Montreal. Information and postoperative care: vaginoplasty [Internet]. Montreal: GrS Montreal; 2017 March [cited 2019 May 20]. Available from: https://www.grsmontreal.com/DATA/TEXTEDOC/8X11WEB-Vaginoplastie-2013-ASC---En-V55.pdf.

92. Gatti C, Del Rossi C, Lombardi L, Caravaggi F, Casolari E, Casadio G. Sexuality and psychosocial functioning in young women after colovaginoplasty. J Urol. 2010 Oct;184(4 Suppl):1799–803. doi:10.1016/j.juro.2010.03.078.

93. Macdonald N, Sullivan AK, French P, White JA, Dean G, Smith A, et al. Risk factors for rectal lymphogranuloma venereum in gay men: results of a multicentre case-control study in the UK. Sex Transm Infect. 2014;90:262–8. doi:10.1136/sextrans-2013-051404.

94. de Vries HJ, van der Bij AK, Fennema JS, Smit C, de Wolf F, Prins M, et al. Lymphogranuloma venereum proctitis in men who have sex with men is associated with anal enema use and high-risk behavior. Sex Transm Dis. 2008;35(2):203–8.

95. Ndimbie OK, Kingsley LA, Nedjar S, Rinaldo CR. Hepatitis C virus infection in a male homosexual cohort: risk factor analysis. Genitourin Med. 1996;72:213–16.

96. Moss AR, Osmond D, Bacchetti P, Chermann JC, Barre-Sinoussi F, Carlson J. Risk factors for AIDS and HIV seropositivity in homosexual men. Am J Epidemiol. 1987;125(6):1035–47.

97. Schreeder MT, Thompson SE, Hadler SC, Berquist KR, Zaidi A, Maynard JE, et al. Hepatitis B in homosexual men: prevalence of infection and factors related to transmission. J Infect Dis. 1982;14(1):7–15.

98. Li P, Fan S, Yuan T, Ouyang L, Gong H, Ding Y, et al. Rectal douching and anal human papillomavirus among young men who have sex with men in China. Sex Transm Dis. 2021;48(8):550–6. doi:10.1097/OLQ.0000000000001392.

99. Schilder AJ, Druyts EF, Orchard TR, Gilbert M, Kwag M, Chan K, et al. Pre-coital douching (PD), sexuality and the association with risk among men who have sex with men (MSM) in Vancouver: preliminary data from the ManCount Survey. Paper presented at: 18th Annual Canadian Conference on HIV/AIDS Research; 2009 Apr 24; Vancouver, BC, Canada.

100. Reeders D, Li P, Yuan T, Feng A, Zhao H, Zou H. Much a-douche about nothing? Rectal douching, HIV, and sexually transmitted infection risks among men who have sex with men. Sex Transm Dis. 2020;47(10):663–4. doi:10.1097/OLQ.0000000000001224.

101. Hassan A, Blumenthal JS, Dube MP, Ellorin E, Corado K, Moore DJ, et al. Effect of rectal douching/enema on rectal gonorrhoea and chlamydia among a cohort of men who have sex with men on HIV pre-exposure prophylaxis. Sex Transm Infect. 2018;94:508–14. doi:10.1136/sextrans-2017–053484.

102. Achterbergh R, van der Helm JJ, van den Boom W, Heijman T, Stolte IG, van Rooijen MS, et al. Is rectal douching and sharing douching equipment associated with anorectal chlamydia and gonorrhoea? A cross-sectional study among men who have sex with men. Sex Transm Infect. 2017 Sep;93(6):431–7. doi:10.1136/sextrans-2016-052777.

103. Schmelzer M, Schiller LR, Meyer R, Rugari SM, Case P. Safety and effectiveness of large-volume enema solutions. Appl Nurs Res. 2004;17(4):265–74. doi:10.1016/j.apnr.2004.09.010.

104. Chertow GM, Brady HR. Hyponatraemia from tap-water enema. Lancet. 1994;344:748.

105. Jalanka J, Salonen A, Salojärvi J, Ritari J, Immonen O, Marciani L, et al. Effects of bowel cleansing on the intestinal microbiota. Gut. 2015 Oct;64(10):1562–8. doi:10.1136/gutjnl-2014-307240.

106. Drago L, Toscano M, De Grandi R, Casini V, Pace F. Persisting changes of intestinal microbiota after bowel lavage and colonoscopy. Eur J Gastroenterol Hepatol. 2016;28(5):532–7. doi:10.1097/MEG.0000000000000581.

107. Crouch PC [Internet]. San Francisco: San Francisco AIDS Foundation; 2017 Mar 29 [cited 2019 May 20]. Anal douching safety tips. Available from: https://www.sfaf.org/collections/beta/anal-douching-safety-tips/.

108. Makadon HJ, Mayer, KH, Potter J, Goldhammer H. The Fenway guide to lesbian, gay, bisexual, and transgender health. 1st ed. Philadelphia: American College of Physicians; 2008.

109. Singh D, Marrazzo JM. Sexually transmitted infections and associated conditions among women who have sex with women. Open Infect Dis J. 2009;3:128–34.

110. Apers L, Vanden Berghe W, De Wit S, Kabeya K, Callens S, Buyze J, et al. Risk factors for HCV acquisition among HIV-positive MSM in Belgium. J Acquir Immune Defic Syndr. 2015 Apr;68(5):585–93.

111. Urbanus AT, van de Laar TJ, Stolte IG, Schinkel J, Heijman T, Coutinho RA, et al. Hepatitis C virus infections among HIV-infected men who have sex with men: an expanding epidemic. AIDS. 2009;23:F1–7. doi:10.1097/QAD.0b013e32832e5631.

112. Rice CE, Maierhofer C, Fields KS, Ervin M, Lanza ST, Turner AN. Beyond anal sex: sexual practices in men who have sex with men and associations with HIV and other sexually transmitted infections. J Sex Med. 2016;13(3):374–82. doi:10.1016/j.jsxm.2016.01.001.

113. Cohen CE, Giles A, Nelson M. Sexual trauma associated with fisting and recreational drugs. Sex Transm Infect. 2004;80:469–70. doi:10.1136/sti.2004.011171.

114. Adkins BD, Barlow AB, Jack A, Schultenover SJ, Desouki MM, Coogan AC, et al. Characteristic findings of cervical Papanicolaou tests from transgender patients on androgen therapy: challenges in detecting dysplasia. Cytopathology. 2018;29:281–7. doi:10.1111/cyt.12525.

115. Rahn DD, Carberry C, Sanses TV, Mamik MM, Ward RM, Meriwether KV, et al.; Society of Gynecologic Surgeons Systematic Review Group. Vaginal estrogen for genitourinary syndrome of menopause: a systematic review. Obstet Gynecol. 2014;124(6):1147–56. doi:10.1097/AOG.0000000000000526.

116. Hoffmann JN, You HM, Hedberg EC, Jordan JA. McClintock MK. Prevalence of bacterial vaginosis and Candida among postmenopausal women in the United States. J Gerontol B Psychol Sci Soc Sci. 2014 Nov;69(8 Suppl 2):S205–14. doi:10.1093/geronb/gbu105.

117. Dorr MB, Nelson AL, Mayer PR, Ranganath RP, Norris PM, Helzner EC, et al. Plasma estrogen concentrations after oral and vaginal estrogen administration in women with atrophic vaginitis. Fertil Steril. 2010;94(6):2365–8. doi:10.1016/j.fertnstert.2010.03.076.

118. Labrie F, Cusan L, Gomez JL, Côté I, Bérubé R, Bélanger P, et al. Effect of one-week treatment with vaginal estrogen preparations on serum estrogen levels in postmenopausal women. Menopause. 2009;16(1):30–6. doi:10.1097/gme.0b013e31817b6132.

119. Mitchell CM, Reed SD, Diem S, Larson JC, Newton KM, Ensrud KE, et al. Efficacy of vaginal estradiol or vaginal moisturizer vs placebo for treating postmenopausal vulvovaginal symptoms: a randomized clinical trial. JAMA Intern Med. 2018;178(5):681–90. doi:10.1001/jamainternmed.2018.0116.

120. Simonetta C, Burns EK, Guo MA. Vulvar dermatoses: a review and update. Mo Med. 2015;112(4):301–7.

121. Hoang MP, Reutter J, Papalas JA, Edwards L, Selim MA. Vulvar inflammatory dermatoses: an update and review. Am J Dermatopathol. 2014;36(9):689–704.

122. McMurray SL, Overholser E, Patel T. A transgender woman with anogenital lichen sclerosus. JAMA Dermatol. 2017;153(12):1334–5. doi:10.1001/jamadermatol.2017.3071.
123. Chamli A, Souissi A [Internet]. Treasure Island (FL): StatPearls Publishing; 2019 Jan [cited 2019 Mar 25]. Lichen sclerosus. Available from: https://www.statpearls.com/kb/viewarticle/24256/.
124. Simpson RC, Thomas KS, Leighton P, Murphy R. Diagnostic criteria for erosive lichen planus affecting the vulva: an international electronic-Delphi consensus exercise. Br J Dermatol. 2013;169:337–43. doi:10.1111/bjd.12334.
125. Kortekangas-Savolainen O, Kiilholma P. Treatment of vulvovaginal erosive and stenosing lichen planus by surgical dilatation and methotrexate. Acta Obstet Gynecol Scand. 2007;86:339–43. doi:10.1080/00016340601110721.
126. Suzuki V, Haefner HK, Piper CK, O'Gara C, Reed BD. Postoperative sexual concerns and functioning in patients who underwent lysis of vulvovaginal adhesions. J Low Geni Tract Dis. 2013;17(1):33–7.
127. Lee A, Fischer G. Diagnosis and treatment of vulvar lichen sclerosus: an update for dermatologists. Am J Clin Dermatol. 2018;19:695–706. doi:10.1007/s40257-018-0364-7.
128. Armstrong HL, Reissing ED. Chronic vulvo-vaginal pain in lesbian, bisexual and other sexual minority women. J Sex Med. 2012;9(3 Suppl):166–7. doi:10.1111/j.1743-6109.2012.02758.x.
129. Harlow BL, Stewart EG. A population-based assessment of chronic unexplained vulvar pain: have we underestimated the prevalence of vulvodynia? J Am Med Womens Assoc. 2003;58(2):82–8.
130. Reissing ED, Binik YM, Khalifé S, Cohen D, Amsel R. Vaginal spasm, pain, and behavior: an empirical investigation of the diagnosis of vaginismus. Arch Sex Behav. 2004;33(1):5–17.
131. Ter Kuile MM, Van Lankveld JJ, Vlieland CV, Willekes C, Weijenborg PT. Vulvar vestibulitis syndrome: an important factor in the evaluation of lifelong vaginismus? J Psychosom Obstet Gynaecol. 2005 Dec;26(4):245–9. doi:10.1080/01674820500165935.
132. Rosen NO, Dawson SJ, Brooks M, Kellogg-Spadt S. Treatment of vulvodynia: pharmacological and non-pharmacological approaches. Drugs. 2019 Apr;79(5):483–93. doi:10.1007/s40265-019-01085-1.
133. Blair KL, Pukall CF, Smith KB, Cappell J. Differential associations of communication and love in heterosexual, lesbian, and bisexual women's perceptions and experiences of chronic vulvar and pelvic pain. J Sex Marital Ther. 2015;41(5):498–524. doi:10.1080/0092623X.2014.931315.
134. van der Sluis WB, Bouman MB, Gijs L, van Bodegraven AA. Gonorrhoea of the sigmoid neovagina in a male-to-female transgender. Int J STD AIDS. 2015;26(8):595–8. doi:10.1177/0956462414544725.

135. Riss S, Weiser FA, Schwameis K, Riss T, Mittlböck M, Steiner G, et al. The prevalence of hemorrhoids in adults. Int J Colorectal Dis. 2012;27:215–20. doi:10.1007/s00384-011-1316-3.

136. Peery AF, Sandler RS, Galanko JA, Bresalier RS, Figueiredo JC, Ahnen DJ, et al. Risk factors for hemorrhoids on screening colonscopy. PLoS One. 2015;10(9):e0139100. doi:10.1371/journal.pone.0139100.

137. Johanson JF, Sonnenberg A. Constipation is not a risk factor for hemorrhoids: a case-control study of potential etiological agents. Am J Gastroenterol. 1994;89(11):1981–6.

138. Lawrence A, McLaren ER. External hemorrhoid. StatPearls [Internet]. 2019 [cited 2019 Jun 13]. Accessed from: https://www.ncbi.nlm.nih.gov /books/NBK500009/.

139. Fargo MV, Latimer KM. Evaluation and management of common anorectal conditions. Am Fam Physician. 2012;85(6):624–30.

140. Zuber TJ. Hemorrhoidectomy for thrombosed external hemorrhoids. Am Fam Physician. 2002;65:1629–32.

141. Banov L Jr, Knoepp LF Jr, Erdman LH, Alia RT. Management of hemorrhoidal disease. J S C Med Assoc. 1985;81(7):398–401.

142. Lund JN, Scholefield JH. Aetiology and treatment of anal fissure. Br J Surg. 1996;83:1335–44.

143. Cox DR, Rao A, Ee E. Syphilis as an atypical cause of perianal fissure. J Surg Case Reps. 2018 Nov;2018(11):rjy320. doi:10.1093/jscr/rjy320.

144. Madalinski MH. Identifying the best therapy for chronic anal fissure. World J Gastrointest Pharmacol Ther. 2011;2(2):9–16. doi:10.4292/wjgpt.v2.i2.9.

145. Vasilevsky CA, Gordon PH. The incidence of recurrent abscesses or fistula-in-ano following anorectal suppuration. Dis Colon Rectum 1984;27:126–30.

146. Becker A, Koltun L, Sayfan J. Simple clinical examination predicts complexity of perianal fistula. Colorectal Dis. 2006;8:601–4. doi:10.1111/j.1463-1318.2006.01025.x.

147. Assi R, Hashim PW, Reddy VB, Einarsdottir H, Longo WE. Sexually transmitted infections of the anus and rectum. World J Gastroenterol. 2014;20(41):15262–8. doi:10.3748/wjg.v20.i41.15262.

148. Ansari P. Pruritus ani. Clin Colon Rectal Surg. 2016;29:38–42. doi:10.1055/s-0035-1570391.

149. Felt-Bersma RJ, Bartelsman JF. Haemorrhoids, rectal prolapse, anal fissure, peri-anal fistulae and sexually transmitted diseases. Best Pract Res Clin Gastroenterol. 2009;23:575–92. doi:10.1016/j.bpg.2009.04.010.

150. Kairaluoma MV, Kellokumpu IH. Epidemiologic aspects of complete rectal prolapse. Scand J Surg. 2005;94:207–10.

151. Chun AB, Rose S, Mitrani C, Silvestre AJ, Wald A. Anal sphincter structure and function in homosexual males engaging in anoreceptive intercourse. Am J Gastroenterol. 1997;92(3):465–8.

152. Markland AD, Dunivan GC, Vaughan CP, Rogers RG. Anal intercourse and fecal incontinence: evidence from the 2009–2010 National Health and Nutrition Examination Survey. Am J Gastroenterol. 2016;111(2):269–74. doi:10.1038/ajg.2015.419.
153. Geynisman-Tan J, Kenton K, Leader-Cramer A, Dave B, Bochenska K, Mueller M, et al. Anal penetrative intercourse as a risk factor for fecal incontinence. Female Pelvic Med Reconstr Surg. 2018;24(3):252–5. doi:10.1097/SPV.0000000000000408.
155. Hollows K. Anodyspareunia: a novel sexual dysfunction? An exploration into anal sexuality. Sex Relationship Ther. 2007;22(4):429–43. doi:10.1080/14681990701481409.
155. Damon W, Rosser BR. Anodyspareunia in men who have sex with men: prevalence, predictors, consequences and the development of DSM diagnostic criteria. J Sex Marital Ther. 2005;31:129–41. doi:10.1080/00926230590477989.
156. Public Health Agency of Canada. Canadian Guidelines on Sexually Transmitted Infections [Internet]. 2010 [cited 2019 Mar 28]. Available from: https://www.canada.ca/en/public-health/services/infectious-diseases/sexual-health-sexually-transmitted-infections/canadian-guidelines/sexually-transmitted-infections.html.
157. Patton ME, Kidd S, Llata E, Stenger M, Braxton J, Asbel L, et al. Extragenital gonorrhea and chlamydia testing and infection among men who have sex with men – STD Surveillance Network, United States, 2010–2012. Clin Infect Dis. 2014 Jun;58(11):1564–70.
158. Gratrix J, Singh AE, Bergman J, Egan C, McGinnis J, Drews SJ, et al. Prevalence and characteristics of rectal chlamydia and gonorrhea cases among men who have sex with men after the introduction of nucleic acid amplification test screening at 2 Canadian sexually transmitted infection clinics. Sex Transm Dis. 2014 Oct;41(10):589–91.
159. van Liere GA, van Rooijen MS, Hoebe CJ, Heijman T, de Vries HJ, Dukers-Muijrers NH. Prevalence of and factors associated with rectal-only chlamydia and gonorrhoea in women and in men who have sex with men. PLoS One. 2015 Oct;10(10):e0140297.
160. Huffam S, Chow EP, Fairley CK, Hocking J, Peel J, Chen M. Chlamydia infection in individuals reporting contact with sexual partners with chlamydia: a cross-sectional study of sexual health clinic attendees. Sex Transm Infect. 2015 Sep;91(6):434–9.
161. Danby CS, Cosentino LA, Rabe LK, Priest CL, Damare KC, Macio IS, et al. Patterns of Extragenital Chlamydia and Gonorrhea in Women and Men Who Have Sex With Men Reporting a History of Receptive Anal Intercourse. Sex Transm Dis. 2016 Feb;43(2):105–9.
162. Workowski KA, Bachmann LH, Chan PA, Johnston CM, Muzny CA, Park I, et al; Centers for Disease Control and Prevention. Sexually

transmitted infections treatment guidelines, 2021. MMWR Recomm Rep. 2021 Jul;70(4):1–187.

163. Schachter J, McCormack WM, Chernesky MA, Martin DH, Van Der Pol B, Rice PA, et al. Vaginal swabs are appropriate specimens for diagnosis of genital tract infection with Chlamydia trachomatis. J Clin Microbiol. 2003 Aug;41(8):3784–9.

164. Public Health Ontario. Chlamydia trachomatis and Neisseria gonorrhoeae – implementation of nucleic acid amplification testing (NAAT) for rectal and pharyngeal sites [Internet]. Toronto: Ontario Agency for Health Protection and Promotion; 2018 Apr [cited 2019 Mar 19]. Available from: https://www.publichealthontario.ca/-/media/documents/lab/lab-sd-128-ct-gc-naat-implementation.pdf?la=en.

165. Dukers-Muijrers NH, Schachter J, van Liere GA, Wolffs PF, Hoebe CJ. What is needed to guide testing for anorectal and pharyngeal Chlamydia trachomatis and Neisseria gonorrhoeae in women and men? Evidence and opinion. BMC Infect Dis. 2015;15:533.

166. Trebach JD, Chaulk CP, Page KR, Tuddenham S, Ghanem KG. Neisseria gonorrhoeae and Chlamydia trachomatis among women reporting extragenital exposures. Sex Transm Dis. 2015;42(5):233–9.

167. Poteat T. Transgender people and sexually transmitted infections (STIs). In: Deutsch MB, editors. Guidelines for the Primary and gender-affirming care of transgender and gender nonbinary people [Internet]. San Francisco: University of California San Francisco; 2016 [cited 2019 Mar 27]. Available from: http://transhealth.ucsf.edu/trans?page=guidelines-stis.

168. Chow EP, Camilleri S, Ward C, Huffam S, Chen MY, Bradshaw CS, et al. Duration of gonorrhoea and chlamydia infection at the pharynx and rectum among men who have sex with men: a systematic review. Sex Health. 2016 Jun;13(3):199–204.

169. World Health Organization. WHO guidelines for the treatment of chlamydia trachomatis [Internet]. Geneva: WHO; 2016 [cited 2019 Mar 17]. Available from: http://apps.who.int/iris/bitstream/10665/246165/1/9789241549714-eng.pdf.

170. Kropp RY, Wong T, Canadian LGV Working Group. Emergence of lymphogranuloma venereum in Canada. CMAJ. 2005 Jun 21;172(13):1674–6.

171. Ward H, Martin I, Macdonald N, Alexander S, Simms I, Fenton K, et al. Lymphogranuloma venereum in the United Kingdom. Clin Infect Dis. 2007 Jan;44(1):26–32.

172. Martin-Iguacel R, Llibre JM, Nielsen H, Heras E, Matas L, Lugo R, et al. Lymphogranuloma venereum proctocolitis: a silent endemic disease in men who have sex with men in industrialised countries. Eur J Clin Microbiol Infect Dis. 2010 Aug;29(8):917–25.

173. Pallawela SN, Sullivan AK, Macdonald N, French P, White J, Dean G, et al. Clinical predictors of rectal lymphogranuloma venereum infection: results from a multicentre case-control study in the U.K. Sex Transm Infect. 2014 Jun;90(4):269–74.

174. de Vrieze NH, de Vries HJ. Lymphogranuloma venereum among men who have sex with men. An epidemiological and clinical review. Expert Rev Anti Infect Ther. 2014 Jun;12(6):697–704.

175. Koper NE, van der Sande MA, Gotz HM, Koedijk FD; Dutch STI Clinics. Lymphogranuloma venereum among men who have sex with men in the Netherlands: regional differences in testing rates lead to underestimation of the incidence, 2006–2012. Euro Surveill. 2013 Aug 22;18(34):pii:20561.

176. Haar K, Dudareva-Vizule S, Wisplinghoff H, Wisplinghoff F, Sailer A, Jansen K, et al. Lymphogranuloma venereum in men screened for pharyngeal and rectal infection, Germany. Emerg Infect Dis. 2013 Mar;19(3):488–92.

177. Foschi C, Marangoni A, D'Antuono A, Nardini P, Compri M, Bellavista S, et al. Prevalence and predictors of Lymphogranuloma venereum in a high risk population attending a STD outpatients clinic in Italy. BMC Res Notes. 2014;7:225.

178. Hughes G, Alexander S, Simms I, Conti S, Ward H, Powers C, et al.; LGV Incident Group. Lymphogranuloma venereum diagnoses among men who have sex with men in the U.K.: interpreting a cross-sectional study using an epidemic phase-specific framework. Sex Transm Infect. 2013 Nov;89(7):542–7.

179. Public Health Ontario [Internet]. Toronto: Ontario Agency for Health Protection and Promotion; [cited 2019 May 18]. Chlamydia trachomatis – lymphogranuloma venereum (LGV) PCR. Available from: https://www .publichealthontario.ca/en/laboratory-services/test-information-index /chlamydia-trachomatis-lgv-pcr.

180. Public Health Ontario [Internet]. Toronto: Ontario Agency for Health Protection and Promotion; [cited 2019 May 18]. Chlamydia trachomatis – culture. Available from: https://www.publichealthontario.ca/en /laboratory-services/test-information-index/ chlamydia-trachomatis-culture.

181. Fairley CK, Hocking JS, Zhang L, Chow EP. Frequent Transmission of Gonorrhea in Men Who Have Sex with Men. Emerg Infect Dis. 2017 Jan;23(1):102–4.

182. Jin F, Prestage GP, Mao L, Kippax SC, Pell CM, Donovan B, et al. Incidence and risk factors for urethral and anal gonorrhoea and chlamydia in a cohort of HIV-negative homosexual men: the Health in Men Study. Sex Transm Infect. 2007 Apr;83(2):113–19.

183. Templeton DJ, Jin F, McNally LP, Imrie JC, Prestage GP, Donovan B, et al. Prevalence, incidence and risk factors for pharyngeal gonorrhoea in a community-based HIV-negative cohort of homosexual men in Sydney, Australia. Sex Transm Infect. 2010 Apr;86(2):90–6.
184. Hutt DM, Judson FN. Epidemiology and treatment of oropharyngeal gonorrhea. Ann Intern Med. 1986 May;104(5):655–8.
185. Chow EP, Lee D, Tabrizi SN, Phillips S, Snow A, Cook S, et al. Detection of Neisseria gonorrhoeae in the pharynx and saliva: implications for gonorrhoea transmission. Sex Transm Infect. 2016 Aug;92(5):347–9.
186. Lunny C, Taylor D, Hoang L, Wong T, Gilbert M, Lester R, et al. Self-collected versus clinician-collected sampling for chlamydia and gonorrhea screening: a systematic review and meta-analysis. PLoS One. 2015;10(7):e0132776. doi:10.1371/journal.pone.0132776.
187. Public Health Ontario. Chlamydia trachomatis and Neisseria gonorrhoeae – implementation of nucleic acid amplification testing (NAAT) for rectal and pharyngeal sites [Internet]. Toronto: Ontario Agency for Health Protection and Promotion; 2018 Apr [cited 2019 Mar 19]. Available from: https://www.publichealthontario.ca/-/media/documents/lab/lab-sd-128-ct-gc-naat-implementation.pdf?la=en.
188. Bodsworth NJ, Price R, Davies SC. Gonococcal infection of the neovagina in a male-to-female transsexual. Sex Transm Dis. 1994 Jul-Aug;21(4):211–12.
189. Haustein UF. [Pruritus of the artificial vagina of a transsexual patient caused by gonococcal infection]. Hautarzt. 1995 Dec;46(12):858–9.
190. van der Sluis WB, Bouman MB, Gijs L, van Bodegraven AA. Gonorrhoea of the sigmoid neovagina in a male-to-female transgender. Int J STD AIDS. 2015 Jul;26(8):595–8.
191. Chow EP, Camilleri S, Ward C, Huffam S, Chen MY, Bradshaw CS, et al. Duration of gonorrhoea and chlamydia infection at the pharynx and rectum among men who have sex with men: a systematic review. Sex Health. 2016 Jun;13(3):199–204.
192. St Cyr S, Barbee L, Workowski KA, Bachmann LH, Pham C, Schlanger K, et al. Update to CDC's treatment guidelines for gonococcal infection, 2020. MMWR Morb Mortal Wkly Rep. 2020 Dec;69(50):1911–16. doi:10.15585/mmwr.mm6950a6.
193. Public Health Agency of Canada [Internet]. Ottawa: Government of Canada; [updated 2020; cited 2021 Jan 3]. National surveillanace of antimicrobial susceptibilities of Neisseria gonorrhoeae annual summary 2018. Available from: https://www.canada.ca/en/public-health/services/publications/drugs-health-products/national-surveillance-antimicrobial-susceptibilities-neisseria-gonorrhoeae-annual-summary-2018.html.

194. World Health Organization. Global action plan to control the spread and impact of antimicrobial resistance in Neisseria gonorrhoeae [Internet]. Geneva: WHO Press; 2012. https://apps.who.int/iris/bitstream/handle/10665/44863/9789241503501_eng.pdf.

195. Lefebvre B, Martin I, Demczuk W, Deshaies L, Michaud S, Labbé AC, et al. Ceftriaxone-Resistant Neisseria gonorrhoeae, Canada, 2017. Emerg Infect Dis. 2018 Feb;24(2):381–3.

196. Public Health England. UK case of Neisseria gonorrhoeae with high-level resistance to azithromycin and resistance to ceftriaxone acquired abroad [Internet]. London, England: PHE; 2018 Mar [cited 2019 Mar 30]. Available from: https://assets.publishing.service.gov.uk/government/uploads/system/uploads/attachment_data/file/694655/hpr1118_MDRGC.pdf.

197. Public Health Agency of Canada [Internet]. Ottawa: Government of Canada; 2021 June 24 [cited 2022 Jan 2]. Report on sexually transmitted infections in Canada, 2018. Available from: https://www.canada.ca/en/public-health/services/publications/diseases-conditions/report-sexually-transmitted-infections-canada-2018.html.

198. Public Health Agency of Canada. Syphilis among gay, bisexual, Two-Spirit and other men who have sex with men: a resource for population-specific prevention [Internet]. Ottawa: Government of Canada; 2015 Mar [cited 2019 Mar 19]. Available from: https://www.catie.ca/sites/default/files/Syphilis-among-gay-bisexual-two-spirit-and-other-MSM.pdf.

199. Campos-Outcalt D, Hurwitz S. Female-to-female transmission of syphilis: a case report. Sex Transm Dis. 2002 Feb;29(2):119–20.

200. Agénor M, Muzny CA, Schick V, Austin EL, Potter J. Sexual orientation and sexual health services utilization among women in the United States. Prev Med. 2017 Feb;95:74–81.

201. Lewis J, Seña AC. Syphilis. In: Bachmann L, editor. Sexually transmitted infections in HIV-infected adults and special populations. Cham: Springer; 2017. p. 89–110.

202. Larsen SA, Steiner BM, Rudolph AH. Laboratory diagnosis and interpretation of tests for syphilis. Clin Microbiol Rev. 1995;8(1):1–21.

203. Toronto Public Health. Syphilis laboratory interpretation [Internet]. Toronto: City of Toronto; 2018 [cited 2019 Jun 29]. Available from: https://www.toronto.ca/wp-content/uploads/2018/02/8528-tph-syphilis-lab-interpretation-guideline-Jan-2018.pdf.

204. Public Health Ontario [Internet]. Toronto: Ontario Agency for Health Protection and Promotion; 2019 Feb 12 [cited 2019 Jun 18]. Syphilis chancre direct fluorescence. Available from: https://www.publichealthontario.ca/en/ServicesAndTools/LaboratoryServices/Pages/Syphilis_Chancre_Direct_Fluorescence.aspx.

205. Hobbs E, Vera JH, Marks M, Barritt AW, Ridha BH, Lawrence D. Neurosyphilis in patients with HIV. Pract Neurol. 2018;18(3):211–18. doi:10.1136/practneurol-2017-001754.

206. Public Health Agency of Canada. Canadian Guidelines on Sexually Transmitted Infections 2016 Updates Summary. 2016 [cited 2019 Mar 16]. Available from: https://www.canada.ca/en/public-health/services/infectious-diseases/sexual-health-sexually-transmitted-infections/canadian-guidelines/2016-updates-summary.html.

207. Marra CM, Maxwell CL, Smith SL, Lukehart SA, Rompalo AM, Eaton M, et al. Cerebrospinal fluid abnormalities in patients with syphilis: association with clinical and laboratory features. J Infect Dis. 2004 Feb;189(3):369–76.

208. Ghanem KG, Moore RD, Rompalo AM, Erbelding EJ, Zenilman JM, Gebo KA. Lumbar puncture in HIV-infected patients with syphilis and no neurologic symptoms. Clin Infect Dis. 2009 Mar;48(6):816–21.

209. Dumaresq J, Langevin S, Gagnon S, Serhir B, Deligne B, Tremblay C, et al. Clinical prediction and diagnosis of neurosyphilis in HIV-infected patients with early Syphilis. J Clin Microbiol. 2013 Dec;51(12):4060–6.

210. Hook EW 3rd. Syphilis. Lancet. 2017 Apr 15;389(10078):1550–7.

211. Manhart LE, Holmes KK, Hughes JP, Houston LS, Totten PA. Mycoplasma genitalium among young adults in the United States: an emerging sexually transmitted infection. Am J Public Health. 2007;97(6):1118–25. doi:10.2105/AJPH.2005.074062.

212. Gottesman T, Yossepowitch O, Samra Z, Rosenberg S, Dan M. Prevalence of Mycoplasma genitalium in men with urethritis and in high risk asymptomatic males in Tel Aviv: a prospective study. Int J STD AIDS. 2017;28(2):127–32. doi:10.1177/0956462416630675.

213. Hjorth SV, Björnelius E, Lidbrink P, Falk L, Dohn B, Berthelsen L, et al. Sequence-based typing of Mycoplasma genitalium reveals sexual transmission. J Clin Microbiol. 2006;44(6):2078–83.

214. Lis R, Rowhani-Rahbar A, Manhart LE. Mycoplasma genitalium infection and female reproductive tract disease: a meta-analysis. Clin Infect Dis. 2015;61(3):418–26. doi:10.1093/cid/civ312.

215. Haggerty CL, Totten PA, Astete SG, Ness RB. Mycoplasma genitalium among women with nongonococcal, nonchlamydial pelvic inflammatory disease. Infect Dis Obstet Gynecol. 2006;2006:30184. doi:10.1155/IDOG/2006/30184.

216. Falk L, Fredlund H, Jensen JS. Symptomatic urethritis is more prevalent in men infected with Mycoplasma genitalium than with Chlamydia trachomatis. Sex Transm Infect. 2004;80(4):289–93. doi:10.1136/sti.2003.006817.

217. Francis SC, Kent CK, Klausner JD, Rauch L, Kohn R, Hardick A, et al. Prevalence of rectal Trichomonas vaginalis and Mycoplasma genitalium

in male patients at the San Francisco STD clinic, 2005–2006. Sex Transm Dis. 2008;35(9):797–800. doi:10.1097/OLQ.0b013e318177ec39.

218. Public Health Agency of Canada [Internet]. Ottawa: Governement of Canada; PHAC; 2019 [cited 2019 Mar 29]. Section 5–1: Management and treatment of specific infections – Mycoplasma genitalium infections. Available from: https://www.canada.ca/en/public-health/services /infectious-diseases/sexual-health-sexually-transmitted-infections /canadian-guidelines/sexually-transmitted-infections/canadian -guidelines-sexually-transmitted-infections-49.html.

219. Mena LA, Mroczkowski TF, Nsuami M, Martin DH. A randomized comparison of azithromycin and doxycycline for treatment of Mycoplasma genitalium-positive urethritis in men. Clin Infect Dis. 2009;48(12):1649–54. doi:10.1086/599033.

220. Hartmann M. Genital mycoplasmas. J Dtsch Dermatol Ges. 2009;7(4):371–7. doi:10.1111/j.1610-0387.2008.06965.x.

221. Zhang N, Wang R, Li X, Liu X, Tang Z, Liu Y. Are Ureaplasma spp. a cause of nongonococcal urethritis? A systematic review and meta-analysis. PLoS One. 2014;9(12):e113771. doi:10.1371/journal.pone.0113771.

222. Shimada Y, Ito S, Mizutani K, Sugawara T, Seike K, Tsuchiya T, et al. Bacterial loads of Ureaplasma urealyticum contribute to development of urethritis in men. Int J STD AIDS. 2014;25(4):294–8. doi:10.1177/0956462413504556.

223. Taylor-Robinson D, Csonka GW, Prentice MJ. Human intra-urethral inoculation of ureplasmas. Q J Med. 1977;46(183):309–26.

224. Kletzel HH, Rotem R, Barg M, Michaeli J, Reichman O. Ureaplasma urealyticum: the role as a pathogen in women's health, a systematic review. Curr Infect Dis Rep. 2018;20(9):33. doi:10.1007 /s11908-018-0640-y.

225. Anderson TA, Schick V, Herbenick D, Dodge B, Fortenberry JD. A study of human papillomavirus on vaginally inserted sex toys, before and after cleaning, among women who have sex with women and men. Sex Transm Infect. 2014 Nov;90(7):529–31.

226. Public Health Agency of Canada [Internet]. Ottawa: Government of Canada; [updated 2017 Oct 4; cited 2019 Mar 24]. Human papillomavirus (HPV). Available from: https://www.canada.ca/en/public-health /services/infectious-diseases/sexual-health-sexually-transmitted -infections/human-papillomavirus-hpv.html.

227. Gallagher KE, LaMontagne DS, Watson-Jones D. Status of HPV vaccine introduction and barriers to country uptake. Vaccine. 2018 Aug 6;36(32 Pt A):4761–67.

228. Lacey CJ, Lowndes CM, Shah KV. Chapter 4: Burden and management of non-cancerous HPV-related conditions: HPV-6/11 disease. Vaccine. 2006 Aug 31;24 Suppl 3:S3/35–41.

229. Nyitray AG, Chang M, Villa LL, Carvalho da Silva RJ, Baggio ML, Abrahamsen M, et al. The natural history of genital human papillomavirus among HIV-negative men having sex with men and men having sex with women. J Infect Dis. 2015 Jul 15;212(2):202–12.

230. Llata E, Stenger M, Bernstein K, Guerry S, Kerani R, Pugsley R, et al.; SSuN GW Working Group. Prevalence of genital warts among sexually transmitted disease clinic patients-sexually transmitted disease surveillance network, United States, January 2010 to December 2011. Sex Transm Dis. 2014 Feb;41(2):89–93.

231. Nyitray AG, Carvalho da Silva RJ, Baggio ML, Lu B, Smith D, Abrahamsen M, et al. Age-specific prevalence of and risk factors for anal human papillomavirus (HPV) among men who have sex with women and men who have sex with men: the HPV in men (HIM) study. J Infect Dis. 2011 Jan 1;203(1):49–57.

232. Goldstone S, Palefsky JM, Giuliano AR, Moreira ED Jr, Aranda C, Jessen H, et al. Prevalence of and risk factors for human papillomavirus (HPV) infection among HIV-seronegative men who have sex with men. J Infect Dis. 2011 Jan 1;203(1):66–74.

233. Matsuki S, Kusatake K, Hein KZ, Anraku K, Morita E. Condylomata acuminata in the neovagina after male-to-female reassignment treated with CO_2 laser and imiquimod. Int J STD AIDS. 2015 Jun;26(7):509–11.

234. Yang C, Liu S, Xu K, Xiang Q, Yang S, Zhang X. Condylomata gigantea in a male transsexual. Int J STD AIDS. 2009 Mar;20(3):211–12.

235. Schlecht HP, Fugelso DK, Murphy RK, Wagner KT, Doweiko JP, Proper J, et al. Frequency of occult high-grade squamous intraepithelial neoplasia and invasive cancer within anal condylomata in men who have sex with men. Clin Infect Dis. 2010 Jul 1;51(1):107–10.

236. Labanca T, Mañero I. Vulvar condylomatosis after sex reassignment surgery in a male-to-female transsexual: complete response to imiquimod cream. Gynecol Oncol Rep. 2017;20:75–7. doi:10.1016/j.gore.2017.03.010.

237. Matsuki S, Kusatake K, Hein KZ, Anraku K, Morita E. Condylomata acuminata in the neovagina after male-to-female reassignment treated with CO_2 laser and imiquimod. Int J STD AIDS. 2015;26(7):509–11. doi:10.1177/0956462414542476.

238. de Sanjosé S, Serrano B, Tous S, Alejo M, Lloveras B, Quirós B, et al.; RIS HPV TT, VVAP and Head and Neck study groups. Burden of human papillomavirus (HPV)-related cancers attributable to HPVs 6/11/16/18/31/33/45/52 and 58. JNCI Cancer Spectrum. 2018 Nov;2(4):pky045.

239. Marrazzo JM, Koutsky LA, Kiviat NB, Kuypers JM, Stine K. Papanicolaou test screening and prevalence of genital human papillomavirus among women who have sex with women. Am J Public Health. 2001;91:947–52.

240. Ferris DG, Batish S, Wright TC, Cushing C, Scott EH. A neglected lesbian health concern: cervical neoplasia. J Fam Pract. 1996;43(6):581–4.
241. O'Hanlan KA, Crum CP. Human papillomavirus-associated cervical intraepithelial neoplasia following lesbian sex. Obstet Gynecol. 1996 Oct;88(4 Pt 2):702–3.
242. Harder Y, Erni D, Banic A. Squamous cell carcinoma of the penile skin in a neovagina 20 years after male-to-female reassignment. Br J Plast Surg. 2002;55(5):449–51.
243. Sturt RJ, Muller HK, Francis GD. Molluscum contagiosum in villages of the West Sepik District of New Guinea. Med J Aust. 1971;2(15):751–4.
244. Koning S, Bruijnzeels MA, van Suijlekom-Smit LWA, van der Wouden JC. Molluscum contagiosum in Dutch general practice. Br J Gen Pract. 1994;44:417–19.
245. Braue A, Ross G, Varigos G, Kelly H. Epidemiology and impact of molluscum contagiosum: a case series and critical review of the literature. Pediatr Dermatol. 2005;22(4):287–94.
246. Foulds IS. Molluscum contagiosum: an unusual complication of tattooing. Br Med J (Clin Res Ed). 1982;285:607.
247. Rich JD, Dickinson BP, Flaxman AB, Mylonakis E. Local spread of molluscum contagiosum by electrolysis. Clin Infect Dis. 1999;28:1171.
248. Choong KY, Roberts LJ. Molluscum contagiosum, swimming and bathing: a clinical analysis. Australas J Dermatol. 1999;40:89–92.
249. Trozak DJ, Tennenhouse DJ, Russell JJ. Dermatology skills for primary care: an illustrated guide. Totowa (NJ): Humana Press; 2006.
250. Gupta R, Warren T, Wald A. Genital herpes. Lancet. 2007 Dec 22;370(9605):2127–37.
251. Mertz GJ, Benedetti J, Ashley R, Selke SA, Corey L. Risk factors for the sexual transmission of genital herpes. Ann Intern Med. 1992 Feb 1;116(3):197–202.
252. Corey L, Wald A, Patel R, Sacks SL, Tyring SK, Warren T, et al.; Valacyclovir HSV Transmission Study Group. Once-daily valacyclovir to reduce the risk of transmission of genital herpes. N Engl J Med. 2004 Jan 1;350(1):11–20.
253. Wald A, Langenberg AG, Link K, Izu AE, Ashley R, Warren T, et al. Effect of condoms on reducing the transmission of herpes simplex virus type 2 from men to women. JAMA. 2001 Jun 27;285(24):3100–6.
254. Stanberry LR, Spruance SL, Cunningham AL, Bernstein DI, Mindel A, Sacks S, et al.; GlaxoSmithKline Herpes Vaccine Efficacy Study Group. Glycoprotein-D-adjuvant vaccine to prevent genital herpes. N Engl J Med. 2002 Nov 21;347(21):1652–61.
255. Elfering L, van der Sluis WB, Mermans JF, Buncamper ME. Herpes neolabialis: herpes simplex virus type 1 infection of the neolabia in a transgender woman. Int J STD AIDS. 2017 Jul;28(8):841–3.

256. Benedetti J, Corey L, Ashley R. Recurrence rates in genital herpes after symptomatic first-episode infection. Ann Intern Med. 1994 Dec 1;121(11):847–54.

257. Engelberg R, Carrell D, Krantz E, Corey L, Wald A. Natural history of genital herpes simplex virus type 1 infection. Sex Transm Dis. 2003 Feb;30(2):174–7.

258. Reeves WC, Corey L, Adams HG, Vontver LA, Holmes KK. Risk of recurrence after first episodes of genital herpes: relation to HSV type and antibody response. N Engl J Med. 1981;305(6):315–19.

259. Lafferty WE, Coombs RW, Benedetti J, Critchlow C, Corey L. Recurrences after oral and genital herpes simplex virus infection: influence of site of infection and viral type. N Engl J Med. 1987;316:1444–9.

260. Benedetti JK, Zeh J, Corey L. Clinical reactivation of genital herpes simplex virus infection decreases in frequency over time. Ann Intern Med. 1999;131:14–20.

261. Mujugira A, Magaret AS, Celum C, Baeten JM, Lingappa JR, Morrow RA, et al.; Partners in Prevention HSV/HIV Transmission Study Team. Daily acyclovir to decrease herpes simplex virus type 2 (HSV-2) transmission from HSV-2/HIV-1 coinfected persons: a randomized controlled trial. J Infect Dis. 2013 Nov 1;208(9):1366–74.

262. Celum C, Wald A, Lingappa JR, Magaret AS, Wang RS, Mugo N, et al.; Partners in Prevention HSV/HIV Transmission Study Team. Acyclovir and transmission of HIV-1 from persons infected with HIV-1 and HSV-2. N Engl J Med. 2010 Feb 4;362(5):427–39.

263. Public Health Agency of Canada [Internet]. Ottawa: Government of Canada; 2010 [updated 2018 Jan; cited 2019 Mar 11]. Section 3: Laboratory diagnosis of sexually transmitted infections of PHAC Canadian guidelines on sexually transmitted infections. Available from: https://www.canada.ca/en/public-health/services/infectious-diseases/sexual-health-sexually-transmitted-infections/canadian-guidelines/sexually-transmitted-infections/canadian-guidelines-sexually-transmitted-infections-18.html.

264. Wilton J, Knowles Z [Internet]. Toronto: CATIE; 2018 [cited 2019 Mar 12]. HIV testing technologies. Available from: http://www.catie.ca/en/fact-sheets/testing/hiv-testing-technologies.

265. Public Health Agency of Canada [Internet]. Ottawa: Government of Canada; 2018 Mar [cited 2019 Mar 27]. Canadian immunization guide: part 4 – active vaccines: hepatitis A vaccine. Available from: https://www.canada.ca/en/public-health/services/publications/healthy-living/canadian-immunization-guide-part-4-active-vaccines/page-6-hepatitis-a-vaccine.html.

266. CATIE [Internet]. Toronto: CATIE: 2016 [cited 2019 Mar 27]. Hepatitis A fact sheet. Available from: https://www.catie.ca/en/fact-sheets/sti/hepatitis-a.

267. Lee HK, Kim KA, Lee JS, Kim NH, Bae WK, Song TJ. Window period of anti-hepatitis A virus immunoglobulin M antibodies in diagnosing acute hepatitis A. Eur J Gastroenterol Hepatol. 2013 Jun;25(6):665–8.

268. Public Health Agency of Canada [Internet]. Ottawa: Government of Canada; 2014 [cited 2019 Mar 27]. Primary care management of hepatitis B – quick reference (HBV-QR) Available from: https://www.canada .ca/en/public-health/services/reports-publications/primary-care -management-hepatitis-b-quick-reference.html.

269. Aberg JA, Gallant JE, Ghanem KG, Emmanuel P, Zingman BS, Horberg MA; Infectious Diseases Society of America. Primary care guidelines for the management of persons infected with HIV: 2013 update by the HIV medicine association of the Infectious Diseases Society of America. Clin Infect Dis. 2014 Jan;58(1):e1–34.

270. Public Health Agency of Canada [Internet]. Ottawa: Government of Canada; 2017 Mar [updated 2017 Jun 29; cited 2019 Mar 27]. Canadian immunization guide: part 4 – active vaccines: hepatitis B vaccine. Available from: https://www.canada.ca/en/public-health/services /publications/healthy-living/canadian-immunization-guide-part-4 -active-vaccines/page-7-hepatitis-b-vaccine.html#a7.

271. CATIE [Internet]. Toronto: CATIE; [ited 2019 Mar 27]. Hepatitis C basics. Available from: https://www.catie.ca/en/basics/hepatitis-c.

272. Fisher MJ, Richardson D. Consider acute hepatitis C, syphilis, and HIV in MSM with hepatitis. BMJ. 2011 Aug;343 aug16 2:d5169.

273. Garg S, Taylor LE, Grasso C, Mayer KH. Prevalent and incident hepatitis C virus infection among HIV-infected men who have sex with men engaged in primary care in a Boston community health center. Clin Infect Dis. 2013 May;56(10):1480–7.

274. van der Helm JJ, Prins M, del Amo J, Bucher HC, Chêne G, Dorrucci M, et al.; CASCADE Collaboration. The hepatitis C epidemic among HIV-positive MSM: incidence estimates from 1990 to 2007. AIDS. 2011 May 15;25(8):1083–91.

275. Zhang L, Zhang D, Yu B, Wang S, Liu Y, Wang J, et al. Prevalence of HIV infection and associated risk factors among men who have sex with men (MSM) in Harbin, P. R. China. PLoS One. 2013;8(3):e58440.

276. Schmidt AJ, Rockstroh JK, Vogel M, An der Heiden M, Baillot A, Krznaric I, et al. Trouble with bleeding: risk factors for acute hepatitis C among HIV-positive gay men from Germany – a case-control study. PLoS One. 2011 Mar 8;6(3):e17781.

277. Urbanus AT, Van De Laar TJ, Geskus R, Vanhommerig JW, Van Rooijen MS, Schinkel J, et al. Trends in hepatitis C virus infections among MSM attending a sexually transmitted infection clinic; 1995–2010. AIDS. 2014 Mar 13;28(5):781–90.

278. Hagan H, Jordan AE, Neurer J, Cleland CM. Incidence of sexually transmitted hepatitis C virus infection in HIV-positive men who have sex with men. AIDS. 2015 Nov;29(17):2335–45.

279. Public Health Agency of Canada [Internet]. Ottawa: Government of Canada; 2012 [cited 2019 Mar 27]. Hepatitis C fact sheet. Available from: https://www.canada.ca/en/public-health/services/surveillance/blood-safety-contribution-program/bloodborne-pathogens-section/hepatitis/hepatitis-fact-sheet.html.

280. Muzny CA, Rivers CA, Mena LA, Schwebke JR. Genotypic characterization of Trichomonas vaginalis isolates among women who have sex with women in sexual partnerships. Sex Transm Dis. 2012;39(7):556–8. doi:10.1097/OLQ.0b013e31824f1c49.

281. Kellock D, O'Mahony CP. Sexually acquired metronidazole-resistant trichomoniasis in a lesbian couple. Genitourin Med. 1996;72:60–1.

282. Hoffman CM, Fritz L, Radebe O, Dubbink JH, McIntyre JA, Kock MM, et al. Rectal Trichomonas vaginalis infection in South African men who have sex with men. Int J STD AIDS. 2018 Dec;29(14):1444–7. doi:10.1177/0956462418788418.

283. Kelley CF, Rosenberg ES, O'Hara BM, Sanchez T, del Rio C, Sullivan PS. Prevalence of urethral Trichomonas vaginalis in black and white men who have sex with men. Sex Transm Dis. 2012 Sep;39(9):739.

284. van der Veer C, van Rooijen MS, Himschoot M, de Vries HJ, Bruisten SM. Trichomonas vaginalis and Mycoplasma genitalium: age-specific prevalence and disease burden in men attending a sexually transmitted infections clinic in Amsterdam, the Netherlands. Sex Transm Infect. 2016 Feb;92(1):83–5.

285. Peterman TA, Tian LH, Metcalf CA, Satterwhite CL, Malotte CK, DeAugustine N, et al.; RESPECT-2 Study Group. High incidence of new sexually transmitted infections in the year following a sexually transmitted infection: a case for rescreening. Ann Intern Med. 2006 Oct 17;145(8):564–72.

286. Sutton M, Sternberg M, Koumans EH, McQuillan G, Berman S, Markowitz L. The prevalence of Trichomonas vaginalis infection among reproductive-age women in the United States, 2001–2004. Clin Infect Dis. 2007 Nov 15;45(10):1319–26.

287. Peterman TA, Tian LH, Metcalf CA, Malotte CK, Paul SM, Douglas JM Jr; RESPECT-2 Study Group. Persistent, undetected Trichomonas vaginalis infections? Clin Infect Dis. 2009 Jan 15;48(2):259–60.

288. Gatski M, Kissinger P. Observation of probable persistent, undetected Trichomonas vaginalis infection among HIV-positive women. Clin Infect Dis. 2010 Jul 1;51(1):114–15.

289. Krieger JN. Trichomoniasis in men: old issues and new data. Sex Transm Dis. 1995 Mar-Apr;22(2):83–96.

290. Krieger JN, Verdon M, Siegel N, Holmes KK. Natural history of urogenital trichomoniasis in men. J Urol. 1993 Jun;149(6):1455–8.
291. Schwebke JR, Rompalo A, Taylor S, Seña AC, Martin DH, Lopez LM, et al. Re-evaluating the treatment of nongonococcal urethritis: emphasizing emerging pathogens–a randomized clinical trial. Clin Infect Dis. 2011 Jan 15;52(2):163–70.
292. Moodley P, Wilkinson D, Connolly C, Moodley J, Sturm AW. Trichomonas vaginalis is associated with pelvic inflammatory disease in women infected with human immunodeficiency virus. Clin Infect Dis. 2002 Feb;34(4):519–22.
293. Anderson BL, Firnhaber C, Liu T, Swarts A, Siminya M, Ingersoll J, et al. Effect of trichomoniasis therapy on genital HIV viral burden among African women. Sex Transm Dis. 2012 Aug;39(8):638–42.
294. Kissinger P, Amedee A, Clark RA, Dumestre J, Theall KP, Myers L, et al. Trichomonas vaginalis treatment reduces vaginal HIV-1 shedding. Sex Transm Dis. 2009 Jan;36(1):11–16.
295. Howe K, Kissinger PJ. Single-dose compared with multidose metronidazole for the treatment of trichomoniasis in women: a meta-analysis. Sex Transm Dis. 2017 Jan;44(1):29–34.
296. Kissinger P, Muzny CA, Mena LA, Lillis RA, Schwebke JR, Beauchamps L, et al. Single-dose versus 7-day-dose metronidazole for the treatment of trichomoniasis in women: an open-label, randomised controlled trial. Lancet Infect Dis. 2018 Nov;18(11):1251–9.
297. Aragón TJ, Vugia DJ, Shallow S, Samuel MC, Reingold A, Angulo FJ, et al. Case-control study of shigellosis in San Francisco: the role of sexual transmission and HIV infection. Clin Infect Dis. 2007;44:327–34.
298. Weir E. Shigella: wash your hands of the whole dirty business. CMAJ. 2002;167(3):281.
299. Huebner J, Czerwenka W, Gruner E, von Graevenitz A. Shigellemia in AIDS patients: case report and review of the literature. Infection. 1993;21(2):122–4.
300. Lolekha S, Vibulbandhitkit S, Poonyarit P. Response to antimicrobial therapy for shigellosis in Thailand. Rev Infect Dis. 1991 Mar-Apr;13 Suppl 4:S342–6.
301. Hoffmann C, Sahly H, Jessen A, Ingiliz P, Stellbrink HJ, Neifer S, et al. High rates of quinolone-resistant strains of Shigella sonnei in HIV-infected MSM. Infection. 2013;41:999–1003. doi:10.1007/s15010-013-0501-4.
302. Baker KS, Dallman TJ, Ashton PM, Day M, Hughes G, Crook PD, et al. Intercontinental dissemination of azithromycin-resistant shigellosis through sexual transmission: a cross-sectional study. Lancet Infect Dis. 2015;15:913–21. doi:10.1016/S1473-3099(15)00002-X.

303. Bowen A, Grass J, Bicknese A, Campbell D, Hurd J, Kirkcaldy RD. Elevated risk for antibiotic drug-resistant Shigella infection among men who have sex with men, United States, 2011–2015. Emerg Infect Dis. 2016;22(9):1613–16. doi:10.3201/eid2209.160624.

304. Escobedo AA, Almirall P, Alfonso M, Cimerman S, Chacín-Bonilla L. Sexual transmission of giardiasis: a neglected route of spread? Acta Trop. 2014;132:106–11. doi:10.1016/j.actatropica.2013.12.025.

305. López CE, Dykes AC, Juranek DD, Sinclair SP, Conn JM, Christie RW, et al. Waterborne giardiasis: a communitywide outbreak of disease and a high rate of asymptomatic infection. Am J Epidemiol. 1980;112(4):495–507.

306. Nash TE, Herrington DA, Losonsky GA, Levine MM. Experimental human infections with Giardia lamblia. J Infect Dis. 1987;156(6):974–84.

307. Pickering LK, Woodward WE, DuPont HL, Sullivan P. Occurrence of Giardia lamblia in children at day care centers. J Pediatr. 1984;104(4):522–6.

308. Chandy E, McCarthy J. Evidence behind the WHO guidelines: hospital care for children: what is the most appropriate treatment for giardiasis? J Trop Pediatr. 2009;55(1):5–7. doi:10.1093/tropej/fmn073.

309. Showler AJ, Boggild AK. Entamoeba histolytica. CMAJ. 2013;185(12):1064.

310. Brindicci G, Picciarelli C, Fumarola L, Carbonara S, Stano F, Ciracì E, et al. Amoebic hepatic abscesses in an HIV-positive patient. AIDS Patient Care STDS. 2006;20(9):606–11.

311. Salit IE, Khairnar K, Gough K, Pillai DR. A possible cluster of sexually transmitted Entamoeba histolytica: genetic analysis of a highly virulent strain. Clin Infect Dis. 2009;49:346–53. doi:10.1086/600298.

312. Gatti S, Cevini C, Bernuzzi AM, Bruno A, Scaglia M. Symptomatic and asymptomatic amoebiasis in two heterosexual couples. Ann Trop Med Parasitol. 1999;93(8):829–34.

313. Vreden SG, Visser LG, Verweij JJ, Blotkamp J, Stuiver PC, Aguirre A, et al. Outbreak of amebiasis in a family in the Netherlands. Clin Infect Dis. 2000;31(4):1101–4.

314. Abdolrasouli A, de Vries HJ, Hemmati Y, Roushan A, Hart J, Waugh MA. Sexually transmitted penile amoebiasis in Iran: a case series. Sex Transm Infect. 2012;88:585–8. doi:10.1136/sextrans-2012-050577.

315. Morán P, Rojas L, Cerritos R, Zermeño V, Valadez A, de Oca GM, et al. Case report: cutaneous amebiasis: the importance of molecular diagnosis of an emerging parasitic disease. Am J Trop Med Hyg. 2013;88(1):186–90. doi:10.4269/ajtmh.2012.12-0278.

316. Fotedar R, Stark D, Beebe N, Marriott D, Ellis J, Harkness J. Laboratory diagnostic techniques for Entamoeba species. Clin Microbiol Rev. 2007;20(3):511–32. doi:10.1128/CMR.00004-07.

317. Haque, R, Huston CD, Hughes M, Houpt E, Petri WA. Amebiasis. N Engl J Med. 2003 Apr;348(16):1565–73.

318. Public Health Agency of Canada [Internet]. Ottawa: Government of Canada; 2017 [cited 2019 Mar 23]. Supplementary statement for the management of Lymphogranuloma venereum (LGV) cases and contacts: Canadian guidelines on sexually transmitted infections. Available from: https://www.canada.ca/en/public-health/services/infectious-diseases /sexual-health-sexually-transmitted-infections/canadian-guidelines /sexually-transmitted-infections/canadian-guidelines-sexually -transmitted-infections-47.html.

319. Chelsea and Westminster Hospital NHS Foundation Trust [Internet]. London: Chelsea and Westminster Hospital NHS Foundation Trust; 2019 [cited 2019 Mar 22]. Chlamydia treatment. Available from: https://www .chelwest.nhs.uk/services/hiv-sexual-health/chlamydia-treatment.

320. Hager WD, Brown ST, Kraus SJ, Kleris GS, Perkins GJ, Henderson M. Metronidazole for vaginal trichomoniasis. Seven-day vs single-dose regimens. JAMA. 1980 Sep 12;244(11):1219–20.

321. New Zealand Sexual Health Society [Internet]. NewZealand: New Zealand Sexual Health Society; 2017 Sep [cited 2019 Mar 23]. Trichomoniasis management guidelines. Available from: https:// www.nzshs.org/docman/guidelines/management-of-sexual -health-conditions/trichomonas/177-trichomoniasis -guideline/file.

322. van Schalkwyk J, Yudin MH; Infectious Disease Committee. Vulvovaginitis: Screening for and management of trichomoniasis, vulvovaginal candidiasis, and bacterial vaginosis. J Obstet Gynaecol Can. 2015 Mar;37(3):266–74.

323. Nayak S, Acharjya B. VDRL test and its interpretation. Indian J Dermatol. 2012 Jan;57(1):3–8.

324. Fife KH, Barbarash RA, Rudolph T, Degregorio B, Roth R. Valaciclovir versus acyclovir in the treatment of first-episode genital herpes infection. Results of an international, multicenter, double-blind, randomized clinical trial. The Valaciclovir International Herpes Simplex Virus Study Group. Sex Transm Dis. 1997 Sep;24(8):481–6.

325. Spruance SL, Tyring SK, DeGregorio B, Miller C, Beutner K; Valaciclovir HSV Study Group. A large-scale, placebo-controlled, dose-ranging trial of peroral valaciclovir for episodic treatment of recurrent herpes genitalis. Arch Intern Med. 1996 Aug;156(15):1729–35.

326. Tyring SK, Douglas JM, Corey L, Spruance SL, Esmann J; The Valaciclovir International Study Group. A randomized, placebo-controlled comparison of oral valacyclovir and acyclovir in immunocompetent patients with recurrent genital herpes infections. Arch Dermatol. 1998 Feb;134(2):185–91.

327. Bodsworth NJ, Crooks RJ, Borelli S, Vejlsgaard G, Paavonen J, Worm AM, et al.; International Valaciclovir HSV Study Group. Valaciclovir versus aciclovir in patient initiated treatment of recurrent genital herpes: a randomised, double-blind clinical trial. Genitourin Med. 1997 Apr;73(2):1106.

328. Corey L, Adams HG, Brown ZA, Holmes KK. Genital herpes simplex virus infections: clinical manifestations, course, and complications. Ann Intern Med. 1983 Jun;98(6):958–72.

329. European Association For The Study Of The Liver. EASL clinical practice guidelines: management of chronic hepatitis B virus infection. J Hepatol. 2012 Jul;57(1):167–85.

330. National Advisory Committee on Immunization [Internet]. Ottawa: Public Health Agency of Canada; 2017 Feb [cited 2019 Mar 27]. Update on the recommended use of Hepatitis B vaccine. Available from: https://www.canada.ca/en/public-health/services/publications/healthy-living/update-recommended-use-hepatitis-b-vaccine.html.

331. Shah H, Bilodeau M, Burak KW, Cooper C, Klein M, Ramji A, et al.; Canadian Association for the Study of the Liver. The management of chronic hepatitis C: 2018 guideline update from the Canadian Association for the Study of the Liver. CMAJ. 2018 Jun 4;190(22):E677–87.

332. Hull M, Shafran S, Wong A, Tseng A, Giguère P, Barrett L, et al. CIHR Canadian HIV Trials Network Coinfection and Concurrent Diseases Core Research Group: 2016 updated Canadian HIV/hepatitis C adult guidelines for management and treatment. Can J Infect Dis Med Microbiol. 2016;2016:4385643.

333. Tan DHS, Hull MW, Yoong D, Tremblay C, O'Byrne P, Thomas R, et al.; Biomedical HIV Prevention Working Group of the CIHR Canadian HIV Trials Network. Canadian guideline on HIV pre-exposure prophylaxis and nonoccupational postexposure prophylaxis. CMAJ. 2017 Nov 27;189(47):E1448–58.

334. U.S. Department of Health and Human Services [Internet]. Rockville (MD): Office of AIDS Research; [updated 2018 Nov 29; cited 2019 Mar 26]. Guidelines for the prevention and treatment of opportunistic infections in HIV-infected adults and adolescents. Available from: https://aidsinfo.nih.gov/guidelines/html/4/adult-and-adolescent-opportunistic-infection/343/hpv.

335. Martin DH . Nongonococcal urethritis: new views through the prism of modern molecular microbiology. Curr Infect Dis Rep 2008;10:128–32.
336. Kinney RG, Spach DH [Internet]. Seattle: National STD Curriculum; 2019 [cited 2019 Jun 30]. Vaginitis quick reference. Available from: https://www.std.uw.edu/go/syndrome-based/vaginal-discharge/core-concept/all.
337. Deutsch MB, editor. Guidelines for the primary and gender-affirming care of transgender and gender nonbinary people [Internet]. 2nd ed. San Francisco: UCSF; c2016 [cited 2019 Jun 30]. Available from: https://transcare.ucsf.edu/guidelines.
338. Marrazzo JM, Antonio M, Agnew K. Distribution of genital Lactobacillus strains shared by female sex partners. J Infect Dis. 2009;199(5):680–3. doi:10.1086/596632.
339. Marrazzo JM, Thomas KK, Fiedler TL, Ringwood K, Fredricks DN. Risks for acquisition of bacterial vaginosis among women who report sex with women: a cohort study. PLoS One. 2010;5(6):2:11139. doi:10.1371/journal.pone.0011139.
340. Manhart LE, Khosropour CM, Liu C, Gillespie CW, Depner K, Fiedler T, et al. Bacterial vaginosis-associated bacteria in men: association of Leptotrichia/Sneathia spp. with nongonococcal urethritis. Sex Transm Dis. 2013;40(12):944–9. doi:10.1097/OLQ.0000000000000054.
341. Koumans EH, Sternberg M, Bruce C, McQuillan G, Kendrick J, Sutton M, et al. The prevalence of bacterial vaginosis in the United States 2001–2004; associations with symptoms, sexual behaviors, and reproductive health. Sex Transm Dis. 2007;34(11):864–9. doi:10.1097/OLQ.0b013e318074e565.
342. Bradshaw CS, Morton AN, Hocking J, Garland SM, Morris MB, Moss LM, et al. High recurrence rates of bacterial vaginosis over the course of 12 months after oral metronidazole therapy and factors associated with recurrence. J Infect Dis. 2006;193:1478–86.
343. Forcey DS, Vodstrcil LA, Hocking JS, Fairley CK, Law M, McNair RP, et al. Factors associated with bacterial vaginosis among women who have sex with women: a systematic review. PLoS One. 2015 Dec 16;10(12):e0141905. doi:10.1371/journal.pone.0141905.
344. Vodstrcil LA, Walker SM, Hocking JS, Law M, Forcey DS, Fehler G, et al. Incident bacterial vaginosis (BV) in women who have sex with women is associated with behaviors that suggest sexual transmission of BV. Clin Infect Dis. 2015;60(7):1042–53. doi:10.1093/cid/ciu1130.
345. Homayouni A, Bastani P, Ziyadi S, Mohammad-Alizadeh-Charandabi S, Ghalibaf M, Mortazavian AM, et al. Effects of probiotics on the recurrence of bacterial vaginosis: a review. J Low Genit Tract Dis. 2014;18(1):79–86.

346. Amaya-Guio J, Viveros-Carreño DA, Sierra-Barrios EM, Martinez-Velasquez MY, Grillo-Ardila CF. Antibiotic treatment for the sexual partners of women with bacterial vaginosis. Cochrane Database Syst Rev. 2016;10. doi:10.1002/14651858.CD011701.pub2.
347. Marrazzo JM, Thomas KK, Fiedler TL, Ringwood K, Fredricks DN. Relationship of specific vaginal bacteria and bacterial vaginosis treatment failure in women who have sex with women. Ann Intern Med. 2008;149(1):20–8.
348. Marrazzo JM, Thomas KK, Ringwood K. A behavioural intervention to reduce persistence of bacterial vaginosis among women who report sex with women: results of a randomised trial. Sex Transm Infect. 2011;87(5):399–405. doi:10.1136/sti.2011.049213.
349. Beigi RH, Meyn LA, Moore DM, Krohn MA, Hillier SL. Vaginal yeast colonization in nonpregnant women: a longitudinal study. Obstet Gynecol. 2004 Nov;104(5 Pt 1):926–30. doi:10.1097/01.AOG.0000140687.51048.73.
350. Sobel JD. Vulvovaginal candidosis. Lancet. 2007;369:1961–71.
351. Duerr A, Heilig CM, Meikle SF, Cu-Uvin S, Klein RS, Rompalo A, Sobel JD; HER Study Group. Incident and persistent vulvovaginal candidiasis among human immunodeficiency virus-infected women: Risk factors and severity. Obstet Gynecol. 2003 Mar;101(3):548–56. doi:10.1016/S0029-7844(02)02729-1.
352. Eschenbach DA, Patton DL, Meier A, Thwin SS, Aura J, Stapleton A, et al. Effects of oral contraceptive pill use on vaginal flora and vaginal epithelium. Contraception. 2000;62:107–12.
353. Bradshaw CS, Morton AN, Garland SM, Morris MB, Moss LM, Fairley CK. Higher-risk behavioral practices associated with bacterial vaginosis compared with vaginal candidiasis. Obstet Gynecol. 2005;106(1):105–14.
354. Muzny CA, Rivers CA, Parker CJ, Mena LA, Austin EL, Schwebke JR. Lack of evidence for sexual transmission of genital Candida species among women who have sex with women: a mixed methods study. Sex Transm Infect. 2014;90:165–70. doi:10.1136/sextrans-2013-051361.
355. Fong, IW. The value of treating the sexual partners of women with recurrent vaginal candidiasis with ketoconazole. Genitourin Med. 1992;68:174–6.
356. Shihadeh AS, Nawafleh AN. The value of treating the male partner in vaginal candidiasis. Saudi Med J. 2000;21(11):1065–7.
357. Weyers S, Verstraelen H, Gerris J, Monstrey S, Santiago GS, Saerens B, et al. Microflora of the penile skin-lined neovagina of transsexual women. BMC Microbiol. 2009;9:102. doi:10.1186/1471-2180-9-102.
358. Petricevic L, Kaufmann U, Domig KJ, Kraler M, Marschalek J, Kneifel W, et al. Molecular detection of Lactobacillus species in the neovagina of male-to-female transsexual women. Sci Rep. 2014;4:3746. doi:10.1038/srep03746.

359. Toolenaar TA, Freundt I, Wagenvoort JH, Huikeshoven FJ, Vogel M, Jeekel H, et al. Bacterial flora of the sigmoid neovagina. J Clin Microbiol. 1993;31:3314–6.

360. de Haseth KB, Buncamper ME, Özer M, Elfering L, Smit JM, Bouman MB, et al. Symptomatic neovaginal candidiasis in transgender women after penile inversion vaginoplasty: a clinical case series of five consecutive patients. Transgend Health. 2018;3(1):105–8. doi:10.1089/trgh.2017.0045.

361. van der Sluis WB, Bouman MB, Meijerink WJ, Elfering L, Mullender MG, de Boer NK, et al. Diversion neovaginitis after sigmoid vaginoplasty: endoscopic and clinical characteristics. Fertil Steril. 2016 Mar;105(3):834–9.e1. doi:10.1016/j.fertnstert.2015.11.013.

362. Carvalho R, Dilworth P, Docimo S, Cuffari C. Crohn disease of the neovagina and augmented bladder in a child born with cloacal exstrophy. J Pediatr Gastroenterol Nutr. 2009;48(1):106–9. doi:10.1097/MPG.0b013e31815c9341.

363. Froese DP, Haggitt RC, Friend WG. Ulcerative colitis in the autotransplanted neovagina. Gastroenterol. 1991;100:1749–52.

364. Grasman ME, van der Sluis WB, de Boer NK. Neovaginal sparing in a transgender woman with ulcerative colitis. Clin Gastroenterology Hepatol. 2016;14:e73–4.

365. Falk L, Fredlund H, Jensen JS. Signs and symptoms of urethritis and cervicitis among women with or without Mycoplasma genitalium or Chlamydia trachomatis infection. Sex Transm Infect. 2005;81:73–8. doi:10.1136/sti.2004.010439.

366. Edwards T, Burke P, Smalley H, Hobbs G. Trichomonas vaginalis: clinical relevance, pathogenicity and diagnosis. Crit Rev Microbiol. 2016;42(3):406–17. doi:10.3109/1040841X.2014.958050.

367. Critchlow CW, Wölner-Hanssen P, Eschenbach DA, Kiviat NB, Koutsky LA, Stevens CE, et al. Determinants of cervical ectopia and of cervicitis: age, oral contraception, specific cervical infection, smoking, and douching. Am J Obstet Gynecol. 1995;173(2):534–43.

368. Marrazzo JM, Wiesenfeld HC, Murray PJ, Busse B, Meyn L, Krohn M, et al. Risk factors for cervicitis among women with bacterial vaginosis. J Infect Dis. 2006;193:617–24.

369. Samantaray S, Parida G, Rout N, Giri SK, Kar R. Cytologic detection of tuberculous cervicitis: a report of 7 cases. Acta Cytol. 2009;53:594–6.

370. Abou M, Dällenbach P. Acute cervicitis and vulvovaginitis may be associated with Cytomegalovirus. BMJ Case Rep. 2013 Apr;2013 apr19 1:bcr2013008884. doi:10.1136/bcr-2013-008884.

371. Meena V, Bansal CL. Study to evaluate targeted management and syndromic management in women presenting with abnormal vaginal

discharge. J Obstet Gynaecol India. 2016 Oct;66(S1 Suppl 1):534–40. doi:10.1007/s13224-016-0879-x.

372. McClelland RS, Sangaré L, Hassan WM, Lavreys L, Mandaliya K, Kiarie J, et al. Infection with Trichomonas vaginalis increases the risk of HIV-1 acquisition. J Infect Dis. 2007;195:698–702. doi:10.1086/511278.

373. Brunham RC, Gottlieb SL, Paavonen J. Pelvic inflammatory disease. N Engl J Med. 2015; 372:2039–48. doi:10.1056/NEJMra1411426.

374. Weimer AK. Pelvic inflammatory disease in a male patient: the importance of understanding the transgender patient. Proceedings UCLA Healthcare. 2017;21.

375. Jackson SL, Soper DE. Pelvic inflammatory disease in the postmenopausal woman. Infect Dis Obstet Gynecol. 1999;7:248–52.

376. Giesler DM, Casillas MA, Wilson DD, Nodit L. The painful diversity of proctitis in the modern era. Am Surg. 2015;81(12):E408–9.

377. Sigle GW, Kim R. Sexually transmitted proctitis. Clin Colon Rectal Surg. 2015;28(2):70–8. doi:10.1055/s-0035-1547334.

378. Studemeister A. Cytomegalovirus proctitis: a rare and disregarded sexually transmitted disease. Sex Transm Dis. 2011;38(9):876–8. doi:10.1097/OLQ.0b013e31821a5a90.

379. Bissessor M, Fairley CK, Read T, Denham I, Bradshaw C, Chen M. The etiology of infectious proctitis in men who have sex with men differs according to HIV status. Sex Transm Dis. 2013;40(10):768–70. doi:10.1097/OLQ.0000000000000022.

380. Ledouble V, Deflandre J, Delos M, Moerman F, Lismonde JL, Putzeys V. [Acute cytomegalovirus proctitis in an immunocompetent patient]. Rev Med Liege. 2018;73(7):380–3.

381. Carlin EM, Coker RJ, Shafi S, Murphy SM. Group A beta haemolytic streptococcal proctitis in an HIV-positive man. Int J STD AIDS. 1994;5:144–5.

382. Langevin S, Menard DB, Haddad H, Beaudry R, Poisson J, Devroede G. Idiopathic ulcerative proctitis may be the initial manifestation of Crohn's disease. J Clin Gastroenterol. 1992;15(3):199–204.

383. Kishikawa H, Nishida J, Hirano E, Nakano M, Arakawa K, Morishita T, et al. Chronic ischemic proctitis: case report and review. Gastrointest Endosc. 2004;60(2):304–8.

384. Simons R, Candfield S, French P, White JA. Observed treatment responses to short-course doxycycline therapy for rectal lymphogranuloma venereum in men who have sex with men. Sex Transm Dis. 2018;45:406–8.

385. Wray A, Hketarpal S. Balanitis. StatPearls [Internet]. Treasure Island (FL) StatPearls Publishing; 2019 Jan [cited 2019 Mar 25]. Available from: https://www.ncbi.nlm.nih.gov/books/NBK537143/.

386. Pandya I, Shinojia M, Vadukul D, Marfatia YS. Approach to balanitis/ balanoposthitis: current guidelines. Indian J Sex Transm Dis AIDS. 2014;352(2):155–7. doi:10.4103/0253-7184.142415.

387. Peutherer JF, Smith IW, Robertson DH. Necrotising balanitis due to a generalised primary infection with herpes simplex virus type 2. Br J Vener Dis. 1979;55:48–51.

388. Wikström A, von Krogh G, Hedblad MA, Syrjänen S. Papillomavirus-associated balanoposthitis. Genitourin Med. 1994;70:175–81.

389. Babu CS, Vitharana S, Higgins SP. Primary syphilis presenting as balanitis. Int J STD AIDS. 2007;18:497–8.

390. Platsidaki E, Tsimbos I, Vassis P, Tzanetakou V, Rigopoulos D, Kontochristopoulos G. Syphilitic balanitis of Follmann: two case reports. Int J Dermatol. 2019;58:e52–7. doi:10.1111/ijd.14319.

391. Rodrigue RB. Amebic balanitis. JAMA. 1978;239(2):109.

392. Michalowski R. [Trichomonal balano-posthitis: report of 16 cases (athour's transl)]. Ann Dermatol Venereol. 1981;108(10):731–8.

393. Cree GE, Willis AT, Phillips KD, Brazier JS. Anaerobic balanoposthitis. Br Med J (Clin Res Ed). 1982 Mar;284(6319):859–60.

394. Orden B, Manjavacas CG, Martinez R, Franco A. Streptococcal balanitis in a healthy adult male. Eur J Clin Microbiol Infect Dis. 1995;14:920–1.

395. Leverkus M, Mayer J, Bröcker EB, Hamm H. Isolated streptococcal balanoposthitis in an adult patient. Dermatol. 2002;204:153–4.

396. Minami M, Wakimoto Y, Matsumoto M, Matsui H, Kubota Y, Okada A, et al. Characterization of Streptococcus pyogenes isolated from balanoposthitis patients presumably transmitted by penile-oral sexual intercourse. Curr Microbiol. 2010;61:101–5. doi:10.1007/s00284-010-9581-x.

397. Lisboa C, Santos A, Dias C, Azevedo F, Pina-Vaz C, Rodrigues A. Candida balanitis: risk factors. J Eur Acad Derm Vener. 2010;24:820–6. doi:10.1111/j.1468-3083.2009.03533.x.

398. Aridogan IA, Izol V, Ilkit M. Superficial fungal infections of the male genitalia: a review. Crit Rev Microbiol. 2011;37(3):237–44. doi:10.3109/1040841X.2011.572862.

399. Zanwar A, Gupta L, Misra R. Balanitis circinata. Rheumatol. 2018;5:285–6. doi:10.5152/eurjrheum.2018.17153.

400. Charlton OA, Smith SD. Balanitis xerotica obliterans a review of diagnosis and management. Int J Dermatol. 2018. [Epub ahead of print]. doi:10.1111/ijd.14236.

401. Vincent MV, Mackinnon E. The response of clinical balanitis xerotica obliterans to the application of topical steroid-based creams. J Pediatr Surg. 2005;40:709–12. doi:10.1016/j.jpedsurg.2004.12.001.

402. Marcos-Pinto A, Soares-de-Almeida L, Borges-Costa J. Nonvenereal penile dermatoses: a retrospective study. Indian Dermatol Online J. 2018;9(2):96–100. doi:10.4103/idoj.IDOJ_23_17.

403. Zampieri N, Corroppolo M, Camoglio FS, Giacomello L, Ottolenghi A. Phimosis: stretching methods with or without application of topical steroids? J Pediatr. 2005;147:705–6.

404. McConaghy JR, Panchal B. Epididymitis: an overview. Am Fam Physician. 2106;94(9):723–6.

405. Srinath H. Acute scrotal pain. Aust Fam Physician. 2013;42(11):790–2.

406. Voelzke BB, Hagedorn JC. Presentation and diagnosis of Fournier gangrene. Urology. 2018;114:8–13. doi:10.1016/j.urology.2017.10.031.

407. Ha S, Totten S, Pogany L, Wu J, Gale-Rowe M. Hepatitis C in Canada and the importance of risk-based screening. Can Commun Dis Rep. 2016 Mar 3;42(3):57–62.

408. Yaphe S, Bozinoff N, Kyle R, Shivkumar S, Pai NP, Klein M. Incidence of acute hepatitis C virus infection among men who have sex with men with and without HIV infection: a systematic review. Sex Transm Infect. 2012 Nov;88(7):558–64.

409. Burchell AN, Gardner SL, Mazzulli T, Manno M, Raboud J, Allen VG, et al. Hepatitis C virus seroconversion among HIV-positive men who have sex with men with no history of injection drug use: Results from a clinical HIV cohort. Can J Infect Dis Med Microbiol. 2015 Jan-Feb;26(1):17–22.

410. Grad R, Thombs BD, Tonelli M, Bacchus M, Birtwhistle R, Klarenbach S, et al.; Canadian Task Force on Preventive Health Care. Recommendations on hepatitis C screening for adults. CMAJ. 2017 Apr 24;189(16):E594–604.

411. Ooi C. Testing for sexually transmitted infections. Aust Prescr. 2007;30(1):8–13. doi:10.18773/austprescr.2007.005.

412. Centers for Disease Control and Prevention [Internet]. Atlanta (GA): CDC; [last reviewed 2018 Oct 31; cited 2019 Mar 27]. Hepatitis B questions and answers for health professionals. Available from: https://www.cdc.gov/hepatitis/hbv/hbvfaq.htm#general.

413. Centers for Disease Control and Prevention [Internet]. Atlanta (GA): CDC; [last reviewed 2018 Oct 31; cited 2019 Mar 27]. Hepatitis C questions and answers for health professionals. Available from: https://www.cdc.gov/hepatitis/hcv/hcvfaq.htm#section3.

414. Henao-Martínez AF, Johnson SC. Diagnostic tests for syphilis: new tests and new algorithms. Neurol Clin Pract. 2014 Apr;4(2):114–22.

415. Ridzon R, Gallagher K, Ciesielski C, Ginsberg MB, Robertson BJ, Luo CC, et al. Simultaneous transmission of human immunodeficiency virus and hepatitis C virus from a needle-stick injury. N Engl J Med. 1997 Mar 27;336(13):919–22.

416. Marcellin P. Hepatitis C: the clinical spectrum of the disease. J Hepatol. 1999;31 Suppl 1:9–16.
417. National Health Service [Internet]. London, Englasn: NHS; [updated 2016 Jul 11; cited 2019 Mar 13]. How soon do STI symptoms appear? Available from: https://www.nhs.uk/common-health-questions /sexual-health/how-soon-do-sti-symptoms-appear/.
418. Horner PJ, Martin DH. Mycoplasma genitalium Infection in Men. J Infect Dis. 2017 Jul;216 suppl_2:S396–405.
419. Wald A, Langenberg AG, Krantz E, Douglas JM, Handsfield HH, DiCarlo RP, et al. The relationship between condom use and herpes simplex virus acquisition. Ann Intern Med. 2005;143:707–13.
420. Winer RL, Hughes JP, Feng Q, O'Reilly S, Kiviat NB, Holmes KK, et al. Condom use and the risk of genital human papillomavirus infection in young women. N Engl J Med. 2006 Jun;354(25):2645–54.
421. Warner L, Stone KM, Macaluso M, Buehler JW, Austin HD. Condom use and risk of gonorrhea and chlamydia: a systematic review of design and measurement factors assessed in epidemiologic studies. Sex Transm Dis. 2006;33(1):36–51. doi:10.1097/01.olq.0000187908.42622.fd.
422. Pinkerton SD, Abramson PR. Effectiveness of condoms in preventing HIV transmission. Soc Sci Med. 1997;44(9):1303–12.
423. Jennings PR, Bachmann L. A clinician's guide to condoms, spermicides, microbicides, and lubricants. JAAPA. 2005;18(12):61–2.
424. Frezieres RG, Walsh TL, Nelson AL, Clark VA, Coulson AH. Evaluation of the efficacy of a polyurethane condom: results from a randomized controlled clinical trial. Fam Plann Perspect. 1999;31(2):81–7.
425. Petrosky E, Bocchini JA Jr, Hariri S, Chesson H, Curtis CR, Saraiya M, et al; Centers for Disease Control and Prevention (CDC). Use of 9-valent human papillomavirus (HPV) vaccine: updated HPV vaccination recommendations of the advisory committee on immunization practices. MMWR Morb Mortal Wkly Rep. 2015 Mar 27;64(11):300–4.
426. Public Health Agency of Canada [Internet]. Ottawa: Government of Canada; 2015 [updated 2016 Mar 10; cited 2019 Mar 22]. Update on the recommended Human Papillomavirus (HPV) vaccine immunization schedule. Available from: https://www.canada.ca/en/public-health /services/publications/healthy-living/update-recommended-human -papillomavirus-vaccine-immunization-schedule.html.
427. Alimonos K, Nafziger AN, Murray J, Bertino JS Jr. Prediction of response to hepatitis B vaccine in health care workers: whose titers of antibody to hepatitis B surface antigen should be determined after a three-dose series, and what are the implications in terms of cost-effectiveness? Clin Infect Dis. 1998 Mar;26(3):566–71.

428. Nashibi R, Alavi SM, Yousefi F, Salmanzadeh S, Moogahi S, Ahmadi F, et al. Post-vaccination immunity against hepatitis B virus and predictors for non-responders among medical staff. Jundishapur J Microbiol. 2015 Mar 21;8(3):e19579.

429. Bakker M, Bunge EM, Marano C, de Ridder M, De Moerlooze L. Immunogenicity, effectiveness and safety of combined hepatitis A and B vaccine: a systematic literature review. Expert Rev Vaccines. 2016 Jul;15(7):829–51.

430. Geretti AM, Doyle T. Immunization for HIV-positive individuals. Curr Opin Infect Dis. 2010 Feb;23(1):32–8.

431. Cruciani M, Mengoli C, Serpelloni G, Lanza A, Gomma M, Nardi S, et al. Serologic response to hepatitis B vaccine with high dose and increasing number of injections in HIV infected adult patients. Vaccine. 2009 Jan 1;27(1):17–22.

432. Lopes VB, Hassing RJ, de Vries-Sluijs TE, El Barzouhi A, Hansen BE, Schutten M, et al. Long-term response rates of successful hepatitis B vaccination in HIV-infected patients. Vaccine. 2013 Feb 4;31(7):1040–4.

433. Gray RH. Male circumcision for HIV and STI prevention: a reflection. Clin Chem. 2019;65(1):15–18. doi:10.1373/clinchem.2018.286542.

434. Yuan T, Fitzpatrick T, Ko NY, Cai Y, Chen Y, Zhao J, et al. Circumcision to prevent HIV and other sexually transmitted infections in men who have sex with men: a systematic review and meta-analysis of global data. Lancet Glob Health. 2019;7:e436–47.

435. Gray RH, Serwadda D, Kong X, Makumbi F, Kigozi G, Gravitt PE, et al. Male circumcision decreases acquisition and increases clearance of high-risk human papillomavirus in HIV-negative men: a randomized trial in Rakai, Uganda. J Infect Dis. 2010;201(10):1455–62. doi:10.1086/652184.

436. Gray RH, Kigozi G, Serwadda D, Makumbi F, Nalugoda F, Watya S, et al. The effects of male circumcision on female partners' genital tract symptoms and vaginal infections in a randomized trial in Rakai, Uganda. Am J Obstet Gynecol. 2009;200(1):42.e1–7. doi:10.1016/j. ajog.2008.07.069.

437. Pintye J, Drake AL, Unger JA, Matemo D, Kinuthia J, McClelland RS, et al. Male partner circumcision associated with lower Trichomonas vaginalis incidence among pregnant and postpartum Kenyan women: a prospective cohort study. Sex Transm Infect. 2017;93(2):137–43. doi:10.1136/sextrans-2016-052629.

438. Tobian AA, Serwadda D, Quinn TC, Kigozi G, Gravitt PE, Laeyendecker O, et al. Male circumcision for prevention of HSV-2 and HPV infections and syphilis. N Engl J Med. 2009 Mar;360(13):1298–309. doi:10.1056/NEJMoa0802556.

439. Homfray V, Tanton C, Miller RF, Beddows S, Field N, Sonnenberg P, et al. Male circumcusion and STI acquisition in Britain: evidence from a national probability sample survey. PLoS One. 2015 Jun;10(6):e0130396. doi:10.1371/journal.pone.0130396.

440. Van Howe RS. Sexually transmitted infections and male circumcision: a systematic review and meta-analysis. ISRN Urol. 2013 Apr;2013:109846. doi:10.1155/2013/109846.

441. Hoang T, Date AA, Ortiz JO, Young TW, Bensouda S, Xiao P, et al. Development of rectal enema as microbicide (DREAM): preclinical progressive selection of a tenofovir prodrug enema. Eur J Pharm Biopharm. 2019;138:23–9. doi:10.1016/j.ejpb.2018.05.030.

442. McCormack S, Dunn DT, Desai M, Dolling DI, Gafos M, Gilson R, et al. Pre-exposure prophylaxis to prevent the acquisition of HIV-1 infection (PROUD): effectiveness results from the pilot phase of a pragmatic open-label randomised trial. Lancet. 2016;387:53–60. doi:10.1016 /S0140-6736(15)00056-2.

443. Newcomb ME, Moran K, Feinstein BA, Forscher E, Mustanski B. Pre-exposure prophylaxis (PrEP) use and condomless anal sex: evidence of risk compensation in a cohort of young men who have sex with men. J Acquir Immune Defic Syndr. 2018;77:358–64.

444. Molina JM, Charreau I, Chidiac C, Pialoux G, Cua E, Delaugerre C, et al.; ANRS IPERGAY Study Group. Post-exposure prophylaxis with doxycycline to prevent sexually transmitted infections in men who have sex with men: an open-label randomised substudy of the ANRS IPERGAY trial. Lancet Infect Dis. 2018;18:308–17. doi:10.1016 /S1473-3099(17)30725-9.

445. Bolan RK, Beymer MR, Weiss RE, Flynn RP, Leibowitz AA, Klausner JD. Doxycycline prophylaxis to reduce incident syphilis among HIV-infected men who have sex with men who continue to engage in high-risk sex: a randomized controlled pilot study. Sex Transm Dis. 2015;42(2):98–103. doi:10.1097/OLQ.0000000000000216.

446. Public Health England [Internet]. London, England: Government of UK; 2017 Nov 3 [cited 2019 May 20]. Position statement on doxycycline as post-exposure prophylaxis for sexually transmitted infections. Available from: https://www.gov.uk/government/publications/doxycycline -as-post-exposure-prophylaxis-for-stis-phe-response.

447. Siguier M, Molina JM. Doxycycline prophylaxis for bacterial sexually transmitted infections: promises and perils. ACS Infect Dis. 2018;4:660–3. doi:10.1021/acsinfecdis.8b00043.

448. Torres TS, Hoagland B, Bezerra DRB, Garner A, Jalil EM, Coelho LE, et al. Impact of COVID-19 pandemic on sexual minority populations in Brazil: an analysis of social/racial disparities in maintaining

social distancing and a description of sexual behaviour. AIDS Behav. 2020;25:73–84. doi:10.1007/s10461-020-02984-1.

449. Chow EPF, Hocking JS, Ong JJ, Phillips TR, Schmidt T, Buchanan A, et al. Changes in PrEP use, sexual practice, and use of face mask during sex among MSM during the second wave of COVID-19 in Melbourne, Australia. J Acquir Immune Defic Syndr. 2021;86(2):153–6. doi:10.1097 /QAI.0000000000002575.

450. Delcea C, Chiril VI, S uchea AM. Effects of COVID-19 on sexual life: a meta-analysis. Sexologies. 2021;30:e49–54. doi:10.1016/j. sexol.2020.12.001.

451. Hammoud MA, Maher L, Holt M, Degenhardt L, Jin F, Murphy D, et al. Physical distancing due to COVID-19 disrupts sexual behaviours among gay and bisexual men in Australia: implications for trends in HIV and other sexually transmissible infections. J Acquir Immune Defic Syndr. 2021;85(3):309–15. doi:10.1097/QAI.0000000000002462.

452. Reyniers T, Rotsaert A, Thunissen E, Buffel V, Masquillier C, Van Landeghem E, et al. Reduced sexual contacts with non-steady partners and less PrEP use among MSM in Belgium during the first weeks of the COVID-19 lockdown: results of an online survey. Sex Transm Infect. 2021;97(6):414–19. doi:10.1136/sextrans-2020-054756.

453. Rogers BG, Tao J, Darveau SC, Maynard M, Almonte A, Napoleon S, et al. The impact of COVID-19 on sexual behaviour and psychosocial functioning in a clinical sample of men who have sex with men using HIV pre-exposure prophylaxis. AIDS Behav. 2021;1–7. doi:10.1007 /s10461-021-03334-5.

454. Hammoud MA, Grulich A, Holt M, Maher L, Murphy D, Jin F, et al. Substantial decline in use of HIV preexposure prophylaxis following introduction of COVID-19 physical distancing protocols in Australia: results from a prospective observational study of gay and bisexual men. J Acquir Immune Defic Syndr. 2021;86(1):22–30. doi:10.1097 /QAI.0000000000002514.

455. Jongen VW, Zimmerman HML, Boyd A, Hoornenborg E, van den Elshout MAM, Davidovich U, et al. Transient changes in pre-exposure prophylaxis use and daily sexual behaviour after the implementation of COVID-19 restrictions among men who have sex with men. J Acquir Immune Defic Syndr. 2021;87(5):1111–18. doi:10.1097 /QAI.0000000000002697.

456. Pampati S, Emrick K, Siegler AJ, Jones J. Changes in sexual behaviour, PrEP adherence, and access to sexual health services because of the COVID-19 pandemic among a cohort of PrEP-using MSM in the South. J Acquir Immune Defic Syndr. 2021;81(1):639–43. doi:10.1097 /QAI.0000000000002640.

457. Walsh AR, Sullivan S, Stephenson R. Are male couples changing their sexual agreements and behaviours during the COVID-19 pandemic? AIDS Behav. 2021;1–6. doi:10.1007/s10461-021-03256-2.
458. Holloway IW, Garner A, Tan D, Ochoa AM, Santos M, Howell S. Associations between physical distancing and mental health, sexual health and technology use among gay, bisexual and other men who have sex with men during the COVID-19 pandemic. J Homosex. 2021;68(4):692–708. doi:10.1080/00918369.2020.1868191.
459. Walsh AR, Stephenson R. Positive and negative impacts of the COVID-19 pandemic on relationship satisfaction in male couples. Am J Men Health. 2021;15(3):1–14. doi:10.1177/15579883211022180.
460. Hill BJ, Anderson B, Lock L. COVID-19 pandemic, pre-exposure prophylaxis (PrEP) care, and HIV and STI testing among patients receiving care in three HIV epidemic priority states. AIDS Behav. 2021; 25(5):1361–5. doi:10.1007/s10461-021-03195-y.
461. Rao A, Rucinski K, Jarrett BA, Ackerman B, Wallach S, Marcus J, et al. Perceived interruptions to HIV prevention and treatment services associated with COVID-19 for gay, bisexual, and other men who have sex with men in 20 countries. J Acquir Immune Defic Syndr. 2021;87(1): 644–51. doi:10.1097/QAI.0000000000002620.
462. van Bilsen WPH, Zimmerman HML, Boyd A, Coyer L, van der Hoek L, Kootstra NA, et al. Sexual behaviour and its determinants during COVID-19 restrictions among men who have sex with men in Amsterdam. J Acquir Immune Defic Syndr. 2021;86(3):288–96. doi:10.1097/QAI.0000000000002581.
463. Hyndman I, Nugent D, Whitlock GG, McOwan A, Girometti N. COVID-19 restrictions and changing sexual behaviours in HIV-negative MSM at high risk of HIV infection in London, UK. Sex Transm Infect. 2021Nov;97(7):521–4. doi:10.1136/sextrans-2020-054768.
464. de Sousa AFL, Queiroz AAFLN, Lima SVMA, Almeida PD, de Oliveira LB, Chone JS, et al. Chemsex practice among men who have sex with men (MSM) during social isolation from COVID-19: multicentric online survey. Cad Saúde Pública. 2020;36(12):e00202420. doi:10.1590/0102-311X00202420.
465. Starks TJ, Jones SS, Sauermilch D, Benedict M, Adebayo T, Cain D, et al. Evaluating the impact of COVID-19: a cohort comparison study of drug use and risky sexual behaviour among sexual minority men in the U.S.A. Drug Alc Dep. 2020;216:108260. doi:10.1016/j.drugalcdep.2020.108260.
466. Stephenson R, Chavanduka TMD, Rosso MT, Sullivan SP, Pitter RA, Hunter AS, et al. Sex in the time of COVID-19: results of an online survey of gay, bisexual, and other men who have sex with men's

experience of sex and HIV prevention during the US COVID-19 epidemic. AIDS Behav. 2021;25(1):40–8. doi:10.1007/s10461-020-03024-8.

467. de Sousa AFL, de Oliveira LB, Queiroz AAFLN, de Carvalho HEF, Schneider G, Camargo ELS, et al. Casual sex among men who have sex with men (MSM) during the period of sheltering in place to prevent the spread of COVID-19. Int J Environ Res Public Health. 2021;18:3266. doi:10.3390/ijerph18063266.

468. Shilo G, Mor Z. COVID-19 and the changes in the sexual behaviour of men who have sex with men: results of an online survey. J Sex Med. 2020;17(10):1827–34. doi:10.1016/j.jsxm.2020.07.085.

469. Maatouk I, Assi M, Jaspal R. Emerging impact of the COVID-19 outbreak on sexual health in Lebanon. Sex Transm Infect. 2021;97(4):318. doi:10.1136/sextrans-2020-054734.

470. Martinez-García L. Rodríguez-Domínguez M, Lejarraga C, Rodríguez-Jiménez MC, González-Alba JM, Puerta T, et al. The silent epidemic of lymphogranuloma venereum inside the COVID-19 pandemic in Madrid, Spain, March 2020 to February 2021. Euro Surveill. 2021;26(18):2100422. doi:10.2807/1560-7917.ES.2021.26.18.2100422.

471. Sacchelli L, Viviani F, Orioni G, Rucci P, Rosa S, Lanzoni A, et al. Sexually transmitted infections during the COVID-19 outbreak: comparison of patients referring to the service of sexually transmitted diseases during the sanitary emergency with those referring during the common practice. J Eur Acad Dermatol Venerol. 2020;34(10):e553–6. doi:10.1111/jdv.16694.

472. Jiang H, Xie J, Xiong Y, Zhou Y, Lin K, Yan Y, et al. HIV self-testing partially filled the HIV testing gap among men who have sex with men in China during the COVID-19 pandemic: results from an online survey. J Int AIDS Soc. 2021;24(5):e25737. doi:10.1002/jia2.25737.

473. Chow EPF, Bradshaw CS, Williamson DA, Hall S, Chen MY, Phillips TR, et al. Changing from clinician-collected to self-collected throat swabs for oropharyngeal gonorrhea and chlamydia screening among men who have sex with men. J Clin Micro. 2020; 58(9):e01215–20. doi:10.1128/JCM.01215-20.

474. Kersh EN, Shukla M, Raphael BH, Habel M, Park I. At-home specimen self-collection and self-testing for STI screening demand accelerated by the COVID-19 pandemic: a review of laboratory implementation issues. J Clin Microbiol. 2021 Oct 19;59(11):e0264620. doi:10.1128/JCM.02646-20.

7 HIV

QUANG NGUYEN

Introduction

The early 1980s saw the onslaught of the AIDS epidemic. It was ruthless and unrelenting. And it attacked the most vulnerable segments of society. In Canada, AIDS nearly wiped out an entire generation of gay men. Fuelled in large part by societal biases, the AIDS crisis was perpetuated by an innate culture of fear and discrimination against the 2SLGBTQ community. As AIDS quickly spread, so did the panic and hysteria. The early days of gay and sexual liberation swiftly became scapegoats for the religious right. Soon AIDS and homosexuality would become synonymous. And as countless gay men were being infected by the merciless virus, they would also be unjustly blamed as its cause.

At the start of the epidemic, a diagnosis of HIV was terminal. Back then, little was known about the risks of HIV transmission, and drug therapies were nowhere in sight. The crisis was met with indifference at all levels of government and complacency within the medical establishment. Yet the arrival of AIDS also unified and strengthened 2SLGBTQ communities across Canada. In the face of political and medical impotence, 2SLGBTQ networks began to rally and mobilize in unparalleled ways. AIDS groups initially came together to engage in social service delivery and education outreach. As the crisis intensified, more militant activism was needed to lobby for clinical trials, medical treatment, and drug funding. The collective response to AIDS became inextricably rooted in the fight for basic health and human rights, a movement that would soon spur important changes to the medical system for all Canadians.

Science has remarkably transformed HIV infection into a manageable chronic disease. With the advent of less toxic and simpler antiretroviral therapy (ART, sometimes now referred to as combination ART or cART), people are now living longer with HIV. In Canada, cardio-vascular disease, diabetes, chronic kidney and liver disease, and mental health disorders are just some of the co-morbid conditions of an aging HIV population. Primary care practitioners (PCPs) with expertise in treating chronic illnesses are well equipped to care for persons living with HIV/AIDS (PLWHA). Preventive medicine that incorporates routine immunizations, regular cancer screening, and ongoing behavioural counselling remains an essential part of HIV primary care. Biomedical strategies such as HIV pre-exposure prophylaxis (PrEP) and post-exposure prophylaxis (PEP) have already become standards of care in HIV prevention. As HIV medicine continues to evolve, PCPs will play an increasingly critical role in the long-term care of HIV-positive patients.

Much has been written about HIV/AIDS. This chapter only scratches the surface. Its intention is to serve as a quick and practical HIV resource guide. The first part takes a more narrative approach. It briefly chronicles the early days of the HIV epidemic and highlights key political, social, and medical events that changed the course of the 2SLGBTQ movement in Canada. The latter part systematically focuses on the science of HIV. It briefly reviews the basic biology of the disease and then informs key recommendations for HIV primary care, including the initial management, treatment, and prevention of HIV. Because of the rapidly changing nature of HIV medicine, readers can appreciate that parts of this chapter may become quickly obsolete. Readers are urged to stay up-to-date with the latest clinical guidelines related to HIV care. Pertinent website information is listed at the end of this chapter. For further optimal management of ART and HIV-associated complications, consultation with an HIV expert is encouraged.

For readers, it is prudent not to think of HIV mainly in medical terms as it discounts and diminishes the social and political impact that HIV has had and continues to have on Canadian history. This chapter provides readers with a glimpse of the past struggles of those afflicted and affected by HIV. In turn, it urges readers to realize that the intersection between sociopolitical advocacy and clinical medicine will remain a vital force in advancing the health care rights of all 2SLGBTQ patients in Canada.

The Start of an Epidemic

In 1981, a new and deadly disease was emerging in North America. By June of that year, the US Centers for Disease Control (CDC) reported a form of atypical pneumonia found among five gay men in Los Angeles, California.[1] By July, the *New York Times* heralded the arrival of a "gay cancer" identified in 41 men in the United States.[2] The lung infection was *pneumocystis carinii* pneumonia and the cancer was Kaposi sarcoma, both uncommon illnesses seen mainly in people with severely compromised immune systems. Soon, similar clusters of the rare conditions were reported among gay men in other major US cities. Though the disease was first thought to be confined to gay men, the CDC later came out with its 4-H list of high-risk groups: homosexuals, hemophiliacs, heroin addicts, and Haitians. The disease soon found its way across the general population but not without leaving behind a stigmatized imprint on the most marginalized in society. Initially dubbed as gay-related immunodeficiency disease (GRID), the illness was renamed in 1982 as acquired immunodeficiency syndrome (AIDS). By 1983, the retrovirus that caused AIDS was isolated, and in 1986, it was introduced to the world as human immunodeficiency virus (HIV).

Although 1981 marked the official arrival of HIV into North American consciousness, the first documented AIDS case was in 1959, retrospectively diagnosed from a blood sample taken from a patient in the Congo.[3] Genetic analyses suggest that HIV may have arrived in the United States around 1968.[4] In Canada, the first AIDS case was retrospectively confirmed in a Montreal man in 1979.[5] Sporadic AIDS cases have been documented before the 1980s, and in hindsight, the AIDS epidemic likely surfaced in the 1970s, undetected and already infecting thousands of people worldwide.

The first formal account of AIDS in Canada was published in the *Canada Diseases Weekly Report* in March 1982.[6] The majority of AIDS cases were initially reported in the three largest cities: Toronto, Montreal, and Vancouver. AIDS was heavily concentrated in gay men but was later seen in hemophiliacs, people who inject drugs (PWID), and those from HIV-endemic countries. Cis women surfaced as a target population in the late 1980s, and more recently, Black, Indigenous, and transfeminine people have been identified as high-risk groups for HIV infection.[7,8] Because of its non-discriminant and inimical nature, HIV continues to remain unconfined to geographic, socioeconomic, and racial boundaries.

In Canada, the dawn of the AIDS epidemic ushered in a period of uncontrolled panic and confusion. Despite revelations that HIV was transmitted through unprotected sex and contact with infected blood, early Canadian media heightened the growing hysteria. They remained focused on individual identities rather than unsafe acts. In doing so, it deepened the AIDS stigma against sexual and gender minorities and reinforced the heteronormative values of an already heterosexist society. By the end of the first decade, 4964 cumulative AIDS cases were reported across the country, with the majority being gay men.[9] Soon the AIDS epidemic became not only a nationwide health issue but also a social one that would demand both a political and a medical response.

HIV Political Landscape

The 1980s saw an upsurge in social and political conservatism in North America. In Canada, the arrival of AIDS coincided with the 1984 federal election of Prime Minister Brian Mulroney and his Progressive Conservative Party. The initial response to the AIDS crisis was one of inaction and prejudicial attitudes that permeated all levels of government. The Mulroney administration mainly worked under a public health paradigm. Its main objective was to prevent the spread of the disease rather than fund much needed research for HIV treatment and social services for PLWHA. Meanwhile, at the provincial level, Nova Scotia and British Columbia were proposing to turn former island leper colonies into isolation camps for those sick with AIDS. BC was also attempting to pass a parliamentary bill that would allow the province to quarantine anyone living with HIV.[10] In Alberta, the government was already enacting legislation to detain and isolate persons who "repeatedly and knowingly" put others at risk of AIDS.[11] And across the country, under the support of the Canadian Medical Association, physicians were looking to break confidentiality by disclosing the HIV status of HIV-positive patients to their sexual partners.[12] As AIDS activist Tim McCaskell once wrote, "the abrogation of civil rights of HIV positive people at such a high level was certainly a political issue," one that would set the stage for a powerful social movement within the 2SLGBTQ community for decades to come.[13]

Around the same time, a nascent political force was growing in the United States. In 1980, Ronald Reagan won the US presidency after unreserved endorsements from the evangelical right. Reagan's landslide victory marked the pernicious rise of the Moral Majority, an ultra-right-wing group whose religious ideologies blurred the lines between church and state.[13] While Reagan embraced its traditional conservative principles, the group steadily became an unyielding force that would influence US social policymaking. As the AIDS crisis intensified, so did the malicious attacks from the evangelical right against those living with the fatal disease. The epidemic soon became a vehicle for US politicians and religious leaders to proselytize and propagate anti-gay sentiments, further broadening the AIDS stigma. Some called for the criminalization of homosexual acts while others declared AIDS as divine punishment for society's gay sexual immorality. Pat Buchanan, a conservative political columnist, referred to AIDS as "nature's revenge on homosexuals" while Jerry Falwell, the infamous Southern Baptist pastor and leader of the Moral Majority, claimed it "the wrath of God upon homosexuals" and "proof of society's moral decay."[14,15] Republican senator Jesse Helms viewed gay men as "morally sick wretches" and believed that there was "not one single case of AIDS in this country that cannot be traced in origin to sodomy."[16] In fact, the 1980s saw the disturbing emergence of another epidemic, one that was socially and politically motivated and involved the repeated systematic assault against the 2SLGBTQ community.

The Reagan administration was firmly shaped by ultra-conservative values under the guise of economic restraint. The government slashed taxes, cut social services, and promoted a right-wing social agenda. In 1987, the Helms Amendment was set in motion to decrease federal AIDS funding and prohibit public education programs that "promoted, encouraged or condoned homosexual sex."[17] Despite AIDS activists advocating for more explicit language to be used in public education and the dissemination of condoms with safer sex campaigns, sex education soon became abstinence-based and aligned with the views of the Moral Majority. During that same year, Reagan instituted a travel ban that prohibited foreigners with HIV from entering the United States under the false pretenses of preserving public safety and economic stability. The ban was met with much protest in San Francisco at the International AIDS conference in 1990, which resulted in the scientific assembly being held outside the United States for more than two decades thereafter. In 2010, the travel ban was lifted by President Barack Obama and the International AIDS conference returned to Washington, DC, in 2012. During the first half of his tenure, Reagan remained steadfastly silent on the AIDS crisis. Only during his second term did Reagan finally mention AIDS in the public forum. Sadly, for the countless people who died of AIDS, any political action by the Reagan government came too late.

The introduction of the Charter of Rights and Freedoms in the early 1980s allowed Canada to forge its own path away from the counter-resistance of the Christian Right. At the time, the country was under a constitutional crisis, with Quebec demanding sovereignty and the western provinces wanting better political representation. Under the Liberal leadership of Prime Minister Pierre Trudeau, the reforms to the Canadian Constitution under the Charter were made to help mollify Quebec sovereigntists and western regionalists by strengthening the pan-Canadian identity.[18] Despite addressing equality rights, the Charter neglected to include protection rights for those experiencing discrimination on the basis of gender identity and expression, as well as sexual orientation. The paradoxical omission was significant as it occurred during the peak of the AIDS crisis where thousands of 2SLG-BTQ community members were dying, all needing access to social services and medical treatment. Nonetheless, the Charter did eventually allow for substantial social and political movements that would later advance human rights protections to the larger 2SLGBTQ community. Notable imminent victories would include the legalization of same-sex marriage in 2005 under Liberal Prime Minister Paul Martin, as well as the revisions to the Canadian Human Rights Act to include sexual orientation in 1996 and, more recently, gender identity and gender expression in 2017 as protected grounds for all Canadians.

At the same time, the guaranteed 2SLGBTQ rights entrenched in the Canadian Constitution were in great contrast to the social conservative politics at play in the United States. In 1986, Georgia enacted anti-sodomy laws that reinforced the moral attacks on the 2SLGBTQ community by fundamentalist Christians. The law was overturned in 2003 by the US Supreme Court but not before being exploited by anti-gay opponents to further their homophobic and heterosexist agenda during the AIDS crisis. In Canada, homosexuality was decriminalized in 1967, by then Justice Minister Pierre Trudeau, who notably affirmed that there was "no place for the state in the bedrooms of the nation."[19] With the Charter in effect, along with the deregulation of homosexuality, any countermeasure attempts to oppose and attack the 2SLGBTQ AIDS movement were subsequently met with multiple defeats in Canada.

With the election of Prime Minister Justin Trudeau in 2016, the political legacy of the Trudeau family had come full circle. In 2017, Justin Trudeau offered a historic and long overdue national apology for the federal government's previous mistreatment of its 2SLGBTQ public servants. In that same year, on World AIDS Day, his government announced that it would dedicate another $36.7 million in research and projects to help eradicate AIDS nationwide.[20] Throughout the course of the AIDS epidemic, Canada firmly distinguished itself as a beacon for progressive values. In doing so, it has become a leader in championing 2SLGBTQ rights and AIDS advocacy worldwide.

HIV Social Movement

In February 1981, four bathhouses in Toronto were raided by law enforcement. Covertly known as "Operation Soap," the event prompted the gay community to vehemently take to the streets and demonstrate against civil rights violations and police harassment. Often viewed as the Canadian equivalent to the 1969 US Stonewall Riots, the Toronto bathhouse raids signified a pivotal shift in the gay rights movement in Canada.[21] Similar raids on gay establishments followed in major cities across the country and were equally greeted by mass protests from the community. A new era of gay liberation and renewed sexual freedom soon emerged in North America. But then came AIDS. All of a sudden, the important contributions of gay activists were being undermined. As pioneer activists died of AIDS, the gay sexual revolution quickly became the target of religious zealotry and would be wrongly accused of causing the epidemic. Among those who lived, many would embark on another movement, one that would eventually see them fighting for the fundamental rights of those living with the fatal disease.

The early arrival of AIDS in Canada forced 2SLGBTQ communities to extensively mobilize and care for their own. The grass-roots organization of 2SLGBTQ networks led to the creation of numerous community-based AIDS groups across Canada. The groups were formed mainly from existing activists, including transgender and lesbian advocates, from the early days of gay liberation. In the face of political and medical inertia, the 2SLGBTQ community and its allies took on the principal role of offering social, psychological, and spiritual support to dying friends and family. As people succumbed to AIDS, important ethical and medicolegal issues arose that challenged existing health systems. These included the hospital visitation rights of same-sex partners, their right to be involved in medical decision making, and the rights of persons wanting to die with dignity during end-of-life treatment. Ironically, the AIDS crisis paved the way for major advancements in gay rights, in addition to basic health and human rights for all Canadians.

Three distinct AIDS groups emerged across Canada during the AIDS epidemic. First were the conventional AIDS service organizations (ASOs) like AIDS Vancouver and the AIDS Committee of Toronto (ACT). These ASOs were well financed through government and corporations. They were more depoliticized and were often criticized for being too bureaucratic. Their priorities were aimed at social services delivery, as well as HIV outreach and prevention education. They were tasked with providing counselling support, hospice services, food and housing assistance, financial and legal aid, and spiritual care. Their education campaigns highlighted safer sex practices through condom distribution and were in stark contrast to the abstinence-based approach of the Christian Right.[17,22]

Second were the AIDS groups formed by PLWHA. These groups often branched away from the constraints of existing ASOs and were more politically inclined to advocate for issues neglected by ASOs.[23]

In 1983, during the National Lesbian and Gay Conference in Denver, a small group of PLWHA formed the Denver Principles, a defining moment in AIDS activism. The activists bravely identified themselves as "people with AIDS" and condemned those who would label them as "victims." They outlined a set of basic human rights for all people living with AIDS, articulating the need for fair access to medical care without discrimination, the capacity to make informed decisions around treatment, the right to privacy and respect, the chance to live fulfilling human lives, and the opportunity to die with dignity.[24] The declaration signified the beginning of the AIDS self-empowerment movement and, for many in the 2SLGBTQ community, the birth of AIDS activism. Today, the Denver Principles continue to resonate throughout the practice of medicine, inspiring many to change the way they think about illness and lending a collective voice to other patient groups, most notably to the breast cancer survivors' movement.[25]

The last of the AIDS groups were more militant in nature. They criticized the mass media for its promulgation of societal prejudices and stigmatization of AIDS. They excoriated the government for its inaction in social services delivery and AIDS research funding. And they confronted the pharmaceutical industry for its inaccessible and often unethical scientific practices. Through their radical demonstrations and civil disobedience, they were able to demand patient representation at all levels of HIV/AIDS policymaking. Modelled under the AIDS Coalition to Unleash Power (ACT UP), a radical protest group with roots in New York City, many factions of ACT UP came to exist in Canada. In Toronto, AIDS Action Now! (AAN!) was formed in early 1987, a similar militant group that would soon galvanize the AIDS movement and bring fundamental changes to the HIV/AIDS national landscape.[17,23]

Multiple regional and linguistic differences existed between the AIDS groups in Canada. In Vancouver, the AIDS epidemic emerged under an intolerant right-wing provincial government that restricted funding allocation to AIDS groups. At the time, Vancouver had the highest incidence of AIDS per capita in the country.[15] In response to the political indifference, AIDS Vancouver was created in 1983 and became the first community-based ASO in Canada. In 1986, the first Canadian PLWHA group was formed within AIDS Vancouver. The group eventually broke away from its parent ASO and received its own federal funding to become the PWA Society of Vancouver. An ACT UP chapter would also emerge from the city. Over the years, financial disputes and varying political views created a strain among the AIDS organizations in Vancouver.[23]

Meanwhile in Montreal, the Comité Sida Aide Montreal (CSAM) became a mainstream ASO in 1983. It was followed by a PLWHA splinter group in 1987 and the appearance of an ACT UP group in 1990. At the time, the Quebec government had a very strong decentralized healthcare system that limited provincial funding to the AIDS crisis. Linguistic and cultural barriers further fractured the AIDS response in Quebec. CSAM was predominantly being accessed by gay anglophones while many gay francophones were still unconvinced that AIDS was real. HIV was also affecting large Haitian communities in the city, which added to the diverse mix of people that the AIDS organizations needed to support. In turn, divisions within the community and between AIDS organizations undercut any collective political action.[15,23]

In contrast, the AIDS organizations in Toronto were able to interact cohesively by learning to respect and appreciate the important work of individual member activists from all AIDS groups. As a result, they wielded significant influence over government policies relating to HIV/AIDS.[23] ACT was created in 1983 and four years later, the PWA Foundation of Toronto was formed. With both AIDS groups working together to help educate and care for the community, the more radical AAN! was able to realize its political agenda. The unified response to the AIDS crisis also extended to minority groups. Targeted community services were being offered by the Black Coalition for AIDS Prevention (Black CAP) and by the Asian Community AIDS Services (ACAS) in Toronto.

In the late 1980s, AAN! became a powerful political force in Canada. With its militant activism, the group managed to make AIDS a nationwide political issue. AAN! highly criticized the lack of government leadership in the testing and regulation of new HIV drugs. The group's first priority was to advocate for fair access to clinical drug trials and experimental HIV treatment. In 1988, AAN! demonstrated in front of the Toronto General Hospital. The members sported coffins and demanded that pentamidine, a drug already approved in the United States for the treatment of *Pneumocystis carinii* infection, immediately be released in Canada. They would later set up the Pentamidine Project and eventually gain access to the drug from the United States.[26,27] That same year, AAN! members protested at the Conference on Clinical Trials in HIV Disease in London, Ontario. There they advocated for easy access to potential life-saving drugs for all PLWHA. AAN! demanded quick entry into clinical trials for PLWHA without fear of discrimination or coercion. Members also condemned the unethical practice of enrolling patients in double-blinded trials where many would die receiving placebo drugs and proposed the use of open arm treatment groups. In addition, the group requested a national surveillance system that would monitor the long-term efficacy and toxicity of new HIV drugs. Endorsed by the Medical Research Council of Canada, AAN! successfully challenged the restrictive and often exploitative ways that big pharma was conducting research. The radical group would soon pave the way for changes in how the country would regulate, fast-track, approve, and monitor other lifesaving drugs in Canada.[13,27]

Another priority of AAN! was to gain access to government funding and establish a treatment registry for knowledge exchange. In May 1988, during the National AIDS conference in Ottawa, AAN! members burned a life-size effigy of federal Health Minister Jake Epp on national television. The event politicized AIDS and shamed the Mulroney government for its lack of commitment to AIDS policy. Shortly after, the government announced over $100 million of federal funding to combat AIDS and its intention to create a national AIDS strategy.[22,27] The strategic plan came to fruition in June 1990 and was made permanent in 1998 under the Liberal government of Prime Minister Jean Chrétien. The plan included the government's renewal of the Clinical Trials Network, a commitment to improve the way drug companies conducted research, and the continuation of the Treatment Information System for AIDS/HIV (TISAH).[13,28] The TISAH was a key victory for AAN! The national database gave patients equal access to current HIV treatment information and provided clinicians with a platform for HIV knowledge exchange. The TISAH would later become part of the Community AIDS Treatment Information Exchange, otherwise known today as CATIE.

Financial access to HIV medications was one of AAN!'s most enduring achievements. Despite the advent of ART, people were still dying of AIDS because of their inability to afford the lifesaving drugs in Canada. In the early 1990s, the group was enmeshed in a battle against Premier Bob Rae and his New Democratic Party (NDP), insisting on a province-wide compassionate drug plan. In November 1994, AAN! activists protested at an NDP conference in Hamilton and threatened to burn an effigy of Rae on World AIDS Day. On November 30th, one day before the planned rally, the Government of Ontario officially announced that it would legislate a catastrophic drug plan for all Ontarians.[13,22] The publicly funded drug plan would subsidize the cost of medications that exceeded a person's ability to pay. Soon similar plans were adopted by other regions in Canada. The Ontario drug plan is known as the Trillium Drug Program, and its success today remains a lasting legacy from AIDS activists to all Canadians.

Throughout the course of the HIV epidemic, community activists unwaveringly viewed HIV as a human rights issue. Unlike other communicable diseases, HIV was a unique and complex biopsychosocial phenomenon that needed its own laws and health policies. This concept of HIV exceptionalism challenged society's prejudicial views on AIDS and criticized the outdated public health models that called for the intrusion into the private lives of PLWHA. As a result, HIV exceptionalism brought on new health initiatives and public policies that would allow for more protected patient rights to privacy, confidentiality, and autonomy in Canada.[29]

HIV Medical Response

Initial efforts by the scientific community to determine the cause of AIDS were significantly skewed. Early speculations attributed the disease to the "homosexual lifestyle." Causal theories included the repeated use of recreational drugs and amyl nitrate inhalants, as well as the continual exposure to semen through ingestion or condomless anal sex.[15] In 1981, the CDC gave the deadly disease a name: GRID. Sadly, it further perpetuated the discrimination and social stigma attached to gay men and AIDS. The medical community was in part to blame for the heightened media frenzy that helped to validate the anti-gay sentiments of the Christian Right. GRID would eventually be renamed AIDS but still invoked much skepticism within the 2SLGBTQ community, especially among gay men who had endured years of being medically pathologized for their sexual orientation.

An early priority for scientists was the hunt for patient zero, the primary source for the AIDS outbreak in North America. In 1984, a Canadian flight attendant by the name of Gaetan Dugas became the face of patient zero. For three decades, Dugas was hypersexualized and vilified by many in the arts, sciences, and media. Through genetic testing, evolutionary biologists in 2016 were able to prove that Dugas was not the first HIV-infected person in North America.[30] It was later discovered that the CDC had initially labelled Dugas as "Patient O," meaning a patient "outside" California, and the letter O was misread as zero in subsequent research. Despite being exonerated, the belief that Dugas was patient zero persists today and is a reminder of the human fallibility of science.

Nonetheless, the AIDS crisis did lead to breakthrough discoveries in virology and new advancements in other scientific fields. In 1983, scientists elucidated the cause of AIDS, a retrovirus that would later become known as HIV. The discovery of HIV validated the biomedical model of AIDS and, in some ways, helped to destigmatize and "de-homosexualize" the disease in future scientific research.[31] Immunologists would assist in the development of HIV antibody testing and facilitate the invention of lifesaving ART. Epidemiologists would characterize the virus by outlining its natural history, tracking its spread in communities, and defining risk factors for its transmission. Sociologists would conduct behavioral research and advise on interventions to help mitigate high-risk acts. And medical clinicians, with the arrival of combination ART, would be able to treat, monitor, and provide comprehensive care to PLWHA. In many ways, the AIDS epidemic helped build capacity across various professions and expedited the bridging of academic sciences with clinical medicine.

Despite the scientific progress seen in the early days of the epidemic, the medical response to AIDS in Canada was somewhat fragmented. Appropriate and swift action was hampered by the lack of coordination and collaboration between governments, public health authorities, medical institutions, and the pharmaceutical industry. In turn, it led to conflicting events and, at times, undesirable consequences. In British Columbia and Nova Scotia, provincial governments were looking to quarantine thousands of PLWHAs under the pretence of public health. This was in stark contrast to Toronto, where the public health department was refusing to shut down bathhouses while working with the gay community to inform and educate members about safer sex behaviours. Meanwhile, the Canadian Red Cross Society was instituting a blanket ban on blood donation by gay men, a criterion that would later be added to Health Canada regulations.[32] And across the country, medical institutions were largely responding with discriminatory health care practices.

It was not uncommon for AIDS patients to be treated inconsistently by the medical profession. Some clinicians were avoiding AIDS patients because of their underlying homophobic views while others were simply terrified of contracting the disease. In hospitals, workers were refusing to empty bedpans and serve food to AIDS patients while same-sex partners were being denied hospital visitation rights. For patients who lived outside major urban areas, HIV referral networks and community supports were limited. The lack of transportation and home care resources and existing linguistic and cultural barriers further exacerbated the problem. Even when HIV drugs were available, there was no way to keep abreast of the current therapies and no means to access the costly medications for patients. At the time, clinical drug trials were being conducted by big pharma under minimal government oversight. Access to trial drugs was unequal and often unethical. And there was no standard protocol in place to help train health care professionals in HIV medicine. Indeed, it was a period when many AIDS patients felt abandoned and betrayed by the medical community, people whom they had entrusted to take care of them during their most vulnerable time of need.[13,27,31]

Nonetheless, the early AIDS crisis was also a period marked by many notable medical contributions and enduring partnerships. Across Canada, pockets of brave medical professionals and AIDS activists assembled their resources and expertise to deliver a unified response to the crisis. Their solutions were community driven and often diverged from the political mainstay. In 1980, Gays in Health Care was formed by a group of health care workers in Toronto who met regularly to discuss topics important to 2SLGBTQ health, including AIDS. Around the same time, the Hassle Free Clinic became a popular medical site for gay men to access HIV prevention education in the city. Despite being illegal at the time, the clinic would soon offer anonymous HIV testing to all its patrons. In 1983, members from Gays in Health Care and the Hassle Free Clinic, along with those from the 2SLGBTQ newspaper *The Body Politic*, came together to address issues around blood donation, the emerging AIDS crisis, and the need for ongoing support for PLWHA. From their meeting emerged what today is known as the AIDS Committee of Toronto.[33]

During the peak of the AIDS epidemic, only a small network of doctors was treating the majority of AIDS patients in Canada. In 1997, St. Paul's Hospital in Vancouver opened Ward 10C, the country's first AIDS unit dedicated to caring for patients with the disease. The unit was eventually repurposed and renamed as the Urban Health Infection Unit, broadening its services to patients with addictions and other infections. At the same time, community physicians across the country were being burdened by an overarching medical system that could not accommodate the needs of their dying AIDS patients. Many doctors knew little about the disease and would often rely on patients themselves for current HIV knowledge. As a result, the Toronto HIV Primary Care Physicians Group was founded in 1987. The doctors provided compassionate care to PLWHA and would regularly meet to discuss HIV-related topics. One of its co-founders, Dr. Philip Berger, went on to establish a mentoring program that supported other physicians caring for PLWHA. In October 1988, the group announced that it was dispensing clean injection equipment to PWID, a contentious move that later paved the way for legal needle-exchange programs across Canada.[28]

In 1992, British Columbia established the BC Centre for Excellence in HIV/AIDS. Under the leadership of Dr. Julio Montaner, the centre provided comprehensive care to PLWHA and helped inform HIV public policies and programs in the province. The centre also created its own set of recommendations for primary HIV care and treatment; clinical practice guidelines that today are accessed and adopted by clinicians all across Canada. Montaner would also become a key player in the research and development of ART. In 1996, during the World AIDS Conference in Vancouver, Montaner announced the arrival of combination triple-drug therapy, a seminal moment that would transform AIDS into the manageable chronic disease it is today. Montaner would go on to become president of the International AIDS Society and later be recognized globally for his HIV treatment as prevention (TasP) strategy.

Another lasting contribution that emerged from the AIDS crisis was compassionate end-of-life care for the terminally ill. Early in the epidemic, as AIDS patients were rapidly succumbing to their illness, many were being shunned by family, friends, and even by those in the medical community. In Toronto, AIDS activists were outraged and repulsed by the human tragedy experienced by AIDS patients in health care institutions. In response, Casey House was established in 1988 and became the first free-standing hospice in Canada dedicated to helping PLWHA die with dignity.

With the advent of ART, HIV-positive persons are now living longer. In turn, a new shift in the medical response to HIV is needed in Canada. PCPs will inevitably play a significant role in this multidisciplinary response. The strength of primary care stems from its central role in the prevention and diagnosis of HIV, as well as its ability to address the multi-morbidities associated with long-term HIV infection. PCPs are uniquely trained for the job as they already have the expertise in managing cardiovascular disease, diabetes, chronic kidney and liver disease, and mental health disorders, all important conditions frequently seen in the HIV population.

HIV in Canada

Approximately 37.7 million people are living with HIV worldwide.[34] In Canada, an estimated one in seven Canadians is unaware of their HIV status.[35] The incidence of new HIV infections in Canada remains high, with 2,122 new HIV cases reported in 2019 (5.6 cases per 100,000 people), with Saskatchewan having the highest provincial diagnosis rate (16.9 per 100,000). Of new infections, nearly 40 per cent were among MSM, who themselves accounted for 56 per cent of all adult male cases in Canada. Indigenous people accounted for almost 25 per cent of new HIV diagnoses but represent only about 5 per cent of the total Canadian population, signifying a high burden of disease among this vulnerable population. Because of limitations to the surveillance system, national HIV estimates for both MSM and Indigenous people may be underreported.[36]

In Canada, provinces and territories have their own legislation for the mandatory reporting of HIV infection. Each regional health authority voluntarily submits HIV and AIDS cases to the National HIV/AIDS Surveillance System (HASS) run by the Public Health Agency of Canada (PHAC). Unfortunately, no standard protocol exists as to what supplementary information should be submitted to HASS. In turn, varying degrees of data collection are seen nationwide. Limitations to HASS include the potential for underreporting, duplication, and missing information, as well as delays and differences in data collection. For example, HIV exposure data are reported by all jurisdictions in Canada except Quebec, while race and ethnicity data are not reported in Quebec and British Columbia, and only reported as Indigenous or non-indigenous in Saskatchewan.[36]

Recent studies suggest that transfeminine people are at high risk of HIV infection yet limited HIV-related data exist for this priority group.[8] Research and surveillance data that do exist frequently come from small sample sizes and are often aggregated with MSM data. At present, many jurisdictions in Canada do not collect HIV epidemiological data on transgender and non-binary persons.[37] This obvious omission continues to highlight the "informational and institutional erasure" of certain sexual and gender minorities from the Canadian healthcare system.[38]

HIV Basics

HIV Nomenclature

There are two distinct types of HIV: HIV-1 and HIV-2. HIV-1 is more pathogenic and accounts for the vast majority of HIV infections worldwide, including in Canada. HIV-2 is endemic to West Africa but through travel and migration, it has been detected in other regions of the world. HIV-2 infection has a slower clinical progression to AIDS than HIV-1 infection. HIV-2 infection is treatable but is inherently resistant to some classes of HIV drugs.[39] Most jurisdictions in Canada employ fourth-generation HIV assays that incorporate both HIV-1 and HIV-2 antibody testing. Current optimal treatment for HIV-2 infection is unclear, and HIV expert consultation is recommended. Given the severity of HIV-1 and its contribution to the current global HIV pandemic, the majority of scientific research has been conducted on HIV-1. The remainder of this chapter will focus mainly on HIV-1.

There are four distinct groups of HIV-1: group M, N, O, and P. Each group emerged from an independent zoonotic transmission of simian immunodeficiency virus (SIV) from monkey to human. Group M is responsible for the current global HIV pandemic and composes 95 per cent of all HIV-1 cases.[40] The other groups are mainly found in West Central Africa. With time, HIV-1 can mutate, leading to genetic variability. Consequently, group M can be further divided into nine clades or subtypes, A-D, F-H, and J-K, as well as circulating recombinant forms. Geographic variations exist among group M strains. Globally, subtype C is the predominant HIV-1 strain. However, subtype B is the most researched, as it is the most prevalent in North America and other high-income countries. Though rare, superinfections can occur when two or more HIV strains are transmitted to the same person.[41,42]

HIV Life Cycle

HIV is a retrovirus that damages and weakens the immune system by infecting and destroying T helper cells, also known as CD4 cells. Since the virus cannot replicate on its own, it requires the host cell to multiply and spread. Current anti-HIV drugs block the various stages of the HIV life cycle. See figure 7.1.

Latent HIV Reservoirs

Upon integration into the CD4 cell genome, HIV can enter a long quiescent state and develop latent HIV reservoirs. In turn, HIV can persist indefinitely despite active ART viral suppression. ART tends to have no effect on viral reservoirs. Adherence to HIV medications is therefore critical as quiescent cells can reactivate at any time. Despite the success of ART in maintaining virologic suppression, latent HIV reservoirs continue to thwart the discovery of any HIV cure.

HIV Natural History

The clinical course of HIV infection is characterized by a depletion in CD4 cells along with an increase in plasma HIV levels, eventually leading to AIDS. There are three main stages of HIV infection: early HIV infection, chronic HIV infection, and AIDS.

Early HIV infection starts from initial infection to the development of detectable HIV antibodies, known as *seroconversion*. The antibodies are usually detected at 4 to 12 weeks by current HIV serologic

Figure 7.1. Diagram of the HIV Life Cycle and Corresponding HIV Drug Classes

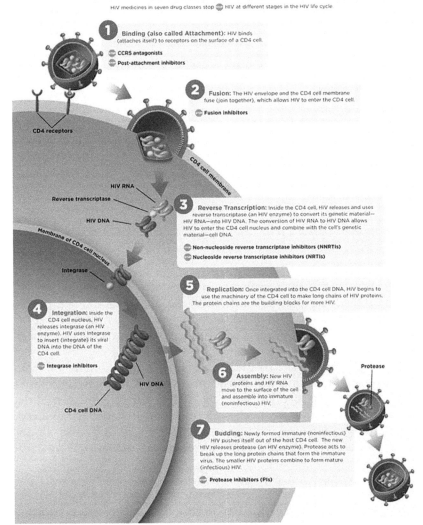

The HIV Life Cycle

HIV medicines in seven drug classes stop HIV at different stages in the HIV life cycle

There are seven major classes of HIV medications. CCR5 antagonists, post-attachment inhibitors, and fusion inhibitors prevent HIV entry into the CD4 cell. Nucleoside reverse transcriptase inhibitors (NRTIs or "nukes") provide chain-terminating proteins that block HIV replication. Non-nucleoside reverse transcriptase inhibitors (NNRTIs or "non-nukes") prevent HIV replication by inhibiting reverse transcriptase. Integrase strand inhibitors (INSTIs) block the integration of viral DNA into the host genome. And protease inhibitors (PIs) prevent the cleavage and maturation of HIV. Familiarity with the HIV drug classes facilitates appropriate ART selection.

Source: US Department of Health and Human Services.[43]

Table 7.1. Signs and Symptoms Associated with Acute HIV Infection

Signs and Symptoms	Frequency (%)
Fever	96
Adenopathy	74
Pharyngitis	70
Rash	70
Myalgia or arthralgia	54
Diarrhea	32
Headache	32
Nausea or vomiting	27
Hepatosplenomegaly	14
Weight loss	13
Thrush	12
Neurologic symptoms	12

Source: Adapted from the US Department of Health and Human Services. 2004.[45]

assays. During this time, patients can present with an acute retroviral syndrome. Described as a flu-like illness, the signs and symptoms are generally non-specific and self-limiting and can last days to weeks. Approximately 40 to 90 per cent of patients will experience clinical symptoms.[44,45] See table 7.1.

The early detection and treatment of acute HIV infection can improve patient health and limit the spread of disease. Clinicians can markedly suppress viral load by initiating ART in a timely manner. Early HIV treatment reduces acute clinical symptoms, lessens HIV-induced inflammation, enhances immune reconstitution of CD4 cells, limits the size of latent reservoirs, and minimizes the risk of onward HIV transmission.[39,46]

After seroconversion, a stage of chronic HIV infection ensues. Also known as *clinical latency*, HIV continues to multiply at low levels while CD4 cells gradually decline. The majority of HIV-positive patients are asymptomatic. Even with minimum immunosuppression, some patients can still display non-specific generalized lymphadenopathy. Without treatment, HIV advances to AIDS in 8 to 10 years.

AIDS is the final stage of HIV infection. AIDS is defined as a CD4 cell count of less than 200 cells/µL or the presence of any AIDS-defining illness regardless of CD4 cell count.[47] See Table 7.2. Without treatment, the median survival of patients living with AIDS is two to three years.

Table 7.2. AIDS-Defining Illnesses

Bacterial	*Mycobacterium avium complex* or Mycobacterium kansasii, disseminated or extrapulmonary *Mycobacterium tuberculosis*, pulmonary or extrapulmonary *Mycobacterium* other species or unidentified species, disseminated or extrapulmonary Pneumonia, recurrent *Salmonella septicemia*, recurrent
Viral	Cytomegalovirus disease, other than liver, spleen, or nodes *Cytomegalovirus* retinitis, with loss of vision Herpes simplex virus, chronic ulcers (>1 month), bronchitis, pneumonitis, or esophagitis Progressive multifocal leukoencephalopathy
Fungal	Candidiasis of the esophagus, bronchi, trachea, or lungs (not oral thrush) *Coccidioidomycosis*, disseminated or extrapulmonary Cryptococcosis, extrapulmonary Histoplasmosis, disseminated or extrapulmonary *Pneumocystis jiroveci pneumonia*
Protozoan	Cryptosporidiosis, chronic intestinal (>1 month) Isosporiasis, chronic intestinal (>1 month) Toxoplasmosis of the brain
Neoplastic	Cervical cancer, invasive Kaposi sarcoma Lymphoma, Burkitt's Lymphoma, immunoblastic Lymphoma, primary brain
Other	Encephalopathy, HIV-related Wasting syndrome, HIV-related

Source: Adapted from the Centers for Disease Control. 2008.[47]

A minority of HIV-positive patients possess high CD4 cell counts and low viremia for many years without ART. Long-term non-progressors have detectable viremia of less than 5000 copies/mL while elite controllers have persistent undetectable viremia. Elite controllers appear to carry a mutation of the CCR5-delta-32 surface marker that prevents HIV from binding to CD4 cells. Long-term non-progressors compose about 1 per cent of all HIV-positive patients worldwide while elite controllers compose much less.[48]

HIV Routes of Transmission

HIV can be found in blood, semen, anorectal and vaginal fluids, and breastmilk. It spreads by entering the bloodstream through broken skin and mucosal membranes. HIV infection can occur during sex, injection drug use (IDU), blood transfusions, occupational exposures, and perinatal transmission. Sharing sex toys without proper disinfection or the use of condoms is also a risk factor. HIV cannot be transmitted through saliva, sweat, tears, urine, or feces. In Canada, HIV is mainly transmitted through sex and the sharing of drug equipment.

HIV in the MSM population

MSM is a term used to capture the broad range of men who engage in sexual activity with other men irrespective of their sexual orientation. In Canada, MSM continue to be disproportionately affected by HIV. Individual risk factors for HIV infection in MSM include unprotected anal intercourse (UAI) or "bareback sex," multiple sex partners, a high number of lifetime sex partners, and IDU.[49-51] The use of recreational drugs has been associated with higher sexual risk behaviour in MSM.[49,51] Club drugs such as methylenedioxy-methamphetamine ("MDMA," "E," "ecstasy," "molly"), gamma-hydroxybutyrate ("G," "GHB," "liquid E"), ketamine ("K," "special K," "vitamin K"), and benzodiazepines ("benzos," "tranks," "roofies") are often consumed at dance clubs, house parties, and raves.[52,53] Sex-associated drugs such as methamphetamine ("crystal meth," "tina," "ice"), mephedrone ("bath salts"), amyl nitrate ("poppers"), and phosphodiesterase type 5 inhibitors (Viagra and Cialis) are thought to facilitate high-risk sex, known as party and play ("PnP") or chemical sex ("chemsex").[52,53] Crystal meth and poppers have consistently been associated with higher rates of HIV infection and other sexually transmitted infections (STIs).[51] Crystal meth use in MSM is 10 times the rate in the general population.[54] For more information on substance abuse in the 2SLGBTQ population see chapter 9.

MSM of colour experience higher rates of racism, poverty, economic instability, incarceration, and internalized homophobia, all of which can potentiate their risk of acquiring HIV infection. They also are less likely to test for HIV.[55,56] With the advent of social-spatial smartphone applications (apps), MSM are now able to access larger networks for sex. Popular mobile apps include Grindr, Jack'd, and Scruff. Some studies show that online sex-seeking by MSM may lead to increased rates of high-risk behaviours and STIs while other data suggest the online behaviour may actually lead to higher rates of STI testing and condom use.[57-60]

The theory of syndemics has been used to explain the high rates of HIV transmission in MSM. Syndemics can be defined as the multiple interrelated epidemics experienced in MSM that can reinforce and compound their risk for HIV infection. The framework also stresses the synergistic effects of social inequities that make MSM more vulnerable to HIV infection.[61] Concurrent syndemic conditions such as polysubstance use, mental illness, and familial violence can be attributed to the intersecting social disparities of poverty, poor access to health care, and stigma.[61,62] As a result, HIV infection should not be seen solely as a discrete biological entity but one that is derived from social, structural, and political forces demanding a multidimensional approach. Clinicians should therefore be aware of the co-existing biopsychosocial needs of MSM. In doing so, they can help address the multiple syndemic factors that currently impede the effectiveness of HIV prevention efforts in MSM.

MSM are adopting various strategies to reduce HIV transmission. Biomedical approaches with scientific support include HIV PrEP and PEP, as well as HIV viral load suppression in HIV-positive patients. At times, other behavioural practices are used in MSM as a risk-reduction approach to HIV prevention.[63,64] Withdrawing before ejaculation during UAI is one such practice. Another practice is negotiated safety, a term used to describe an agreement between regular partners that sets the sexual boundaries allowed in open relationships. Examples include agreeing to UAI only with the main partner, simply having oral sex with casual partners, and consistently using condoms for anal sex outside the primary relationship. Other behavioural strategies include serosorting, in which MSM seek partners of similar HIV serostatus to have UAI, and strategic positioning, in which the HIV-negative partner takes on the insertive role during UAI. Such behavioural practices can only work if open and honest communication is achieved. Regular HIV testing is critical as the effectiveness of these risk-reduction strategies depends on persons having accurate knowledge of their HIV status.

PCPs should inquire about high-risk behaviours in MSM patients in a respectful and non-judgmental manner. They should appreciate the various strategies that MSM employ to mitigate HIV risk. Condoms are effective at reducing both HIV and STI risks. HIV PrEP, PEP, and undetectable viral loads greatly reduce HIV transmission but have no effect on the transmission of other STIs. An HIV-negative patient who strategically positions himself as the insertive partner during UAI should be reminded that he is still at risk for STIs and HIV infection. For the patient who negotiates safety, he should be advised that he is not necessarily safe from STIs and HIV infection, especially when both partners are not forthcoming with their sexual experiences outside the primary relationship. And for the HIV-positive patient who serosorts, he should be informed that he is not only putting himself at risk for other STIs but also the rare possibility of superinfection. PCPs should routinely offer MSM patients HIV and STI screening, risk reduction education, HIV PrEP with condom use, and, if needed, referral to counselling and addiction services in a timely manner.

HIV in the Transgender Population

In Canada, the lack of research and surveillance data has made it challenging to understand the true burden of HIV in the transgender population. Global estimates suggest that HIV rates among transfeminine people are high, with a pooled prevalence of 19.1 per cent among studies of transfeminine people worldwide.[8] Alarmingly, the odds of HIV infection among transfeminine people are 49 times that of the general population.[8] The World Health Organization now considers transgender persons as a key population in its global HIV response.

Multiple factors put transfeminine people at high risk of HIV infection. Similar to MSM, individual risk factors include UAI, multiple sex partners, IDU, and other recreational drug use.[8,65] Syndemic factors include the widespread stigma, discrimination and transphobia that transfeminine people face through societal rejection, economic marginalization, and poor medical access.[66] Evidence also suggest that transfeminine people who have sex with cisgender MSM are at high risk of HIV infection.[8,67] In addition, a high proportion of transfeminine people engage in sex work. Many trade sex for housing and other basic needs, also known as "survival sex," while others are financially incentivized for participating in UAI. The pooled HIV prevalence for transfeminine people who engage in sex work was 27.3 per cent compared to 14.7 per cent in those who did not.[8] Transfeminine sex workers were four times at higher risk of HIV infection when compared to cisgender female sex workers.[8] For some transfeminine people, sex work may be the only means to validate their femininity and seek gender affirmation from sex partners, leaving them less able to negotiate risk reduction strategies during sex. In addition, transfeminine people on hormone therapy may find it difficult to maintain an erection and may forgo condom use altogether.[65]

Little is known about the HIV infection rates of transmasculine people. Current estimates put their HIV prevalence rate at 0 to 3 per cent.[68] Besides the shared individual, social and structural risks seen in transfeminine people, a number of other factors put transmasculine people at risk of HIV infection. Similar to transfeminine people, some transmasculine individuals engage in sex work and survival sex.[68,69]

Transmasculine people are also having sex with cisgender MSM who are at high risk of HIV infection.[69,70] For those on testosterone therapy, an increase in sex drive and a new attraction to cisgender men may occur. For some transmasculine people, the opportunity to have sex with cisgender men is a powerful way to assert their male queer identity, and to them, it may seem more important than negotiating condom use.[71] Transmasculine people on testosterone therapy can also experience vaginal or "front hole" dryness which can put them at risk for STIs and HIV infection.[72] In urban centres, trans MSM may use drugs and engage in unprotected genital sex with cisgender MSM as a way to integrate into the MSM community.

Transgender persons living with HIV tend to present late for HIV care. PCPs should realize that many transgender people will prioritize their gender-related health concerns over seeking HIV treatment. Studies suggest that adherence to hormone therapy is associated with increased adherence to ART in the clinical setting.[73] Providers should therefore be ready to integrate ART with gender-affirming care and hormone therapy. As with MSM, PCPs should regularly inquire about high-risk behaviours in transgender patients. PCPs should obtain a sexual history without making cisnormative assumptions about the anatomy and sexual practices of the patient. Current research is limited around the risk of HIV transmission for surgically constructed genitalia. As with MSM, the syndemics of HIV infection should be addressed. Similarly, PCPs should routinely offer HIV and STI screening, HIV risk reduction education, HIV PrEP with condom use, and, if needed, referral to counselling and addiction services in a timely manner.

HIV Treatment Cascade

The HIV treatment cascade, otherwise known as the HIV continuum of care, is a framework that outlines the stages of HIV care. The cascade consists of early HIV diagnosis, linkage and retention to care, access and adherence to ART, and virologic suppression. In 2014, the United Nations adapted the cascade and proposed its global 90–90–90 HIV Strategy for 2020: 90 per cent of people living with HIV worldwide will be diagnosed, 90 per cent of those diagnosed will receive ART, and 90 per cent of those receiving ART will achieve viral suppression. In 2018, an approximate 62,050 persons were living with HIV in Canada, of whom an estimated 87 per cent were diagnosed. Of those diagnosed, 85 per cent were on ART, and 94 per cent were virally suppressed.[35] The collection of data along the continuum of care can help identify gaps in

HIV services and, in turn, target future interventions to improve HIV prevention and care in Canada.

HIV in Primary Care

With the advent of ART, PCPs are now able to provide comprehensive and longitudinal HIV care. The scope of HIV primary care will depend on the individual comfort level of each provider. PCPs are not expected to initiate ART or manage complex HIV-related complications if they are uncomfortable doing so. Those who feel they are working outside their scope of practice should consider co-managing patients with an HIV expert. Consultation with an HIV pharmacist is encouraged when dealing with ART resistance, toxicity, and drug–drug interactions.

This section aims to provide readers with a framework on how to care for HIV-positive patients in the primary care setting. It incorporates HIV primary care and therapeutic guidelines obtained largely from Canada, the United States, and Europe. The various guidelines are broadly consistent, with a few minor differences. In Canada, the BC Centre of Excellence in HIV/AIDS has published both primary care (BCE-PC) and therapeutic (BCE-TH) guidelines for the management of adult HIV infection, although the latter requires an update of its first-line therapies.[74,75] Links to other HIV guidelines, including those from the US Department of Health and Human Services (DHHS), the Infectious Diseases Society of America (IDSA), the International Antiviral Society-USA Panel (IAS-US), and the European AIDS Clinical Society (EACS), are readily accessible online.[39,76-78] Recommendations on how to care for HIV-positive children and pregnant persons are not addressed in this chapter but can be found in the pediatric and perinatal HIV guidelines published by the DHHS. Information on HIV and fertility is discussed later in the chapter.

Since HIV medicine is rapidly evolving, some of the information in this section will likely become obsolete. Readers should note that although the ensuing HIV recommendations are intended to help clinicians optimize HIV patient care, they ultimately do not replace clinical judgment and medical expertise.

New HIV Patient

INITIAL COUNSELLING
Counselling patients with a new diagnosis of HIV infection may require more than one visit. Patients are oftentimes shocked to receive their diagnosis and may fail to focus on what is being said during the

office visit. PCPs need to be mindful of not just the medical but also the psychological, social, and legal ramifications involved with a new HIV diagnosis. It is important to emphasize that HIV is no longer a fatal disease but one that has evolved into a treatable chronic condition just like diabetes and hypertension. With access to newer, simpler, and less toxic combination ART, HIV patients are now living longer and healthier lives.[79-81] PCPs should identify the psychosocial needs of their newly infected HIV patients. With a new diagnosis, patients will instantly need to confront and live with the societal stigma attached to HIV. Gay patients who had difficulty coming to terms with their sexuality in the past may feel overwhelmed by having to "come out" again to family and friends with their new diagnosis. PCPs should participate in active listening and be ready to validate the experiences and feelings of their patients. It is important to ensure that patients have a safety plan, if need be, upon leaving the office. If patients have no support system, prompt follow-up visits with the provider or interdisciplinary team for emotional support may be warranted, as well as a referral to a counsellor or support group offered by community ASOs.

Counselling also involves assessing patients' HIV knowledge and offering education around safer sex practices and harm reduction. This should be done in a non-judgmental and culturally sensitive manner. PCPs should provide risk reduction counselling to HIV-positive patients to mitigate high risk behaviors that can lead to other STIs, onward HIV transmission, and the possibility of superinfection. Emphasis on partner notification and testing is also important, as well as alerting patients to the involvement of local public health authorities in contact tracing.

The legal implications around HIV non-disclosure should be reviewed. In Canada, the criminalization of HIV is complex and somewhat archaic and is at odds with HIV medical advancements and public health initiatives. Currently, HIV-positive persons who do not disclose their HIV serostatus to sex partners can be charged with aggravated sexual assault, a serious offence that can lead to life imprisonment and registration on the sex offender list. As a result, HIV criminalization further stigmatizes HIV and subsequently deters people from getting tested and accessing treatment. In 2014, prominent Canadian scientists released a consensus statement on HIV transmissibility that refuted the criminal justice system's current misuse of the law against PLWHA.[82] In 2018, the statement was further supported at the 22nd International AIDS Conference in the Netherlands, as HIV experts from around the world announced a global consensus statement on HIV and the law. The experts affirmed that for PLWHA who have a low to undetectable viral load, the probability for HIV transmission during a single sex encounter ranged from negligible to none.[83] An announcement by the Ontario government in December 2017 did show a moderate shift away from the over-criminalization of HIV non-disclosure. The province asserted in prosecutorial guidelines that it will no longer seek HIV non-disclosure charges against HIV-positive persons who are on ART and who have been virally suppressed for at least six months.[84] Changes to the criminal code itself are still pending. Despite this small victory, PCPs are encouraged to provide HIV non-disclosure information to all HIV-positive patients. If needed, PCPs should refer patients to legal counsel for specific legal advice since the laws are still in favour of HIV criminalization across Canada.

HISTORY AND PHYSICAL EXAMINATION

The BCE-PC guidelines provide a comprehensive review of the HIV-related history and physical exam for all HIV-positive patients. The history should generally include past and current co-morbidities, as well as a family history. Current medication and vaccination history should be recorded. Lifestyle behaviors such as diet, exercise, and substance use should be assessed along with financial, immigration, and housing status. A sexual and gender history should be documented. Screening for neurocognitive impairment and mental health disorders should be noted.

A specific HIV-related history should also be obtained. This includes date of confirmatory HIV testing, symptoms of current or prior acute HIV infection, and any diagnoses of opportunistic infections (OIs) or AIDS-related conditions. If the HIV patient is new to the practice, it is necessary to document the patient's most recent CD4 count and HIV viral load, as it may indicate an urgent need for OI prophylaxis. A record of the patient's current and previous ART regimens, as well as any resistance testing and prior adverse reactions to ART, should be noted.

A comprehensive HIV-specific physical exam should be performed. Except in cases of acute or advanced HIV, the physical exam is often unremarkable, although persistent generalized lymphadenopathy can occur.

INITIAL AND FOLLOW-UP BLOODWORK

Baseline bloodwork is indicated for all new HIV-positive patients. This includes laboratory tests specific to HIV and other underlying co-morbid conditions. See table 7.3.

Table 7.3. Baseline and Routine Bloodwork in HIV-Positive Persons on ART

Laboratory Test	At Baseline before ART Initiation	2–8 Weeks after ART Initiation or Modification	First 2 Years after ART Initiation or Modification	After 2 Years on ART with Stable Viral Suppression	Comments
HIV-Specific Tests					
CD4 count	X		Every 3–6 months	Every 12 months if CD4 count 300–500 cells/µL	CD4 monitoring is optional if CD4 count >500 cells/µL after 2 years on ART with stable viral suppression; repeat if treatment failure
HIV viral load	X	X	Every 3–6 months	Every 6 months	Repeat if treatment failure
HIV resistance testing	X				Repeat if treatment failure; some experts routinely order INSTI resistance testing
HIV-Related Tests					
HLA-B5701	X				Prevent hypersensitivity reaction with abacavir
Glucose-6-phosphate dehydrogenase (G6PD)	X				If of Mediterranean, North African or South-East Asian descent; avoid dapsone if G6PD deficient
Hepatitis A serology	X				Immunize if non-immune
Hepatitis B serology (HBsAg, HBsAb, HBcAb)	X				Immunize if non-immune; perform hepatitis B DNA testing if HBsAg negative, HBsAb negative and HBcAb positive
Hepatitis C serology	X				Repeat annually if at high risk*
Other STI testing (chlamydia, gonorrhea, syphilis)	X				Repeat if clinically indicated
Toxoplasma serology	X				If negative, avoid cat feces and uncooked meat

(Continued)

Table 7.3. (Continued)

Laboratory Test	At Baseline before ART Initiation	2–8 Weeks after ART Initiation or Modification	First 2 Years after ART Initiation or Modification	After 2 Years on ART with Stable Viral Suppression	Comments
Co-morbid Tests					
Complete blood count	X		Every 6 months	Every 6 months	
Liver function (AST, ALT, bilirubin)	X	X	Every 3–6 months	Every 3–6 months	Assess for underlying hepatic inflammation or dysfunction
Lipid profile	X		Annually	Annually	Repeat every 6 months if abnormal on last test; assess for underlying dyslipidemia
Blood glucose (A1c or fasting glucose)	X		Annually	Annually	Repeat every 3 months if abnormal on last test; assess for underlying diabetes
Renal function (Cr, eGFR, electrolytes)	X	X	Every 3–6 months	Every 3–6 months	Monitor serum phosphate in patients who are on TDF or TAF
Urinalysis	X		Annually	Annually	Repeat every 6 months if on TDF or TAF; if proteinuria present, quantify with spot urine for ACR or spot urine for PCR[†]
Pregnancy test	X				Repeat if clinically indicated

Source: Adapted from the US Department of Health and Human Services[39] and the Infectious Diseases Society of America.[76]

ACR = albumin creatinine ratio, ALT = alkaline aminotransferase, ART = antiretroviral therapy, AST = aspartate aminotransferase, CMV = cytomegalovirus, Cr = creatinine, eGFR = estimated glomerular filtration rate, HBcAb = hepatitis B core antibody, HBsAb = hepatitis B surface antibody, HBsAg = hepatitis B surface antigen, INSTI = integrase strand inhibitor, MSM = men who have sex with men, PCR = protein creatinine ratio, PWID = people who inject drugs, STIs = sexually transmitted infections, TAF = tenofovir alafenamide, TDF = tenofovir disoproxil fumarate

* High risk for hepatitis C infection includes MSM, PWID, and recent incarceration.

† Proteinuria and glucosuria, in the absence of high serum glucose and presence of low serum phosphate, can be a marker of proximal tubular dysfunction from tenofovir toxicity; spot urine for ACR assesses for glomerular dysfunction while spot urine for PCR assesses for both glomerular and tubular dysfunction.

HIV-Specific Tests

CD4 COUNT

The absolute CD4 count is used to stage HIV infection. It is an indicator of immune function and disease progression. A CD4 count of less than 200 cells/μL signifies AIDS and requires OI prophylaxis. The CD4 count can fluctuate because of acute illness, immunosuppressive drugs and diurnal variation.[39] Patients on ART should expect an average increase of 50 to 100 cells/μL during the first year on treatment. About 15 to 20 per cent of patients who start ART at low baseline CD4 counts can have a reduced immunologic response despite achieving virologic suppression.[39] The DHHS guidelines recommend assessing CD4 count upon entry into care and then every three to six months during the first two years on ART. Patients who consistently achieve viral suppression after two years on ART and whose CD4 count is between 300 and 500 cell/μL can have their CD4 count monitored annually; testing is optional in those with a CD4 count greater than 500 cells/μL.[39,76] Alternatively, recent IAS-US guidelines recommend that the CD4 count be monitored every six months and be discontinued once patients have achieved both an undetectable viral load and a CD4 count above 250 cell/μL for at least one year.[77]

HIV VIRAL LOAD

The HIV viral load is used to monitor treatment response to ART. The goal of ART is to suppress and maintain the virus at undetectable levels. Most HIV RNA assays have a quantifiable lower limit of detection of 50 copies/mL or less. Acute illness or recent vaccination can temporarily increase the viral load and should be interpreted accordingly. Knowledge of pre-treatment viral load is important as some ART options, such as rilpivirine-based regimens, are not indicated for baseline viral levels of more than 100,000 copies/mL. Viral suppression is usually achieved within 12 to 24 weeks of ART initiation. If not, problems with adherence and drug resistance should be considered. The DHHS guidelines recommend checking HIV viral load upon entry into care and two to eight weeks following treatment initiation or modification of ART. For patients suppressed on ART, HIV RNA levels can be measured every three to four months and can be extended to every six months if viral suppression is consistently achieved after two years on ART.[39,76] Alternatively, recent IAS-US guidelines recommend that HIV viral load be monitored within the first six weeks of ART initiation and then every three months until undetectable for at least one year. The viral load can then be checked every six months thereafter.[77]

HIV RESISTANCE TESTING

HIV resistance testing is used to guide ART selection. Genotype testing can identify mutations that are resistant to a particular drug or drug category. Identifying resistant drug mutations is best done during early HIV infection. With time, mutant virus may revert to wild-type virus, although the process may take years. Without ART, levels of resistant virus can decline below the levels of detection of current assays. Therefore, a negative resistance test in a patient with chronic HIV infection should be interpreted with caution as potential archived viral resistance can lead to future treatment failure.[39] Generally, resistance testing can be performed once viral levels exceed 500 copies/mL and can be done retrospectively on stored viral load samples. The DHHS guidelines recommend performing genotype resistance testing upon initial entry into care and for patients experiencing virologic failure. For patients who have deferred ART, repeat resistance testing before ART initiation can look for potential superinfection. At present, baseline INSTI resistance testing is not recommended unless patients fail an INSTI-based regimen. However, with the increased use of INSTIs, some HIV experts are now routinely ordering the test before ART selection.[39] For patients who fail ART and have multi-drug resistance, all historical genotypes should be taken into account before selecting a new regimen. The online Stanford HIV Drug Resistance Database can be used to interpret complex genotype results.[85] In such cases, a referral to a specialist is highly recommended.

HIV-RELATED TESTS

HLA-B5701 screening identifies patients who are at risk for abacavir hypersensitivity reaction. Abacavir is an NRTI drug. Patients who test positive should never be given abacavir. The reaction generally appears within six weeks of taking the drug and can lead to multi-organ failure. First-line combination ART regimens such as Triumeq contain abacavir.

G6PD screening is recommended in patients of Mediterranean, North African, or South-East Asian background. G6PD deficiency is a genetic condition that can cause hemolytic anemia in patients who are exposed to certain oxidative drugs. Examples are dapsone and sulfonamides, drugs that are often used in OI prophylaxis.

Toxoplasma serologic testing identifies patients with prior exposure to *Toxoplasma gondii*. Since toxoplasma encephalitis is one of the most common AIDS-related central nervous system infections, patients at higher risk for reactivation (CD4 count <100 cells/μL) can be identified at baseline.[74]

CMV serologic testing identifies patients with prior exposure to *Cytomegalovirus*. Seronegative patients require blood transfusions with CMV-negative or leukocyte-reduced blood products. CMV screening is not indicated in MSM or PWIDs as they are presumed to be CMV-positive.[76]

Hepatitis A virus (HAV) screening is recommended. Hepatitis A can be transmitted through anal-oral sex or "rimming." It is a self-limiting illness and does not result in chronic infection. Patients who are non-immune to HAV should be vaccinated.

Hepatitis B virus (HBV) screening is recommended. Hepatitis B is highly infectious and can be transmitted through IDU, unprotected sex, and vertical transmission. Worldwide prevalence of HIV-HBV co-infection is estimated at 5 to 25 per cent, with higher rates in Asia and Africa.[86] Hepatitis B screening should include hepatitis B surface antigen (HBsAg), hepatitis B surface antibody (HBsAb), and hepatitis B core antibody (HBcAb). Patients who test negative for both HBsAg and HBsAb but positive for HBcAb should receive HBV DNA testing to look for occult HBV infection. Patients who are non-immune to HBV should be vaccinated.

Hepatitis C virus (HCV) screening is recommended. In Canada, prevalence of HIV-HCV co-infection from different studies ranges from 20 to 90 per cent.[74] Patients who have positive HCV antibodies should have subsequent HCV RNA testing, either to evaluate for chronic HCV disease or to assess for ongoing risk of HCV re-infection. An estimated 6 to 13 per cent of HCV co-infected patients do not develop HCV antibodies.[74,86] In turn, HIV-positive patients who are HCV seronegative but who have a history of IDU or unexplained transaminitis should be screened with HCV RNA testing.

STI screening for syphilis, gonorrhea, and chlamydia should be performed upon entry into care and routinely thereafter based on risk.

CO-MORBID TESTS

A complete blood count (CBC), serum electrolytes, renal and liver function tests (LFTs), lipid profile, glucose level, and urinalysis should be performed at baseline and routinely thereafter. These standard tests screen for co-morbid conditions. They also aid in initial ART selection. Clinicians can identify patients who may require renal or hepatic dosing and avoid certain ART regimens in those with significant organ damage.

Serologies for measles, mumps, and rubella (MMR) and varicella zoster virus (VZV) are often recommended at baseline to assess for immunity. Patients who are non-immune to MMR and VZV should be vaccinated when their CD4 count is more than 200 cell/μL.

A tuberculin skin test (TBST) or interferon-gamma release assay (IGRA) is recommended in all HIV-positive patients who do not have a history of tuberculosis (TB) or prior positive TBST. The IGRA is preferred in patients who received the Bacillus Calmette-Guerin (BCG) vaccine in the past. A TBST result of more than 5 mm is positive in HIV-positive patients. Patients who test positive require a chest X-ray to rule out active TB. Patients with active M. tuberculosis should be referred to a TB specialist. Patients with latent disease should be treated according to current TB guidelines. Patients with advanced HIV may get false-negative readings, and testing should be repeated once their CD4 count is >200 cells/µL. Annual testing should be considered in patients who have ongoing exposure risks. Regular screening is important as TB can manifest at any CD4 count level.[76]

Morning serum testosterone levels can be considered in men with advanced HIV infection who are at risk for hypogonadism. Symptoms include fatigue, weight loss, decreased libido, depression, and reduced bone mass. Androgen replacement therapy may be considered.[76]

IMMUNIZATION SUMMARY

An important component of HIV primary care is to ensure that patients are appropriately immunized. See table 7.4.

All live vaccines are contraindicated in patients with CD4 counts less than 200 cells/µL. Vaccine responses are often lower in HIV-positive patients, especially those with low CD4 counts. Immunization can be deferred until viral suppression and immune reconstitution (CD4 > 200 cells/µL) are achieved with ART. Vaccines can cause viral blips and should not be given immediately before viral load testing. For HIV-positive patients who require the HBV vaccine, a dose of 40 µg should be administered at intervals of 0, 1, and 6 months for the Recombivax vaccine and at intervals of 0, 1, 2, and 6 months for the Engerix-B vaccine.[89,90]

In Canada, vaccines are generally provided free by local public health authorities. Regional differences exist in the accessibility and funding of certain vaccines. Consultation with local public health departments can help clinicians keep abreast of important immunization updates. It may be necessary to advocate for vaccines on a compassionate basis through pharmaceutical companies. The human papilloma virus (HPV) vaccine is one such example that is recommended in HIV-positive MSM but may not be covered regardless of age in certain jurisdictions.

Table 7.4. Routine Immunizations for HIV-Positive Persons

Vaccine	Comments
Non-live Vaccine	
Hepatitis A	2 doses if non-immune
Hepatitis B*	3 or 4 doses if non-immune, consider double dosing
Human papilloma virus[†]	3 doses
Influenza	1 dose annually, live vaccine contraindicated
Meningococcal[‡]	1 dose of Men-C-ACYW, repeat at least 8 weeks after
Pneumococcal	1 dose of PCV13 initially, followed by one dose of PPV23 at least 8 weeks after; if already vaccinated with PPV23, give PCV13 at least 1 year after PPV23; repeat PPV23 at 5 years
Tetanus toxoid	1 dose, substitute 1-time dose of Tdap, repeat every 10 years
Live Vaccine	
Measles, mumps, rubella	2 doses if non-immune, contraindicated in CD4 count <200 cells/µL
Varicella	2 doses if non-immune, contraindicated in CD4 count <200 cells/µL
Zoster[§]	1 dose, insufficient data, contraindicated in CD4 count <200 cell/µL

Source: Adapted from the Infectious Diseases Society of America,[76] Public Health Agency of Canada,[87,90] and National Advisory Committee on Immunization.[88,91]

HPV = human papilloma virus vaccine (Gardasil 4 or 9), Men-C-ACYW = quadrivalent meningococcal conjugate vaccine (Menactra or Menveo), NACI = Canadian National Advisory Committee on Immunization, PCV13 = 13-valent pneumococcal conjugate vaccine (Prevnar), PPV23 = 23-valent pneumococcal polysaccharide vaccine (Pneumovax), Tdap = tetanus, diphtheria, acellular pertussis vaccine (Adacel)

* Consider hepatitis B vaccine dose of 40 µg at intervals of 0, 1, 6 months (Recombivax) or at intervals 0, 1, 2, 6 months (Engerix-B).

[†] Administer HPV4 or HPV 9 vaccine as recommended by NACI.

[‡] Administer Men-C-ACYW vaccine as recommended by NACI.

[§] There are insufficient data regarding the safety and efficacy of zoster vaccine for HIV-positive persons.

Cancer Screening

Routine cancer screening is recommended in all HIV-positive patients. See table 7.5. Insufficient data exist in regards to cancer screening in HIV-positive transgender populations. Generally, screening should be done based on the patient's organ-specific anatomy irrespective of gender identity. For more information see chapter 11.

HIV-positive patients do not have higher rates of breast, colorectal, and prostate cancer compared to the general population.[74] Screening for these cancers should therefore follow provincial and territorial guidelines regardless of HIV serostatus. Breast cancer screening should be considered in transmasculine people who have not undergone chest surgery and transfeminine people above the age of 50 who are on hormone therapy for more than five years.[92] Limited research exists on how to screen transmasculine people post-mastectomy. For transmasculine people who have undergone chest surgery, ultrasound or magnetic resonance imaging (MRI) may be appropriate modalities for evaluating new chest wall complaints. Although there remains no evidence to support screening with the clinical breast exam, a diagnostic chest wall and axillary exam may be considered in cases of a new palpable mass. The Canadian Task Force on Preventive Health Care (CTFPHC) recommends against screening for prostate cancer using the prostate specific antigen (PSA) test and digital rectal exam (DRE).[93] Clinicians are reminded that the prostate is intact in transfeminine people post-vaginoplasty. Either a diagnostic DRE or neovaginal exam can be performed if a prostate exam is clinically indicated.[74]

The prevalence of abnormal cervical Papanicolaou (Pap) tests among HIV-positive patients is 10 times that in the general population.[74] HIV-positive cis women should have a cervical Pap test upon entry into care and annually thereafter (although some guidelines suggest a second pap at six months after the first, then annually). After three consecutive normal results, cervical pap testing can be performed every three years. If results are abnormal, patients should be sent for colposcopy.[94] The same recommendation may be inferred for HIV-positive transmasculine people with a cervix and transfeminine people with a neocervix, although data are limited. At present, there are no established guidelines to recommend cancer screening in HIV-positive transfeminine people with a neovagina and transmasculine people post-hysterectomy. In such cases, it may be reasonable for patients who are severely immunocompromised, or who have a history of cervical dyplasia or cancer, or a prior history of HPV infection, to undergo a vault smear. However, the use and effectiveness of vault smears have not been established.[92]

Table 7.5. Cancer Screening in HIV-Positive Persons

Cancer	Screening Test	Recommendation
Anal	DRE Anal Pap	Screen every 1–3 years in MSM Consider anal pap test if available but not standard of care* Refer for HRA if anal pap results abnormal
Breast	Mammogram	Follow provincial guidelines Screen in trans women >50 years old and on estrogen >5 years Screen in trans men >50 years old, include trans men post-chest surgery if at high risk[†]
Cervical	Pap test	Screen in cis women annually, after 3 consecutive normal results screen every 3 years thereafter Screen in trans men with cervix[‡] Refer for colposcopy if Pap results abnormal
Colorectal	FOBT	Follow provincial guidelines Refer for colonoscopy if at high risk or if FOBT results abnormal[§]
Liver	Liver ultrasound	Screen every 6 months for HCC in HBV+ or HCV+ persons with cirrhosis[‖]
Lung	Chest X-ray Low dose CT	Screen at baseline Consider low dose CT if 55–74 years old, current smoker or have quit in the past 15 years, and who have ≥30 pack-year smoking history[#]
Prostate	DRE PSA test	Both routinely not recommended**

Source: Adapted from British Columbia Centre for Excellence in HIV/AIDS,[75] the Infectious Diseases Society of America,[76] European AIDS Clinical Society,[78] Canadian Cancer Society,[92] and Canadian Task Force on Preventive Health Care.[93,99]

CT = computed tomography, DRE = digital rectal exam, FOBT = fecal occult blood test, HBV = hepatitis B virus, HCC = hepatocellular carcinoma, HCV = hepatitis C virus, HRA = high resolution anoscopy, MSM = men who have sex with men, Pap = Papanicolaou, PSA = prostate specific antigen

* No consensus guidelines available for anal pap screening in Canada.

† Consider ultrasound or MRI for screening high-risk trans men post-chest surgery.

‡ No consensus guidelines available for vault smear screening in both trans men post-hysterectomy and trans women post-vaginoplasty.

§ Immunochemical-based FOBT is more sensitive than guaiac-based FOBT; availability of tests varies among provinces and territories.

‖ Consider routine HCC screening in HBV co-infected persons with a history of transaminitis, who are of Asian or African descent, or who have a family history of HCC.

Low-dose CT of chest should be done at designated specialty facilities.

** Not recommended by the Canadian Task Force on Preventive Health Care.

For clarity, cytology requisitions should note the patient's gender identity, anatomical site, and use of any cross-sex hormones.

The incidence of anal cancer in HIV-positive MSM is 46 per 100,000 and currently exceeds the rate of cervical cancer in cis women before the introduction of cervical cancer screening.[86,95] At present, there are no valid clinical trials to conclusively link widespread anal Pap screening to decreased mortality rates. The IDSA guidelines suggest anal Pap tests for all HIV-positive persons who have a history of receptive anal sex or abnormal cervical Pap tests, and those with a history of genital warts, although the recommendation is weak.[76] Anal Pap smears have a high sensitivity (84 per cent) but low specificity (39 per cent) and abnormal results should be sent for biopsy under high resolution anoscopy.[96] In Canada, there are no consensus guidelines for anal cancer screening. Because of resource and physician constraints, screening programs for anal cancer in at-risk populations are currently unavailable. A digital rectal exam (DRE) is cost-effective and recommended for detecting anal cancer in all HIV-positive patients but it may not detect pre-cancerous lesions.[96,97] Administration of the HPV vaccine and smoking cessation counselling are effective ways to prevent anal cancer in HIV-positive patients.[96]

HIV infection is an independent risk factor for lung cancer.[98] A baseline chest X-ray is recommended in all HIV-positive patients and may be used for comparison in the case of future respiratory complaints. Clinicians should have a low threshold for ordering a chest X-ray or computed tomography (CT) scan in HIV-positive patients who smoke and present with severe respiratory symptoms.[74,76] The CTFPHC currently recommends annual screening for lung cancer using low-dose CT scan for any persons ages 55–74 years old who currently smoke or have quit in the past 15 years and who have at least a 30-pack/year smoking history. The recommendation is weak and screening should only be performed at designated specialty sites.[99] The same recommendation may be inferred for HIV-positive patients although insufficient data exist. Notwithstanding, the use of low-dose CT scan in lung cancer screening has been associated with higher rates of false positive results in HIV-positive patients with a CD4 count less than 200 cell/μL and in turn, results in such cases should be carefully interpreted.[100]

HIV-positive patients co-infected with HBV and/or HCV develop cirrhosis more quickly compared to hepatitis-infected patients without HIV. All HIV co-infected patients with cirrhosis should be routinely screened for hepatocellular carcinoma (HCC) with liver ultrasound every six months. Serum AFP is no longer used for HCC screening because of poor sensitivity and specificity.[74] In HBV co-infected patients without cirrhosis, the EACS guidelines recommend HCC screening in patients with a past history of elevated transaminases or who are at high risk for HCC, such as those of Asian or African descent or who have a family history of HCC.[78] Concurrent management with a liver specialist is strongly recommended.

Prophylaxis for Opportunistic Infections

The CD4 count determines when prophylaxis for OIs is needed and when it can be discontinued.[94] See table 7.6. Recent IAS-US guidelines recommend against the prophylaxis of *Mycobacterium avium complex* (MAC) in HIV-positive patients who are virally suppressed while on ART, irrespective of CD4 count.[76] Those with advanced HIV who present with signs and symptoms of OIs should be admitted to hospital for further expert evaluation.

HIV Treatment

Initiating Treatment

The goal of HIV treatment is to restore immune function and maintain viral suppression. ART is recommended for all HIV patients irrespective of CD4 count or viral load. ART initiation in the setting of acute HIV infection is also recommended. HIV suppression reduces ongoing immune activation and chronic inflammation, both linked to cardiovascular and end-organ damage. It also minimizes community viral load and prevents onward HIV transmission.[39,46]

Clinicians should be familiar with the eligibility requirements and levels of ART coverage that exist for patients as it may affect what ART regimen is prescribed. For refugee claimants, Indigenous persons, military personnel, and war veterans, drug coverage is facilitated by the federal government through the following programs, respectively: Interim Federal Health (IFH), Non-Insured Health Benefits (NIHB), Canadian Forces Health Services (CFHS), and Veterans Affairs Canada (VAC). For the remainder of Canadians, individual provinces and territories regulate the way ART is approved, prescribed, dispensed, and funded. An excellent summary of the HIV drug reimbursement programs across Canada can be found on both the Toronto General Hospital Immunodeficiency Clinic and the Canadian Treatment Action Council (CTAC) websites.[101,102]

ART is a lifelong commitment. Poor drug adherence can cause resistance to ART and complicate future HIV treatment. Clinicians should

Table 7.6. Prophylaxis for Opportunistic Infections in HIV-Positive Persons

Infection	Indication	Prophylaxis	Comments
Pneumocystis jirovecii pneumonia (PJP)	CD4 count <200 cells/μL **or** CD4% <14% **or** CD4 count of 200–250 cells/μL if monitoring not possible every 3 months	TMP-SMX 1 double **or** single strength tablet daily*	Discontinue when CD4 count >200 cells/μL for >3 months while on ART
Toxoplasma gondii (Toxo)	CD4 count <100 cells/μL **and** Toxo serology positive	TMP-SMX 1 double strength tablet daily†	Discontinue when CD4 count >200 cells/μL for >3 months while on ART
Mycobacterium avium complex (MAC)	CD4 count <50 cells/μL **and** no active MAC infection	Azithromycin 1200 mg weekly **or** 600 mg twice weekly **or** Clarithromycin 500 mg twice daily‡	Discontinue when CD4 count >100 cells/μL for >3 months while on ART or discontinue when virally suppressed while on ART irrespective of CD4 count
Cytomegalovirus (CMV)	CD4 count <50 cells/μL **and** CMV serology positive	Eye exam for CMV retinitis	Refer to ophthalmologist; MSM and PWID presumed to be CMV positive
Mycobacterium tuberculosisis (TB)	Positive TBST ≥ 5 mm **or** positive IGRA **or** prior untreated LTBI **or** contact with infectious TB case	Isoniazid 300 mg daily **or** 900 mg twice weekly **and** pyridoxine 25 mg daily for 9 months§	Rule out active TB with CXR, consider IGRA if history of BCG vaccine, repeat TBST if initially done at CD4 count <200 cells/μL

Source: Adapted from International Antiviral Society-USA[77] and US Department of Health and Human Services.[94]

ART = antiretroviral therapy, BCG = Bacillus Calmette-Guerin, CXR = chest X-ray, IGRA = interferon-gamma release assay, LTBI = latent tuberculosis infection, MSM = men who have sex with men, PWID = people who inject drugs, TBST = tuberculin skin test, TMP-SMX = trimethroprim-sulfamethoxazole

*Alternative: Dapsone 100 mg daily (if not G6PD deficient), Atovaquone 1500 mg daily or aerosolized Pentamidine 300 mg monthly

† Alternative: Dapsone 50 mg daily + Pyrimethamine 50 mg weekly + Leucovorin 25 mg weekly or Atovaquone 1500 mg daily

‡ Alternative: Rifabutin 300 mg daily (rule out active TB and ART drug–drug interactions)

§ Alternative: Rifampin 600 mg daily for 4 months or Rifabutin 300 mg daily for 4 months; refer to specialist for multi-drug resistant TB

assess the patient's willingness to begin treatment and identify factors that may lead to ART failure. Concerns may include non-adherence, short- and long-term side effects, pill burden, dosing frequency, drug interactions, caloric requirements, and financial costs. Psychosocial barriers may include unstable housing, employment status, mental health, and substance use, as well as stigma around taking ART. Connecting patients to counselling, case management and HIV support services is a key component in HIV primary care. In some cases, deferring ART until patients are ready to adhere to treatment is warranted.[39,74]

ART selection should be individualized and based on the results of pre-treatment bloodwork and a careful examination for potential ART toxicity, drug–drug interactions, and co-morbidities. Patients with a history of HIV multi-drug resistance should be referred to an HIV specialist.

Recommended Initial ART Regimens

There are currently seven HIV drug classes. Refer back to figure 7.1. In general, ART regimens for HIV treatment comprise two NRTIs as the "nuke backbone," along with one of the following as the base: an INSTI, a boosted-PI, or an NNRTI. See figure 7.2.

Numerous ART drugs may be used to initiate HIV therapy. See table 7.7. Two of the drugs, ritonavir (RTV or r) and cobicistat (COBI or c), are used to pharmacokinetically boost certain PIs and INSTIs. Fusion inhibitors, CCR5 antagonists, and post-attachment inhibitors are mainly used in

Figure 7.2. HIV ART Regimens

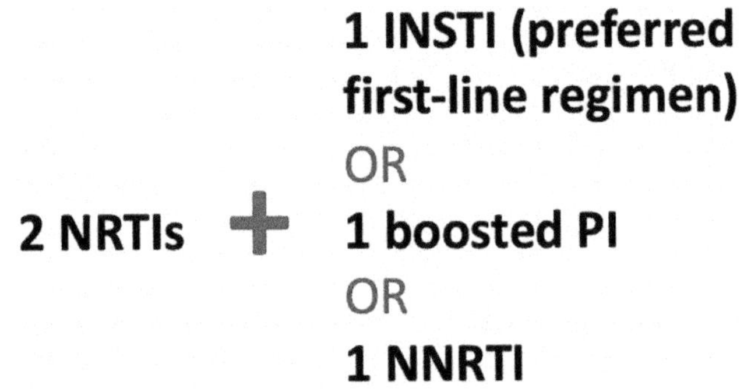

2 NRTIs ➕ **1 INSTI (preferred first-line regimen)**
OR
1 boosted PI
OR
1 NNRTI

Regimens generally consist of two nucleoside reverse transcriptase inhibitors (NRTIs) combined with one of the following: integrase strand inhibitor (INSTI) or boosted-protease inhibitor (PI) or non-nucleoside reverse transcriptase inhibitor (NNRTI).

Table 7.7. Commonly Used HIV Antiretroviral Drugs and Their Common Side Effects

Drug Name	Brand Name	Food Intake	Side Effects	Comments
NRTIs				
Abacavir (ABC)*	Ziagen	None	Minimal. Serious: hypersensitivity reaction including rash, nausea, diarrhea	Use only if HLA-B5701 negative; may not be ideal for persons with high cardiovascular risk
Emtricitabine (FTC)	Emtriva	None	Minimal	Has anti-HBV activity, must use with another anti-HBV agent to avoid HBV resistance; FTC is co-formulated with TDF or TAF
Lamivudine (3TC)	Epivir	None	Minimal	Has anti-HBV activity, must use with another anti-HBV agent to avoid HBV resistance
Tenofovir (TDF or TAF)	Viread or Vemlidy	None	Minimal. May get nausea, diarrhea, headache, hepatotoxicity. TDF: proximal renal tubular dysfunction, bone mass loss	TDF better lipid and BMI profile; TAF less renal and bone toxicity; both have anti-HBV activity; avoid TDF/FTC if CrCl <60mL/min and TAF/FTC if CrCl <30mL/min
INSTIs				
Bictegravir (BTG)[†]	Biktarvy	None	Common: headache, insomnia. May get nausea, diarrhea, rash. Other: may increase serum Cr, worsen mood	High barrier to resistance; may increase BMI; may cause false increase in

Drug Name	Brand Name	Food Intake	Side Effects	Comments
				serum Cr; take 2 hours before or 6 hours after cations; limited data in pregnancy.
Dolutegravir (DTG)[†]	Tivicay	None	Common: headache, insomnia. May get nausea, diarrhea, rash. Other: may increase serum Cr, worsen mood	High barrier to resistance; may increase BMI; may cause false increase in serum Cr; take 2 hours before or 6 hours after cations
Elvitegravir (EVG)	Vitekta	Take with food	Common: nausea. May get headache, insomnia, diarrhea, dyslipidemia. Other: may worsen mood	Requires boosting; low barrier to resistance; may increase BMI; take 2 hours before or 6 hours after cations; avoid in pregnancy
Raltegravir (RAL)	Isentress	None	Minimal. May get headache, insomnia, nausea. Other: hypersensitivity rash, myopathy, rhabdomyolysis, worsen mood	Low barrier to resistance; may increase BMI; take 2 hours before or 6 hours after cations
NNRTIs				
Efavirenz (EFV)	Sustiva	On empty stomach at bedtime	Common: rash, insomnia, headache, dyslipidemia. Other: worsen mood, hepatotoxicity, prolong QT, teratogenic	Low barrier to resistance; avoid if underlying psychiatric illness; avoid in pregnancy; caution with QT drugs, effective in high VL baseline

(Continued)

Table 7.7. (Continued)

Drug Name	Brand Name	Food Intake	Side Effects	Comments
Rilpivirine (RPV)	Edurant	Take with > 400 kcal meal	Minimal. May get rash, headache, insomnia, hepatotoxicity. Other: may worsen mood, prolong QT	Low barrier to resistance; caution with H2-RAs; PPIs contraindicated; avoid if VL > 100,000 copies/mL or CD4 count < 200 cells/µmL; caution with QT drugs, small pill size and easy to swallow
PIs				
Atazanaivr (ATV)	Reyataz	Take with food	Common: hyperbilirubinemia, jaundice, rash, diarrhea, nausea, dyslipidemia. Other: nephrolithiasis	Requires boosting; high barrier to resistance, may switch if jaundice and bilirubin > 5x ULN; avoid acid-reducing drugs, avoid in CKD; caution with QT drugs
Darunavir (DRV)	Prezista	Take with food	Common: rash, diarrhea, nausea, dyslipidemia, headache. Other: hypersensitivity rash	Requires boosting; high barrier to resistance, contains sulfa moiety, use with caution in persons with known sulfa allergy; caution with QT drugs
Boosters				
Cobiscistat (COBI/c)[†]	Tybost	Take with food	Common: may increase serum Cr	Potent CYP3A4 inhibitor; may cause false

Drug Name	Brand Name	Food Intake	Side Effects	Comments
				increase in serum Cr; avoid if CrCl < 70 mL/min
Ritonavir (RTV/r)		Take with food	Common: diarrhea, nausea, dyslipidemia	Potent CYP3A4 inhibitor; capsule formulation must be refrigerated

Source: Adapted from US Department of Human Health Services[39] and European AIDS Clinical Society.[78]

CKD = chronic kidney disease, Cr = creatinine, CrCl = creatinine clearance, CYP = cytochrome P450, HBV = hepatitis B virus, INSTI = integrase strand inhibitor, MI = myocardial infarct, NNRTI = non-nucleoside reverse transcriptase inhibitor, NRTI = nucleoside/tide reverse transcriptase inhibitor, PI = protease inhibitor, TAF = tenofovir alafenamide fumarate, TDF = tenofovir disoproxil fumarate, ULN = upper limit of normal, VL = viral load

* Abacavir has been associated with cardiovascular disease and MI events in some cohort studies.

† False rise in serum Cr can occur because of inhibition of tubular renal secretion of Cr without affecting true glomerular function.

treatment-experienced patients with multi-drug resistance and should be prescribed by a specialist.

Many ART drugs now come in fixed-dose combinations for ease of treatment. See table 7.8.

The DHHS guidelines recommend several ART regimens as first-line treatment.[39] See table 7.9. The preferred ART regimen for most ART-naive patients consist of two NRTIs plus one unboosted INSTI. An unboosted INSTI-based regimen is generally more tolerable and can be taken with or without food. This includes either a dolutegravir (DTG)-based or bictegravir (BTG)-based regimen. The added benefits of these two drugs include their high barrier to resistance and low potential for drug–drug interactions as neither drug requires pharmacokinetic enhancers that inhibit the CYP3A4 system. Current evidence also supports the dual regimen of DTG/3TC (Dovato) as first-line treatment for HIV patients who have a confirmed viral load of <500,000 copies/mL, no HBV co-infection, and no genotype resistance. Since HIV medicine is rapidly evolving, readers should refer to the various HIV treatment guidelines for up-to-date recommendations on initial HIV therapy.

Table 7.8. Commonly Used HIV Combination Drugs

Brand Name	Drug Names
Atripla	EFV/TDF/FTC
Biktarvy	BTG/TAF/FTC
Complera	RPV/TDF/FTC
Descovy	TAF/FTC
Dovato	DTG/3TC
Evotaz	ATV/c
Genvoya	EVG/c/TAF/FTC
Juluca	DTG/RPV
Kivexa	ABC/3TC
Odefsey	RPV/TAF/FTC
Prezcobix	DRV/c
Stribild	EVG/c/TDF/FTC
Symtuza	DRV/c/TAF/FTC
Triumeq	DTG/ABC/3TC
Truvada	TDF/FTC

3TC = lamivudine, ABC = abacavir, c = cobicistat, BTG = bictegravir, DRV = darunavir, DTG = dolutegravir, EFV = effavirenz, EVG = elvitigravir, FTC = emitricitabine, RPV = rilpivirine, TAF = tenofovir alafenamide, TDF = tenofovir disoproxyl fumarate

Table 7.9. Preferred ART Regimens for HIV Treatment-Naive Persons*

ART Regimen	Brand Name	No. Pills	Comments
BTG/TAF/FTC	Biktarvy	1	
DTG/ABC/ 3TC	Triumeq	1	HLA-B5701 negative for ABC, no HBV co-infection.
DTG + TDF/FTC or TAF/FTC	Tivicay + Truvada or Descovy	2	Higher pill burden.
DTG/3TC	Dovato	1	Viral load <500,000, no HBV co-infection, no genotype resistance.

Source: Adapted from US Department of Human Health Services. 2021.[39]

3TC = lamivudine, ABC = abacavir, ART = antiretroviral therapy, BID = twice daily, BTG = bictegravir, c = cobicistat, DTG = dolutegravir, EVG = elvitegravir, FTC = emtricitabine, r = ritonavir, RAL = raltegravir, TAF = tenofovir alafenamide fumarate, TDF = tenofovir disoproxil fumarate

* Refer to DHHS guidelines for most recent up-to-date recommendations and alternatives for initial ART therapy in HIV treatment-naive patients.

In acute HIV infection, where resistance data are unavailable, empiric treatment with darunavir (DRV) boosted with RTV is often recommended since PI-based regimens have a high genetic barrier to resistance.[39] A DTG- or BTG-based regimen can also be considered in rapid ART initiation.[77] Abacavir (ABC) should be avoided unless HLA-B5701 results are negative. Modification to the ART regimen can be considered once resistance testing is completed.

ART Drug Considerations

Differences between the various NRTIs should be considered when selecting a dual-NRTI backbone. Tenofovir alafenamide fumarate (TAF) has less renal and bone toxicity than tenofovir disoproxil fumarate (TDF). Both TAF and TDF are converted to tenofovir, TAF mostly intracellularly while TDF mostly in plasma. Systemic exposure to tenofovir may lead to renal proximal tubular dysfunction and loss of bone mass in a small number of patients. TDF-based regimens are therefore best avoided in patients with pre-existing renal and bone disease.[103,104] An advantage of TDF is its association with lower lipid profiles and its effect on weight suppression when compared to TAF. TAF has been associated with increased BMI, especially in HIV treatment with DTG and its use in HIV PrEP.[105–107] Although still debatable, ABC may be associated with an increased risk of cardiovascular disease (CVD) and should be avoided in patients with high risk for CVD.[74] On the other hand, ABC does not require renal dosing. But unlike TAF and TDF, ABC has no activity against HBV. Emtricitabine (FTC) and lamivudine (3TC) have minimal side-effects and either one is often used as part of the dual-NRTI backbone in combination ART.

NNRTIs and first-generation INSTIs, such as raltegravir (RAL) and elvitegravir (EVG), have a low genetic barrier to resistance. Resistance to one of these drugs may confer cross resistance to the entire drug class. In contrast, second-generation INSTIs like DTG and BTG, and boosted-PIs like boosted-DRV both have a high genetic resistance barrier. Resistance to these drugs tends to develop more slowly, requires the accumulation of multiple mutations, and when transmitted, is often clinically insignificant.[74] Genetic resistance is not commonly seen in patients experiencing virologic failure while on these drugs. DTG-, BTG-, and DRV-based regimens are therefore preferred in patients who have drug adherence issues or in the setting where ART is initiated when genotype testing is unavailable, such as in acute HIV infection.

INSTI-based regimens have been associated with weight gain, especially with DTG.[106,108] There also may be a small increased risk of neural tube defects in patients taking DTG during pregnancy. Whether or not an INSTI-based class effect exists is still unknown. EVG should be avoided during pregnancy since concentrations of the drug have been shown to decline after the first trimester. A pregnancy test should be considered and a discussion around the possible risk for birth defects should be done before initiating an INSTI-based regimen in patients who may be pregnant.[39] For more information on HIV and fertility, please see box 7.1.

Older boosted-PI regimens are known for their high rates of metabolic and gastrointestinal side-effects. Body fat re-distribution because of lipodystrophy is a common side effect. Current PI-based regimens containing atazanavir (ATV) and DRV are lipid neutral with limited GI toxicity. Unlike DRV, ATV is known to cause benign hyperbilirubinemia leading to higher discontinuation rates. Patients with a sulfa allergy should avoid DRV as the drug contains a sulfanomide moiety. Caution should be taken when PIs are used with drugs associated with QT prolongation such as methadone, macrolides, and quinolones. Baseline and routine ECGs should be performed if QT prolongation is a concern.[74]

NNRTI-based regimens can benefit some patients. Efavirenz (EFV) when used with TDF/FTC (Atripla) was the first combination pill initially on the market. It has excellent virologic efficacy in patients with high viremia. It is also known for its higher rates of drug toxicity, including neuropsychiatric and metabolic side-effects. Rilpivirine (RPV) when used with TDF/FTC (Complera) or TAF/FTC (Odefsey) has fewer side effects and better lipid profiles than EFV. RPV-based combination pills are smaller and may benefit patients who have swallowing difficulties. Because of higher rates of virologic failure, patients with baseline CD4 counts less than 200 cells/mL and viral loads more than 100,000 copies/mL should avoid RPV. RPV-based regimens should be taken with a large meal and not combined with acid-reducing medications or drugs associated with QT prolongation. As with PIs, baseline and routine ECGs should be performed if QT prolongation is a concern.[74]

ART Side Effects and Drug Interactions

The common ART drugs and their side-effects were listed in table 7.7. Many medications used in primary care can interact with these common ART drugs. See table 7.10. Several excellent resources are available online to help manage ART toxicities and drug interactions. These include the interactive *HIV Drug Interaction Checker* by the University of Liverpool, the online *HIV InSite Database of Antiretroviral Drug Interactions* by the University of California San Francisco, and the online *HIV/*

Table 7.10. Common ART Drug–Drug Interactions in Primary Care

Common Drug Classes	Drug Examples	Comments
Acid reducers	PPIs	**Avoid PPI with RPV and unboosted ATV**; take boosted ATV 12 hours apart from PPI.
	H2-RAs	Take RPV and boosted ATV 12 hours apart from H2-RA.
	Cation-containing antacids	**Avoid with RAL**; take antacids 6 hours before or after ATV, RPV, DTG, EVG/c, BTG.
Analgesics/ narcotics/ opioid substitutions	Acetaminophen	No significant interactions.
	Anti-inflammatoires	Monitor for renal toxicity in prolonged use with TDF.
	Morphine, hydromorphone	No significant interactions.
	Codeine, oxycodone, hydrocodone, tramadol	Can ↑ drug levels with PIs and EVG/c, start low and titrate to effect; consider dose reduction.
	Fentanyl	
	Buprenorphine	**Avoid with PIs and EVG/c.**
	Methadone	**Avoid with unboosted ATV**; consider dose reduction with boosted ATV. Opioid withdrawal common with EFV, consider dose increase.
Anti-convulsants	Carbamazepine, phenobarbital, phenytoin	**Avoid with PIs, RPV, EFV, EVG/c**; consider valproic acid, lamotrigine, topiramate, levetiracetam with routine drug level monitoring.
Anti-diabetics	Metformin	Can ↑ drug levels with DTG and BTG; limit dose to 500 mg twice daily.
	Saxagliptin, linagliptin	Can ↓ drug levels with EFV, titrate to effect; consider sitagliptin.
	Liraglutide	Monitor for QT prolongation with PIs, RPV.
	Repaglinide	Can ↑ drug levels with PIs and EVG/c, start low and titrate to effect.
	Canagliflozin	Can ↓ drug levels with ritonavir-boosted PIs and EFV, titrate to effect; consider empagliflozin.
	Gliclazide, glyburide	Can ↑ drug levels with EFV, start low and titrate to effect; can ↓ drug levels with ritonavir-boosted PIs and EVG/c, titrate to effect.

(Continued)

Table 7.10. (Continued)

Common Drug Classes	Drug Examples	Comments
Anti-infectives	Antifungals: ketoconazole, voriconazole	**Avoid voriconazole with PIs, EFV; avoid ketoconazole with EFV**; consider fluconazole.
	Macrolides: clarithromycin	**Avoid with PIs, RPV, EVG/c**; consider azithromycin.
Cardiac/ anti-hypertensives	ACE-inhibitors	No significant interactions.
	ARBs: candesartan, irbesartan, losartan	Can ↑ drug levels with PIs and EGV/c, start low and titrate to effect; consider valsartan.
	Beta-blockers: bisoprolol, metoprolol, propranolol	Can ↑ drug levels with PIs and EVG/c, start low and titrate to effect; consider atenolol.
	Calcium channel blockers	Can ↑ drug levels with PIs and EVG/c, start low and titrate to effect; consider 50% dose reduction; consider ECG with ATV.
	Diuretics: hydrochlorothiazide, furosemide, spironolactone	No significant interactions.
	Anti-arrhythmics: amiodarone, digoxin	Can ↑ drug levels with PIs and EVG/c, start low and titrate to effect; monitor drug toxicity; consider routine drug levels and ECG.
Corticosteroids	Inhaled/intranasal: budesonide, fluticasone	**Avoid with PIs and EVG/c if possible**; consider inhaled/intranasal beclomethasone.
	Systemic or injectable: prednisone	**Avoid injectable prednisone with PIs and EVG/c**; monitor for adrenal insufficiency if taking oral prednisone with PIs and EVG/c.
PDE5-inhibitors	Sildenafil	Can ↑ drug levels with PIs and EVG/c; limit dose to 25 mg every 48 hours.
	Tadalafil	Can ↑ drug levels with PIs and EVG/c; limit dose to 10 mg every 72 hours.
	Vardenafil	**Avoid with PIs and EVG/c.**

Psychotropics	Citalopram, escitalopram, sertraline, fluoxetine, mirtazapine, venlafaxine, trazodone	Can ↑ drug levels with PIs and EVG/c, start low and titrate to effect; can ↓ drug levels with EFV, titrate to effect.
	Duloxetine	No significant interactions.
	Bupropion	Can ↓ drug levels with ritonavir-boosted PIs and EFV, titrate to effect.
	Amitriptyline, nortriptyline	Can ↑ drug levels with PIs and EVG/c, start low and titrate to effect.
	Lurasidone	**Avoid lurasidone with EVG/c and PIs.**
	Quetiapine, risperidone, ziprasidone, aripiprazole	Can ↑ drug levels with PIs and EVG/c, start low and titrate to effect.
	Clozapine, olanzapine	**Can ↓ drug levels with ritonavir-boosted PIs and EVG/c, titrate to effect.**
Sedatives	Midazolam, triazolam	**Avoid with PIs, NNRTIs and EVG/c.**
	Alprazolam, clonazepam, diazepam, zopiclone	Consider switching to low dose lorazepam, oxazepam, temazepam with PIs and EVG/c.
Statins	Atorvastatin	**Avoid with ATV/c;** can ↑ drug levels with PIs and EVG/c; limit dose to 20 mg .
	Lovastatin, simvastatin	**Avoid with PIs and EVG/c.**
	Rosuvastatin	Can ↑ drug levels with PIs and EVG/c; limit dose to 10mg.
	Pravastatin	Can ↑ drug levels with PIs and EVG/c, start low and titrate to effect.
	Pitavastatin	No significant interactions.

Source: Adapted from US Department of Human Health Services,[39] and University Health Network/Toronto General Hospital Immunodeficiency Clinic.[111]

ART = antiretroviral therapy, ATV = atazanavir, DTG = dolutegravir, ECG = electrocardiogram, EFV = efavirenz, EVG/c = elvitegravir/ cobicistat, H2-RA = H2-receptor antagonist, INR = international normalized ratio, INSTI = integrase strand inhibitor, NNRTI = non-nucleoside reverse transcriptase inhibitor, NRTI = nucleoside/tide reverse transcriptase inhibitor, OST = opioid substitution therapy, PDE = phosphodiesterase, PI = protease inhibitor, PPI = proton pump inhibitor, RAL = raltegravir, RPV = rilpivirine, SSRI = serotonin re-uptake inhibitor, TAF = tenofovir alafenamide, TCA = tricyclic antidepressant

HCV Drug Therapy Guide by the Toronto University Health Network and Toronto General Hospital.[109-111]

Treatment Monitoring

Once ART is initiated, blood work should be done to monitor for ART toxicity and treatment efficacy. Routine blood work is also important to monitor for age-related HIV co-morbidities.

Short-term clinical side effects can occur in the first couple of weeks after ART initiation. Patients should be advised not to discontinue ART. In general, only basic symptom management is needed. If side effects worsen or affect multiple organ systems, ART should then be discontinued and referral to an HIV expert is recommended. A small number of patients can develop an immune-mediated reaction that can occur weeks to months after ART initiation. Known as immune reconstitution inflammatory syndrome (IRIS), the reaction is more common in patients with very low pre-treatment CD4 counts (CD4 < 50 cells/mL). As the immune system reconstitutes, it can produce a severe inflammatory response to a currently treated OI or unmask a latent one. Clinical presentation often includes fever, lymphadenopathy, and symptoms related to the OI. A prompt referral to an HIV specialist is warranted for diagnostic clarification and optimal management.[112]

HIV Co-morbid Conditions

Patients with long-term HIV infection are at high risk for chronic co-morbid conditions. The causes are multifactorial and include premature aging due to chronic immune activation and inflammation, long-term ART toxicity, and conventional risk factors such as age, gender and smoking.[39,113] Monitoring should be more frequent in HIV-positive patients with existing co-morbidities as they are at risk for ART toxicity. Regardless of co-morbidity, HIV-positive patients should receive ongoing counselling on modifiable risk factors with attention to weight management through diet and exercise, smoking cessation, avoidance of hepatotoxic and nephrotoxic drugs, and minimization of alcohol and salt intake. Attention to strict blood pressure and glucose control, especially in those with chronic diabetes and renal disease, is also advisable.

Cardiovascular Disease and Dyslipidemia

Cardiovascular disease (CVD) is a leading cause of morbidity and mortality in the aging HIV population. Persons with HIV have an approximately two-fold greater risk of acute myocardial infarction compared to non-HIV patients.[114] Despite viral suppression with ART, low levels of HIV immune activation and inflammation have been linked to vascular dysfunction and the formation of extensive coronary plaques.[115,116] HIV-positive patients tend to have a high prevalence of dyslipidemia irrespective of ART. Exposure to ABC may be associated with CVD and older generation PIs, such as lopinavir (LPV), have been linked to higher rates of dyslipidemia and CVD events.[74]

Current cardiovascular risk calculators do not incorporate HIV infection and may underestimate risk levels.[74,117] Whether or not to aggressively treat dyslipidemia in HIV-positive patients remains unclear. For risk stratification, the Framingham risk score is the recommended tool to assess CVD risk.[74] Treatment of HIV-positive patients with dyslipidemia should be based on current Canadian guidelines. If statin therapy is required, the potential for drug–drug interactions should be considered as some statins may be contraindicated or may require dose modification with certain ART drugs. The DHHS and BCE-PC guidelines recommend routine lipid screening for all HIV patients. Also, see the section ART Drug Considerations, above.

Glucose Intolerance and Diabetes

HIV-positive patients are at high risk for abnormal glucose metabolism. The incidence of diabetes in patients who are taking older-generation PIs and NRTIs is more than 4 times higher than the general population.[118] Some studies suggest that HbA1c levels may underestimate glycemic levels in HIV-positive patients with diabetes.[119] The diagnosis and treatment of diabetes should still follow current Canadian guidelines. In general, metformin is a safe first-line anti-diabetic drug. When taken with DTG or BTG, metformin should be limited to 1000 mg/day.[120] The DHHS and BCE-PC guidelines recommend routine diabetes screening for all HIV patients.

Liver Disease

HIV-positive patients co-infected with HBV and/or HCV progress more rapidly to cirrhosis compared to non-HIV patients with viral hepatitis. Patients co-infected with HBV should consider a dual-NRTI backbone comprising TDF or TAF with 3TC or FTC. Monotherapy with 3TC or FTC can lead to HBV resistance and virologic failure.[74] Patients co-infected with HCV should consider an INSTI-based ART regimen because of its minimal drug interactions with current HCV therapies.[39,77] Prevalence rates of non-alcoholic fatty liver disease (NAFLD) in HIV-positive patients are 30 to 40 per cent higher than in the general population. Lipid-neutral ART regimens should be considered in HIV-positive patients with NAFLD. Expert consultation is strongly recommended in HIV co-infected patients and in those whose NAFLD has progressed to non-alcoholic steatohepatitis (NASH).[78]

HIV-positive MSM have higher rates of HCV transmission through sexual contact. Risk factors include multiple sex partners, concurrent STIs, group sex, engagement in UAI, and use of illicit drugs during sex.[95] Any injury to the anorectal mucosa can facilitate HCV transmission. Damage can occur from the use of anal enemas and sex toys, the presence of ulcerative STIs, and engagement in rough UAI during chemsex.[95] About 50 to 85 per cent of HCV co-infected patients will develop chronic HCV infection. Survival outcomes are poorer among HCV co-infected patients compared to those with HCV mono-infection.[74]

The DHHS and BCE-PC guidelines recommend routine liver monitoring for all HIV patients. All HIV co-infected patients with documented liver cirrhosis should be screened for HCC every six months with ultrasound. Patients with chronic liver disease may require hepatic dosing of their ARVs.[39]

Kidney Disease

Chronic kidney disease (CKD) is common in HIV-positive patients with prevalence rates of 4.7 to 9.7 per cent in North America and Europe.[121] With the advent of ART, HIV-associated nephropathy is rare. Co-morbid conditions such as diabetes and hypertension, as well as nephrotoxic drugs such as tenofovir, have contributed to the rise in other CKD-related conditions.

Urinalysis is a simple test to monitor for kidney damage. Proteinuria >1+ on urinalysis should be quantified with either a spot urine albumin-to-creatinine ratio (uACR) or a urine protein-to-creatinine ratio (uPCR). A spot uACR mainly detects glomerular disease whereas a spot uPCR detects total urinary protein caused by both glomerular and tubular disease.[78,121] The uACR is used to stage CKD. When tenofovir toxicity is suspected, the uPCR is preferred by some experts.[78,122] Urine glucose, in the absence of high serum blood glucose and the presence of low serum phosphate, can also be a marker for tenofovir toxicity.[121] A renal ultrasound is often performed to identify other causes of renal injury. Treatment with TDF and TAF is not recommended in patients with eGFR less than 60 mL/min and less than 30 mL/min, respectively. Patients with ongoing significant proteinuria and declining renal function should be referred to a nephrologist.

Regimens that contain DTG, BTG, RPV, and COBI may increase the serum creatinine by inhibiting proximal renal tubular secretion of creatinine. The result is a decrease in estimated glomerular filtration rate (eGFR) without affecting true GFR. A potential 15 to 30 per cent rise in serum creatinine may occur in the first four weeks of treatment, creating a new baseline value.[39,104,122]

The DHHS and BCE-PC guidelines recommend routine renal monitoring in all HIV patients with some minor differences. Serum phosphate is recommended by the DHHS in patients who are on a TAF- or TDF-based regimen while the BCE-PC recommends the test at consistent intervals regardless of ART regimen. The BCE-PC also recommends regular interval screening with uACR. It may be more practical for clinicians to conduct a urinalysis first, and if the result is abnormal, a quantifiable spot urine test can be done thereafter.[121] Patients with chronic kidney disease may require renal dosing of their ARVs.[39]

Bone Disease

Studies suggest that after two years on ART, HIV-positive patients may have a 2 to 6 per cent reduction in their bone mass. Patients on a TDF-based or boosted-PI-based regimen showed the greatest risk for bone mass loss. In turn, these regimens should be avoided in patients with underlying osteopenia or osteoporosis.[123]

A dual-energy X-ray absorptiometry (DEXA) scan should be performed in all HIV-positive post-menopausal women and men aged 50 years or older.[123] In HIV-positive men 40 to 49 years old and premenopausal women >40 years old, the fracture risk assessment tool (FRAX) without DEXA may be used to calculate the risk for fragility fractures.[123] Secondary causes of osteoporosis should be considered including vitamin D deficiency, thyroid disease, hyperparathyroidism, hypogonadism, renal disorders, and chronic malnutrition or malabsorption.[123] Patients should be counselled on diet, weight bearing exercises and smoking cessation. If indicated, calcium and vitamin D supplementation or bisphosphonate therapy should be initiated.

Other Treatment Considerations

Switching ART

Indications for ART modification in the setting of viral suppression include acute drug toxicity (neuropsychiatric effects with EFV), avoidance of long-term toxicity (renal tubular dysfunction with TDF), potential drug–drug interactions (ART with future HCV therapy), planned pregnancy (teratogenicity of DTG), exacerbation of co-morbid conditions (ABC with CVD risk), and simplification of drug regimen (minimize pill burden, dosing frequency, caloric restriction).[78] In the absence of virologic failure and archived resistance, patients can easily switch out from one drug to another within the same drug class or genetic resistance barrier without risk of treatment failure. An example would be switching from EFV to RPV or RAL. Caution should be taken when patients are switched to a regimen that has a lower genetic barrier to resistance, especially in cases of prior viro-logic failure and poor drug adherence. An example would be switch-ing from a boosted-PI regimen to an NNRTI- or INSTI-based regimen (other than DTG and BTG).[39] The abrupt discontinuation of TDF or TAF should be avoided in patients with chronic HBV as it can cause severe liver injury due to HBV reactivation.[39] HIV viral load testing should be repeated at least two to eight weeks after regimen modifica-tion to ensure viral suppression.

Virologic failure is the inability to suppress and maintain HIV RNA levels below 200 copies/mL. Causes of virologic failure may include drug toxicity, drug–drug or drug–food interactions, and psychoso-cial factors that can affect adherence such as mental health, poly-substance use, neurocognitive decline, and economic instability.[39] Resistance testing should be done once virologic failure has been confirmed. This should be performed when the patient is still on the failing regimen or within one month of stopping therapy. Resis-tance testing is less dependable once ART is discontinued for greater than four weeks as resistance mutations can revert to wild type, at which time results should be interpreted with caution.[39] HIV-positive patients who experience virologic failure will require consultation with an HIV expert, especially patients with multi-drug resistance. Switching ART in the context of virologic failure is outside the scope of this chapter.

In certain clinical settings, switching ART may not be indicated. An example would be during a viral blip where an isolated HIV viral load is detectable but subsequently becomes suppressed with repeat testing. Blips can happen during an acute illness or after administra-tion of a vaccine. In 15 to 20 per cent of patients who initiate ART at very low CD4 counts, a suboptimal immunologic response can occur despite viral suppression. In such cases, switching to a different ART regimen has not been shown to improve CD4 cell recovery and is not recommended.[39,74]

HIV Treatment and Recreational Drug Use

Recreational drugs are often consumed by HIV-positive patients on ART. In one large UK study, more than half of HIV-positive MSM reported the use of illicit drugs in the past three months and almost a quarter used at least three types of drugs.[124] Use of recreational drugs in the context of chemsex is associated with high risk behaviours including UAI, multiple sex partners, and sexual disinhibition. Active substance use is also associated with mood disorders and can be a predictor of poor adherence to ART.[39,125]

Limited data exist on the interactions between recreational drugs and ART. Since some ART drugs are metabolized by the CYP450 system, potential drug–drug interactions can be postulated. Both RTV and COBI are known inhibitors of the CYP3A4 and CYP2D6 systems. These boosting drugs can potentially cause dangerous levels of illicit drugs to accumulate in the body, leading to severe side effects and overdose. Serious reactions can potentially occur when these boosters are concomitantly used with cocaine, crystal meth, MDMA, LSD, GHB, ketamine, erectile dysfunction agents, and certain benzodiazepines.[111,126,127] In contrast, NNRTIs are known inducers of the CYP3A4 system. With the exception of RPV, NNRTIs can potentially cause levels of illicit drugs to dramatically decrease in the body, leading to significant withdrawal symptoms and the need for more uptake of the illicit drug. Such interactions can occur when NNRTIs are used with LSD, ketamine, and erectile dysfunction agents.[111,126] Alcohol, cannabis, opioids, and amyl nitrates have less potential to interact with ART.[111,127]

Clinicians should screen all HIV-positive patients for active substance use and offer opioid substitution therapy (OST) as needed. Methadone is a common OST drug that can interact with NNRTIs, causing a significant decrease in methadone levels. Severe opiate withdrawal symptoms can ensue, and increases to methadone doses may be required. In contrast, buprenorphine is an OST drug that appears to have limited interactions with ART. Similarly, naltrexone is often used to treat alcohol dependence and does not appear to have any major interactions with ART.[39] See chapter 9 for more information on substance abuse.

HIV Treatment and Cross-Sex Hormone Therapy

A dearth of research is available on how cross-sex hormones affect ART in the transgender population. HIV-positive transgender patients may be reluctant to engage in care because of myriad psychosocial and economic challenges that can lead them to delay HIV treatment. In Canada and the United States, studies have reported up to 60 per cent of transfeminine people are accessing cross-sex hormones outside the health care system.[128] Clinicians can link HIV-positive transgender patients to HIV care by integrating hormone therapy with ART.[73,128]

Spironolactone and cyproterone acetate are the anti-androgens most commonly prescribed in Canada as part of a feminizing hormone regimen. There are no significant drug interactions between anti-androgens and ART but data are limited.[128] Since cyproterone acetate can be associated with rare fulminant hepatitis, patients who are already on ART should be regularly monitored for liver toxicity. Of note, androgen blockers may not be required in HIV-positive transfeminine people since an estimated 25 per cent of HIV-positive cis men are reported to be hypogonadal.[128] It may be useful to check testosterone levels before deciding to start androgen blockers in such patients. As spironolactone is also a potassium-sparing diuretic, routine electrolyte and renal monitoring should be done in patients who are on sulfamethoxazole and trimethoprim (Septra) for OI prophylaxis, as the combination of both drugs can cause severe hyperkalemia.[129]

Studies on the pharmacokinetic effects of ART and estrogen have mainly involved ethinyl estradiol, a component of oral contraceptives (OCPs), and have all been conducted in cis women.[128] To date, the only potential interactions between ethinyl estradiol and ART have been with amprenavir and fosamprenavir, both older ART agents not frequently used in HIV therapy. The DHHS guidelines recommend against the use of these two ART agents with OCPs as it may result in virologic failure.[39] In Canada, 17-B estradiol is the most common form of estrogen prescribed for feminizing hormone therapy. Although data are limited, it appears that 17-B estradiol has no significant interactions with ART.[128]

Data are also lacking around the use of ART with testosterone therapy in transmasculine people. Testosterone appears to be relatively safe as it has been administered with ART for years to HIV-positive cis men with hypogonadism.[130] Since testosterone is known to potentially cause vaginal atrophy, it may put transmasculine people who have receptive vaginal or "front hole" sex at higher risk for HIV infection, although data are lacking.

Both estradiol and testosterone are independent risk factors for CVD. Both have thrombogenic effects and can cause liver inflammation. Since persons with HIV already have higher rates of CVD, HIV-positive transgender patients should routinely be monitored for co-morbid conditions and counselled on reducing modifiable risk factors. In the case of transfeminine people, transdermal estrogen is preferred in those with significant risk for CVD.

Low bone mass has been reported in HIV patients in general and in some transfeminine people before hormone initiation.[124] Since sex hormones have an important effect on bone metabolism, HIV-positive transgender patients should remain on cross-sex hormones post-gonadectomy.

HIV Treatment and COVID-19

In December 2019, the severe acute respiratory syndrome coronavirus 2 (SARS-CoV-2), known to cause coronavirus disease 2019 (COVID-19), rapidly emerged from China into a new global pandemic. Its broad clinical spectrum ranges from asymptomatic and uncomplicated symptoms to severe multi-organ failure and death. Although still inconclusive at the time of publication, data suggest that HIV may be an independent risk factor for negative clinical outcomes to COVID-19 infection.[131-134]

In the general population, disease severity from COVID-19 has been associated with older age, male sex, and underlying medical conditions such as diabetes, hypertension, cardiovascular disease, pulmonary disease, liver disease and obesity.[135-137] Since PLWHA often present with various co-morbidities, they may be at greater risk for serious COVID-19 sequelae. Racialized communities of color have been disproportionately affected by COVID-19.[131,138] The CDC estimates that Black and Hispanic persons experience approximately a three-fold higher rate of hospitalizations and a two-fold higher rate of deaths to COVID-19 compared to White non-Hispanic persons.[139] Health and economic disparities, as well as community and workplace exposure, are probable factors that underscore the need for further research.[140,141]

Current data on the use of the COVID-19 vaccine in PLWHA are limited. At present, it is recommended that all PLWHA be vaccinated against COVID-19. Since it is not a live vaccine, it may be administered to PLWHA irrespective of CD4 count and HIV viral load. The vaccine is predicted to be safe and to produce a similar immune response in PLWHA compared to those without HIV infection. However, for those with a CD4 count of <200 cells/mm^3 or who have uncontrolled HIV, counselling on the unknown safety and efficacy of the vaccine may be warranted. Immunization against influenza and pneumococcal disease should be updated. In addition, PLWHA should continue to follow local public health guidelines around social distancing, mask-wearing, and proper hand hygiene in order to prevent COVID-19 infection and transmission.[142-144]

HIV care delivery may be interrupted because of health care constraints during the COVID-19 pandemic. It is imperative that patients maintain an adequate supply of their HIV medications during this period. Regimen switches should be postponed unless for reasons of toxicity or treatment failure. Telemedicine appointments may replace face-to-face encounters, if warranted. And for patients who are stable on ART with sustained viral suppression, routine laboratory monitoring may be delayed.[142,145] Because of social distancing restrictions, some PLWHA may experience increased social isolation and psychological distress. In turn, this may worsen underlying mental health, substance use and malnutrition, as well as exacerbate structural burdens that may already exist such as poverty, food insecurity, unstable housing, health access, and societal stigma.[140,141] PCPs should be able to recognize these unique concerns and connect patients to counseling, case management, and social support services within the community.

HIV Treatment and the Aging Population

Old age and existing co-morbidities can impact the pharmacokinetics of drugs and contribute to polypharmacy. Routine medication reviews should be conducted to identify unnecessary drugs, avoid serious medication interactions, allow for dose adjustments, and ensure drug adherence. The Beers and STOPP criteria are tools that can be used to reduce inappropriate drug prescribing in the aging HIV population.[146,147]

Older HIV-positive patients tend to have a slower and lower CD4 cell recovery with ART. Because of their high incidence of co-morbidities, modifications to ART may be required.[39] For instance, switching older patients out of a TDF-based regimen may be prudent if they are at high risk for falls or have renal impairment. Clinicians should regularly assess older patients for neurocognitive deficits that may stem from chronic HIV infection or a mood disorder. Risk factors for HIV-associated neurocognitive disorder (HAND) are likely multifactorial and include older age, advanced HIV, high viral load, psychiatric illness, substance use, and vascular factors. Chronic immune activation and inflammation in the brain has been posited to be the main cause of HAND.[148] In such cases, brain imaging and a referral to a neuropsychiatric specialist may be warranted.

The devastating impact of AIDS on the older generation of HIV-positive gay men is seldom acknowledged. These long-term HIV survivors likely experienced unimaginable loss during the early days of the epidemic. For many of these patients, survivor's guilt can complicate their grief.[149] The traumatic effects of witnessing friends and loved ones die of AIDS in the past can often resurface as older patients try to manage their multi-morbidities and begin to question their own mortality. In turn, PCPs should regularly monitor HIV long-term survivors for psychiatric co-morbidities including mood and anxiety disorders, as well as substance use.[113,150] PCPs should be ready to provide emotional support to older HIV-positive patients and refer them to counselling and addiction services as needed. PCPs should also be comfortable in reviewing the spiritual care needs of their patients and discuss advanced care planning with them. In doing so, PCPs can help older HIV-positive patients age with dignity and respect. For more information on caring for older 2SLGBTQ adults, see chapter 13.

Box 7.1. Fertility Considerations for Individuals and Couples with HIV

Author: Ian Armstrong

HIV and antiretroviral therapy may have a marginal impact on fertility via reduced ovarian reserve,[151] hypogonadism,[152] and lower sperm quality.[153]

- Numerous medical advances have been employed to prevent horizontal transmission.
  - For serodiscordant couples attempting to conceive naturally, current evidence suggests there is no risk of transmitting HIV sexually if the HIV-positive partner has maintained an undetectable viral load for at least six months.[154]
  - For couples attempting to conceive using intrauterine insemination or in vitro fertilization, current evidence suggests there is no risk of acquiring HIV from semen that has undergone "sperm washing."[155]
  - HIV pre-exposure prophylaxis (PrEP) can also be used to mitigate risk from exposure to HIV[156] during natural or assisted fertilization, or surrogacy.
- Antiretroviral therapy has been shown to reduce risk of vertical transmission.
  - AIDSinfo guidelines recommend a multi-pronged approach to preventing vertical transmission,[157] including the following:
    - Viral suppression during pregnancy
    - If parental HIV viral load is high or unknown near delivery, scheduled C-section and/or intrapartum IV antiretroviral therapy

- Short course of neonatal post-exposure prophylaxis
- Careful and context-specific counselling on risks and benefits of breastfeeding, with the awareness that HIV-positive individuals can transmit HIV via breast milk even while maintaining an undetectable viral load[158]
  o Individuals attempting to conceive should consult their HIV specialist for up-to-date information on antiretroviral therapy regimens recommended for use during pregnancy.
    - Although most antiretroviral regimens are not associated with congenital defects,[157] with the possible exception of dolutegravir,[159] ongoing research is attempting to clarify whether in utero antiretroviral exposure may have mild neurodevelopmental impacts.[160,161]

HIV Prevention

Treatment as Prevention

Treatment as prevention (TasP) refers to the concept that HIV treatment can reduce community viral load and prevent HIV transmission. The CDC states that PLWHA who continually maintain viral suppression while on ART have "effectively no risk of transmitting HIV to their HIV-negative sexual partners."[162] Several landmark studies clearly support the benefits of TasP and the growing evidence that "undetectable = untransmittable" (U = U).[154,163,164] They also underscore the need for strict ART adherence and routine viral load monitoring during HIV care.

HIV Pre-exposure Prophylaxis

HIV PrEP has become an exceedingly important tool in the HIV prevention armamentarium. PrEP refers to taking HIV medication daily to prevent HIV infection. Truvada (TDF/FTC) for PrEP has been shown to reduce HIV transmission rates in MSM, transgender women, PWIDs, and heterosexual persons by 44 to 75 per cent in randomized clinical trials.[165–168] According to the CDC, Truvada can be 99 per cent effective in preventing HIV infection when taken consistently for sex and at least 74 per cent effective for injection drug use.[169] In most cases, transgender and gender non-binary persons have been underrepresented in PrEP studies. PrEP does not protect against other STIs and should be used in combination with other prevention strategies, which include condom use, risk-reduction counselling, TasP, and routine screening for STIs and syndemic conditions.[170] Truvada for PrEP was approved in Canada in 2016.

More recent, Descovy (TAF/FTC) has been shown to be as effective as Truvada for the prevention of HIV in MSM and transgender women. As expected, PrEP studies have shown that the TAF component of Descovy improves renal function and bone mineral density, while the TDF component of Truvada lent to better weight and lipid outcomes. Truvada may significantly lower lipid profiles, including HDL, but total cholesterol to HDL ratios remain comparable to Descovy. Descovy may increase BMI levels but whether this increase mirrors the expected weight gain in the general population is still debatable. However, studies do suggest that TAF may be associated with weight gain, especially when used in an INSTI-based regimen for HIV treatment.[105–107,171] Descovy for PrEP was approved in Canada in late 2020. Because of limited data, Descovy is currently not recommended for use in PWID and persons who engage in vaginal or front hole sex.

The 2017 CDC guidelines recommend PrEP to sexually active MSM who are at substantial risk for HIV infection which include having a partner who is HIV positive, a diagnosis of recent bacterial STIs, inconsistent condom use with partners of unknown status, multiple sex partners, and commercial sex work.[172] The 2017 Canadian PrEP guidelines extend the recommendation to transfeminine people and further note that in serodiscordant relationships, PrEP need only be offered when the HIV-positive partner is not on ART or has a detectable viral load.[170] Patients with recurrent use of PEP should also be offered PrEP. The HIV Incidence Risk Index for Men Who Have Sex with Men (HIRI-MSM) is a validated screening tool that was adapted by the Canadian guidelines to help identify MSM who may benefit from PrEP. See table 7.11. According to the guidelines, PrEP should be offered to patients with a HIRI-MSM risk score of ≥11.[170] No PrEP data currently exist for cis women and transmasculine people who have condomless genital sex with MSM and transfeminine people. The decision to start PrEP in these patients should be made on an individual basis taking into consideration individual risk factors and local HIV prevalence rates. At present, PrEP use among PWID is off-label in Canada and should not be considered unless access to harm reduction interventions is scaled up and readily available.[170]

Guidelines for PrEP recommend baseline bloodwork and routine monitoring. See table 7.12. The Canadian guidelines are generally consistent with those of the CDC.[173] PrEP should be prescribed to patients with a documented negative HIV test. Before PrEP initiation,

Table 7.11. HIV Incidence Risk Index for MSM

1. How old are you today (years)?	<18 years	Score 0	_____
	18–28 years	Score 8	
	29–40 years	Score 5	
	41–48 years	Score 2	
	49 years or more	Score 0	
2. How many men have you had sex with in the last 6 months?	>10 male partners	Score 7	_____
	6–10 male partners	Score 4	
	0–5 male partners	Score 0	
3. How many of your male sex partners were HIV positive?	>1 positive partner	Score 8	_____
	1 positive partner	Score 4	
	<1 positive partner	Score 0	
4. In the last 6 months, how many times did you have receptive anal sex (you were the bottom) with a man without a condom?	1 or more times	Score 10	_____
	0 times	Score 0	
5. In the last 6 months, how many times did you have insertive anal sex (you were the top) without a condom with a man who was HIV-positive?	5 or more times,	Score 6	_____
	0–4 times	Score 0	
6. In the last 6 months, have you used methamphetamines such as crystal or speed?	Yes	Score 5	_____
	No	Score 0	
7. In the last 6 months, have you used poppers (amyl nitrate)?	Yes	Score 3	_____
	No	Score 0	
	Add down entries in right-hand column to calculate total score*		_____

Source: Adapted from Canadian PrEP guideline. 2017.[170]

* PrEP should be offered to patients with a HIRI-MSM risk score ≥11.

Table 7.12. HIV Pre-exposure Prophylaxis (PrEP) Recommendations

Indication	• Persons who are at high risk for HIV infection
Baseline Evaluation	• HIV testing with fourth-generation assay • Assessment for signs and symptoms of acute HIV infection • Serum Cr and urinalysis, CBC optional • Hepatitis A serology, vaccinate if non-immune • Hepatitis B serology (HBsAg, HBsAb, HBcAb), vaccinate if non-immune • Hepatitis C serology • STIs screening, including gonorrhea, chlamydia, syphilis • Urine pregnancy test in cis women (and trans men if appropriate) • Discuss daily adherence, risks and benefits of PrEP
Preferred Drug Regimen	• TDF/FTC (Truvada) or TAF/FTC (Descovy)* once daily • TDF/FTC if eGFR >60mL/min • TAF/FTC if eGFR >30mL/min • Maximum prescription no more than 90 days
Follow-Up Monitoring	• At 4 weeks: HIV testing[†] and serum Cr • Every 3 months thereafter: HIV testing, serum Cr, STI screening, and pregnancy test (if appropriate) • Annually: hepatitis C serology • At each visit: assess for signs and symptoms of acute HIV infection, drug adherence and toxicity, continued need for PrEP, and counsel on other HIV prevention strategies[‡]

Source: Adapted from Canadian guideline on HIV pre-exposure prophylaxis and nonoccupational postexposure prophylaxis. 2017.[170]

CBC = complete blood count, Cr = creatinine, eGFR = estimated glomerular filtration rate, FTC = emtricitabine, HBcAb = hepatitis B core antibody, HBsAb = hepatitis B surface antibody, HBsAg = hepatitis B surface antigen, STIs = sexually transmitted infections, TAF = tenofovir alafenamide, TDF = tenofovir disoproxil fumarate

* Currently not approved for use in people who inject drugs and people who engage in vaginal or front hole sex

† Patients who test HIV-positive or who show early signs of acute HIV infection during PrEP should either discontinue PrEP or be given boosted-DRV and DTG with Truvada while waiting for results of HIV RNA testing; urgent referral to an HIV expert is warranted.

‡ PrEP does not protect against STIs and should be used in combination with other HIV prevention strategies including condom use, behaviour counselling, and routine screening for STIs and syndemic conditions.

a fourth-generation HIV test should be used to detect undiagnosed HIV infection. In patients with a recent high-risk exposure, HIV RNA testing may be useful to rule out acute HIV infection.[170,174] Patients who have signs and symptoms of acute HIV infection within the past 12 weeks and who received a negative HIV test should also be considered for HIV RNA testing.[173] Initial HBV screening is important as the anti-HBV activity of Truvada and Descovy may cause HBV flare-ups if PrEP were to be stopped abruptly. Truvada may be given to patients with a CrCl greater than 60 mL/min and Descovy to those with a CrCl greater than 30 mL/min. PrEP is generally well tolerated. It should be given no more than three months at a time to allow for routine drug toxicity monitoring, STI testing, and adherence; behavioural counselling; and assessment for acute HIV infection. Patients who test positive for HIV or who show early signs of acute HIV infection while on PrEP should either discontinue PrEP or be given an intensified ART regimen, with the addition of boosted-DRV and DTG, while waiting for confirmatory results of HIV RNA testing.[170,174] In such cases, an urgent referral to an HIV expert is highly recommended. Resistance to PrEP is rare and has been mainly noted when PrEP was initiated during undiagnosed acute HIV infection. However, a small number of confirmed cases of HIV transmission have been reported in North America and Europe despite strict daily adherence to PrEP.[175–177]

Patients should be advised that PrEP may take longer to accumulate in different regions of the body and that its protective effect may not be immediate. The CDC advises that PrEP should be taken daily for about 7 days before it can provide protection for receptive anal sex and about 21 days for receptive vaginal or front hole sex, keeping in mind that Descovy is currently not recommended for the latter.[173,178,179] Pharmokinetic data have suggested that TAF may exhibit lower tenofovir levels in rectal and genital mucosa than TDF, leading to some debate around the use of Descovy in PrEP.[180,181] Whether achieving maximal drug concentrations at these sites correlates to maximal HIV protection is still unclear. Limited research also exists on the effectiveness of PrEP in transgender patients with surgically constructed genitalia. Transmasculine people who are on testosterone therapy may experience vaginal atrophy, which can put them at risk for HIV infection when engaging in vaginal or front hole sex. Whether vaginal atrophy has an effect on PrEP remains unknown.

According to the Canadian guidelines, there is insufficient data to recommend pericoital or "on-demand" PrEP, although it has been used off-label in Canada.[170] Conversely, the 2018 IAS-US guidelines do recommend on-demand PrEP with Truvada as a substitute for daily PrEP in MSM who have infrequent sex. Sometimes known as the "2-1-1" regimen, a double dose of Truvada can be taken 2 to 24 hours before sex with additional single doses at 24 hours and 48 hours after sex. For each new sex encounter, re-initiation of PrEP with a double dose of Truvada applies unless the last dose was taken within seven days, in which case only one dose is necessary.[77] Because of limited data, Descovy is currently not recommended for on-demand PrEP.

The discussion around what medication to prescribe for HIV PrEP depends on several factors, including patient co-morbidities and financial status. Some experts favor Truvada for its robust and decade-long data showing efficacy among different populations, including cis women, as well as its safety history among long-term users. Since a generic version of Truvada is now available in Canada, it also has become the cheaper option for PrEP. At present, many provinces and territories in Canada provide coverage for Truvada for PrEP, while Descovy for PrEP is currently covered only through private health insurance. Moving forward, more advocacy is needed to ensure better financial access to HIV PrEP nationwide.

HIV Post-exposure Prophylaxis

HIV post-exposure prophylaxis (PEP) is the use of ART to prevent HIV infection in both occupational and non-occupational settings. PEP is another important HIV prevention tool in 2SLGBTQ primary care, especially in patients with a recent high-risk exposure to HIV infection. PEP should be offered to patients who have recently engaged in condomless vaginal or anal sex with a sex partner of unknown HIV status from a prevalent HIV group (MSM, transfeminine people, PWID) or with a sex partner known to be HIV-positive with a detectable viral load. The Canadian guideline on non-occupational PEP recommends immediate PEP initiation no later than 72 hours after the exposure event. PEP should be taken for 28 days. Emergency contraception counselling may be needed in trans men exposed to sperm. If there is potential for pregnancy, a DTG-based regimen should be avoided because of its potential teratogenic effects. Baseline PEP blood work and follow-up monitoring is recommended. See table 7.13. All HIV testing should be done with a fourth-generation assay. For patients presenting with acute HIV infection symptoms or who later test positive for HIV, PEP should not be withheld or discontinued. In such cases, HIV RNA testing should be performed and a prompt referral to an HIV expert is warranted. Patients already on HIV PrEP do not require PEP after a potential HIV exposure. Although the Canadian guideline suggests follow-up HIV testing at three months only, the CDC guideline recommends additional HIV testing at four to six weeks.[170,182] Patients who repeatedly go on PEP should be considered for PrEP.

Table 7.13. HIV Non-occupational Post-exposure Prophylaxis (PEP) Recommendations

Indication	• Persons with a recent high-risk exposure to HIV infection
Baseline Evaluation	• HIV testing with fourth-generation assay • Assessment for signs and symptoms of acute HIV infection* • Hepatitis A serology, vaccinate if non-immune • Hepatitis B serology (HBsAg, HBsAb, HBcAb), vaccinate if non-immune • Hepatitis C serology • STIs screening for gonorrhea, chlamydia, syphilis • Complete blood count • Alanine aminotransferase • Serum creatinine • Urine pregnancy test in cis women (and trans men if appropriate)
Preferred Drug Regimen	• TDF/FTC (Truvada) once daily + DTG (Tivicay) once daily OR • TDF/FTC (Truvada) once daily + RAL (Isentress) twice daily OR • TDF/FTC (Truvada) once daily + DRV (Prezista) once daily + ritonavir (Norvir) once daily • PEP must be initiated within 72 hours after exposure • PEP must be taken for 28 days
Follow-Up Monitoring	• At 2 weeks: repeat serum ALT and Cr if abnormal at baseline or symptomatic • At 3 months: repeat HIV testing, hepatitis C serology, and STIs screening† • At 6 months: consider repeat HIV testing if hepatitis C infection was acquired from recent exposure • At each visit: assess for signs and symptoms of acute HIV infection, drug adherence and toxicity, and counsel on other HIV prevention strategies including condom use, behavior counseling, routine screening for syndemic conditions, and future consideration of PrEP

Source: Adapted from Canadian guideline on HIV pre-exposure prophylaxis and nonoccupational postexposure prophylaxis. 2017.[170]

ALT = alanine aminotransferase, Cr = creatinine, DRV = darunavir, DTG = dolutegravir, FTC = emtricitabine, HBcAb = hepatitis B core antibody, HBsAb = hepatitis B surface antibody, HBsAg = hepatitis B surface antigen, PEP = post-exposure prophylaxis, PrEP = pre-exposure prophylaxis, RAL = raltegravir, STIs = sexually transmitted infections, TDF = tenofovir disoproxil fumarate

* At baseline, if acute HIV infection is suspected, PEP should not be withheld; confirm with HIV RNA testing and refer to an HIV expert.

† While on PEP, if acute HIV infection is suspected or HIV test is positive, PEP should be continued; confirm with HIV RNA testing and refer to an HIV expert.

Future of HIV Treatment and Prevention

Key developments in HIV medicine are currently underway. New anti-HIV drugs are being studied and show great promise. Injectable lenacapavir, an HIV capsid inhibitor, and GSK3640254, a HIV maturation inhibitor, represent two experimental classes of drugs that are being investigated.[183–186] Other new drug classes include the HIV post-attachment inhibitor fostemsavir (Rukobia) and the injectable monoclonal antibody ibalizumab (Trogarzo), both approved in the United States for treatment-experienced patients with HIV multi-drug resistance.[187–190] Doravirine (Pifeltro), a unique NNRTI with potential for better lipid profiles and fewer side effects, was recently approved in Canada.[191,192] Also approved is Cabenuva, the combination of RPV and the novel long-acting INSTI cabotegravir (CGV), an injectable treatment option for HIV patients who struggle with daily ART adherence.[193,194] The move to combination dual-drug therapy is also making its mark in the treatment landscape. The DHHS guidelines currently include three dual-drug regimens that may be considered in treatment-naive patients who cannot take ABC, TAF, or TDF.[39] More recently, the dual regimens of DTG/3TC (Dovato) for initial HIV treatment and DTG/RPV (Juluca) for simplification therapy were approved in Canada.[195–197] In the domain of HIV prevention, on-demand PrEP and injectable CGV are actively being investigated, along with the continuing search for an HIV vaccine and cure.[198]

Conclusion

Four decades later, the global response to HIV/AIDS forges stalwartly ahead. In Canada, ART remains the cornerstone of HIV treatment. Once a fatal disease, HIV infection has now become a chronic yet manageable condition. Despite scientific advances, a cure for HIV remains elusive as Canadians continue to be infected by the virus. Emergent strategies in education and prevention, as well as shifting discourses on health systems and policies, are urgently needed to mitigate the burden of HIV in our country.

The early response to AIDS was one of fear and blame, marked by undercurrents of religious righteousness and broken morality. The outcome was discriminatory and stigmatizing, and punctuated by unfathomable loss. Today, these injustices still remain. MSM and trans-feminine people continue to be disproportionately affected by HIV and face innumerable social, structural, and medical barriers. Many remain economically vulnerable and socially isolated, while others suffer from racial-, gender-, and sexual-based violence. McCaskell appropriately referred to HIV/AIDS as a lens that magnifies all social problems.[13] His statement loudly rings true today as it reminds us that HIV is as much of a social and political phenomenon as it is a medical one.

The advent of AIDS left an indelible mark on Canadian 2SLGBTQ history. AIDS advanced gay rights and mobilized 2SLGBTQ communities in ways not previously seen. What emerged from a period of darkness and despair was a triumphant spirit of hope and solidarity. It paved the way for changes in science and politics, health care policies and practices, and basic human rights. By referencing the past, we pay tribute to the lives lost and the advances made by AIDS activists who have come before us. It teaches us courage, compassion, and tolerance. And it reminds us that social change is always possible when enough dedicated people come together to willingly fight for it.

In Canada, HIV-related inequities still exist. The criminalization of HIV non-disclosure continues to minimize prevention efforts, leading to the incarceration of 2SLGBTQ persons based on disproven risk assumptions. The blood donation ban against MSM continues to expose the discriminatory screening policies of the Canadian Blood Services. And the "institutional erasure" of transgender and non-binary persons continues to silence 2SLGBTQ minorities in the health care system. As clinicians, we have the unique ability to challenge these societal injustices and asymmetric systems by serving as strong social and political advocates for our 2SLGBTQ patients. By using our medical expertise and professional influence, we can lend our voices to the fight for 2SLGBTQ health care rights nationwide. In doing so, we can collectively reshape the future course of HIV in Canada.

HIV Resources for the Care of HIV-Positive Persons

Topic/Organization	Resource Title	Website Link
Primary Care Guidelines		
BC Centre for Excellence in HIV/ AIDS (BC-CfE)	Primary Care Guidelines for the Management of HIV/ AIDS in British Columbia	http://www.cfenet.ubc.ca/sites /default/files/uploads/primary -care-guidelines/primary-care -guidelines_015-09-15.pdf
Infectious Diseases Society of America (IDSA)	Primary Care Guidelines for the Management of Persons Infected with HIV: 2013 Update by the HIV Medicine Association of the Infectious Diseases of America	http://www.idsociety.org /Guidelines/Patient_Care /IDSA_Practice_Guidelines /Infections_By_Organism -28143/HIV/AIDS/Primary _Care_Management_of_HIV -Infected_Patients/

Topic/Organization	Resource Title	Website Link
Adult Treatment Guidelines		
US Department of Health and Human Services (DHHS)	Guidelines for the Use of Antiretroviral Agents in Adults and Adolescents Living with HIV	https://aidsinfo.nih.gov /guidelines/html/1 /adult-and-adolescent-arv/0
BC Centre of Excellence in HIV/ AIDS	Therapeutic Guidelines for Antiretroviral (ARV) Treatment of Adult HIV Infection, September 2015	http://www.cfenet.ubc.ca /sites/default/files/uploads /Guidelines/bccfe-art -guidelines-Oct_14_2015. pdf
International Antiviral Society (IAS)	Antiretroviral Drugs for Treatment and Prevention of HIV Infection in Adults: 2018 Recommendations of the International Antiviral Society-USA Panel	https://jamanetwork.com /journals/jama/fullarticle /2688574
	Antiretroviral Drugs for Treatment and Prevention of HIV Infection in Adults: 2016 Recommendations of the International Antiviral Society-USA Panel	https://jamanetwork.com /journals/jama/fullarticle /2533073
European AIDS Clinical Society (EACS)	EACS Guidelines, Version 9.0, October 2017	http://www.eacsociety.org/files /guidelines_9.0-english.pdf
Opportunistic Infections Guidelines		
BC Centre of Excellence in HIV/ AIDS (BC-CfE)	Therapeutic Guidelines for Opportunistic Infections	http://www.cfenet.ubc.ca/sites /default/files/uploads/docs /Opportunistic_Infection _Therapeutic_ Guidelines2009.pdf
US Department of Health and Human Services (DHHS)	Guidelines for the Prevention and Treatment of Opportunistic Infections in HIV-Infected Adults and Adolescents	https://aidsinfo.nih.gov /guidelines/html/4/adult-and -adolescent-opportunistic -infection/0

(Continued)

(Continued)

Topic/Organization	Resource Title	Website Link
Pediatric and Perinatal Guidelines		
US Department of Health and Human Services (DHHS)	Guidelines for the Use of Antiretroviral Agents in Pediatric HIV Infection Recommendations for the Use of Antiretroviral Drugs in Pregnant Women with HIV Infection and Interventions to Reduce Perinatal HIV Transmission in the United States	https://aidsinfo.nih.gov /guidelines/html/2 /pediatric-arv/0 https://aidsinfo.nih.gov /guidelines/html/3/perinatal/0
Immunizations		
National Advisory Committee on Immunizations (NACI)	NACI Recommendations, Statements and Updates	https://www.canada.ca/en /public-health/services /immunization/national -advisory-committee-on -immunization-naci.html
Cancer Screening		
Canadian Cancer Society	Cancer Screening Information and Considerations for LGBTQ Clients	http://convio.cancer.ca/site /PageServer?pagename =SSL_ON_HCP_HCPGen _LGBTQClients#.Wq4vnL YZPeQ
Canadian Task Force on Preventive Health Care (CTFPHC)	Published Guidelines	https://canadiantaskforce .ca/guidelines /published-guidelines
BC Centre for Excellence in HIV/ AIDS (BC-CfE)	Primary Care Guidelines for the Management of HIV/ AIDS in British Columbia	http://www.cfenet.ubc.ca/sites /default/files/uploads/primary -care-guidelines/primary-care -guidelines_015-09-15.pdf
Infectious Diseases Society of America (IDSA)	Primary Care Guidelines for the Management of Persons Infected with HIV: 2013 Update by the HIV Medicine Association of the Infectious Diseases of America	http://www.idsociety.org /Guidelines/Patient_Care /IDSA_Practice_Guidelines /Infections_By _Organism-28143/HIV/AIDS /Primary_Care_Management _of_HIV-Infected_Patients/
European AIDS Clinical Society (EACS)	EACS Guidelines, Version 9.0, October 2017	http://www.eacsociety.org/files /guidelines_9.0-english.pdf

Topic/Organization	Resource Title	Website Link
Drug Coverage		
Toronto General Hospital Immunodeficiency Clinic	Drug Reimbursement Information: Reimbursement Status of Antiretrovirals in Canada	https://hivclinic.ca/drug-information/drug-reimbursement-information/
Canadian Treatment Action Council	Tx Map	https://ctac.ca/tx-map/
Drug Interactions and Side-Effects		
University of Liverpool	HIV Drug Interaction Checker	https://www.hiv-druginteractions.org/
University Hospital Network and Toronto General Hospital	HIV/HCV Drug Therapy Guide Database of Antiretroviral Drug Interactions	https://hivclinic.ca/drug-information/drug-interaction-tables/
University of California, San Francisco	American Geriatrics Society 2015 Updated Beers Criteria for Potentially Inappropriate Medication Use in Older Adults	http://arv.ucsf.edu/insite?page=ar-00-02
American Geriatrics Society	STOPP/START criteria for potentially inappropriate prescribing in older people: version 2	http://onlinelibrary.wiley.com/doi/10.1111/jgs.13702/abstract;jsessionid=7BA8BBFDFFB7B9F1E948D74BE6A3CBA4.f03t04
British Geriatrics Society		https://www.ncbi.nlm.nih.gov/pmc/articles/PMC4339726/
Co-morbid Conditions *Dyslipidemia*		
Canadian Cardiovascular Society (CCS)	2016 Guidelines for the Management of Dyslipidemia for the Prevention of Cardiovascular Disease in the Adult	http://www.onlinecjc.ca/article/S0828-282X(16)30732-2/abstract
Diabetes		
Canadian Diabetes Association (CDA)	The Canadian Diabetes Association 2013 Clinical Practice Guidelines for the Prevention and Management of Diabetes	http://guidelines.diabetes.ca
Hypertension		
Hypertension Canada	Hypertension Canada Guidelines: Diagnosis and Assessment, Prevention and Treatment	http://guidelines.hypertension.ca

(Continued)

(Continued)

Topic/Organization	Resource Title	Website Link
Liver		
American Association for the Study of Liver Diseases (AALD)	Practice Guidelines – Various	https://www.aasld.org /publications/practice -guidelines-0
European AIDS Clinical Society (EACS)	EACS Guidelines, Version 9.0, October 2017	http://www.eacsociety.org/files /guidelines_9.0-english.pdf
European Association for the Study of the Liver (EASL)	EASL Clinical Practice Guidelines – Various	http://www.easl.eu/research /our-contributions /clinical-practice-guidelines
US Department of Health and Human Services (DHHS)	Guidelines for the Use of Antiretroviral Agents in Adults and Adolescents Living with HIV, Appendix B. Antiretroviral Dosing Recommendations in Patients with Renal or Hepatic Insufficiency	https://aidsinfo.nih.gov /guidelines/html/1/adult -and-adolescent-arv/44/arv -dosing-for-renal-or-hepatic -insufficiency
Renal		
Infectious Diseases Society of America (IDSA)	Clinical Practice Guideline for the management of Chronic Kidney Disease in Patients infected with HIV: 2014 Update by the HIV Medicine Association of the Infectious Diseases Society of America	https://www.ncbi.nlm.nih.gov /pmc/articles/PMC4271038/
US Department of Health and Human Services (DHHS)	Guidelines for the Use of Antiretroviral Agents in Adults and Adolescents Living with HIV, Appendix B. Antiretroviral Dosing Recommendations in Patients with Renal or Hepatic Insufficiency	https://aidsinfo.nih.gov /guidelines/html/1/adult -and-adolescent-arv/44/arv -dosing-for-renal-or-hepatic -insufficiency
Bone		
Infectious Diseases Society of America (IDSA)	Recommendations for Evaluation and Management of Bone Disease in HIV	https://www.ncbi.nlm.nih.gov /pmc/articles/PMC4400413/

Topic/Organization	Resource Title	Website Link
HIV Prevention		
HIV Pre-Exposure Prophylaxis (PrEP)		
Canadian Guidelines	Canadian Guideline on HIV Preexposure Prophylaxis and Nonoccupational Postexposure Prophylaxis	http://www.cmaj.ca/content /cmaj/189/47/E1448.full.pdf
Centers for Disease Control and Prevention (CDC)	Preexposure Prophylaxis for the Prevention of HIV Infections in the United States – 2014 Clinical Practice Guideline	https://www.cdc.gov/hiv/pdf /prepguidelines2014.pdf
HIRI-MSM	HIV Incidence Risk Index for Men who have Sex with Men	http://voices-tmc.net/tmc2014 /library/54-008.pdf, https:// www.aidsunited.org/data/files /Site_18/PrEP/MSM_Risk _Index.pdf
HIV Post-Exposure Prophylaxis (PEP)		
Canadian Guidelines	Canadian Guideline on HIV Preexposure Prophylaxis and Nonoccupational Postexposure Prophylaxis	http://www.cmaj.ca/content /cmaj/189/47/E1448.full.pdf
Centers for Disease Control and Prevention (CDC)	Updated Guidelines for Antiretroviral Postexposure Prophylaxis after Sexual, Injection Drug Use, or Other Nonoccupational Exposure to HIV – United States, 2016	https://stacks.cdc.gov/view /cdc/38856
General Resource		
CATIE	Canada's Source for HIV and Hepatitis C Information	http://www.catie.ca/en/about /milestones
US Department of Health and Human Services	AIDSInfo Offering Information on HIV/AIDS Prevention, Treatment, and Research	https://aidsinfo.nih.gov

References

1. Centers for Disease Control. Pneumocystis pneumonia – Los Angeles. MMWR Morb Mortal Wkly Rep. 1981;30(21):250–2.
2. Altman L. Rare cancer seen in 41 homosexuals. The New York Times. 1981 Jul 3 [cited 2017 Jul 15]. Avaialbe from: http://www.nytimes .com/1981/07/03/us/rare-cancer-seen-in-41-homosexuals.html.
3. Zhu T, Korber BT, Nahmias AJ, Hooper E, Sharp PM, Ho DD. An African HIV-1 sequence from 1959 and implications for the origin of the epidemic. Nature. 1998;391(6667):594–7.
4. Robbins KE, Lemey P, Pybus OG, Jaffe HW, Youngpairoj AS, Brown TM, et al. U.S. Human immunodeficiency virus type 1 epidemic: date of origin, population history, and characterization of early strains. J Virol. 2003;77(11):6359–66.
5. Public Health Agency of Canada [Internet]. Ottawa: Government of Canada; 2015 [cited 2018 Jul 15]. Chapter 2: Population-specific HIV/AIDS status report: people living with HIV/AIDS – epidemiological profile of HIV and AIDS in Canada. Available from: https://www.canada.ca/en /public-health/services/hiv-aids/publications/population-specific-hiv -aids-status-reports/people-living-hiv-aids/chapter-2-epidemiological -profile-hiv-aids-canada.html.
6. Canada Diseases Weekly Report. Pneumocystis carinii pneumonia in a homosexual male – Ontario. CDWR. 1982 8(13):65–7.
7. Bourgeois AC, Edmunds M, Awan A, Jonah L, Varsaneux O, Siu W. HIV in Canada – surveillance report, 2016. Can Commun Dis Rep. 2017;43(12):248–56.
8. Baral SD, Poteat T, Strömdahl S, Wirtz AL, Guadamuz TE, Beyrer C. Worldwide burden of HIV in transgender women: a systematic review and meta-analysis. Lancet Infect Dis. 2013;13(3):214–22.
9. Public Health Agency of Canada [Internet]. Ottawa: Government of Canada; 2014; [cited 2017 Aug 15]. HIV and AIDS in Canada: surveillance report to December 31, 2014. Available from: https://www.canada.ca /en/public-health/services/publications/diseases-conditions/hiv-aids -canada-surveillance-report-december-31-2014.html.
10. Manon Tremblay, editor. Queer mobilizations: social movement activism and Canadian public policy. Vancouver: UBC Press; 2015.
11. Cappon P, Adrien A, Hankins C, Remis R, Roy E. HIV: the debate over isolation as a measure of personal control. Can J Public Health. 1991;82(6):404–8.
12. Duffin J. AIDS, memory and the history of medicine: musings on the Canadian response. Genitourin Med. 1994;70(1):64–9.

13. McCaskell T. Queer progress: from homophobia to homonationalism. Toronto: Between the Lines; 2016.
14. CBC Digital Archives [Internet]. Toronto: Canadian Broadcasting Corporation; 1983 [cited 2018 Mar 23]. Ministers debate AIDS and the politics of plague – CBC Archives. Available from: http://www.cbc.ca/archives/entry/ministers-debate-aids-and-the-politics-of-plague.
15. Smith RA. Encyclopedia of AIDS: a social, political, cultural, and scientific record of the HIV epidemic. New York: Penguin Books; 2001.
16. Neuman J. Former Sen. Jesse Helms dies at 86. LA Times [Internet]. 2008 Jul 5 [cited 2018 Mar 3]. Available from: http://www.latimes.com/news/la-me-helms5-2008jul05-story.html.
17. Stein M. Rethinking the gay and lesbian movement. New York: Routledge; 2012.
18. FitzGerald M, Rayter S. Queerly Canadian: an introductory reader in sexuality studies. Toronto: Canadian Scholars' Press; 2012.
19. MacNeil J. "No place for the state:" The day Ottawa got out of the nation's bedrooms. The Globe and Mail [Internet]; 2016 [updated 2016 Feb 29; cited 2018 Mar 20]. Available from: https://www.theglobeandmail.com/opinion/editorials/no-place-for-the-state-the-day-ottawa-got-out-of-the-nations-bedrooms/article28956096/.
20. Public Health Agency of Canada [Internet]. Ottawa: Government of Canada; 2017 [cited 2018 Jan 30]. Minister Petitpas Taylor marks World AIDS Day with investments of $36.4 million in projects to help eliminate AIDS. Available from: https://www.canada.ca/en/public-health/news/2017/12/minister_petitpastaylormarks worldaidsdaywithinvestmentsof364mill.html.
21. Bradburn J [Internet]. Ottawa: Historica Canada; 2013 Feb 3 [edited 2018 Jul 17; cited 2018 Oct 2]. Toronto bathhouse raids (1981). Available from: https://www.thecanadianencyclopedia.ca/en/article/toronto-feature-bathhouse-raids. Published February 2013.
22. Warner T. Never going back: a history of queer activism in Canada. Toronto: University of Toronto Press; 2002.
23. Rayside DM, Lindquist EA. AIDS activism and the state in Canada. Stud Polit Econ. 1992(39):37–76.
24. UNAIDS [Internet]. Geneva, Switzerland: United Nations; 1983; [cited 2018 Mar 3]. The Denver principles. Available from: http://data.unaids.org/pub/externaldocument/2007/gipa1983denverprinciples_en.pdf.
25. Smith MC, editor. Group politics and social movements in Canada. 2nd ed. Toronto: University of Toronto Press; 2014.
26. Rau K [Internet]. Ottawa: Historica Canada; 2014 [updated 2015 Jul 17; cited 2018 Jan 29]. Lesbian, gay, bisexual and transgender rights in

Canada. Available from: http://www.thecanadianencyclopedia.ca/en
/article/lesbian-gay-bisexual-and-transgender-rights-in-canada/.

27. Silversides A. AIDS activist: Michael Lynch and the politics of
community. Toronto: Between the Lines; 2003.

28. Berger P. Canada's national AIDS strategy neglects role of physicians.
CMAJ. 1990;143(4):309–11.

29. Smith JH, Whiteside A. The history of AIDS exceptionalism. J Int AIDS
Soc. 2010;13(1):47.

30. Worobey M, Watts TD, McKay RA, Suchard MA, Granade T, Teuwen DE,
et al. 1970s and "Patient 0" HIV-1 genomes illuminate early HIV/AIDS
history in North America. Nature. 2016;539(7627):98–101.

31. Fan HY, Conner RF, Villarreal LP. AIDS: science and society. 5th ed.
Massachusetts: Jones and Bartlett Publishers; 2007.

32. Canadian Blood Services [Internet]. Ottawa: Canadian Blood Services;
2018 [cited 2018 Oct 2]. About men who have sex with men. Available
from: https://blood.ca/en/blood/am-i-eligible/about-msm.

33. AIDS Committee of Toronto [Internet]. Toronto: Aids Committee of
Toronto; 2016 [cited 2017 Jul 15]. History of ACT. Available from:
http://www.actoronto.org/about-act/our-organization/history.

34. UNAIDS [Internet]. Geneva, Switzerland: United Nations; [cited 2021
Aug 15]. Fact sheet – latest statistics on the status of the AIDS epidemic.
Available from: http://www.unaids.org/en/resources/fact-sheet.

35. Public Health Agency of Canada [Internet]. Ottawa: Government of Canada;
[updated 2021 Jun 28; cited 2021 Aug 15]. Summary estimates of HIV
incidence, prevalence and Canada's progress on meeting the 90-90-90 HIV
targets. Available from: https://www.canada.ca/en/public-health/services
/publications/diseases-conditions/summary-estimates-hiv-incidence
-prevalence-canadas-progress-90-90-90.html#s4.

36. Public Health Agency of Canada [Internet]. Ottawa: Government of
Canada; [updated 2021 Jun 29; cited 2021 Aug 15]. Canada communicable
disease report: HIV in Canada – surveillance report, 2019. Available from:
https://www.canada.ca/en/public-health/services/reports-publications
/canada-communicable-disease-report-ccdr/monthly-issue/2021-47
/issue-1-january-2021/hiv-surveillance-report-2019.html.

37. Bourgeois AC, Edmunds M, Awan A, Jonah L [Internet]. Ottawa:
Government of Canada; 2017 [updated 2018 Jul 17; cited 2018 Jul 22]. HIV
in Canada – supplementary tables, 2016. CDWR. Available from:
https://www.canada.ca/en/public-health/services/reports-publications
/canada-communicable-disease-report-ccdr/monthly-issue/2017-43/ccdr
-volume-43-12-december-7-2017/hiv-2016-supplementary-tables.html.

38. Bauer GR, Hammond R, Travers R, Kaay M, Hohenadel KM, Boyce M.
"I don't think this is theoretical; this is our lives": how erasure impacts

health care for transgender people. J Assoc Nurses AIDS Care: JANAC. 2009;20(5):348–61.

39. Panel on Antiretroviral Guidelines for Adults and Adolescents [Internet]. Bethesda (MD): National Institutes of Health; [updated 2018 Oct 25; cited 2018 Nov 9 and 2021 Oct 20]. Guidelines for the use of antiretroviral agents in adults and adolescents living with HIV. Available from: https://aidsinfo.nih.gov/guidelines/html/1 /adult-and-adolescent-arv/0.

40. Fields BN, Knipe DM, Howley PM. Fields virology. 6th ed. Philadelphia: Wolters Kluwer Health/Lippincott Williams & Wilkins; 2013.

41. Hemelaar J, Gouws E, Ghys PD, Osmanov S, WHO-UNAIDS Network for HIV Isolation and Characterisation. Global trends in molecular epidemiology of HIV-1 during 2000–2007. AIDS. 2011;25(5):679–89.

42. Hemelaar J. The origin and diversity of the HIV-1 pandemic. Trends Mol Med. 2012;18(3):182–92.

43. US Department of Health and Human Services [Internet]. Washington (DC): National Institutes of Health; [cited 2018 Nov 9]. HIV overview: The HIV life cycle. Available from: http://aidsinfo.nih.gov /education-materials/fact-sheets/19/73/the-hiv-life-cycle.

44. Kinloch-de Loës S, de Saussure P, Saurat JH, Stalder H, Hirschel B, Perrin LH. Symptomatic primary infection due to human immunodeficiency virus type 1: review of 31 cases. Clin Infect Dis. 1993;17(1):59–65.

45. Panel on Clinical Practices for Treatment of HIV Infection. Guidelines for the use of antiretroviral agents in HIV-1 infected adults and adolescents [Internet]. Bethesda (MD): National Institutes of Health; 2004 Mar 23 [cited 2017 Aug 22]. Available from: https://aidsinfo.nih.gov /ContentFiles/AdultandAdolescentGL03232004003.pdf.

46. Günthard HF, Saag MS, Benson CA, del Rio C, Eron JJ, Gallant JE, et al. Antiretroviral Drugs for Treatment and Prevention of HIV Infection in Adults: 2016 Recommendations of the International Antiviral Society-USA Panel. JAMA. 2016;316(2):191–210.

47. Centers for Disease Control and Prevention [Internet]. Atlanta (GA): CDC; [updated 2008 Nov 20; cited 2017 Aug 22]. A ppendix A: AIDS-defining conditions. MMWR. Available from: https://www.cdc.gov/mmwr /preview/mmwrhtml/rr5710a2.htm.

48. Saksena NK, Rodes B, Wang B, Soriano V. Elite HIV controllers: myth or reality? AIDS Rev. 2007;9(4):195–207.

49. Koblin BA, Husnik MJ, Colfax G, Huang Y, Madison M, Mayer K, et al. Risk factors for HIV infection among men who have sex with men. AIDS. 2006;20(5):731–9.

50. Rosenberg ES, Sullivan PS, Dinenno EA, Salazar LF, Sanchez TH. Number of casual male sexual partners and associated factors among men who

have sex with men: results from the National HIV Behavioral Surveillance system. BMC Public Health. 2011;11:189.

51 Hirshfield S, Remien RH, Humberstone M, Walavalkar I, Chiasson MA. Substance use and high-risk sex among men who have sex with men: a national online study in the USA. AIDS Care. 2004;16(8):1036–47.

52. Colfax G, Guzman R. Club drugs and HIV infection: a review. Clin Infect Dis. 2006;42(10):1463–9.

53. Sewell J, Miltz A, Lampe FC, Cambiano V, Speakman A, Phillips AN, et al.; Attitudes to and Understanding of Risk of Acquisition of HIV (AURAH) Study Group. Poly drug use, chemsex drug use, and associations with sexual risk behaviour in HIV-negative men who have sex with men attending sexual health clinics. Int J Drug Policy. 2017 May;43:33–43.

54. Grov C, Parsons JT, Bimbi DS, Sex and Love v3.0 Research Team. In the shadows of a prevention campaign: sexual risk behavior in the absence of crystal methamphetamine. AIDS Educ Prev. 2008;20(1):42–55.

55. Vosvick M, Fritz S, Henry D, Prybutok V, Sheu S, Poe J. Correlates and racial/ethnic differences in bareback sex among men who have sex with men with unknown or negative HIV serostatus. AIDS Behav. 2016;20(12):2798–811.

56. Millett GA, Peterson JL, Flores SA, Hart TA, Jeffries WL 4th, Wilson PA, et al. Comparisons of disparities and risks of HIV infection in black and other men who have sex with men in Canada, UK, and USA: a meta-analysis. Lancet. 2012;380(9839):341–8.

57. Beymer MR, Weiss RE, Bolan RK, Rudy ET, Bourque LB, Rodriguez JP, et al. Sex on demand: geosocial networking phone apps and risk of sexually transmitted infections among a cross-sectional sample of men who have sex with men in Los Angeles County. Sex Transm Infect. 2014;90(7):567–72.

58. Goedel WC, Halkitis PN, Duncan DT. Behavior- and partner-based HIV risk perception and sexual risk behaviors in men who have sex with men (MSM) who use geosocial-networking smartphone applications in New York City. J Urban Health. 2016;93(2):400–6.

59. Rice E, Holloway I, Winetrobe H, et al. Sex risk among young men who have sex with men who use Grinder, a smartphone geosocial networking application. J AIDS Clin Res. 2012;S4:005. doi:10.4172 /2155-6113.S4-005.

60. Rendina HJ, Jimenez RH, Grov C, Ventuneac A, Parsons JT. Patterns of lifetime and recent HIV testing among men who have sex with men in New York City who use Grindr. AIDS Behav. 2014;18(1):41–9.

61. Singer M, Clair S. Syndemics and public health: reconceptualizing disease in bio-social context. Med Anthropol Q. 2003;17(4):423–41.
62. Stall R, Mills TC, Williamson J, Hart T, Greenwood G, Paul J, et al. Association of co-occurring psychosocial health problems and increased vulnerability to HIV/AIDS among urban men who have sex with men. Am J Public Health. 2003;93(6):939–42.
63. Otis J, McFadyen A, Haig T, Blais M, Cox J, Brenner B, et al.; Spot Study Group. Beyond condoms: risk reduction strategies among gay, bisexual, and other men who have sex with men receiving rapid HIV testing in Montreal, Canada. AIDS Behav. 2016;20(12):2812–26.
64. Card KG, Lachowsky NJ, Cui Z, Sereda P, Rich A, Jollimore J, et al. Seroadaptive Strategies of gay & bisexual men (GBM) with the highest quartile number of sexual partners in Vancouver, Canada. AIDS Behav. 2017;21(5):1452–66.
65. Hoffman BR. The interaction of drug use, sex work, and HIV among transgender women. Subst Use Misuse. 2014;49(8):1049–53.
66. Reisner SL, Poteat T, Keatley J, Cabral M, Mothopeng T, Dunham E, et al. Global health burden and needs of transgender populations: a review. Lancet. 2016;388(10042):412–36.
67. Operario D, Burton J, Underhill K, Sevelius J. Men who have sex with transgender women: challenges to category-based HIV prevention. AIDS Behav. 2008;12(1):18–26.
68. Herbst JH, Jacobs ED, Finlayson TJ, McKleroy VS, Neumann MS, Crepaz N; HIV/AIDS Prevention Research Synthesis Team. Estimating HIV prevalence and risk behaviors of transgender persons in the United States: a systematic review. AIDS Behav. 2008;12(1):1–17.
69. Bauer GR, Travers R, Scanlon K, Coleman TA. High heterogeneity of HIV-related sexual risk among transgender people in Ontario, Canada: a province-wide respondent-driven sampling survey. BMC Public Health. 2012(1);12:292.
70. Scheim AI, Travers R. Barriers and facilitators to HIV and sexually transmitted infections testing for gay, bisexual, and other transgender men who have sex with men. AIDS Care. 2017;29(8):990–5.
71. Rowniak S, Chesla C, Rose CD, Holzemer WL. Transmen: the HIV risk of gay identity. AIDS Educ Prev. 2011;23(6):508–20.
72. Sevelius J. "There's no pamphlet for the kind of sex I have": HIV-related risk factors and protective behaviors among transgender men who have sex with nontransgender men. J Assoc Nurses AIDS Care: JANAC. 2009;20(5):398–410.
73. Sevelius JM, Patouhas E, Keatley JG, Johnson MO. Barriers and facilitators to engagement and retention in care among transgender women living with human immunodeficiency virus. Ann Behav Med. 2014;47(1):5–16.

74. Primary Care Guidelines Panel. Primary care guidelines for the management of HIV/AIDS in British Columbia [Internet]. Vancouver: British Columbia Centre for Excellence in HIV/AIDS; 2011 Mar [2015 Aug; 2017 Aug 27]. Available from: http://www.cfenet.ubc.ca /sites/default/files/uploads/primary-care-guidelines/primary-care -guidelines_015-09-15.pdf.

75. Committee for Drug Evaluation and Therapy. Therapeutic guidelines for antiretroviral (ARV) treatment of adult HIV infection. Vancouver: British Columbia Centre for Excellence in HIV/AIDS; 2015 Sept [cited 2017 Aug 27]. Available from: http://www.cfenet.ubc.ca/sites/default/files /uploads/Guidelines/bccfe-art-guidelines-Oct_14_2015.pdf.

76. Aberg JA, Gallant JE, Ghanem KG, Emmanuel P, Zingman BS, Horberg MA; Infectious Diseases Society of America. Primary care guidelines for the management of persons infected with HIV: 2013 update by the HIV medicine association of the Infectious Diseases Society of America. Clin Infect Dis. 2014 Jan;58(1):e1–34.

77. Saag MS, Benson CA, Gandhi RT, Hoy JF, Landovitz RJ, Mugavero MJ, et al. Antiretroviral Drugs for Treatment and Prevention of HIV Infection in Adults: 2018 Recommendations of the International Antiviral Society-USA Panel. JAMA. 2018;320(4):379–96.

78. European AIDS Clinical Society [Internet]. Brussels, Belgium: EAC Society; 2017 Oct [cited 2018 Jan 29]. EACS guidelines, version 9.0. Available from: http://www.eacsociety.org/guidelines/eacs-guidelines/eacs-guidelines. html.

79. Trickey A, May MT, Vehreschild JJ, Obel N, Gill MJ, Crane HM, et al.; Antiretroviral Therapy Cohort Collaboration. Survival of HIV-positive patients starting antiretroviral therapy between 1996 and 2013: a collaborative analysis of cohort studies. Lancet HIV. 2017;4(8):e349–56.

80. Samji H, Cescon A, Hogg RS, Modur SP, Althoff KN, Buchacz K, et al.; North American AIDS Cohort Collaboration on Research and Design (NA-ACCORD) of IeDEA. Closing the gap: increases in life expectancy among treated HIV-positive individuals in the United States and Canada. PLoS One. 2013;8(12):e81355.

81. Teeraananchai S, Kerr SJ, Amin J, Ruxrungtham K, Law MG. Life expectancy of HIV-positive people after starting combination antiretroviral therapy: a meta-analysis. HIV Med. 2017;18(4):256–66.

82. Loutfy M, Tyndall M, Baril JG, Montaner JS, Kaul R, Hankins C. Canadian consensus statement on HIV and its transmission in the context of criminal law. Can J Infect Dis Med Microbiol. 2014;25(3):135–40.

83. Barré-Sinoussi F, Abdool Karim SS, Albert J, Bekker LG, Beyrer C, Cahn P, et al. Expert consensus statement on the science of HIV in the context of criminal law. J Int AIDS Soc. 2018;21(7):e25161.

84. Ontario Working Group on Criminal Law + HIV Exposure. Ending overcriminalization of people living with HIV in Ontario. Toronto: Ontario Working Group on Criminal Law + HIV Exposure; 2018 Apr 12 [cited 2018 Jul 15]. Available from: http://clhe.ca/owg-criminal-law -hiv-exposure/wp-content/uploads/2018/05/Brief_Ministerial-Meeting _FINAL.pdf.

85. Stanford University [Internet]. Stanford, California: Stanford University; 1998 [updated 2018; cited 2018 Oct 2]. Stanford HIV drug resistance database version 8.6. Available from: https://hivdb.stanford.edu.

86. Goncalves PH, Montezuma-Rusca JM, Yarchoan R, Uldrick TS. Cancer prevention in HIV-infected populations. Semin Oncol. 2016;43(1):173–88.

87. Public Health Agency of Canada [Internet]. Ottawa: Government of Canada; 2015 [updated 2016 Sept 1; cited 2017 Aug 22]. Canadian immunization guide: part 4 – active vaccines – meningococcal vaccine, p. 13. Available from: https://www.canada.ca/en/public-health/services /publications/healthy-living/canadian-immunization-guide-part-4 -active-vaccines/page-13-meningococcal-vaccine.html#p4c12a5c1.

88. National Advisory Committee on Immunization [Internet]. Ottawa: Government of Canada; 2017 May [cited 2017 Aug 22]. Updated recommendations on human papillomavirus (HPV) vaccines: 9-valent HPV vaccine 2-dose immunization schedule and the use of HPV vaccines in immunocompromised populations – An advisory committee statement. Available from: https://www.canada.ca/en/public-health /services/publications/healthy-living/updated-recommendations -human-papillomavirus-immunization-schedule-immunocompromised -populations.html#tab1.

89. Catherine FX, Piroth L. Hepatitis B virus vaccination in HIV-infected people: A review. Hum Vaccin Immunother. 2017;13(6):1–10.

90. Public Health Agency of Canada [Internet]. Ottawa: Government of Canada; 2017 [updated 2017 Jun 29; cited 2018 Oct 2]. Canadian immunization guide: part 4 – active vaccines – hepatitis B vaccine, p. 7. Available from: https://www.canada.ca/en/public-health/services /publications/healthy-living/canadian-immunization-guide-part-4 -active-vaccines/page-7-hepatitis-b-vaccine.html#tab3.

91. National Advisory Committee on Immunization [Internet]. Ottawa: Government of Canada; 2016 Nov 24 [cited 2018 Oct 2]. Update on the use of herpes zoster vaccine – an advisory committee statement. Available from: https://www.canada.ca/en/public-health/services/publications /healthy-living/update-use-herpes-zoster-vaccine.html#immunocomp.

92. Canadian Cancer Society [Internet]. Toronto: Canadian Cancer Society; [cited 2018 Mar 20]. Cancer screening information and considerations for LGBTQ clients. Available from: https://cancer.ca

/en/cancer-information/find-cancer-early/screening-in-lgbtq-communities.

93. Canadian Task Force on Preventive Health Care [Internet]. Ottawa: Government of Canada; 2014 [cited 2018 Jul 15]. Prostate cancer (2014): Summary of recommendations for clinicians and policy-makers. Available from: https://canadiantaskforce.ca/guidelines/published -guidelines/prostate-cancer/.

94. Panel on Opportunistic Infections in HIV-Infected Adults and Adolescents [Internet]. Bethesda (MD): National Institutes of Health; [cited 2017 Aug 22]. Guidelines for the prevention and treatment of opportunistic infections in HIV-infected adults and adolescents: recommendations from the Centers for Disease Control and Prevention, the National Institutes of Health, and the HIV Medicine Association of the Infectious Diseases Society of America. Available from: https:// clinicalinfo.hiv.gov/en/guidelines/adult-and-adolescent -opportunistic-infection/whats-new-guidelines.

95. van de Laar TJ, Richel O. Emerging viral STIs among HIV-positive men who have sex with men: the era of hepatitis C virus and human papillomavirus. Sex Transm Infect. 2017;93(5):368–73.

96. Medford RJ, Salit IE. Anal cancer and intraepithelial neoplasia: epidemiology, screening and prevention of a sexually transmitted disease. CMAJ. 2015;187(2):111–15.

97. Ong JJ, Fairley CK, Carroll S, Walker S, Chen M, Read T, et al. Cost-effectiveness of screening for anal cancer using regular digital ano-rectal examinations in men who have sex with men living with HIV. J Int AIDS Soc. 2016;19(1):20514.

98. Sigel K, Wisnivesky J, Gordon K, Dubrow R, Justice A, Brown ST, et al. HIV as an independent risk factor for incident lung cancer. AIDS. 2012;26(8):1017–25.

99. Canadian Task Force on Preventive Health Care [Internet]. Ottawa: Government of Canada; 2016 [cited 2018 Jul 15]. Lung cancer (2016): Summary of recommendations for clinicians and policymakers. CTFPHC. Available from: https://canadiantaskforce.ca/guidelines /published-guidelines/lung-cancer/.

100. Sigel K, Wisnivesky J, Shahrir S, Brown ST, Justice A, Kim J, et al. Findings in asymptomatic HIV-infected patients undergoing chest computed tomography testing: implications for lung cancer screening. AIDS. 2014;28(7):1007–14.

101. Immunodeficiency Clinic [Internet]. Toronto: United Health Network; 2017 [cited 2018 Jul 15]. Drug reimbursement information. Available

from: https://hivclinic.ca/drug-information/drug-reimbursement
-information/.

102. Canadian Treatment Action Council [Internet]. Toronto: CTAC; 2016 [cited 2018 Oct 2]. Available from: https://ctac.ca/tx-map/.

103. Wang H, Lu X, Yang X, Xu N. The efficacy and safety of tenofovir alafenamide versus tenofovir disoproxil fumarate in antiretroviral regimens for HIV-1 therapy: meta-analysis. Medicine (Baltimore). 2016;95(41):e5146.

104. Cohen SD, Kopp JB, Kimmel PL. Kidney diseases associated with human immunodeficiency virus infection. N Engl J Med. 2017;377(24): 2363–74.

105. Ogbuagu O, Ruane PJ, Podzamczer D, Salazar LC, Henry K, Asmuth DM, et al.; DISCOVER study team. Long-term safety and efficacy of emtricitabine and tenofovir alafenamide vs emtricitabine and tenofovir disoproxil fumarate for HIV-1 pre-exposure prophylaxis: week 96 results from a randomised, double-blind, placebo-controlled, phase 3 trial. Lancet HIV. 2021;8(7):e397–e407.

106. Lake JE, Trevillyan J. Impact of Integrase inhibitors and tenofovir alafenamide on weight gain in people with HIV. Curr Opin HIV AIDS. 2021;16(3):148–51.

107. Sax PE, Erlandson KM, Lake JE, Mccomsey GA, Orkin C, Esser S, et al. Weight gain following initiation of antiretroviral therapy: risk factors in randomized comparative clinical trials. Clin Infect Dis. 2020;71(6):1379–89.

108. Kolakowska A, Maresca AF, Collins IJ, Cailhol J. Update on adverse effects of HIV integrase inhibitors. Curr Treat Options Infect Dis. 2019;11(4):372–87.

109. Liverpool Drug Interactions [Internet]. Liverpool, England: Department of Pharmacology, University of Liverpool; 2018 [cited 2018 Oct 18]. Available from: https://www.hiv-druginteractions.org.

110. Center for HIV Information [Internet]. San Francisco: University of California; 2018 [cited 2018 Oct 2] HIV InSite: Antiretroviral (ARV) drug interactions database. Available from: https://hividgm.ucsf.edu /hiv-insite.

111. Immunodeficiency Clinic [Internet]. Toronto: United Health Network; 2018 [cited 2018 Oct 2]. HIV/HCV drug therapy guide – drug interaction tables. Available from: https://hivclinic.ca/drug-information/drug -interaction-tables/.

112. Müller M, Wandel S, Colebunders R, Attia S, Furrer H, Egger M; IeDEA Southern and Central Africa. Immune reconstitution inflammatory syndrome in patients starting antiretroviral therapy for HIV

infection: a systematic review and meta-analysis. Lancet Infect Dis. 2010;10(4):251–61.

113. Wing EJ. HIV and aging. Int J Infect Dis. 2016;53:61–8.

114. Triant VA, Lee H, Hadigan C, Grinspoon SK. Increased acute myocardial infarction rates and cardiovascular risk factors among patients with human immunodeficiency virus disease. J Clin Endocrinol Metab. 2007;92(7):2506–12.

115. Hsue PY, Deeks SG, Hunt PW. Immunologic basis of cardiovascular disease in HIV-infected adults. J Infect Dis. 2012;205 Suppl 3:S375–82.

116. Post WS, Budoff M, Kingsley L, Palella FJ Jr, Witt MD, Li X, et al. Associations between HIV infection and subclinical coronary atherosclerosis. Ann Intern Med. 2014;160(7):458–67.

117. Dubé MP, Stein JH, Aberg JA, Fichtenbaum CJ, Gerber JG, Tashima KT, et al.; Adult AIDS Clinical Trials Group Cardiovascular Subcommittee; HIV Medical Association of the Infectious Disease Society of America. Guidelines for the evaluation and management of dyslipidemia in human immunodeficiency virus (HIV)-infected adults receiving antiretroviral therapy: recommendations of the HIV Medical Association of the Infectious Disease Society of America and the Adult AIDS Clinical Trials Group. Clin Infect Dis. 2003;37(5):613–27.

118. Brown TT, Cole SR, Li X, Kingsley LA, Palella FJ, Riddler SA, et al. Antiretroviral therapy and the prevalence and incidence of diabetes mellitus in the multicenter AIDS cohort study. Arch Intern Med. 2005;165(10):1179–84.

119. Slama L, Palella FJ Jr, Abraham AG, Li X, Vigouroux C, Pialoux G, et al. Inaccuracy of haemoglobin A1c among HIV-infected men: effects of CD4 cell count, antiretroviral therapies and haematological parameters. J Antimicrob Chemother. 2014;69(12):3360–7.

120. Song IH, Zong J, Borland J, Jerva F, Wynne B, Zamek-Gliszczynski MJ, et al. The Effect of Dolutegravir on the Pharmacokinetics of Metformin in Healthy Subjects. J Acquir Immune Defic Syndr. 2016;72(4):400–7.

121. Lucas GM, Ross MJ, Stock PG, Shlipak MG, Wyatt CM, Gupta SK, et al.; HIV Medicine Association of the Infectious Diseases Society of America. Clinical practice guideline for the management of chronic kidney disease in patients infected with HIV: 2014 update by the HIV Medicine Association of the Infectious Diseases Society of America. Clin Infect Dis. 2014;59(9):e96–138.

122. Holt SG, Gracey DM, Levy MT, Mudge DW, Irish AB, Walker RG, et al. A consensus statement on the renal monitoring of Australian patients receiving tenofovir based antiviral therapy for HIV/HBV infection. AIDS Res Ther. 2014;11:35.

123. Brown TT, Hoy J, Borderi M, Guaraldi G, Renjifo B, Vescini F, et al. Recommendations for evaluation and management of bone disease in HIV. Clin Infect Dis. 2015;60(8):1242–51.

124. Daskalopoulou M, Rodger A, Phillips AN, Sherr L, Speakman A, Collins S, et al. Recreational drug use, polydrug use, and sexual behaviour in HIV-diagnosed men who have sex with men in the UK: results from the cross-sectional ASTRA study. Lancet HIV. 2014;1(1):e22–31.

125. Garin N, Zurita B, Velasco C, Feliu A, Gutierrez M, Masip M, et al. Prevalence and clinical impact of recreational drug consumption in people living with HIV on treatment: a cross-sectional study. BMJ Open. 2017;7(1):e014105.

126. Pebody R [Internet]. London, Englan: NAM Publications; 2015 Nov [cited 2018 Jan 29]. Factsheet: interactions between HIV treatment and recreational drugs. aidsmap. Available from: https://www.aidsmap.com/Interactions-between-HIV-treatment-and-recreational-drugs/page/3009725.

127. Bracchi M, Stuart D, Castles R, Khoo S, Back D, Boffito M. Increasing use of 'party drugs' in people living with HIV on antiretrovirals: a concern for patient safety. AIDS. 2015;29(13):1585–92.

128. Radix A, Sevelius J, Deutsch MB. Transgender women, hormonal therapy and HIV treatment: a comprehensive review of the literature and recommendations for best practices. J Int AIDS Soc. 2016;19(3 Suppl 2):20810.

129. Antoniou T, Hollands S, Macdonald EM, Gomes T, Mamdani MM, Juurlink DN; Canadian Drug Safety and Effectiveness Research Network. Trimethoprim-sulfamethoxazole and risk of sudden death among patients taking spironolactone. CMAJ. 2015;187(4):E138–43.

130. Williamson C. Providing care to transgender persons: a clinical approach to primary care, hormones, and HIV management. J Assoc Nurses AIDS Care: JANAC. 2010;21(3):221–9.

131. Bhaskaran K, Rentsch CT, MacKenna B, Schultze A, Mehrkar A, Bates CJ, et al. HIV infection and COVID-19 death: a population-based cohort analysis of UK primary care data and linked national death registrations within the OpenSAFELY platform. Lancet HIV. 2021;8(1):e24–e32.

132. Boulle A, Davies MA, Hussey H, Ismail M, Morden E, Vundle Z, et al. Risk factors for coronavirus disease 2019 (COVID-19) death in a population cohort study from the Western Cape Province, South Africa. Clin Infect Dis. 2021 Oct 5;73(7):e2005–15. doi:10.1093/cid/ciaa1198.

133. Dandachi D, Geiger G, Montgomery MW, Karmen-Tuohy S, Golzy M, Antar AAR, Llibre JM, Camazine M, Díaz-De Santiago A, Carlucci PM, Zacharioudakis IM, Rahimian J, Wanjalla CN, Slim J, Arinze F, Kratz AMP, Jones JL, Patel SM, Kitchell E, Francis A, Ray M, Koren

DE, Baddley JW, Hill B, Sax PE, Chow J. Characteristics, comorbidities, and outcomes in a multicenter registry of patients with human immunodeficiency virus and coronavirus disease 2019. Clin Infect Dis. 2021 Oct 5;73(7):e1964–72. doi:10.1093/cid/ciaa1339.

134. Geretti AM, Stockdale AJ, Kelly SH, Cevik M, Collins S, Waters L, Villa G, Docherty A, Harrison EM, Turtle L, Openshaw PJM, Baillie JK, Sabin CA, Semple MG. Outcomes of Coronavirus Disease 2019 (COVID-19) Related Hospitalization Among People With Human Immunodeficiency Virus (HIV) in the ISARIC World Health Organization (WHO) Clinical Characterization Protocol (UK): A Prospective Observational Study. Clin Infect Dis. 2021 Oct 5;73(7):e2095–106. doi:10.1093/cid/ciaa1605.

135. Docherty AB, Harrison EM, Green CA, Hardwick HE, Pius R, Norman L, et al.; ISARIC4C investigators. Features of 20133 UK patients in hospital with covid-19 using the ISARIC WHO Clinical Characterisation Protocol: prospective observational cohort study. BMJ. 2020;369:m1985.

136. Richardson S, Hirsch JS, Narasimhan M, Crawford JM, McGinn T, Davidson KW, et al.; the Northwell COVID-19 Research Consortium. Presenting characteristics, co-morbidities, and outcomes among 5700 patients hospitalized with COVID-19 in the New York City area. JAMA. 2020;323(20):2052–9.

137. Wu Z, McGoogan JM. Characteristics of and Important Lessons From the Coronavirus Disease 2019 (COVID-19) Outbreak in China: Summary of a Report of 72314 Cases From the Chinese Center for Disease Control and Prevention. JAMA. 2020;323(13):1239–42.

138. Meyerowitz EA, Kim AY, Ard KL, Basgoz N, Chu JT, Hurtado RM, et al. Disproportionate burden of coronavirus disease 2019 among racial minorities and those in congregate settings among a large cohort of people with HIV. AIDS. 2020;34(12):1781–7.

139. Centers for Disease Control and Prevention [Internet]. Atlanta (GA): CDC; [updated 2021 Jul 16; cited 2021 Aug 15]. Risk for COVID-19 infection, hospitalization, and death by race/ethnicity. Available from: https://www.cdc.gov/coronavirus/2019-ncov/covid-data/investigations-discovery/hospitalization-death-by-race-ethnicity.html.

140. Shiau S, Krause KD, Valera P, Swaminathan S, Halkitis PN. The burden of COVID-19 in people living with HIV: a syndemic perspective. AIDS Behav. 2020;24(8):2244–9.

141. Cooper TJ, Woodward BL, Alom S, Harky A. Coronavirus disease 2019 (COVID-19) outcomes in HIV/AIDS patients: a systematic review. HIV Med. 2020;21(9):567–77.

142. Office of AIDS Research Advisory Council [Internet]. Bethesda (MD): National Institutes of Health; 2021 Feb 26 [cited 2021 Aug 15]. Guidance

for COVID-19 and people with HIV. Available from: https://clinicalinfo
.hiv.gov/en/guidelines/covid-19-and-persons-hiv-interim-guidance/
interim-guidance-covid-19-and-persons-hiv.

143. CDET Committee [Internet]. Vancouver: British Columbia Centre for
Excellence in HIV/AIDS; 2020 Nov [updated 202 Dec; cited 2021 Aug 15].
Statement on the use of COVID-19 MRNA vaccines (Pfizer and Moderna)
in pesons living with HIV. Available from: http://bccfe.ca/therapeutic
-guidelines/healthcare-providers/therapeutic-guidelines/
bc-centre-excellence-hivaids-cdet-committee-statement.

144. British HIV Association [Internet]. London, England: 2021 Jan 15 [cited
2021 Aug 15]. BHIVA; BHIVA, DAIG, EACS, GESIDA, Polish Scientific
AIDS Society and Portuguese Association for the clinical study of AIDS
(APECS). Statement on risk of COVID-19 for people living with HIV
(PLWH) and SARS-CoV-2 vaccine advice for adults living with HIV.
Available from: https://www.bhiva.org/joint-statement-on-risk-of
-COVID-19-for-PLWH-and-SARS-CoV-2-vaccine-advice.

145. CDET Committee [Internet]. Vancouver: British Columbia Centre for
Excellence in HIV/AIDS; 2020 Nov [cited 2021 Aug 15]. BC-CfE CDET
interim recommendations for COVID-19 vaccines in persons living
with HIV. Available from: http://bccfe.ca/therapeutic-guidelines
/bc-cfe-cdet-statement-use-of-covid19-vaccines-persons-living-hiv.

146. American Geriatrics Society 2015 Beers Criteria Update Expert Panel.
American Geriatrics Society 2015 updated beers criteria for potentially
inappropriate medication use in older adults. J Am Geriatr Soc.
2015;63(11):2227–46.

147. O'Mahony D, O'Sullivan D, Byrne S, O'Connor MN, Ryan C, Gallagher P.
STOPP/START criteria for potentially inappropriate prescribing in older
people: version 2. Age Ageing. 2015;44(2):213–18.

148. Clifford DB. HIV-associated neurocognitive disorder. Curr Opin Infect
Dis. 2017;30(1):117–22.

149. Demmer C. Dealing with AIDS-related loss and grief in a time of
treatment advances. Am J Hosp Palliat Care. 2001;18(1):35–41.

150. Sangarlangkarn A, Appelbaum JS. Caring for Older Adults with the
Human Immunodeficiency Virus. J Am Geriatr Soc. 2016;64(11):2322–9.

151. Wessman M, Korsholm AS, Bentzen JG, Andersen AN, Ahlström MG,
Katzenstein TL, Weis N. Anti-müllerian hormone levels are reduced in
women living with human immunodeficiency virus compared to control
women: a case-control study from Copenhagen, Denmark. J Virus Erad.
2018 Apr 1;4(2):123–7.

152. Bhatia R, Murphy AB, Raper JL, Chamie G, Kitahata MM, Drozd
DR, et al.; Centers for AIDS Research (CFAR) Network of Integrated
Clinical Systems (CNICS). Testosterone replacement therapy among

HIV-infected men in the CFAR Network of Integrated Clinical Systems. AIDS. 2015;29(1):77–81.

153. Savasi V, Parisi F, Oneta M, Laoreti A, Parrilla B, Duca P, et al. Effects of highly active antiretroviral therapy on semen parameters of a cohort of 770 HIV-1 infected men. PLoS One. 2019;14(2):e0212194.

154. Rodger AJ, Cambiano V, Bruun T, Vernazza P, Collins S, van Lunzen J, et al.; PARTNER Study Group. Sexual activity without condoms and risk of HIV transmission in serodifferent couples when the HIV-positive partner is using suppressive antiretroviral therapy. JAMA. 2016;316(2):171–91.

155. Zafer M, Horvath H, Mmeje O, van der Poel S, Semprini AE, Rutherford G, Brown J. Effectiveness of semen washing to prevent human immunodeficiency virus (HIV) transmission and assist pregnancy in HIV-discordant couples: a systematic review and meta-analysis. Fertil Steril. 2016 Mar;105(3):645–55.e2.

156. Baeten JM, Donnell D, Ndase P, Mugo NR, Campbell JD, Wangisi J, et al.; Partners PrEP Study Team. Antiretroviral prophylaxis for HIV prevention in heterosexual men and women. N Eng J Med. 2012;367:399–410.

157. AIDSinfo [Internet]. Bethesda (MD): National Institutes of Health; [updated 2018 Dec 7; cited 2019 Jun 14]. Recommendations for the use of antiretroviral drugs in pregnant women with HIV infection and interventions to reduce perinatal HIV transmission in the United States. Available from: https://aidsinfo.nih.gov/guidelines/html/3/perinatal/0.

158. Shapiro RL, Hughes MD, Ogwu A, Kitch D, Lockman S, Moffat C, et al. Antiretroviral regimens in pregnancy and breast-feeding in Botswana. N Eng J Med. 2010;362(24):2282–94.

159. Zash R, Holmes L, Makhema J, Diseko M, Jacobson DL, Mayondi G, et al. Surveillance for neural tube defects following antiretroviral exposure from conception. Paper presentation at: 22nd IAS Conference; 2018 Jul 23–27, Amsterdam, Netherlands.

160. Rice ML, Zeldow B, Siberry GK, Purswani M, Malee K, Hoffman HJ, et al. Evaluation of risk for late language emergence after in utero antiretroviral drug exposure in HIV-exposed uninfected infants. Ped Infect Dis J. 2013;32(10):e406–13.

161. Smith ML, Puka K, Sehra R, Read SE, Bitnun A. Longitudinal development of cognitive, visuomotor and adaptive behavior skills in HIV uninfected children, aged 3–5 years of age, exposed pre- and perinatally to anti-retroviral medications. AIDS Care. 2017;29(10):1302–8.

162. Centers for Disease Control and Prevention [Internet]. Atlanta (GA): CDC; 2020 Dec 14 [2021 Aug 15; cited 2021 Aug 15]. Evidence of HIV

treatment and viral suppression in preventing the sexual transmission of HIV. Available from: https://www.cdc.gov/hiv/risk/art/evidence-of -hiv-treatment.html.

163. Cohen MS, Chen YQ, McCauley M, et al. Antiretroviral Therapy for the Prevention of HIV-1 Transmission. N Engl J Med. 09 2016;375(9):830–9.

164. Bavinton BR, Pinto AN, Phanuphak N, et al. Viral suppression and HIV transmission in serodiscordant male couples: an international, prospective, observational, cohort study. Lancet HIV. 08 2018;5(8):e438–e47.

165. Grant RM, Lama JR, Anderson PL, McMahan V, Liu AY, Vargas L, et al.; iPrEx Study Team. Preexposure chemoprophylaxis for HIV prevention in men who have sex with men. N Engl J Med. Dec 2010;363(27):2587–99.

166. Choopanya K, Martin M, Suntharasamai P, Sangkum U, Mock PA, Leethochawalit M, et al.; Bangkok Tenofovir Study Group. Antiretroviral prophylaxis for HIV infection in injecting drug users in Bangkok, Thailand (the Bangkok Tenofovir Study): a randomised, double-blind, placebo-controlled phase 3 trial. Lancet. Jun 2013;381(9883):2083–90.

167. Baeten JM, Donnell D, Ndase P, Mugo NR, Campbell JD, Wangisi J, et al.; Partners PrEP Study Team. Antiretroviral prophylaxis for HIV prevention in heterosexual men and women. N Engl J Med. Aug 2012;367(5):399–410.

168. Sharma M, Tan DH. HIV pre-exposure prophylaxis. CMAJ. Oct 2014;186(15):E588.

169. Centers for Disease Control and Prevention [Internet]. Atlanta (GA): CDC; 2021 Aug 6 [cited 2021 Aug 15]. PrEP effectiveness. Available from: https://www.cdc.gov/hiv/basics/prep/prep-effectiveness.html.

170. Tan DH, Hull MW, Yoong D, Tremblay C, O'Byrne P, Thomas R, et al.; Biomedical HIV Prevention Working Group of the CIHR Canadian HIV Trials Network. Canadian guideline on HIV pre-exposure prophylaxis and nonoccupational postexposure prophylaxis. CMAJ. 2017;189(47):E1448–58.

171. Mayer KH, Molina JM, Thompson MA, Anderson PL, Mounzer KC, De Wet JJ, et al. Emtricitabine and tenofovir alafenamide vs emtricitabine and tenofovir disoproxil fumarate for HIV pre-exposure prophylaxis (DISCOVER): primary results from a randomised, double-blind, multicentre, active-controlled, phase 3, non-inferiority trial. Lancet. 2020;396(10246):239–54.

172. Centers for Disease Control and Prevention. Pre-exposure prophylaxis for the prevention of HIV infection in the United States – 2017 update [Internet]. Atlanta (GA): CDC; 2017 [cited 2021 Aug 15]. Available from: https://www.cdc.gov/hiv/pdf/risk/prep/cdc-hiv-prep-guidelines -2017.pdf.

173. Centers for Disease Control and Prevention. Preexposure prophylaxis for the prevention of HIV infection in the United States – 2014 clinical practice guideline [Internet]. Atlanta (GA): CDC; 2014 [cited 2017 Aug 22]. Available from: https://www.cdc.gov/hiv/pdf/guidelines /PrEPguidelines2014.pdf.

174. Günthard HF, Saag MS, Benson CA, del Rio C, Eron JJ, Gallant JE, et al. Antiretroviral drugs for treatment and prevention of HIV infection in adults: 2016 recommendations of the International Antiviral Society-USA Panel. JAMA. 2016;316(2):191–210.

175. Knox DC, Anderson PL, Harrigan PR, Tan DH. Multidrug-Resistant HIV-1 Infection despite Preexposure Prophylaxis. N Engl J Med. 2017;376(5):501–2.

176. Hoornenborg E, Prins M, Achterbergh RCA, et al. Acquisition of wild-type HIV-1 infection in a patient on pre-exposure prophylaxis with high intracellular concentrations of tenofovir diphosphate: a case report. Lancet HIV. 2017;4(11):e522-e8.

177. Cohen S, Sachdev D, Lee S, et al. Acquisition of TDF-susceptible HIV despite high level adherence to daily TDF/FTC PrEP as measured by dried blood spot (DBS) and segmental hair analysis: a case report. ID Week; 2018; San Francisco.

178. Centers for Disease Control and Prevention [Internet]. Atlanta (GA): CDC; 2018 Jul 23 [cited 2018 Jan 29]. PrEP. Available from: https://www .cdc.gov/hiv/basics/prep.html.

179. Seifert SM, Chen X, Meditz AL, Castillo-Mancilla JR, Gardner EM, Predhomme JA, et al. Intracellular tenofovir and emtricitabine anabolites in genital, rectal, and blood compartments from first dose to steady state. AIDS Res Hum Retroviruses. 2016;32(10–11):981–91.

180. Garrett KL, Cottrell ML, Prince HM, Sykes C, Schauer A, Peery A, Rooney J, McCallister S, Gay C, Kashuba A. Concentrations of TFV and TFVdp in female mucosal tissues after a single dose of TAF. Paper presented at: CROI Conference; 2016 Feb 22–25; Boston, MA [cited 2021 Aug 15]. Available from: http://www.croiconference.org/sessions/concen trations-tfv-and-tfvdp-female-mucosal-tissues-after-single-dose-taf.

181. Thurman AR, Schwartz JL, Cottrell ML, Brache V, Chen BA, Cochón L, et al. Safety and pharmacokinetics of a tenofovir alafenamide fumarate-emtricitabine based oral antiretroviral regimen for prevention of HIV acquisition in women: a randomized controlled trial. EClinicalMedicine. 2021;36:100893. doi:10.1016/j.eclinm.2021.100893

182. Centers for Disease Control and Prevention. Announcement: updated guidelines for antiretroviral postexposure prophylaxis after sexual, injection-drug use, or other nonoccupational exposure to HIV – United States, 2016. MMWR Morb Mortal Wkly Rep. 2016;65(17):458.

183. Piscaglia M, Cossu MV, Passerini M, Petri F, Gerbi M, Fusetti C, Capetti A, Rizzardini G. Emerging drugs for the treatment of HIV/AIDS: a review of 2019/2020 phase II and III trials. Expert Opin Emerg Drugs. 2021 Sep;26(3):219–30.

184. Pene Dumitrescu T, Joshi SR, Xu J, Zhan J, Johnson M, Butcher L, et al. A phase I evaluation of the pharmacokinetics and tolerability of the HIV-1 maturation inhibitor GSK3640254 and tenofovir alafenamide/ emtricitabine in healthy participants. Antimicrob Agents Chemother. 2021 May;65(6):e02173–20. doi:10.1128/AAC.02173-20.

185. Pene Dumitrescu T, Joshi SR, Xu J, Greene TJ, Johnson M, Butcher L, et al. Phase I evaluation of pharmacokinetics and tolerability of the HIV-1 maturation inhibitor GSK3640254 and dolutegravir in healthy adults. Br J Clin Pharmacol. 2021 Sep;87(9):3501–7. doi:10.1111/bcp.14759.

186. Thornhill J, Orkin C. Long-acting injectable HIV therapies: the next frontier: Republication. Curr Opin HIV AIDS. 2021;16(2):98–105.

187. Kozal M, Aberg J, Pialoux G, Cahn P, Thompson M, Molina JM, et al.; BRIGHTE Trial Team. Fostemsavir in Adults with Multidrug-Resistant HIV-1 Infection. N Engl J Med. 2020;382(13):1232–43.

188. Lataillade M, Lalezari JP, Kozal M, Aberg JA, Pialoux G, Cahn P, et al. Safety and efficacy of the HIV-1 attachment inhibitor prodrug fostemsavir in heavily treatment-experienced individuals: week 96 results of the phase 3 BRIGHTE study. Lancet HIV. 2020;7(11):e740–51.

189. Emu B, Fessel J, Schrader S, Kumar P, Richmond G, Win S, et al. Phase 3 Study of ibalizumab for multidrug-resistant HIV-1. N Engl J Med. 2018;379(7):645–54.

190. Blair HA. Ibalizumab: A Review in Multidrug-Resistant HIV-1 Infection. Drugs. 2020;80(2):189–96.

191. Molina JM, Squires K, Sax PE, Cahn P, Lombaard J, DeJesus E, et al.; DRIVE-FORWARD trial group. Doravirine versus ritonavir-boosted darunavir in antiretroviral-naive adults with HIV-1 (DRIVE-FORWARD): 96-week results of a randomised, double-blind, non-inferiority, phase 3 trial. Lancet HIV. 2020;7(1):e16–26.

192. Gatell JM, Morales-Ramirez JO, Hagins DP, Thompson M, Arastéh K, Hoffmann C, et al. Doravirine dose selection and 96-week safety and efficacy versus efavirenz in antiretroviral therapy-naive adults with HIV-1 infection in a Phase IIb trial. Antivir Ther. 2019;24(6):425–35.

193. Orkin C, Oka S, Philibert P, Brinson C, Bassa A, Gusev D, et al. Long-acting cabotegravir plus rilpivirine for treatment in adults with HIV-1 infection: 96-week results of the randomised, open-label, phase 3 FLAIR study. Lancet HIV. 2021;8(4):e185–96.

194. Swindells S, Lutz T, van Zyl L, Porteiro N, Stoll M, Mitha E, et al. Long-acting cabotegravir + rilpivirine for HIV-1 treatment: ATLAS

week 96 results. AIDS. 2021 Jul;Publish Ahead of Print: doi:10.1097/
QAD.0000000000003025.

195. Cahn P, Madero JS, Arribas JR, Antinori A, Ortiz R, Clarke AE, et al.
Durable efficacy of dolutegravir plus lamivudine in antiretroviral
treatment-naive adults with HIV-1 infection: 96-week results from the
GEMINI-1 and GEMINI-2 randomized clinical trials. J Acquir Immune
Defic Syndr. 2020;83(3):310–18.

196. van Wyk J, Ajana F, Bisshop F, De Wit S, Osiyemi O, Portilla Sogorb
J, et al. Efficacy and safety of switching to dolutegravir/lamivudine
fixed-dose 2-drug regimen vs continuing a tenofovir alafenamide-
based 3- or 4-drug regimen for maintenance of virologic suppression
in adults living with human immunodeficiency virus type 1: phase
3, randomized, noninferiority TANGO study. Clin Infect Dis.
2020;71(8):1920–9.

197. Llibre JM, Hung CC, Brinson C, Castelli F, Girard PM, Kahl LP, et
al. Efficacy, safety, and tolerability of dolutegravir-rilpivirine for the
maintenance of virological suppression in adults with HIV-1: phase 3,
randomised, non-inferiority SWORD-1 and SWORD-2 studies. Lancet.
2018;391(10123):839–49.

198. Stellbrink HJ, Hoffmann C. Cabotegravir: its potential for antiretroviral
therapy and preexposure prophylaxis. Curr Opin HIV AIDS.
2018;13(4):334–40.

8 Mental Health

CHRISTOPHER MCINTOSH

Introduction

In the 18 years since Peterkin and Risdon's *Caring for Lesbian and Gay People: A Clinical Guide* was published, what has changed about 2SLG-BTQ mental health? Perhaps one of the most salient considerations is that *2SLGBTQ people* have changed. Statisticians and sociologists use the term *age cohort* to describe a particular group of people defined by their date of birth. Sometimes, in popular media, larger age cohorts are referred to as *generations.* Age cohort effects are relevant in working in 2SLGBTQ mental health because your patient's life and the stresses they may have been exposed to are highly influenced by the social milieu of their cohort, which has changed dramatically over the lifetime of 2SLGBTQ people in Canada. For example, consider the following two life narratives:

Patrick, a gay man now age 86, was born in 1935. He has his first memories of being a child during World War II and developing as an adolescent and a young adult during the postwar years of the 1950s and 1960s, when gender roles were rigid and the expectations of forming a heterosexual family were strong. He marries a woman and has two children, but he represses his sexual feelings for men and becomes an alcoholic, causing a breakdown in his marriage. He attends a treatment program and achieves sobriety, recognizing his true sexual orientation in the process. He comes out to his family, and he and his wife divorce in an ugly battle in which his sexual orientation and alcoholism are used against him to exclude him from child custody. He moves to an urban centre and discovers his sexuality in a more complete way in his mid- to late 30s during the sexual revolution of the 1970s. He finds community with other urban gay men, banding together to fight police oppression in the early 1980s, only to lose many of those friends to the AIDS epidemic. This grief precipitates a relapse of alcoholism. He recovers again and reconciles with his young adult children. He meets his husband at a support group for gay fathers and they move in together, legally marrying in the 2000s. Their marriage breaks down after 10 years because of conflict over whether their relationship will continue to remain monogamous. He moves back to his small town to be more involved in his grandchildren's lives and does his best to maintain his friendships over the Internet, though he is beginning to have cognitive issues. His functioning declines to the point that he enters a nursing home, and he fears that he will have to go back into the closet because of the negative attitudes of staff and co-residents.

Now consider Lindsay, a 15-year-old-girl, born in 2006. She is raised by two loving heterosexual parents who have many gay and lesbian friends in their social circle. She lives in a time when there is nothing unusual at all about girls and boys socializing together and having similar and shared interests. Gender role expectations in her family are not rigid, with her mother having been a "tomboy" in her youth and her father having been a stay-at-home father for part of her early childhood. This allows her to have little conflict about dressing and acting how she feels, which is neither girly nor butch but more androgynous. Simultaneously, she is coming of age sexually in a time where teenagers have unprecedented access to pornography via the Internet and the hyper-masculine and hyper-feminine body ideals promulgated there. Lindsay finds herself attracted to both boys and girls, though in different ways. Her dates with boys have been a challenge because they have brought to the fore conflicted feelings she has about her body, especially her breasts. In response to one date that went badly, she feels frozen out from the peer group of this boy and experiences bullying from several girls about her androgynous appearance. She decides to change her look to a more conventionally feminine appearance to fit in better, but this produces feelings of depression that she does not understand, and she begins using cannabis heavily to feel numb. Her parents express worries about her school marks sliding, but she reacts angrily, seeing their comments as intrusive and overbearing.

While there are separate chapters in this volume that will deal with older adults and substance use, one can see from these contrasting examples of life narratives of two 2SLGBTQ people from different age cohorts that very different stressors may affect mental health in the breadth of the 2SLGBTQ population alive today.

Do members of the 2SLGBTQ communities suffer disproportionately from mental health disorders? Despite multiple complexities in research methods, we now have an established research literature that says yes, for those with a minority sexual orientation, rates of mental health disorders can be elevated, with adjusted odds ratios ranging from 1.5 to 2.5 for issues of depression, anxiety disorders, suicide attempts and suicidal ideation, and substance use disorders.[1] While there are less data about severe, persistent mental illness (SPMI) such as schizophrenia and bipolar disorder, what data we have also suggests significantly elevated rates, as well as poor access to 2SLGBTQ-friendly mental health services.[2] The research base on transgender and gender non-binary (TNB) individuals individuals is growing and suggests this population is at even greater risk, with one Ontario study identifying that 35 per cent of respondents had seriously considered and 11 per cent had attempted suicide in the previous year.[3]

Helping your 2SLGBTQ patients with their mental health problems requires you to keep two priorities in mind. One, ensure that your practice and your therapeutic relationship building skills are such that your patients will feel comfortable disclosing to you their sexual orientation and gender identity. Two, keep in mind the above-mentioned elevated risks so that you do proper mental health screening for your patients.

This chapter is structured using the typical headings of a history taking. Each heading will describe tips for eliciting this part of the history from the patient but will also incorporate other important considerations. While the chapter will endeavour to be applicable to the 2SLGBTQ population broadly, it will also conclude with a section specifically discussing mental health considerations in work with transgender patients.

Taking the History

Setting the Stage with Identifying Data

Asking basic information about the patient before getting to the clinical problem is a standard way of orienting the clinician to some context of the patient's life circumstances. However, in working with 2SLGBTQ patients, one of the easiest mistakes to make is with these opening questions. Age and occupational status are important in situating the patient in their cohort and socioeconomic class. Relationship status must be asked in a particular way, or your therapeutic relationship with your 2SLGBTQ patients may be over before it begins. "Who lives with you at home?" is an ordinary question that can be asked of anybody and invites the partnered 2SLGBTQ patient to come out to you right off the bat, if they feel comfortable doing so, with an answer like "my wife" or "my boyfriend." Even if the answer is "no one" or "my partner" or "my roommate," asking the question in this way sends the right signal and allows the patient the space to come out subsequently in the interview by using gendered pronouns in reference to their partner or when you later ask directly about their sexual orientation, gender identity, and relationship history. Asking "Are you married?" in the identifying data sends the opposite signal: the patient will assume you are expecting a heterosexual response – and yes, this is still true even after more than a decade of equal marriage in Canada. Another point about pronouns: asking about preferred pronouns will go a long way in helping your TNB patients feel similarly comfortable.

History of Presenting Concerns

Give the patient space to relate their problem in their own way before diving in with close-ended questions. This is important advice for interviewing any patient, but as identified above and elsewhere in this book, 2SLGBTQ people may have had bad experiences with previous health care providers.

DEPRESSION AND ANXIETY DISORDERS
Depressed mood. Lack of interest in previously pleasurable activities. Sleep disturbance. Change in appetite, concentration, and energy. Rumination and worry. Fears and panic attacks. Agitation and irritability. Feelings of guilt. Thoughts of death or suicide. There may be no particular difference in how you ask 2SLGBTQ patients about the symptoms of depression and anxiety disorders, but what you must attend to are the unique stressors that may be associated with these symptoms.

We are limited in our ability to identify causal explanations for the twofold relative risk of 2SLGBT people for mood and anxiety disorders by the lack of prospective studies. However, clinical experience and the cross-sectional research available has led to theories related to social stress and identity conflict; therefore, asking about these stressors will be an important part of the history taking. One important social stress theory is the minority stress theory,[4] which postulates plausibly that the prejudice and discrimination experienced by sexual and gender identity minorities leads to mental distress.

Meyer identified four types of stressors:

- *Prejudice events:* Outright episodes of discrimination, abuse, or interpersonal violence.
- *Stigma:* Expectations by the individual of rejection and discrimination; the more stigma attached to a particular identity, the

more likely that it could lead to a chronic, stressful vigilance in the stigmatized person.

- *Concealment:* The stress associated with hiding one's sexual orientation or gender identity.
- *Internalized homophobia/transphobia:* Even in the absence of overt prejudice or the successful concealment of one's identity, an internalized redirection of societal anti-2SLGBTQ attitudes towards the self may have a strong impact.

Despite advances in human rights for 2SLGBTQ people in Canada, these stressors remain for many today and must be considered in relation to depression and anxiety disorders.

VIOLENCE AND POST-TRAUMATIC STRESS DISORDER

Police-reported hate crimes related to sexual orientation were substantially more likely to be violent and to result in an injury compared to hate crimes related to religion or ethnoracial group, according to a recent report from Statistics Canada.[5] In a large US sample, Roberts et al.[6] found that those with a minority sexual orientation were twice as likely to have PTSD, and subsequent research by the same investigators showed that this could be partially explained by an increased incidence of traumatic events in childhood, which was itself associated with reported gender non-conformity in childhood.[7]

Clearly, inquiring about traumatic events is an important part of your history taking regarding mental health, but like 2SLGBTQ identity itself, it may be something that patients are reluctant to disclose. Inquiring into the four broad domains of PTSD symptoms will provide you with more information:

- *Re-experiencing:* Nightmares, waking flashbacks, or intrusive memories. Physical or psychological reactions to reminders of the trauma (sometimes called *triggers* although this colloquialism should be avoided as some sufferers' trauma will have involved gun violence).
- *Avoidance:* Avoiding thoughts, memories, and feelings related to the trauma, avoiding places, persons, or conversations related to the trauma.
- *Emotional numbing/mood changes:* Social withdrawal, a general feeling of numbed emotional expression.
- *Hyperarousal:* Insomnia, hypervigilance (fearful expectations of further trauma), irritability, agitation.

Box 8.1. After a Violent Physical Assault

- Refer for urgent physical care, emergency room sexual assault protocols, and documentation and photographing of injuries (when indicated).
- If there is a risk of stalking or retaliation, ensure the patient's immediate safety by recruiting supportive friends or family members or by involving the police. Explore alternative housing options when indicated.
- Encourage the patient to maximize supports after a trauma and to report the incident to the police. Keep a list of 2SLGBTQ community contacts who deal with hate crimes. Encourage the patient to document carefully what has happened, the time and place, and any witnesses who were present while the patient's memory is still fresh and details are clear.
- When counselling in the aftermath of trauma, ask the patient to describe the incident and assault, and note elements of marked distress in reporting the incident. Immediately and actively challenge any assumptions of self-blame or the emergence of increased internalized homophobia or transphobia with respect to the incident (e.g., "This wouldn't have happened if I wasn't so obviously gay/trans").
- Explore feelings of helplessness, anger, shame, fear, and loss.
- Look for increased suicidal ideation or homicidal fantasies and for the increased use of drug or alcohol to cope with the incident.
- Ask about past incidents of violence or trauma, which may make the individual more vulnerable to developing posttraumatic stress disorder. Refer for 2SLGBTQ-affirmative psychological/psychiatric care where appropriate.
- Emphasize survival rather than victimhood. Refer the individual to 2SLGBTQ-affirmative violence support groups.
- Look for the emergence of social withdrawal or the development of mood disorders or anxiety disorders. Refer where appropriate for subspecialty follow-up.
- If the patient is not responding to basic counselling manoeuvres, refer for subspecialty care for consideration of cognitive-behavioural therapy with trauma/phobia desensitization protocols. Short-term prescription of anti-anxiety agents may be indicated.

Source: Adapted from first edition.

BIPOLAR DISORDERS AND PSYCHOTIC DISORDERS

Screening for manic episodes and psychosis is an important part of your mental health assessment of your patient because the presence of these disorders will lead to a different treatment plan. Depending on the availability of psychiatric services in your community, these patients may be mainly managed by specialized care or may be assessed by a specialist and referred back to you to implement treatment recommendations. In either case, it is important to remember that these SPMI, and often their treatments, put your primary care patient at higher risk of chronic medical conditions, such as obesity, metabolic syndrome, coronary artery disease, and hypertension, so it is important to consider screening and preventative management for these conditions, particularly since SPMI may also lead to infrequent attendance for medical care.

The appearance of an SPMI can have considerable consequences for the normal development of your 2SLGBTQ patients. Since 2SLGBTQ people are often marginalized in our society, having an SPMI can lead to further marginalization, including more isolation from family members, and more difficulty with housing and employment. As well, mental illness stigma within the 2SLGBTQ community may make it challenging for your patient to connect with other 2SLGBTQ people for support or to find romantic partners.

In some ways, the development of an SPMI can precipitate an identity crisis not unlike that of a difficult coming out process.[8] A patient may have issues with denial or disavowal of their mental illness and may go through several episodes of illness before there is acceptance of the need for long term mood stabilizing or antipsychotic medication. Even subsequently, the patient may be "closeted" about their illness, keeping it from important people in their life who might otherwise be able to provide social support. Referral for psychotherapy for management of these overlapping coming out issues may be an important consideration for such patients, and it may help with adherence to medication regimens.

BODY IMAGE PROBLEMS AND EATING DISORDERS

Body image, which is how a person feels they look, as opposed to how they actually look, is an important area of discussion with 2SLGBTQ patients. The limited research available in this area has generally focused on examining sociocultural influences (how cultural and subcultural factors may influence disordered eating and/or exercise behaviours) and minority stress factors or both. In general, minority stress factors are associated with elevated risk for eating disorders, but it may be that this is an indirect effect; that is, minority stress puts 2SLGBTQ people at greater risk for trauma, anxiety, and depression, and these lead to an elevated risk of eating disorders.[9]

Theories about gay and lesbian subcultural influences have had mixed support in the literature. For example, the lesbian community is thought to have more acceptance of diverse body shapes, and one would think this would lead to lower rates of eating disorders compared to heterosexual women, but rates are roughly equivalent. Similarly, gay male culture seems to prize a muscular physique, but use of muscle-building supplements and anabolic steroids is not elevated compared to heterosexual men, although use of weight-loss supplements is. Even so, gay and bisexual men do describe strong pressure to have a certain body type to attract attention on peer-to-peer mobile dating applications, which have become a popular way of meeting people for dates and sexual encounters.[10]

It is possible that ethnoracial minority LGB and transgender individuals of all ethnicities do have elevated rates of disordered eating and exercise behaviours compared to white LGB and cisgender individuals, but this research is at present limited by small sample sizes.[9] Trans individuals have been known to develop disordered eating behaviours, especially restricting food, to try to reduce muscularity in transfeminine individuals and halt menstruation in transmasculine individuals.

Past Mental Health History

This section of the mental health history is about past diagnoses, past mental health providers, and history of previous treatments, hospitalizations, and suicide attempts. Ask whether your 2SLGBTQ patients have had homophobic or transphobic experiences in accessing previous mental health care as many have.

It is important to recognize that the history of psychiatry and the 2SLGBTQ community is fraught. Homosexuality was listed as a mental disorder starting in the second edition of the *Diagnostic and Statistical Manual of Mental Disorders (DSM)* and until 1973.[11] At the time, pro-homosexual rights activist groups recognized that while progress had been made in some countries on the legal front, with the decriminalization of homosexuality in England in 1967 and Canada in 1968, the categorization of homosexuality as a mental illness was a major barrier to greater social acceptance of gay and lesbian people.

After protests disrupted the 1970 and 1971 annual meetings of the American Psychiatric Association (APA), a panel discussion at the 1972 meeting included a closeted psychiatrist who wore a disguise and called himself Dr. H. Anonymous (later revealed to be Dr. John Fryer). In 1973 the APA removed homosexuality from the *DSM*, though it retained a condition that reflected distress about being homosexual until 1987.

Transgender activists have had similar, though somewhat different, issues with a mental disorder diagnosis and the stigma associated with it. The difference being that many trans people (though not all) need medical treatment with hormone therapies and/or surgery, and in most medical systems, treatment requires a medical diagnosis. Thus removing the diagnosis completely might impact access to care. The APA revamped its trans-related diagnosis in 2012, changing the name from gender identity disorder to gender dysphoria and explicitly indicating that transgender identity per se is not considered a mental disorder; it is the associated distress that is considered a focus of clinical attention. The World Health Organization's International Classification of Diseases, 11th edition (ICD-11)[12] has moved its trans-related diagnosis, now called gender incongruence, from its mental health section and into a section called "Conditions Related to Sexual Functioning." As the diagnosis of gender incongruence has become the new standard, this diagnostic term will be used in the remainder of this chapter.

Another important consideration in the 2SLGBTQ population is whether there has been past exposure to sexual orientation change efforts (SOCE), also known as *conversion therapy*. While every major mental health organization has issued statements opposing SOCE, and many North American jurisdictions have passed legislation outlawing conversion therapy for minors,[13] your 2SLGBTQ patients may very well have had some exposure to SOCE, especially if they come from certain religious backgrounds (e.g., evangelical Christianity) or if they are immigrants from countries where homosexuality remains highly stigmatized and/or outlawed (see below). SOCE has been known to produce profound negative effects on a 2SLGBTQ person's self-esteem and normal 2SLGBTQ development.[14] At times, a 2SLGBTQ patient who is ashamed of their sexual orientation and/or gender identity may present asking for a referral for conversion therapy. It is important to emphasize to them that SOCE has not been shown to result in a change of sexual orientation and can be psychologically damaging as it is, effectively, a concentrated program of anti-homosexual bias.[13]

Substance History

Even in a society with socialized medicine such as Canada, there are significant barriers to accessing good treatments (psychotherapy, social interventions, medication) for mental health disorders; in contrast, access to mood- and mind-altering substances of abuse is relatively barrier free. Given this reality and the elevated risk of trauma, anxiety, and depression in the 2SLGBTQ community, it is no surprise that use of substances is also elevated as patients may attempt to "self-medicate" their symptoms. Additionally, before the onset of the Internet as a way for 2SLGBTQ people to connect with each other, the entrance point to the 2SLGBTQ community was often through gay and lesbian bars, so the use of alcohol to socialize was normalized.

The Q in 2SLGBTQ stands for "queer," and although for some this is an umbrella term for several sexual and gender identities, for others the meaning is more specific. Queer-identified people tend to prize the counter-cultural aspect of being 2SLGBTQ and may be skeptical of efforts to integrate 2SLGBTQ identities into the broader culture through, for example, promotion of equal marriage. As such, queer-identified people may see substance use as part of that countercultural aspect of their identity, and this may affect their movement along the stages of change towards taking action on a substance use disorder. For more details on substance issues in the 2SLGBTQ community, please see chapter 9 in this volume.

Legal History

Recent data from the United States indicate that a disproportionate number of 2SLGBTQ people are incarcerated in that country, with the rates being slightly higher for men and much higher for women.[15] Unfortunately, there is little data on sexual orientation or gender identity among incarcerated people in Canada or other countries, and it is difficult to know how broadly applicable these American data are given that the United States is such an anomaly when it comes to incarcerating its citizens (it does so at a rate seven times that of Canada or the European average, for example).[16] The study also found that 2SLGBTQ inmates were more likely to be exposed to physical and/or sexual assault by inmates or correctional staff.

Worldwide, same-sex sexual acts continue to be criminalized in 74 countries, one-third of which are members of the United Nations, mostly in Asia, Africa, and the Caribbean. In 13 countries, such acts can be punished by death.[17] This is an important consideration for the health care and legal issues of 2SLGBTQ refugees.

Trans prisoners have had the right to be incarcerated at a prison that is consistent with their gender identity in Ontario since 2015, and recently this policy was also adopted for federal Canadian prisons.

Family and Developmental History

This part of the history taking may be an opportunity to confirm that your patient is 2SLGBTQ if they haven't yet disclosed this information to you, and it will give you a better understanding of your patient as a whole person.

"I'd like to ask about your life, growing up" opens the topic, and asking about what they may have been told about their mother's pregnancy, their birth, and their early development milestones sets the stage. We do not have good data on associations between developmental or intellectual disorders and 2SLGBTQ identity, with perhaps one exception: autism spectrum disorder (ASD). There is a higher prevalence of ASD among individuals presenting for transgender-related health care.[18]

Review of the patient's early memories and early school experiences may indicate a history of gender non-conforming behaviour in childhood. Not all 2SLGB or even trans individuals experience this, but the two are consistently strongly correlated in studies (e.g., Cohen 2002).[19] Gender non-conforming behaviour is also associated with a risk for physical and sexual abuse and is a common target for taunts and abuse from bullies (regardless of the youth's sexual orientation or gender identity).

Asking about puberty and early sexual and romantic feelings for others may be where you are best able to elicit a disclosure of 2SLGBTQ experience from your patient. Typically, by this point of the history taking, the patient is more comfortable with you and less anxious and will have noticed the signals alluding to your openness that you established earlier. Asking, "Did you find yourself attracted to boys, girls, both, or neither?" is a simple way of providing another opportunity for the individual to disclose to you.

COMING OUT

An oft-cited difference between the experience of sexual and gender minority people and ethnoracial minority people is that 2SLGBTQ people are, so to speak, "born into the enemy camp." Most typically, 2SLGBTQ people are born into families that are heterosexual and cisgender and to parents who will have this expectation for their offspring. As such, normal 2SLGBTQ development necessitates a process known as *coming out*.

At the time of the writing of the first edition of this book, stage-based models of sexual orientation development were popular (e.g., Cass's six-stage model or Troiden's four-stage model). While these models have some appeal for identifying development tasks that an individual LGBQ person may be dealing with, the idea that people progress in a linear fashion through stages that start with being unaware and confused and culminate in pride in one's identity is not necessarily empirically supported.[20] Therefore, while some experts find utility in the stage model, it can be argued that consideration of coming out and LGBQ identity formation as task-based rather than stage-based is optimal. In this chapter, we will describe the task-based approach whereas the stage-based approach is described in chapter 5, 2SLGBTQ Children and Youth.

Box 8.2. Tasks of LGBQ Coming Out

Feeling different from peers. This is often related to gender non-conformity and develops into feelings of shame or ineptitude in the absence of peer or parental support.

Same-sex attractions. They are typically experienced as more romantic than sexual for women and girls compared to men and boys.

Questioning assumed heterosexuality. This may be a more complicated task for those with a bisexual orientation or from cultures where same-sex attractions are acknowledged but infantilized (i.e., considered reasonable in adolescence, after which one must "grow up" and be heterosexual).

Same-sex behaviour. This is more likely to be at an earlier age, not in the context of a relationship, and before LGBQ identity formation in men compared to women.

Self-identification. Women typically arrive at this task earlier than men; this task may be deferred to reject sexual identity labels or because another identification (religion, culture, race) is given priority.

Disclosure. This involves coming out to others, most importantly to family and friends, though this is an ongoing lifelong task, considering social presumptions of heterosexuality.

Romantic relationships. Young people are arriving at this task earlier than did older cohorts; as with heterosexuals, first relationships may not endure but still provide important developmental opportunities.

Self-acceptance and synthesis. Remaining conflicted, ambivalent, or rejecting of sexuality may lead to poor self-esteem and life satisfaction; synthesis means an integration of sexual identity with other important identities.

Source: Adapted from Cohen and Savin-Williams, 2012[21]

Mental Health in Transgender Health Care

Mental health is an essential element of the holistic consideration of your TNB patients' health care. As mentioned earlier in this chapter, the burden of mental illness in the trans population is high compared to the general population. The World Professional Association for Transgender Health (WPATH), which publishes internationally recognized standards of care (SOC) in transgender health, recommends that the mental health professional working with transgender people should have the minimal credentials shown in box 8.3.

Box 8.3. Recommended Credentials for Mental Health Professionals Working with TNB Adults

1. A master's degree or its equivalent in a clinical behavioural science field. This degree, or a more advanced one, should be granted by an institution accredited by the appropriate national or regional accrediting board. The mental health professional should have documented credentials from a relevant licensing board or equivalent for that country.
2. Competence in using the *DSM* and/or the ICD-11 for diagnostic purposes.
3. The ability to recognize and diagnose coexisting mental health concerns and to distinguish these from gender incongruence.
4. Documented supervised training and competence in psychotherapy or counselling.
5. Knowledge about gender-nonconforming identities and expressions, and assessment and treatment.

Source: Adapted from WPATH SOC version 7[22]

The role of the mental health professional on an interdisciplinary team providing care to transgender patients is manifold and may include clinical assessment for gender incongruence, identification and treatment of co-occurring mental health conditions, family interventions to help ensure family support (a significant factor in positive outcomes for trans people), and supportive treatment through the process of transition.[23] Assessment of eligibility and readiness to proceed with an endocrinological or a surgical intervention for gender transition is also a key role for the mental health practitioner, though in interdisciplinary teams, it is acknowledged that it is also suitable for this assessment to be done by another knowledgeable professional, such as the primary care physician or nurse practitioner, ideally one who has ready access to a mental health professional should there be significant co-occurring mental health concerns.

While the WPATH SOC version 7 discusses specific eligibility criteria in more detail, the focus of our attention here is on a distinction made in the SOC about co-occurring medical and mental health conditions. The SOC indicate that for hormone therapies and "top" surgeries (that is, breast/chest surgeries) that such conditions should be "reasonably well controlled." For "bottom" surgeries (that is gonadal or genital surgeries), such conditions should be "well controlled."

UNCONTROLLED OR POORLY CONTROLLED
As the WPATH SOC do not provide guidance regarding this distinction with respect to either medical or mental health conditions, outwardly this would appear to be unclear. However, perhaps the easiest distinction to make is what is *not* reasonably well controlled. Examples of uncontrolled or poorly controlled mental health conditions could include the following:

- a psychotic disorder that is highly symptomatic and for which the patient is either untreated or is poorly adherent to treatment
- repetitive non-superficial self-harm behaviours that are either untreated or persistent despite treatment
- poorly constrained, highly frequent substance abuse with significant adverse consequences
- profound depression or a severe anxiety disorder (e.g., agoraphobia with hoarding) that has a significant impact on the patient's basic activities of daily living
- any mental health disorder that is having a significantly negative impact on the patient's ability to provide informed consent to treatment

One can imagine why, despite meeting diagnostic criteria for gender incongruence, a patient this impaired would be an unsuitable candidate for either hormone therapy or a breast/chest surgery. Hormone therapies have established effects on the brain and have been known to worsen psychosis in some cis women. This has also been seen in trans individuals with psychotic disorders (and there is at least one case report of the converse: psychosis precipitated by abrupt hormone withdrawal in a trans woman).[24] Breast augmentation and mastectomy surgeries require a level of basic functioning, self-care, and/or personal support to ensure good post-operative recovery.

REASONABLY WELL CONTROLLED

The term *reasonably* implies the use of reason and thoughtfulness. What, then, are the factors that we should think about in considering this? If considered against the description above, one could say that *reasonably well controlled* would mean the following, at the minimum:

- *substantial engagement with treatment* for the conditions of concern, and
- evidence of this treatment bringing the symptoms of concern *under some control.*

How much control? *Reasonably* might also imply that this criterion is contextual and could depend on a few factors, including how much supervision and support the patient has available to them and what condition and treatment we are talking about. That is, a clinician perhaps might want to see more control of symptoms for a top surgery than for initiation of hormone therapy or more control for a depression with psychosis than a depression without psychosis.

Another important part of this reasoning is the consideration of how likely the hormone therapy or top surgery is to *itself improve the patient's functioning*. If the patient's depression or anxiety disorder is substantially perpetuated by the patient's gender incongruence, then it is possible that the hormone therapy or chest surgery will substantially improve the situation or, at least, *reduce harm*.

WELL CONTROLLED

Why do the WPATH criteria make a distinction between chest/breast surgeries ("reasonably well controlled") and gonadal and genital surgeries ("well controlled")?

It is easiest to understand this in consideration of the genital surgeries. Put simply, these surgeries, which include vaginoplasty, metoidioplasty (+/– urethral extension and vaginectomy), and phalloplasty, are complex surgeries with burdensome recovery and rehabilitation expectations, and necessitate vigilance for post-operative complications. A patient preoccupied with mental health symptoms that are not well controlled would be at higher risk for these complications and possible poor surgical outcomes. Poor surgical outcomes are an oft-cited reason for overall dissatisfaction with a gender transition experience. Additionally, these surgeries, compared to the top surgeries, are highly specialized, and patients often travel a long distance from home to obtain them (for example, in Canada, genital surgeries are currently available only at surgical centres in Montreal, Toronto, and Vancouver). They therefore may have less access to their usual social supports.

It is less clear why the SOC also make this distinction for gonadal surgeries (orchiectomy and hysterectomy), which are less burdensome in the post-operative period and less specialized, especially orchiectomy, which typically does not even involve general anaesthesia. It is likely that WPATH will make a finer distinction between gonadal and genital surgeries in the next version of the SOC, version 8, expected to be published in the near future.

In summary, the mental health needs of the 2SLGBTQ population have been established in many studies to be elevated compared to the general population, and our best idea of why is minority stress. Taking a careful history that respects the patient's identity, if disclosed, and signals openness, if not yet disclosed, is important. Also important is an understanding that the patient may have past negative experiences with health care providers. Some individuals may have experienced conversion therapy or other SOCE, with consequences for their self-esteem as a 2SLGBTQ person. This chapter also examined considerations for 2SLGBTQ people in taking a history related to mood, anxiety, psychotic, and eating disorders, and explored the SOC of WPATH as they speak to the management of mental health concerns in the context of trans health care.

References

1. Chakraborty A, McManus S, Brugha TS, Bebbington P, King M. Mental health of the non-heterosexual population of England. Br J Psychiatry. 2011;198(2):143–8. doi:10.1192/bjp.bp.110.082271.
2. Kidd SA, Howison M, Pilling M, Ross LE, McKenzie K. Severe mental illness in LGBT populations: a scoping review. Psychiatr Serv. 2016 Jul;67(7):779–83. doi:10.1176/appi.ps.201500209.
3. Bauer GR, Scheim AI, Pyne J, Travers R, Hammond R. Intervenable factors associated with suicide risk in transgender persons: a respondent driven sampling study in Ontario, Canada. *BMC Public Health* 2015; 15: 525.
4. Meyer IH. Prejudice, social stress, and mental health in lesbian, gay, and bisexual populations: conceptual issues and research evidence. Psychol Bull. 2003;129:674–97.

5. Statistics Canada [Internet]. Ottawa: Government of Canada; 2017 [cited 2021 Oct 2]. Police-reported hate crime in Canada, 2015. Juristat. Available from: http://www.statcan.gc.ca/pub/85-002-x/2017001/article/14832-eng.htm.

6. Roberts AL, Austin SB, Corliss HL, Vandermorris AK, Koenen KC. Pervasive trauma exposure among US sexual orientation minority adults and risk of posttraumatic stress disorder. Am J Public Health. 2010 Dec;100(12):2433–41.

7. Roberts AL, Rosario M, Corliss HL, Koenen KC, Austin SB. Elevated risk of posttraumatic stress in sexual minority youths: mediation by childhood abuse and gender nonconformity. Am J Public Health. 2012 Aug;102(8):1587–93.

8. McIntosh CA. Bipolar disorder: identity crisis. In: Levounis P, Drescher J, Barber, ME, editors. *The LGBT casebook*. Washington (DC): American Psychiatric Publishing; 2012. p. 141–9.

9. Calzo JP, Blashill AJ, Brown TA, Argenal RL. Eating Disorders and Disordered Weight and Shape Control Behaviors in Sexual Minority Populations. Curr Psychiatry Rep. 2017 Aug;19(8):49. doi:10.1007/s11920-017-0801-y.

10. Choi EP, Wong JY, Fong DY. The use of social networking applications of smartphone and associated sexual risks in lesbian, gay, bisexual, and transgender populations: a systematic review. AIDS Care. 2017 Feb;29(2):145–55.

11. American Psychiatric Association. *DSM-II: Diagnostic and statistical manual of mental disorders*. Washington (DC): American Psychiatric Association; 1968.

12. World Health Organization. International classification of diseases for mortality and morbidity statistics. 11th ed. Geveva (Switzerland): World Health Organization; 2018. Available from: https://icd.who.int/browse11/l-m/en.

13. Drescher J, Schwartz A, Casoy F, McIntosh CA, Hurley B, Ashley K, et al. The growing regulation of conversion therapy. J Med Regul. 2016;102(2):7–12.

14. Bialer PA, McIntosh CA, Barber ME. New perspectives on sexual orientation change efforts. J Gay Lesbian Ment Health. 2015;19(1):1–3.

15. Meyer IH, Flores AR, Stemple L, Romero AP, Wilson BD, Herman JL. Incarceration rates and traits of sexual minorities in the United States: national inmate survey, 2011–2012. Am J Public Health. 2017 Feb;107(2):267–73. doi:10.2105/ AJPH.2016.303576

16. Walmsley R. World prison population list. 11th ed. London (England): Institute for Crime and Justice Policy Research; 2016. Available

from: https://www.prisonstudies.org/sites/default/files/resources/downloads/world_prison_population_list_11th_edition_0.pdf.

17. Carroll A. State sponsored homophobia 2016: A world survey of sexual orientation laws: criminalisation, protection and recognition. Geneva (Switzerland): ILGA; 2016.

18. de Vries AL, Noens IL, Cohen-Kettenis PT, van Berckelaer-Onnes IA, Doreleijers TA. Autism spectrum disorders in gender dysphoric children and adolescents. J Autism Dev Disord. 2010 Aug;40(8):930–6. doi:10.1007/s10803-010-0935-9

19. Cohen KM. Relationships among childhood sex-atypical behavior, spatial ability, handedness, and sexual orientation in men. Arch Sex Behav. 2002 Feb;31(1):129–43.

20. Savin-Williams RC. The new gay teenager. Cambridge (MA): Harvard University Press; 2005.

21. Cohen KM, Savin-Williams RC. Coming out to self and others: developmental milestones. In: Levounis P, Drescher J, Barber, ME, editors. *The LGBT casebook*. Washington (DC): American Psychiatric Publishing; 2012. p. 17–23.

22. Coleman E, Bockting W, Botzer M, Cohen-Kettenis P, DeCuypere G, Feldman J, et al. Standards of care for the health of transsexual, transgender, and gender-nonconforming people, version 7. Int J Transgenderism. 2012;13(4):165–232. doi:10.1080/15532739.2011.700873.

23. McIntosh C. Interdisciplinary care for transgender patients. In: Ehrenfeld J, Eckstrand K, editors. Lesbian, gay, bisexual, transgender, and intersex healthcare: a clinical guide to preventative, primary, and specialist care. New York: Springer; 2016. p. 339–49.

24. Summers SM, Onate J. New onset psychosis following abrupt discontinuation of hormone replacement therapy in a trans woman. J Gay Lesbian Ment Health. 2014;18(3):312–19. doi:10.1080/19359705.2014.915463.

9 Substance Abuse

CHRISTOPHER (KIT) FAIRGRIEVE

Background and Epidemiology of Substance Use Disorders

Substance use is often perceived to be a prevalent cultural aspect within the 2SLGBTQ community at large and represents an ongoing source of stereotype and stigmatization for many 2SLGBTQ people. 2SLGBTQ-friendly bars certainly have historical (and ongoing) importance as places for people to congregate in relative safety, although the use of alcohol and other substances as means to facilitate social interaction is hardly unique to the 2SLGBTQ community. Substance use is certainly more prevalent within some settings such as bathhouses,[1] however, and the phenomenon of *chemsex* (in which amyl nitrites, club drugs such as gamma-hydroxybutyrate [GHB], and methamphetamines are used in combination with sexual intercourse)[2] has a particular and longstanding history in the community of men who have sex with men (MSM).[3] Furthermore, it has been reported that past-year substance use, perceived availability, and tolerance of substance use within the 2SLGBTQ community is higher than in the general population.[4] Nonetheless, it should be noted at the outset of this chapter that many 2SLGBTQ people do not use substances.

As reviewed in the first edition of this book, earlier studies on the active prevalence of substance use disorders (SUD) in the "gay and lesbian population" were estimated at 30 per cent, much higher than the estimated 10 to 12 per cent in the general population. These findings were often skewed by the sampling bias of surveying people in bars,[5] however, and newer studies have found that substance use among 2SLGBTQ people, although higher, is likely closer to prevalence rates in the general population than previously estimated.[6] Unfortunately, Canadian data on substance use prevalence among 2SLGBTQ people are fairly sparse, as both the Canadian Tobacco Alcohol and Drugs

Table 9.1. Past-Year[13] and Lifetime Prevalence[14] of Substance Use and SUD by Gender Identity and Sexual Orientation, from the NESARC, 2004–2005 (n = 34,653)

	Past Year Prevalence (%)				Lifetime Prevalence (%)	
	Heavy Drinking	AUD	Other Substance Use	Other SUD	AUD	Other SUD
Women						
Lesbian	20.1	13.3**	12.6**	5.7	58.6**	24.5*
Bisexual	25.0**	15.6**	14.1**	3.0	53.5**	40.4*
Heterosexual	8.4	2.5	3.1	0.4	22.0	8.0
Men						
Gay	18.1	16.8**	16.8**	3.2*	58.7	32.7**
Bisexual	16.4	19.5**	17.7**	5.1*	52.1	25.0**
Heterosexual	8.4	6.1	4.5	0.5	47.7	15.7

AUD = alcohol use disorder; SUD = substance use disorder

*p < .05. **p < .01.

Survey and Canadian Alcohol and Drug Use Monitoring Survey (most recently collected in 2015 and 2012, respectively) categorize substance use rates based on biological sex and age but neither gender identity nor sexual orientation.[7,8] A recent report and literature review by Rainbow Health Ontario found little available Canadian data on the prevalence of SUD within the 2SLGBTQ population,[9] and the data collected in several studies were by convenience samples that may overestimate prevalence as with earlier studies.[10,11]

In the United States, the first version of the National Epidemiological Survey of Alcohol and Related Conditions (NESARC) study was conducted in 2004–5 and included prevalence rates of substance use and SUD by biological sex and sexual orientation. A more recent NESARC survey was conducted in 2012–13, but substance use prevalence by gender identity and sexual orientation has not yet been published.[12] The results of the 2004–2005 survey are summarized in table 9.1 and report that both past-year and lifetime prevalence of substance use and SUD are significantly higher for several subsections of the 2SLGBTQ population.

NESARC data does not report substance use prevalence among transgender people, but a 2008 systematic review on past-year substance use among trans women found that 43.7 per cent reported alcohol use, 20.2 per cent reported cannabis use, and 26.7 per cent reported other illicit substance use. Furthermore, intravenous drug use was reported among 12.0 per cent of trans women, although only 2.0 per cent reported sharing syringes.[15] Conversely, trans men reported relatively lower rates of SUD (13.7 per cent), but fewer studies were included.[15] Furthermore, neither the Canadian nor American surveys reported on substance use prevalence among 2SLGBTQ youth, but it has been found that substance use is almost three times higher in this group, and particularly higher among bisexual youth (3.4 times) and women who have sex with women (WSW, 4 times) compared to heterosexual youth.[16] Similarly, substance use among older adults is a less-studied but increasingly prevalent phenomenon,[17] and higher rates of SUD have been reported among older 2SLGBTQ adults,[18] including increased non-medical use of opioids in combination with risky sexual behaviour among older MSM.[19]

Pathophysiology of Substance Use Disorders

What are SUD and how do they develop? This complex question has been studied at length, and the current understanding is that SUD involves a disorder in the brain's *reward* system, which includes the primitive meso-limbic system acting on higher levels of executive functioning in the prefrontal cortex and mediated by dopamine release at the nucleus accumbens.[20] For people with this disordered reward system, ongoing substance use becomes more important (or *salient*) via down regulation of dopamine receptors and less response from natural reinforcers such as food or sex; ongoing substance use becomes the most salient option.[21] Animal studies have found that pleasurable stimuli such as food and sex increase dopamine release at the nucleus accumbens by 150 per cent and 200 per cent, respectively; by comparison, alcohol and opioids increase dopamine by 200 to 250 per cent, cocaine by 350 per cent and amphetamines by 1000 per cent.[22] Drug salience is also affected by environmental factors, and a recent systematic review found support for the correlation between an insecure childhood attachment pattern and later development of substance use disorder.[23] A more thorough review of the complex and evolving understanding of the neurobiology of the "brain disease model of addiction" by Volkow et al. is recommended for interested readers.[24]

Furthermore, and specifically for SUD in the 2SLGBTQ population, the intersectionality and so-called *syndemics* between the process and experience of identifying as 2SLGBTQ, cultural factors within the 2SLGBTQ community, and personal and cultural factors of resiliency with respect to substance use and other risk exposures are intricate, and interested readers are referred to the excellent discussion in the chapter on substance use disorder by Hall, Reback, and Shoptaw in *The Fenway Guide to Lesbian, Gay, Bisexual and Transgender Health*[25] and in published discussions on syndemic effects within MSM,[26] WSW,[27] and transgender communities.[28]

Screening and Diagnosis of Substance Use Disorder

It has been estimated that 20 to 30 per cent of people presenting to primary care have a SUD[29] and, given the higher prevalence of SUD among 2SLGBTQ people, this number may be higher among 2SLGBTQ patients presenting to care. General screening for substance use and potential SUD is recommended for all patients and can be integrated into a periodic health assessment or into specific assessments for symptoms or diagnoses that may be related to substance use. In the United States, the emerging model for primary care providers is called SBIRT: screening, brief intervention, and (if necessary for persistent SUD) referral to treatment. SBIRT has been extensively studied in the United States and has a robust body of literature in support of its use in the treatment of SUD.[30]

A number of validated screening tools are available, including the well-known CAGE questionnaire for alcohol use disorders (AUD). This is a brief, four-question assessment that acts as its own mnemonic, and a score of two or more yes responses is fairly accurate in identifying "alcoholism."[31] If the CAGE test is positive, the more in-depth Alcohol Use Disorders Identification Test (AUDIT) can then be administered to better evaluate for "hazardous drinking."[32] For other substance use, the 10-question Alcohol, Smoking, and Substance Involvement Screening Tool (ASSIST) can be used,[33] and the Drug Abuse Screening Test (DAST) can be used for a more specific assessment of illicit drug use.[34] Specifically for prescription opioids, the Opioid Risk Tool[35] and Current Opioid Misuse Measure (COMM)[36] are validated screening tools to identify those at risk of opioid misuse or current opioid misuse, respectively.

In addition, criteria from the fifth edition of the *Diagnostic and Statistical Manual of Mental Disorders* (*DSM-5*) can be applied to any substance to make a formal diagnosis of a substance use disorder for people with a positive screening test.[37] Of note, the previous diagnostic categories of *substance abuse* and *substance dependence*, as defined in the previous edition (*DSM-IV*),[38] were revised in 2013 to the current diagnostic framework that includes 11 criteria (see box 9.1) and a spectrum of diagnosis of substance use disorder ranging from mild (2 to 3 criteria), moderate (4 to 5 criteria), or severe (6 or more criteria). Of note, the presence of cravings has been added to the new criteria as a distinct feature of substance use disorder.

Box 9.1. *Diagnostic and Statistical Manual of Mental Disorders,*
5th Edition: Criteria for Substance Use Disorder[37]

A pattern of substance use leading to significant impairment or distress, as manifested by two or more of the following within a 12-month period:

1. Tolerance or markedly increased amounts of the substance to achieve intoxication or desired effect OR markedly diminished effect with continued use of the same amount of substance.
2. Withdrawal symptoms or the use of substances to avoid withdrawal.
3. Use of a substance in larger amounts or over a longer period than was intended.
4. Persistent desire or unsuccessful efforts to cut down or control substance use.
5. Involvement in chronic behaviour to obtain the substance, use the substance, or recover from its effects.
6. Reduction or abandonment of social, occupational, or recreational activities because of substance use.
7. Use of substances even though there are persistent or recurrent physical or psychological problems that are likely to have been caused or exacerbated by the substance.
8. Craving or a strong desire or urge to use a substance.
9. Failure to fulfill major role obligations (work, school, home), such as repeated absences or poor work performance related to substance use; substance-related absences, suspensions, or expulsions from school; neglect of children or household.
10. Frequent use of substances in situations that are physically hazardous.
11. Continued use despite having persistent social or interpersonal problems.

Clinicians may consider providing screening tests to patients in waiting rooms or other settings before general health assessments or assessments specifically related to SUD, and patients should be reassured that such assessments are part of routine care and not an implication of suspected substance use. Screening tests can then be reviewed in the office and can form the basis for a more thorough history taking of substance use, possible related problems, provision of a diagnosis, and discussion of appropriate treatment options if needed. A careful history (see box 9.2) should include a timeline for each substance, including age of first use, age at which use became regular, and age at which use became problematic (such as occupational or health problems); present stage of change (as per the model developed by Prochaska and DiClemente)[39] and goals of care for their substance use (i.e., abstinence versus reduced use, or ongoing use); and treatment history (including pharmaceutical and psychosocial treatments) and related responses to treatment, and preferred treatment options for present care, if any. Patients may not want treatment for their substance use and should instead be supported for their honesty in reporting substance use and encouraged to return if support is wanted. In addition, interventions to reduce harms associated with substance use (such as take-home naloxone distribution for those at risk of opioid overdose) should be offered at every opportunity.

Box 9.2. Focused Substance Use History

- Presenting symptom or concern prompting substance assessment
- Screening tests and results (i.e., which responses were positive?)
- For each reported substance used, inquire about
  - Age of first use
  - Age at which use became heavier and/or more regular (e.g., weekends, daily use)
  - Age at which use became problematic (as per DSM-5 criteria)
  - Physical symptoms associated with use (e.g., chest pain)
  - Medical complications of substance use (e.g., cirrhosis, infectious complications of intravenous drug use, overdose history)
  - Presence of tolerance (i.e., higher amounts needed for same effect) and withdrawal symptoms (physical and psychological)
  - Review of present harms such as overdose risk, blackouts, seizures, impaired driving, occupational risks, childcare, etc.
  - Treatment history (i.e., medications, psychosocial) and related responses to treatment

- – Social factors associated with substance use (particularly with respect to 2SLGBTQ community), including people and places that are either triggering or protective
  - – Present stage of change* and patient goals of care for treatment
- Screen for other substance use (nicotine, alcohol, caffeine, cannabis, opioids, stimulants, sedative-hypnotics, club drugs, steroids, others)
- Medications: inquire about misuse of prescribed medications (i.e., appropriate dose, frequency, and route of administration as prescribed) and consider medication taper or change if substance use disorder is identified (as per provincial college guidelines)
- Collateral information from other providers (with consent)
- Review provincial medication database if available to screen for multiple providers, early refills, and review risk of polypharmacy and unintentional overdose

* Prochaska and DiClemente, 1992[39]

While much of the information will be obtained from history, physical examination and laboratory investigations are an important adjunct to diagnosis of both SUD and related medical comorbidities (see box 9.3). Physical examination should include general assessment for signs of either intoxication or withdrawal, such as autonomic hyperactivity, tremor, diaphoresis, or general malaise. Table 9.2 lists the general signs and symptoms of intoxication (i.e., toxicity state) and withdrawal syndromes by substance.

Cardiorespiratory, abdominal, and neurological examinations are helpful for identifying signs of chronic substance use such as liver dysfunction, but physical findings are by no means diagnostic of SUD. Dermatological exam may reveal injection marks, abscesses or cellulitis, or skin lesions typical of amphetamine use, but permission should be obtained before examination as this experience can be stigmatizing for many people. Appropriate lab investigations include a complete blood count, renal and liver function tests, urine drug screen, and electrocardiogram if cardiac disease is suspected. An increase in mean corpuscular volume (MCV) or liver transaminases (i.e., AST/ALT ratio greater than two, elevated GGT) are suggestive of AUD but are not diagnostic.

Table 9.2. Intoxication and Withdrawal Syndromes by Substance

Substance	Intoxication	Withdrawal
Nicotine	Autonomic hyperactivity, headache, nausea, vomiting	Irritability, anxiety, headache, insomnia, diaphoresis, nausea, hyperphagia
Cannabis	Tachycardia, xerostomia, hyperphagia, nausea, vomiting, psychosis	Irritability, anxiety, insomnia, diaphoresis, headache, anorexia, nausea
Alcohol	Cerebellar dysfunction (ataxia, loss of coordination, slurred speech), anterograde amnesia ("blackouts"), decreased level of consciousness, respiratory depression	Psychomotor agitation, tremor, autonomic hyperactivity, seizures, visual hallucinations, delirium tremens
Gamma-hydroxybutyrate (GHB)	Similar to alcohol	Similar to alcohol
Benzodiazepines	Similar to alcohol	Similar to alcohol (with delayed onset due to longer half-life, i.e., 7–14 days after last use)
Opioids	Respiratory depression, decreased level of consciousness, miosis, hypotension, hypothermia, hyporeflexia	Irritability, autonomic hyperactivity, mydriasis, diaphoresis, chills, nausea, vomiting, diarrhea, myalgias, arthralgias, piloerection
Stimulants	Autonomic hyperactivity, psychosis, psychomotor agitation, anorexia, insomnia	Hypersomnia, hyperphagia, irritability, anxiety, severely decreased mood, anhedonia

---

Box 9.3. Focused Substance Use Physical Examination and Laboratory Investigations

Physical Examination

- General appearance, grooming, signs of acute intoxication or withdrawal (see table 9.2), fever, malaise

- Cardiovascular: heart rate and blood pressure, signs of cardiovascular disease (including pallor or erythema, peripheral edema, etc.), precordial exam for extra heart sounds or murmurs (e.g., tricuspid or mitral valve regurgitation secondary to infective endocarditis)
- Respiratory: respiratory rate and oxygen saturation (especially for acute intoxication), signs of nicotine or other inhaled substance use, signs of chronic obstructive pulmonary disease
- Abdominal: signs of liver dysfunction including jaundice, scleral icterus, telangiectasia, etc.; auscultation for bowel sounds (may be reduced with opioid use), palpation for tenderness and hepatomegaly, percussion for upper border of liver and presence of ascites
- Dermatological: diffuse excoriating skin lesions (typical of amphetamine use), presence of active or healed injection marks (most commonly in antecubital fossae but may be diffuse) and associated cellulitis or abscesses
- Neurological: tremor (suggestive of alcohol or opioid withdrawal), signs of B12 deficiency associated with AUD (peripheral neuropathy, hyporeflexia, pathological reflexes), signs of thiamine deficiency, i.e., Wernicke's encephalopathy (classic triad of lateral nystagmus, ataxia, mental status changes) and/or Korsakoff syndrome (neuropsychiatric changes including retrograde and anterograde amnesia)

Laboratory Investigations

- Complete blood count: anemia (from active GI bleeding, B12 deficiency, chronic disease, etc.), increased white blood count caused by acute infection (especially among people who inject drugs), increased mean corpuscular volume (MCV) often from B12 or folate deficiency in AUD, low platelet count in AUD.
- Renal function tests: volume/hydration status, electrolyte abnormalities
- Liver function tests: elevated GGT and AST/ALT ratio typically greater than 2:1 in alcoholic hepatitis, elevated INR in cirrhosis (alcoholic, hepatitis C, etc.), hepatitis serology
- Electrocardiogram
- Urine drug screening: typically first-line is immunoassay (i.e., dipstick), can be sent for gas chromatography-mass spectrometry if needed to confirm unexpected positive or negative results

Urine drug screening (UDS) is useful, and standard urine-dipped immunoassays should be routinely collected for all patients receiving prescription opioids, stimulants, or sedative/hypnotics (such as benzodiazepines) to screen for concurrent substance use and to ensure that medications are being taken by the patient for whom they are prescribed. Both false positives and false negatives are possible, however, and can be confirmed by gas chromatography-mass spectrometry if needed for unexpected results prior to reviewing with patients. Most substances, including opioids and stimulants, are typically present in urine samples for 48 to 72 hours, while longer-acting substances such as benzodiazepines or methadone can persist for up to 7 to 10 days.[40] Heavy use of cannabinoids can persist for an especially long time, typically up to 28 days. Alcohol is usually metabolized within 12 hours, and serum alcohol levels are rarely useful, but the alcohol metabolite ethyl glucuronide can be added to a standard urine drug screen if needed for more sensitive detection of recent alcohol use (such as for occupational monitoring programs). Local laboratory staff can be helpful with interpreting unusual UDS findings or suggesting appropriate follow-up tests if needed for confirmation.

Providers are encouraged to make UDS a standard part of practice for patients receiving prescription opioids, benzodiazepines, or stimulants, rather than only when illicit substance use is suspected, and it has been found that up to 20 per cent of patients on prescription opioids had an unexpected result for another substance.[41] If illicit substance use is identified, a non-judgmental approach will hopefully foster a good therapeutic alliance that will encourage open disclosure and appropriate treatment options if SUD is present. Efforts to reduce the risk of prescription drug misuse and diversion, such as requiring daily witnessed ingestion of medications, may be necessary if illicit substance use is present. A balance between retaining patients in care and maintaining safe prescribing practices is a frequent challenge in the care of people with SUD, and clinicians are encouraged to seek the support of addiction medicine specialist services if needed to develop a safe and effective treatment plan.

Treatment of Substance Use Disorders

General Treatment Recommendations for Substance Use Disorders

It is important to consider that SUD change over time, and it has been estimated that only 28 per cent of people with a history of AUD report any history of formal treatment,[42] and approximately one third of people will achieve abstinence without intervention.[43] In addition, many people reduce their use over time: A study of the 1995 Ontario Health Survey found that 58 per cent of people who had previously met the criteria for AUD had reduced their consumption to more moderate amounts.[43] A US survey of people with lifetime past history of SUD found remission rates of 84 per cent for nicotine, 91 per cent for alcohol, 97 per cent for cannabis, and 99 per cent for cocaine, with 50 per cent abstinence rates reported after an average of 26, 14, 6, and 5 years after onset of SUD, respectively. Furthermore, rates were lower among men, Black people, those with personality disorders, and those with medical comorbidities related to substance use.[44] A systematic review with follow-up periods of up to three years found lower rates of remission, however, including amphetamines (16 to 45 per cent), opioids (9 to 22 per cent), cocaine (5 to 14 per cent), and cannabis (17 per cent), depending on remission definition. Good health status and higher social functioning were associated with better prognosis, but concurrent psychiatric comorbidity was associated with a worse prognosis.[45] Thus many people with SUD are able to reduce their substance use or achieve abstinence over time, although this process often takes years.

If SUD is identified, a brief office-based intervention by primary care providers can be given to patients to offer feedback and education, increase insight and awareness of the risks associated with their substance use, enhance motivation for change, and review available treatment options. Even brief, one- to three-minute interventions can have a significant impact on substance use.[46] A range of office-based interventions are available specific to various substances, including smoking,[46] alcohol,[47] and other illicit substance use.[48] Furthermore, some 2SLGBTQ-specific tools are also available, such as the US National LGBT Tobacco Control Network, and interventions specific for transgender people[49] and 2SLGBTQ youth.[50]

A range of treatment options beyond the brief intervention are also available, although these vary significantly by region. Perhaps the most ubiquitous option is mutual support programs, primarily 12-step programs such as Alcoholics Anonymous (see section below). Patients may elect for alternative treatment options, particularly if they have had negative experiences with mutual support groups or continue to have cravings or use substances despite active participation in such programs. Formal counselling options may be available, either in group or individual settings. For people seeking or requiring more extensive treatment, a referral to an intensive outpatient program (which typically involves full-day programming in an outpatient setting) may be warranted. Inpatient hospital or residential-based treatment programs may also be available options and have a moderate evidence base,[51] although the cost of private programs and lengthy waitlists for publicly funded programs may be a deterrent for patients. There is evidence that outpatient programs may be as effective as inpatient programs at significantly lower cost,[52-54] and may be preferable for people who need to structure treatment around work, childcare, pets, or other considerations. Unfortunately, completion of a treatment program is often insufficient to maintain abstinence, and sparse follow-up data available for inpatient programs suggest a high rate of relapse.[55] Some people may benefit from longer-term treatment, such as second-stage housing or other programs that offer ongoing care for up to a year or longer. International models of such "therapeutic communities," such as San Patriano in Italy, have been associated with positive outcomes and are currently being adapted in some Canadian settings such as Vancouver.[56]

Formal guidelines on appropriate treatment options have been developed, such as the American Society of Addiction Medicine Criteria, which is based on severity of SUD, potential need for medically supervised withdrawal (such as for alcohol, benzodiazepine, or GHB withdrawal), and presence and severity of concurrent psychiatric diagnoses,[57] but a general guideline would be to work with patients to select an appropriate treatment option that is available and in accordance with their preference and goals of treatment, and then intensify as needed for ongoing symptoms of SUD. See box 9.4 for a review of general diagnostic and treatment considerations.

Box 9.4. Diagnosis and Treatment of Substance Use Disorders

- Diagnosis (as per *DSM*-5 criteria, i.e., mild, moderate or severe) for each substance
- Note inconsistencies between reported use and urine drug screen results or available collateral information

Treatment Plan for Each Substance

- Acute management of intoxication and withdrawal as needed, including referral to addiction medicine specialist or medically supervised withdrawal facility if indicated
- Present stage of change and patient goals of care for treatment

- Brief, office-based intervention (e.g., motivational interviewing) as needed
- Persistent cravings or substance use despite effort to abstain or cut down:
  - Medications (add or increase as needed)
  - Referral to treatment (outpatient and/or inpatient options)
  - Referral to addiction medicine specialist
  - Self-referral to mutual support groups (e.g., 12-step, SMART, etc.)
- Safety considerations:
  - Occupational, driving, and childcare safety considerations
  - May involve a duty to report, consult provincial/territorial Ministry of Health or addiction medicine specialist if needed
  - Access to take-home naloxone and sterile supplies if needed
  - Review overdose risk factors and provide education about lower-risk use practices:
    - Encourage people not to use alone.
    - Use supervised consumption sites where and when available.
    - Don't combine opioids with other sedative-hypnotics including alcohol and benzodiazepines.
    - Use "test doses," i.e., smaller amounts to help determine potency of illicit substances and reduce overdose risk.
    - Non-opioid substances (e.g., stimulants, cannabis) can potentially be adulterated with high-potency synthetic opioids like fentanyl.
- Review infectious complications of intravenous drug use (i.e., abscess, cellulitis, bacteremia, endocarditis, osteomyelitis, etc.) and provide education for lower-risk injecting practices:
  - Avoid sharing or reusing syringes.
  - Use sterile supplies including water and cooking implements.
  - Provide locations and contact information for needle exchange programs.
  - Use an alcohol swab on skin injection site before injection.

Follow-Up Plan

- Consider regular and frequent appointments until more stable.
- Encourage patients to book next appointment while in clinic to avoid running out of medications before follow-up.
- Encourage patients to return sooner if needed for medication review or additional supports.

2SLGBTQ-Specific Treatment Considerations

Many SUD treatment providers report uncertainty about discussing issues related to gender identity and sexuality, even in more urban locations,[58] and few treatment programs provide 2SLGBTQ-specific treatment options.[59] In addition, negative experiences have been reported among 2SLGBTQ people in conventional SUD programs and better outcomes with 2SLGBTQ-focused programs.[60] Within Canada, several local 2SLGBTQ-specific resources are available for treatment of SUD in major centres, such as Rainbow Services at the Centre for Addiction and Mental Health (CAMH) in Toronto, which has a range of treatment options and accepts self-referrals from patients across Canada.[61] Other 2SLGBTQ-affiliated services are recommended through websites such as Rainbow Health Ontario, although many programs are open to 2SLGBTQ patients but are not necessarily 2SLGBTQ specific. Outside Canada, the Pride Institute in Minnesota is a 2SLGBTQ-specific treatment program that accepts Canadian referrals but may be prohibitively expensive for patients without private insurance or considerable financial resources.

Other Treatment Considerations

MUTUAL SUPPORT GROUPS

Twelve-step programs are international organizations of mutual support programs, based on the belief that SUD are a medical and a spiritual disease. Twelve-step programs are distinct and autonomous, so that Alcoholics Anonymous (AA) has no affiliation with Narcotics Anonymous (NA) or other programs, despite the shared 12-step model of AA on which other programs are based. Participation is anonymous, with no required cost, and questions are not asked of new participants unless desired. Furthermore, participation in 12-step programs is not mutually exclusive from engaging in other treatment modalities. Among people with a past-year diagnosis of AUD, 17 per cent reported attending both formal treatment and AA, 5 per cent received formal treatment but did not attend AA, and 3 per cent attended AA but did not engage in formal treatment.[62] Twelve-step programs do not take a formal position on the use of medications to treat SUD, neither advocating nor rejecting their use, and instead recommend that participants consult a health care provider.[63] Nonetheless, many individuals who attend 12-step meetings may express strong opinions on the use of medications, and patients should be encouraged to disregard these and seek 12-step literature on the subject for more support.

Meta-analyses of randomized controlled trials have found no good evidence in favour of 12-step programs,[45] particularly when participation is coerced (such as by the criminal justice system),[64] but a large body of observational studies found significant benefits to attendance.[65,66] Among those attending AA, long-term abstinence was maintained among 67 per cent of people who achieved one year of continuous sobriety, 85 per cent of people who achieved between two and five years, and 90 per cent for those who achieved more than five years.[67] Similar five-year follow-up data exist for opioid use disorder and NA attendance but not for stimulants.[68] Limited data are available for 2SLGBTQ communities, but a 1994 study of lesbian AA members identified concerns about a sense of differentiation, perception of AA as a white, male, heterosexist organization, including sexist language in the literature (which includes a chapter called "To the Wives").[69]

These programs may be unpalatable to people who do not have a goal of abstinence, who bristle at the discussion of SUD as a spiritual malady whose solution lies in forging a connection with a higher power, or who have attended meetings and found them either unhelpful or even harmful and unsafe, as some 2SLGBTQ people may have experienced. Fortunately, many communities have 12-step meetings that are listed as 2SLGBTQ friendly or specific, and it is hoped that 2SLGBTQ people will be welcomed in any meeting they attend. A hallmark feature of 12-step programs is that abstinence is maintained by seeking out and helping others, and many members take this responsibility seriously and practise it without harassment or discrimination. Online meetings are also a useful resource for patients looking for 2SLGBTQ-specific resources.

In addition, many other types of alternative mutual support programs exist but are less well studied than 12-step programs. There are some studies in support of SMART (Self-Management and Recovery Training) meetings, a facilitated, abstinence-based, cognitive-behavioural program that some people may find more palatable than the spirituality and concept of a "higher power" prominent in 12-step programs.[70,71]

PSYCHOTHERAPEUTIC TREATMENT OPTIONS
Cognitive behavioural therapy (CBT) is a therapist-led intervention that has been adapted from the treatment of mood and anxiety disorders and has been shown to have a small but significant effect in reducing substance use.[72] Higher-intensity programs, such as the matrix model developed for treatment of stimulant use disorders among MSM, have been associated with a significant reduction in both stimulant use and high-risk sexual behaviour after one year.[73] The matrix model involves

several treatment modalities including both individual and group CBT, relapse prevention education, mutual support program attendance, and UDS.[74]

Motivational interviewing (MI) is a "collaborative, goal-oriented style of communication with particular attention to the language of change. It is designed to strengthen personal motivation for and commitment to the specific goal by eliciting and exploring the person's own reasons for change within an atmosphere of acceptance and compassion."[75] MI has been shown to be effective in the treatment of SUD,[76] although studies of MI interventions in MSM populations have shown no consistent benefit.[77] MI can support people along the stages of change.[39]

TRAUMA-INFORMED CARE

Seventy-six per cent of Canadian adults report some history of trauma, and the lifetime prevalence of post-traumatic stress disorder (PTSD) is 9.2 per cent, with a current prevalence of 2.4 per cent.[78] Furthermore, the overlap between trauma history, PTSD, and SUD is significant. The Adverse Childhood Events (ACE) study included 10 categories of childhood abuse or neglect and family dysfunction, and found that in study participants who reported four or more categories of events (17 per cent), rates of AUD and intravenous substance use disorder were three and 11 times greater, respectively.[79,80] A study of residential school survivors in BC found that 64 per cent reported a history of PTSD, and 26 per cent reported a substance use disorder.[81] In a study of five Canadian treatment centres for SUD, 90 per cent of women reported a history of abuse-related trauma, and 60 per cent reported other forms of trauma.[82] Recognizing the high prevalence of trauma history and PTSD is essential for providing care to people with SUD.

Trauma-informed care involves an integrated approach to treatment of people with concurrent SUD and trauma experiences, and it has been found to help reduce both substance use and trauma symptoms.[83] Clinicians are encouraged to screen for trauma history and PTSD symptoms among patients being treated for SUD. Manualized programs such as Seeking Safety can be adapted by clinicians into their care and have been shown to be effective for specific populations including military veterans[84] and transgender women living with HIV.[85]

OCCUPATIONAL HEALTH

The occupational risks of substance use and SUD are significant. A 2004 Alberta survey found that 8 per cent of workers reported a history of alcohol-related harms at work, but only 2 per cent had reported them to their employer. Nine per cent of workers also reported driving a motor vehicle within one hour of consuming two or more standard drinks.[86] Mandatory reporting by clinicians is required for patients at risk of impaired driving and for those working in safety-sensitive positions, defined as "one in which drug or alcohol impairment could result in direct and significant risk of injury to the employee, others or the environment."[87] People with SUD working in safety-sensitive positions may be required to participate in intensive monitoring programs to safely return to work, which typically include random UDS screening and ongoing treatment participation. Fortunately, such monitoring programs have high success rates: Physician Health Programs (PHPs) in the United States have been associated with greater than 80 per cent long-term remission rates from SUD,[88] and the Physician Health Program in Ontario reported that 85 per cent of participants achieved sustained remission and completed the five-year program, including 14 per cent of people who had a relapse during that time.[89]

Specific Treatment Options by Substance

ALCOHOL

Alcohol use is highly prevalent in Canada, with 78 per cent of Canadians reporting alcohol use in the past year[8] at a rate 50 per cent above the global average.[90] Alcohol use in Canada is also highly problematic, with an estimated $15 billion spent annually in health care, law enforcement, and lost productivity because of disability and premature death.[91] Eighteen per cent of Canadians over the age of 15 report a lifetime incidence of AUD.[8] It has been also estimated that 14 per cent drink above Canada's low-risk drinking guidelines,[8] which recommend no more than three standard drinks per day for men (two for women), no more than 15 drinks per week for men (10 for women), and non-drinking days to avoid physical dependence.[92] Heavy alcohol consumption is associated with many health risks including cirrhosis,[93] cardiovascular disease, and gastrointestinal and breast cancer.[91] The Canadian Institute for Substance Use Research has also refuted the general belief that moderate drinking has potential health benefits,[94] and have suggested that the cancer risk of alcohol is likely underestimated.[95]

With respect to treatment of AUD, psychosocial treatment and mutual support programs such as AA have long been the mainstay of recommendations for patients. There is good evidence for psychosocial treatment, and the large-scale Project Match trial in the 1990s found similar treatment outcomes for cognitive behavioural therapy, motivational enhancement therapy,* and 12-step facilitation, all of which had a 30 per cent total abstinence rate (i.e., abstinence maintained for the entire study period) and a 65 to 75 per cent cumulative abstinence rate (i.e., ongoing substance use during the study period but 65 to 75 per cent substance-free days reported) over the three-year study period.[96] Thus all three of these modalities have been found to be moderately and fairly equally effective.

A number of pharmacological treatment options also have strong evidence. Naltrexone, an opioid antagonist, has been shown to reduce the amount of alcohol consumed and the number of heavy drinking days, and is thus recommended for patients whose goal is to reduce alcohol consumption rather than abstain.[97] Naltrexone acts by reducing the euphoric effects of alcohol and may be more effective among people who report a more stimulatory effect of alcohol or a paternal history of AUD.[98] Acamprosate acts as a neuromodulator by restoring the balance between the main inhibitory (GABA) and excitatory neurotransmitters (glutamate), thus reducing the intensity of so-called *post-acute withdrawal symptoms*, including anxiety, insomnia, and cravings, that can persist for months or even years after alcohol cessation as a result of excess glutamate produced by the brain in response to the chronic inhibitory effects of alcohol.[99] It has been shown to significantly increase abstinence rates but is less effective than naltrexone for reducing both cravings and heavy drinking. Acamprosate is thus recommended for people for whom alcohol cessation is the goal.[97] Gabapentin has also been shown to both reduce heavy drinking and increase abstinence rates in a dose-dependent manner,[100] likely in a mechanism similar to acamprosate, but has not been approved by Health Canada for AUD, and its use is thus off-label.

A further note should be added about disulfiram (Antabuse), which was the first pharmacotherapeutic option for AUD and often the option best known by clinicians and patients alike. Disulfiram acts by blocking the hepatic enzyme acetalydehyde dehydrogenase, thus causing an accumulation of acetaldehyde and subsequent flushing, increased autonomic activity, nausea and vomiting, by which it is meant to deter people from drinking alcohol. Although disulfiram is approved by Health Canada for the treatment of AUD, it has been found to be largely ineffective in randomized studies,[101] and adherence rates are generally

---

* Of note, motivational enhancement is a standardized four-session intervention that incorporates motivational interviewing strategies; furthermore, 12-step facilitation is distinct from 12-step meetings and involves a formalized, counsellor-led process that incorporates 12-step principles such as 12-step meeting attendance and sponsorship.

poor unless it is being provided in a supervised setting for motivated individuals.[102,103]

In summary, a robust body of evidence supports both psychotherapeutic and pharmacotherapeutic options available for the treatment of AUD. Unfortunately, a 2012 report from the National Center on Addiction and Substance Abuse at Columbia University found that "addiction care is usually provided by unskilled laypersons" and that "most medical professionals who should be providing addiction treatment are not sufficiently trained to diagnose or treat it."[104] Furthermore, mutual support programs and formal psychotherapeutic interventions such as CBT may be insufficient for stabilizing AUD for many people, and adjunct medications are frequently indicated. Awareness and use of these medications is low among clinicians:[105] fewer than one-third of people with AUD ever receive treatment of any kind, and fewer than 10 per cent are offered pharmacotherapy.[106] Clinicians are thus encouraged to offer both pharmacological and psychotherapeutic options to patients at every opportunity depending on their symptoms (such as the presence of cravings) and goals for treatment.

NICOTINE

Tobacco smoking is long-standing and widespread among many cultures, and the associated health risks are now so well established that they are typically mentioned only briefly in any discussion about nicotine use disorders (NUDs). Tobacco use has been found to be a direct cause of numerous diseases, including several types of cancer (respiratory, oral, gastrointestinal, genitourinary, and leukemia, among others), ischemic heart disease, respiratory disease, and cirrhosis.[107-109] Fortunately, as public awareness of the harms of tobacco use has grown, smoking rates of conventional cigarettes have decreased steadily since the 1960s (when 50 per cent of Canadians over the age of 15 smoked) to the present rate of 15 to 20 per cent.[110]

Smoking prevalence among 2SLGBTQ people remains higher than in the general population, however, with an American study of 2016 data reporting current rates of conventional cigarette smoking of 21.8 per cent of lesbian, gay, and bisexual people (LGB, reported jointly) and 21.0 per cent of transgender people, compared to 14.6 per cent of heterosexual/cisgender people.[111] An additional study found higher rates of NUD among bisexual men (45.2 per cent) and women (44.9 per cent) compared to both homosexual and heterosexual men and women, and bisexual people were much more likely to continue smoking over the age of 55.[112] Thus, while the prevalence of cigarette smoking has decreased, 2SLGBTQ people continue to have higher rates of NUD.

In addition, the prevalence of e-cigarette smoking is on the rise, with 13 per cent of Canadians over 15 years old having ever tried an e-cigarette in 2015, up from 9 per cent just two years earlier. This trend is even more striking among youth, with 26 per cent of Canadians ages 15 to 19 reporting e-cigarette use in 2015.[113] In the United States, 22.3 and 27.9 per cent of LGB and transgender people, respectively, reported current e-cigarette use in 2016, compared to 19.7 per cent of heterosexual people.[111] It has been estimated that e-cigarette use will surpass conventional cigarette consumption in the next decade.

Although e-cigarettes may represent a potentially safer option than conventional cigarette smoking,[114] there is also some cause for concern: many young people who have never smoked a cigarette have used e-cigarettes. Among them, 44 per cent of those who have ever smoked an e-cigarette reported an intention to smoke conventional cigarettes, twice the rate reported among youth who had never smoked an e-cigarette.[115] Meanwhile, the perceived risk of smoking has also been found to be decreasing over the past decade.[116]

Although little is known about the potential health outcomes of e-cigarette use, small studies have found signs of obstructive airway disease after e-cigarette exposure.[117] Nicotine vaporization has also been found to produce formaldehyde and other compounds that have been associated with bronchiolitis obliterans.[118] As of 2018, these products remain largely unstudied and unregulated in Canada, and the newly renamed Tobacco and Vaping Products Act has been met with concerns that the potential harm reduction of e-cigarette use (compared to combustible tobacco use) may be offset by increasing rates of nicotine use among previous non-smokers.[119]

Smoking cessation has been associated with numerous health benefits: within one year, the risk of having a myocardial infarction is halved; within 10 years, the risk of lung cancer mortality is half that of continuing smokers; within 15 years, the risk of coronary artery disease is reduced to that of a lifetime non-smoker.[109] Smoking cessation is notoriously challenging, with a recent Ontario study reporting that ex-smokers had attempted an average of over 30 quit attempts.[120] The majority of smokers are motivated to quit in the future, with 70 per cent reporting plans to quit in the next year and 10 to 30 per cent in the next month.[121]

Fortunately, there is strong evidence for the value of both psychosocial and pharmacological interventions for NUDs, which are recommended to be offered in combination to every smoker interested in quitting at every office visit.[46] Every quit attempt should be supported and, although longer counselling sessions are associated with higher rates of smoking cessation, even short interventions of one to three minutes are effective. Support programs, such as the Smokers' Helpline and Smoke Free smartphone application, are free, accessible, and effective ways to support patients interested in quitting. Some programs, such as Leave the Pack Behind, have 2SLGBTQ-specific resources, although a recent review found that more specific resources are needed to engage 2SLGBTQ youth in smoking cessation.[122] Clinicians are encouraged to review local and Internet-based resources for available programs.

There are three first-line pharmacological options for NUD. Nicotine replacement therapy (NRT) has been found to increase quit rates by 80 per cent[123] and can be titrated up to any amount (e.g., adding a second patch if one is insufficient for cravings and withdrawal symptoms). Furthermore, the combination of multiple modalities of NRT (e.g., gum and patch together) is 43 per cent more effective than a single modality. Adverse effects of NRT are fairly minimal (with the exception of local irritation on nicotine patch sites, which can be rotated), and although there is some debate about the safety of NRT following a cardiovascular event,[124] numerous guidelines, including the Ottawa Model for Smoking Cessation, have advocated for its use.[125]

Bupropion, an antidepressant medication, has also been found to be effective for smoking cessation, although the mechanism of action is not well understood. It has been found to be as efficacious as single-modality NRT, thus increasing the rate of smoking cessation by 80 per cent.[123] Potential adverse events include xerostomia, insomnia, vertigo, and agitation. Bupropion can also lower the seizure threshold and should therefore be avoided in patients with a seizure disorder, eating disorder, or intracranial abnormality. Varenicline, a partial nicotine receptor agonist, has been found to have better quit rates than either NRT or bupropion (and roughly equal to combination NRT). Side effects include nausea (30 per cent), insomnia, and vivid dreams. There has also been controversy about the potential for both cardiovascular and neuropsychiatric adverse events, and Health Canada issued a black box warning when varenicline was approved in 2008 that discouraged its use for those with a history of mood disorder or suicidality.[126] Since then, numerous large-scale studies have demonstrated only slight increases in low-grade events such as tachycardia and vivid dreams, and a history of cardiovascular or neuropsychiatric disease should not preclude clinicians from prescribing varenicline.[123,127,128] Nonetheless, optimizing NRT has been found to be as effective with fewer potential complications, and is here recommended as the first-line option. Combinations have also been found to be safe and effective, such as better outcomes with NRT and varenicline compared to varenicline alone.[129]

It is recommended to start pharmacotherapy one week before choosing a quit date, and this run-in time (during which medication doses are gradually titrated) may help to minimize side effects and reduce cravings and withdrawal symptoms on the patient-selected quit date.

OPIOIDS

Natural opiates, such as morphine and codeine, are present in the opium resin collected from the poppy plant, *papaver somniferum*. The broader term *opioid* refers not only to these opiates but also to semi-synthetic opioids such as hydromorphone and entirely synthetic opioids such as methadone and fentanyl. Opioids act primarily on the *mu* receptor to provide analgesia, but can also cause euphoria, sedation, and respiratory depression. Opioids can be very helpful for acute pain but have been found to be largely ineffective for subacute and chronic pain conditions such as headache[130] and lower back pain,[131] and are no longer recommended for either condition.

Despite these recommendations, opioids are prescribed frequently in North America, more than in many other parts of the world, and increasingly over the past 20 years. It has been estimated that up to 30 per cent of adults (and up to 40 per cent of older adults) have chronic pain,[132] but there is insufficient evidence for the effectiveness of long-term opioid therapy (LTOT) for improving chronic pain and function.[133] Furthermore, there is a dose-dependent risk for serious harms,[133] and LTOT has been associated with increased all-cause mortality, including cardiorespiratory and other causes, in addition to increased overdose risk.[134]

The Canadian National Opioid Use Guidelines for Chronic Non-Cancer Pain (CNCP) were updated in 2017 and now recommend optimization of non-opioid pharmacotherapy and non-pharmacological therapy rather than opioid use. If pain and impaired function persist, it is then recommended that a trial of opioids be used and discontinued if pain and function do not improve, given that many patients do not respond to opioids. Furthermore, it is recommended that opioids not be used for people with CNCP with concurrent SUD. For a complete list of recommendations, please refer to the full guidelines.[135]

Several features of opioid prescribing are associated with an increased probability of LTOT: early prescribing patterns for opioid-naive patients, initial prescriptions of more than 10 days (even more so with more than 30 days), and a second opioid prescription. Patients are also more likely to end up on LTOT if taking opioids for more than 5 days (and more so if more than 31 days) or if taking a cumulative dose of more than 700 morphine equivalents.[136]

In addition to the general lack of efficacy and the harms associated with LTOT, there are significant concerns about the widespread misuse and diversion of prescription opioids. In 2013, the United States reported that 37 per cent of overdose deaths were related to prescription opioids, more than the 19 per cent attributed to heroin. Furthermore, there has been an increase in the rate of opioid use disorders, which was estimated to affect 2.5 million people in the United States in 2014.[132] Of note, it has been reported that intravenous heroin use is less common in the 2SLGBTQ community than the general population,[137] although the rate of prescription opioid use is similar.[138]

Unfortunately, many clinicians report a lack of confidence about safe opioid prescribing and identifying opioid misuse and opioid use disorder among their patients.[132] An example of this phenomenon is the previous prescribing practices of long-acting oxycodone, which increased in Ontario by 850 per cent from 1991 to 2007. During this period, the number of oxycodone-related deaths rose by over four times from 1999–2004, and the long-acting oxycodone formulation OxyContin was subsequently removed from the market in 2012.[139] Unfortunately, efforts to reduce prescribing practices and illicit access to prescription opioids resulted in an increase of heroin use in North America, which became a cheaper and more available alternative for people with opioid use disorder.[140,141] The subsequent adulteration of the illicit opioid supply with fentanyl and other high-potency synthetic opioids has driven the present opioid epidemic. In British Columbia, which has the highest overdose death rate in Canada,[142] over 80 per cent of illicit drug overdose deaths in 2017 involved fentanyl or its analogues.[143]

In response to the alarming surge of opioid overdoses, national clinical practice guidelines for the management of opioid use disorders were recently published.[144] Briefly, the recommendations can be summarized as follows: the use of opioid agonist therapy (OAT) is strongly recommended for people with moderate to severe opioid use disorder, preferentially buprenorphine-naloxone if possible rather than methadone, given the similar efficacy and superior safety profile of buprenorphine-naloxone; psychosocial treatment options (including counselling and mutual support programs as previously discussed) should be offered but should not be a requirement for accessing OAT; withdrawal management alone should be avoided and is associated with increased rates of relapse, morbidity, and death; and harm reduction approaches, such as take-home naloxone and sterile syringe distribution, should be offered to everyone with opioid use disorder as needed.

In summary, chronic pain is common, and the use of LTOT is unfortunately also common despite the general lack of efficacy and potential for harms, including opioid use disorder. The risk of opioid overdose is increasing due to the contamination of illicit opioids with fentanyl. Fortunately, there is strong evidence for the use of psychosocial treatment in combination with OAT and harm reduction approaches, such as take-home naloxone. All primary care providers are encouraged to make the assessment and treatment of opioid use disorders a fundamental part of their practice.

STIMULANTS

The use of stimulants has a long and pervasive history. Caffeine consumption is ubiquitous in society but has been found to be safe in moderate amounts.[145] Coca leaves have been chewed for thousands of years for their stimulant effect and were used in beverages and analgesic agents until the early twentieth century. Khat (*Catha edulis*) has been used in Africa and the Middle East as a mild stimulant that contains the alkaloid cathinone. Amphetamines were first synthesized in Japan in 1893 and marketed as a decongestant before recreational use of methamphetamines began among truckers, bikers, and MSM on the west coast of North America. Newer synthetic cathinones such as "bath salts" have recently become more prevalent[146] and are being produced to evade international law and UDS. Stimulants act on catecholamine receptors to cause increase energy, libido, and euphoria but can also cause agitation, paranoia, and even psychosis. In addition, alcohol and cocaine combine to form the metabolite coca-ethylene, which may prolong and intensify the stimulant properties of cocaine while decreasing the sedating effects of alcohol and has been associated with greater cardiotoxicity.[147]

The Canadian Centre on Substance Use and Addiction estimates a past-year prevalence of 1 to 3 per cent for stimulant use other than caffeine. Rates of methamphetamine use are higher among MSM than the general population, with one study reporting that 11 to 17 per cent MSM in San Francisco had used methamphetamines in the previous six months.[148] Methamphetamine use among MSM has also been associated with high-risk sexual behaviour, higher rates of injection, and a 1.5- to 2.9-fold increase in HIV transmission.[149] Of note, snorting and smoking implements have also been associated with an increased risk of blood-borne disease transmission, such as hepatitis B and C.[150]

With respect to pharmacotherapeutic options, meta-analyses have found that numerous classes of medications are ineffective for the treatment of stimulant use disorders including antidepressants,[151] antipsychotics,[152] anticonvulsants,[153] dopamine agonists,[154] and even psychostimulants themselves.[155,156] Stimulants such as methylphenidate have been found to be useful in some trials,[157] and further study may provide more support for the use of stimulants for treating stimulant use disorders; however, at the present time, there is no consistent and convincing evidence in support of psychostimulants or other pharmacotherapy, and none can be recommended with confidence. Of particular interest to the care of 2SLGBTQ patients, one study found that among non-dependent methamphetamine-using and binge-drinking MSM, naltrexone was found to reduce sexual risks and alcohol and methamphetamine use.[158] Other studies of naltrexone have shown benefit for both cocaine[159] and methamphetamine use disorders,[160] but more research is needed before a firm recommendation can be made. Psychosocial treatment options are thus the mainstay of treatment for stimulant use disorders.

Stimulant-specific mutual support groups, such as Cocaine Anonymous and Crystal Meth Anonymous, and non-12-step alternatives like SMART, are often available in larger cities for people whose goal is abstinence. In smaller communities, NA and AA are more common and may provide a less specific but supportive therapeutic community that many people (although not all) find helpful. There is evidence that active 12-step participation (such as sponsorship, setting up at meetings, and so-called step work rather than just meeting attendance) is associated with reduced cocaine use.[161] In addition, both cognitive behavioural therapy and 12-step facilitation have been found to improve abstinence rates in cocaine use disorder.[162] The most evidence-based treatment for stimulant disorders is contingency management, based on a model of operant conditioning in which participants receive a reward (such as a gift certificate) for a specific outcome such as a negative urine drug screen.[163–165] Meta-analysis has shown consistent benefit of contingency management in the treatment of stimulant use disorders.[149] To date, no known studies have investigated the use of contingency management in an office-based setting, and it is hoped that primary care tools for treating stimulant use disorders will be available in the future.

CANNABIS

Cannabis has been used in China since 2700 BC. The main psychoactive component in cannabis is *tetrahydrocannabinol* (THC), which is associated with euphoria, as well as cognitive impairment, decreased motivation, anxiety, and acute psychotic effects. Conversely, the non-psychotropic component cannabidiol (CBD) may have antipsychotic[166] and analgesic properties. There are two types of cannabis receptors: CB1, which is found mainly in the central nervous system, and CB2, which is found mainly in the peripheral nervous and immune systems.

THC binds primarily to the CB1 receptor as a partial agonist, and CBD is a CB1 and CB2 antagonist which buffers the effects of THC and enhances the body's endogenous cannabinoids.[167]

Cannabis is most frequently combusted or vaporized and, when inhaled, has a rapid onset and relatively short half-life, with intoxication typically lasting between one and three hours. Oral cannabinoids, including "edible" products often made in fat-containing foods, have a slower onset but can last for up to 8 to 12 hours with greater risk of cannabis toxicity. Cannabis has also become increasingly potent over the past 20 years, from an average of 4 per cent THC concentration in 1995 to 12 per cent in 2014, and the average THC:CBD ratio increased from 14 in 1995 to 80 in 2014.[168] Higher-potency cannabis preparations such as hash oil (30 to 40 per cent THC) and the waxy "shatter" (80–90 per cent THC) have also become more prevalent. Furthermore, synthetic cannabinoids are also being used increasingly among people who undergo occupational UDS because they are not detected but are highly potent and have a higher risk of psychosis. Health Canada has approved several cannabinoid medications including nabilone (a synthetic cannabinoid made entirely of THC) and nabiximols (which contains a 1:1 ratio of THC and CBD).

Cannabis use is most common among Canadians ages 15 to 24, although rates decreased somewhat from over 30 per cent past-year use in 2008 to 25 per cent in 2015.[8] About 10 per cent of adults over 25 report past-year cannabis use,[7] and 28 per cent of people who have used cannabis in the past three months report daily or almost daily use.[169] The average age of initiation is 14 years old, and cannabis use disorder develops in 18 per cent of people who initiate use under the age of 17. Because the brain develops into the mid-20s, with frontal lobes being among the last to develop, regular use beginning before the age of 17 has been associated with smaller brain volume, altered synaptic pruning, and memory impairment.[170] Adolescents with cannabis use disorder have a significantly lower rate of high school completion.[171] Cannabis use has also been associated with depression, bipolar disorder, anxiety disorders, and psychosis, although the nature of these relationships is not well understood.

Cannabis is widely used to treat medical conditions and alleviate symptoms, and has been studied in many randomized controlled trials (RCTs) in the treatment of nausea and vomiting secondary to chemotherapy, appetite suppression in HIV/AIDS, chronic pain, spasticity caused by multiple sclerosis, mood and anxiety disorders, and sleep disorders. A recent Canadian systematic review of medical cannabinoid use found an average decrease of chronic pain by 0.4 to 0.8 points on a

10-point scale, but larger and longer-term RCTs included in the analysis showed no overall benefit. Cannabinoids were also found to have some evidence for reducing spasticity associated with multiple sclerosis and for reducing nausea and vomiting associated with chemotherapy. Unfortunately, the quality of the studies included was considered to be poor, and the overall benefits of cannabinoids were found to be low. Furthermore, cannabinoids were associated with an increased risk of adverse events including drowsiness, confusion, and loss of balance.[171]

Familiarity with the evidence for the medical use of cannabinoids is very important for primary care providers given that cannabis laws are evolving in Canada. In 2001, the Marihuana Medical Access Regulations made Canada the first nation to allow the growth and personal use of cannabis for medical reasons. In 2013, however, the Marihuana for Medical Purposes Regulations were enacted to allow consumers to buy only government-approved dried cannabis rather than growing their own supply or possessing other cannabinoid products such as oils. In 2015, the Supreme Court of Canada deemed this unconstitutional, and in 2016 these restrictions were lifted to allow people with medical authorization to resume growing their own cannabis if desired.[172] As of 2018, cannabis became legal in Canada, but uncertainty remains about how it is being regulated. The recent proliferation of cannabis "dispensaries" are presently unregulated by Health Canada, and are supplied by cannabis producers that sell untested products for non-medical reasons.[173] The new Cannabis Act also includes legislation to restrict cannabis access to youth and increase public awareness about the health risks associated with cannabis.

As of January 2018, cannabis was legalized for people over the age of 21 in nine US states, and "medical marijuana" is legal in 29 states. Despite fears that legalization would lead to increased access to and prevalence of cannabis use, preliminary studies have found only a non-statistical increase among adolescents[174] and no change in ease of accessibility.[175] Furthermore, states with a medicinal marijuana program had a 25 per cent average decrease in prescription opioid-related mortality, suggesting that cannabis may have a protective effect on hazardous opioid use.[176]

In summary, the expansion of cannabis regulation and legalization in Canada is an evolving process. The use of cannabis in the treatment of some medical conditions is supported, but cannabis has also been associated with numerous potential harms. A recent clinical practice guideline was written for Canadian primary care providers by the authors of the above-mentioned systematic review, which recommends against the use of cannabis for most medical conditions with the exception of chronic and refractory neuropathic pain, chemotherapy-induced nausea and vomiting, and spasticity associated with multiple sclerosis.[177] Therefore, the College of Family Physicians of Canada recommends that physicians sign "declarations" rather than prescriptions for medical marijuana given the lack of evidence to support its use.[178] Additionally, the Centre for Addiction and Mental Health in Toronto has developed a set of Lower-Risk Cannabis Use Guidelines[179] that are summarized as follows: the use of cannabis should be avoided in adolescence, particularly before the age of 16; cannabis should be avoided among pregnant women and those with a personal history or first-degree family history of psychosis or substance use disorder; synthetic and high-THC cannabinoids should be avoided; combusting cannabis and "deep inhalation" methods should be avoided; driving should be avoided within six hours of cannabis use. Primary care providers are encouraged to review the potential risks and benefits of cannabis use regularly with patients, particularly among adolescents and those with concurrent mental health disorders.

BENZODIAZEPINES

Benzodiazepines (BZD) are a class of sedative/hypnotic medications that act on the inhibitory GABA receptor and are commonly prescribed for a number of conditions including mood, anxiety, and sleep disorders. It has been estimated that 15 per cent of Canadians over the age of 65 years are prescribed BZD, and 10 per cent of adult Canadians report past-year use of prescription BZD.[7] Long-term BZD prescribing is common, despite recommendations for short-term use only and evidence that BZDs do not improve sleep architecture or quality. BZDs can also have amnestic effects, which may have medical uses such as in procedural sedation with midazolam,[180] as well as the potential for nefarious uses such as facilitating sexual assault with flunitrazepam (Rohypnol or "roofies"),[181] and are associated with reversible memory loss with chronic use.[182]

Long-term BZD use has also been associated with dementia,[183] psychomotor impairment, fall risk, and an estimated three-fold increased risk of mortality.[184] In addition, BZD use significantly increases the risk of unintentional overdose death among people on opioid therapy. This is concerning because 17 per cent of people with chronic non-cancer pain receiving LTOT report daily BZD use, and 30 per cent report use in the past month. Patients taking both LTOT and BZDs have been found to be more likely to have higher opioid doses, higher pain severity, higher rates of SUD and psychiatric disorders, and higher use of emergency medical services. The high prevalence of BZD use is inconsistent with guidelines for the treatment of both chronic pain and chronic mental illness.[185]

BZD withdrawal can be dangerous, and sudden discontinuation is not recommended. A gradual dose reduction by methods such as the Ashton protocol can be used,[186] and supportive visits and a structured taper every two weeks has been associated with higher rates of BZD cessation after one year.[187] However, if a BZD or other SUD is diagnosed, a faster taper in a medically supervised setting may be required. Readers are encouraged to read the excellent review by Ashton for further discussion and management recommendations.[188]

HALLUCINOGENS

Hallucinogens are a broader class of substances that includes MDMA (3,4-methylenedioxymethamphetamine, or "Ecstasy"), ketamine, psilocybin ("magic") mushrooms, mescaline, LSD, salvia divinorum, dextromethorphan (DM, present in cough syrups), ayahuasca, and many others. Hallucinogens are somewhat unique among other substances of abuse in that they act on serotonin receptors rather than dopamine receptors and for that reason have a fairly low rate of related use disorders. They are by no means without risk of harm, however, and MDMA is related to amphetamine and has been associated with neurotoxic effects with long-term use. Ketamine, a dissociative anaesthetic and N-methyl, D-aspartate (NMDA) antagonist, is used medically in perioperative settings or for procedural sedation and is typically obtained illicitly from veterinary suppliers and associated with dissociative "k-hole" experiences, abdominal cramping, and inflammation of the genito-urinary tract. Regular use is rare, however, and withdrawal syndromes can typically be managed with supportive care if needed. If there is uncertainty about substance ingestion or the risk of a potential toxidrome, emergency medicine and poison control centres should be consulted.

In addition, there has been a recent revival in the interest of studying hallucinogens such as LSD and psilocybin in the treatment of SUD,[189] and recent meta-analysis of the original RCTs in the 1950s and 1960s found a benefit in the treatment of AUD.[190] More recent studies have supported the use of psilocybin in the treatment of both AUD[191] and NUD.[192] In addition, ayahuasca, a traditional plant-based preparation containing the psilocybin analogue DMT, has been found to reduce substance use and improve subjective symptoms of mental health among people with SUD.[193,194] Recently, the use of hallucinogen "microdosing" (typically doses at one-tenth of the usual dose, taken every few days) has been reported in the media but has not yet been established in any clinical trials. Hallucinogens are thus an evolving area of focus for clinical research and a current "hot topic" in addiction medicine.

GHB

GHB is a naturally occurring inhibitory neurotransmitter that acts on both GHB and GABA receptors. It is approved for the treatment of narcolepsy but is mainly obtained and used illicitly. It has also been reported to have anabolic effects on endogenous growth hormone release, and it may be used among image-conscious people to induce an alcohol-like effect without the associated calories. It has a short duration of action, typically lasting 20 to 60 minutes and eliminated in four to eight hours, but withdrawal can last up to 21 days with regular use.[195] As with alcohol and BZD, GHB withdrawal can be life-threatening; can involve seizures, hallucinations, and agitation; and can be treated with BZD or baclofen. Withdrawal in a medically supervised setting with addiction specialist support is recommended.

AMYL NITRITES

Amyl nitrites are a class of vasodilators that are used both medically, as an anti-angina medication, and recreationally for their disinhibitory and muscle-relaxing effects, including anal sphincter tone, and are thus used to facilitate receptive sex.[146] "Poppers," so called because of the popping effect of opening the ampules they once came in, can cause headaches, erectile dysfunction, chemical burns, and even hemolysis among people with G6PD deficiency. Amyl nitrites have been illegal in Canada since 2013 but are frequently obtained by mail-order and remain commonly used. A US survey of MSM found a reported use of 20 per cent in the previous six months.[196] Amyl nitrites should also be distinguished from other types of organic solvent inhalants that are used typically among adolescents and that have not been reported to have significant use among 2SLGBTQ populations.

PRO-ERECTILE DRUGS

Phosphodiesterase (PDE5) inhibitors, initially developed as antihypertensives that cause vasodilation by release of nitric oxide, are used in the treatment of erectile dysfunction and are used among MSM to counteract the effects of other substances such as amphetamines[137] to maintain erections. The use of PDE5 inhibitors among MSM has been associated with HIV and other sexually transmitted infections.[197] Patients should be cautioned about the hypotensive risks of PDE5 inhibitors if used in combination with nitrate medications (such as nitroglycerin) or amyl nitrites.

STEROIDS

Steroid hormones, including testosterone, estrogen, and progesterone, are used medically for many indications, including hormone therapy among transgender people and in the treatment of perimenopausal symptoms, depression, hypogonadism, and HIV-related muscle wasting, among others. Please see chapter 11 for more information on hormone therapy in transgender health. The use of illicit steroids among transgender people may be due to barriers to accessing medical care and is not in itself diagnostic of a steroid use disorder. With respect to the non-medical use of steroids, however, a few considerations are recommended for clinicians. Estrogens increase the risk of venous thromboembolism,[198] and this risk is greatly increased by tobacco smoking.[199] Testosterone has abusive potential for its effects on building muscle mass, and the prevalence of its use has been estimated at 10 per cent among MSM who frequent gyms. Aside from the numerous health risks associated with anabolic steroids, the sharing of syringes was also reported by 25 per cent of those surveyed.[200]

Related Behavioural Disorders

SEXUAL COMPULSIVITY

The American Psychiatric Association did not include sexual compulsivity as a recognized disorder in the *DSM*-5, but it is included in the World Health Organization's International Statistical Classification of Diseases and Related Health Problems (ICD-10).[201] Sexual compulsivity has been reported among 2SLGBTQ populations[202] and has been associated with having a higher number of sexual partners, engaging in unprotected anal sex, disregarding a partner's HIV status, and having sex under the influence of substance use.[203] Screening for sexual compulsivity can be done with the Sexual Compulsivity Scale,[204] and counselling options specific to sexual compulsivity may be available depending on local resources. Mutual support groups such as Sexual Compulsives Anonymous (SCA) and Sex and Love Addicts Anonymous are also available, and SCA literature includes the publication *Secret Shame*, which 2SLGBTQ patients may find particularly helpful.[205]

GAMBLING DISORDERS

Gambling disorders likely have a similar pathophysiology as SUD, and one study of patients in treatment for SUD found a prevalence of 20 per cent for gambling disorders as identified by the South Oaks Gambling Screen. Furthermore, 30 per cent of study participants reported that gambling symptoms were affecting their recovery.[206] Concurrent treatment options may be limited, but mutual support programs such as Gamblers Anonymous are available in many centres or online and can be integrated into SUD treatment.

EATING DISORDERS

Eating disorders (ED) likely have some overlap with SUD, and one study found that the prevalence of ED among patients in residential treatment for SUD was 7 per cent, with 21 per cent of those leaving treatment against medical advice.[207] It is important to screen for the presence of ED among patients with SUD (and for SUD among patients with ED) and provide concurrent treatment when present. Please see chapter 8 for more information on eating disorders among 2SLGBTQ people.

Conclusion

Substance use disorder is a chronic disease that results from changes in the brain's reward pathway. Although the prevalence of SUD among 2SLGBTQ people is not as high as was once thought, it remains higher than in the general population because of a complex constellation of syndemic factors. For that reason, it is perhaps reasonable to inquire more frequently about the presence of substance use and SUD among 2SLGBTQ patients and particularly among people engaging in high-risk behaviour such as bathhouse attendance. The detection and treatment of SUD is often lacking in all aspects of medicine, however, and it is thus recommended that clinicians apply the approach of screening, brief intervention, and referral to treatment to all of their patients with equal vigour. Treatment options, both pharmacologic and psychotherapeutic, are both evidence based and underused, and providers are encouraged to expand their scope of practice to incorporate these tools and seek the advice of local addiction medicine resources as needed. In addition, specialized treatment options may be available for 2SLGBTQ patients with SUD, if desired, and a good knowledge of these resources is also recommended for all primary care providers.

References

1. Garofalo R, Mustanski BS, McKirnan DJ, Herrick A, Donenberg GR. Methamphetamine and young men who have sex with men: understanding patterns and correlates of use and the association with HIV-related sexual risk. Arch Pediatr Adolesc Med. 2007;161(6):591–6.

2. Giorgetti R, Tagliabracci A, Schifano F, Zaami S, Marinelli E, Busardò FP. When "chems" meet sex: a rising phenomenon called "chemsex." Curr Neuropharmacol. 2017;15(5):762–70.

3. Race K. Pleasure consuming medicine: the queer politics of drugs. Raleigh (NC): Duke University Press; 2009.

4. Cochran SD, Grella CE, Mays VM. Do substance use norms and perceived drug availability mediate sexual orientation differences in patterns of substance use? Results from the California Quality of Life Survey II. J Stud Alcohol Drugs. 2012;73(4):675–85.

5. Bux DA. The epidemiology of problem drinking in gay men and lesbians: A critical review. Clin Psychol Rev. 1996;16(4):277–98.

6. Green KE, Feinstein BA. Substance use in lesbian, gay, and bisexual populations: an update on empirical research and implications for treatment. Psychol Addict Behav. 2012;26(2):265–78.

7. Health Canada [Internet]. Ottawa: Government of Canada; 2017 Mar [cited 2021 Oct 3]. Canadian tobacco alcohol and drug (CTADS): 2015 summary. Available from: https://www.canada.ca/en/health-canada /services/canadian-alcohol-drugs-survey/2015-summary.html.

8. Health Canada [Internet]. Ottawa: Government of Canada; [last modified 2014 Apr 8; cited 2021 Oct 3]. Canadian alcohol and drug use monitoring survey. Available from: https://www.canada.ca/en/health-canada /services/health-concerns/drug-prevention-treatment/drug-alcohol-use-statistics/canadian-alcohol-drug-use-monitoring-survey-summary-results-2012.html.

9. Rainbow Health Ontario. LGBTQ people, drug use & harm reduction [Internet]. Toronto: Rainbow Health Ontario; 2015 Jun [cited 21 Oct 3]. Available from https://www.rainbowhealthontario.ca/wp-content /uploads/woocommerce_uploads/2015/06/RHO_FactSheet _LGBTDRUGUSEHARMREDUCTION_E.pdf.

10. Lampinen TM, McGhee D, Martin I. Increased risk of "club" drug use among gay and bisexual high school students in British Columbia. J Adolesc Health. 2006;38(4):458–61.

11. MMyers T, Rowe CJ, Tudiver FG, Kurtz RG, Jackson EA, Orr KW, et al. HIV, substance use and related behaviour of gay and bisexual men: an examination of the talking sex project cohort. Br J Addict. 1992;87(2):207–14.

12. Grant BF, Goldstein RB, Saha TD, Chou SP, Jung J, Zhang H, et al. Epidemiology of DSM-5 Alcohol Use Disorder: Results From the National Epidemiologic Survey on Alcohol and Related Conditions III. JAMA Psychiatry. 2015;72(8):757–66.

13. McCabe SE, Hughes TL, Bostwick WB, West BT, Boyd CJ. Sexual orientation, substance use behaviors and substance dependence in the United States. Addiction. 2009;104(8):1333–45.

14. McCabe SE, West BT, Hughes TL, Boyd CJ. Sexual orientation and substance abuse treatment utilization in the United States: results from a national survey. J Subst Abuse Treat. 2013;44(1):4–12.
15. Herbst JH, Jacobs ED, Finlayson TJ, McKleroy VS, Neumann MS, Crepaz N; HIV/AIDS Prevention Research Synthesis Team. Estimating HIV prevalence and risk behaviors of transgender persons in the United States: a systematic review. AIDS Behav. 2008;12(1):1–17.
16. Marshal MP, Friedman MS, Stall R, King KM, Miles J, Gold MA, et al. Sexual orientation and adolescent substance use: a meta-analysis and methodological review. Addiction. 2008;103(4):546–56.
17. Wu LT, Blazer DG. Illicit and nonmedical drug use among older adults: a review. J Aging Health. 2011;23(3):481–504.
18. Yarns BC, Abrams JM, Meeks TW, Sewell DD. The Mental Health of Older LGBT Adults. Curr Psychiatry Rep. 2016;18(6):60.
19. Benotsch EG, Martin AM, Koester S, Cejka A, Luckman D. Nonmedical use of prescription drugs and HIV risk behavior in gay and bisexual men. Sex Transm Dis. 2011;38(2):105–10.
20. Robinson TE, Berridge KC. The psychology and neurobiology of addiction: an incentive-sensitization view. Addiction. 2000;95 Suppl 2:S91–117.
21. Volkow ND, Fowler JS, Wang GJ. The addicted human brain: insights from imaging studies. J Clin Invest. 2003;111(10):1444–51.
22. Di Chiara G, Imperato A. Drugs abused by humans preferentially increase synaptic dopamine concentrations in the mesolimbic system of freely moving rats. Proc Natl Acad Sci USA. 1988;85(14):5274–8.
23. Unterrainer HF, Hiebler-Ragger M, Rogen L, Kapfhammer HP. Sucht als Bindungsstörung [Addiction as an attachment disorder]. Nervenarzt. 2018 Sep;89(9):1043–8. German. doi:10.1007/s00115-017-0462-4.
24. Volkow ND, Koob GF, McLellan AT. Neurobiologic Advances from the Brain Disease Model of Addiction. N Engl J Med. 2016;374(4):363–71.
25. Makadon HJ, Potter J, Mayer KH, Goldhammer, H, editors. The Fenway guide to lesbian, gay, bisexual and transgender health. 2nd ed. Boston: Fenway Institute; 2015.
26. Herrick AL, Lim SH, Wei C, et al. Resilience as an untapped resource in behavioral intervention design for gay men. AIDS Behav. 2011;15 Suppl 1:S25–29.
27. Coulter RW, Kinsky SM, Herrick AL, Stall RD, Bauermeister JA. Evidence of Syndemics and Sexuality-Related Discrimination Among Young Sexual-Minority Women. LGBT Health. 2015;2(3):250–7.
28. Martinez O, Wu E, Levine EC, Muñoz-Laboy M, Spadafino J, Dodge B, et al. Syndemic factors associated with drinking patterns among Latino men

and Latina transgender women who have sex with men in New York City. Addict Res Theory. 2016;24(6):466–76.

29. Funk M, Wutzke S, Kaner E, Anderson P, Pas L, McCormick R, et al.; World Health Organization Brief Intervention Study Group. A multicountry controlled trial of strategies to promote dissemination and implementation of brief alcohol intervention in primary health care: findings of a World Health Organization collaborative study. J Stud Alcohol. 2005;66(3):379–88.

30. Madras BK, Compton WM, Avula D, Stegbauer T, Stein JB, Clark HW. Screening, brief interventions, referral to treatment (SBIRT) for illicit drug and alcohol use at multiple healthcare sites: comparison at intake and 6 months later. Drug Alcohol Depend. 2009;99(1–3):280–95.

31. Ewing JA. Detecting alcoholism. The CAGE questionnaire. JAMA. 1984;252(14):1905–7.

32. Reinert DF, Allen JP. The Alcohol Use Disorders Identification Test (AUDIT): a review of recent research. Alcohol Clin Exp Res. 2002;26(2):272–9.

33. Group WH; WHO ASSIST Working Group. The alcohol, smoking and substance involvement screening test (ASSIST): development, reliability and feasibility. Addiction. 2002;97(9):1183–94.

34. Skinner HA. The drug abuse screening test. Addict Behav. 1982;7(4):363–71.

35. Webster LR, Webster RM. Predicting aberrant behaviors in opioid-treated patients: preliminary validation of the Opioid Risk Tool. Pain Med. 2005;6(6):432–42.

36. McCaffrey SA, Black RA, Villapiano AJ, Jamison RN, Butler SF. Development of a brief version of the current opioid misuse measure (COMM): The COMM-9. Pain Med. 2019 Jan 1;20(1):113–8. doi:10.1093/pm/pnx311.

37. American Psychiatric Association. Diagnostic and Statistical Manual of Mental Disorders. 5th edition. ed. Washington, DC: American Psychiatric Association; 2013.

38. American Psychiatric Association. Diagnostic and statistical manual of mental disorders. 4th ed. Washington (DC): American Psychiatric Association; 1994.

39. Prochaska JO, DiClemente CC. Stages of change in the modification of problem behaviors. Prog Behav Modif. 1992;28:183–218.

40. Heit HA, Gourlay DL. Urine drug testing in pain medicine. J Pain Symptom Manage. 2004;27(3):260–7.

41. Katz NP, Sherburne S, Beach M, Rose RJ, Vielguth J, Bradley J, et al. Behavioral monitoring and urine toxicology testing in patients

receiving long-term opioid therapy [table of contents]. Anesth Analg. 2003;97(4):1097–102.

42. Russell M, Peirce RS, Chan AW, Wieczorek WF, Moscato BS, Nochajski TH. Natural recovery in a community-based sample of alcoholics: study design and descriptive data. Subst Use Misuse. 2001;36(11):1417–41.

43. Cunningham JA, Lin E, Ross HE, Walsh GW. Factors associated with untreated remissions from alcohol abuse or dependence. Addict Behav. 2000;25(2):317–21.

44. Lopez-Quintero C, Hasin DS, de Los Cobos JP, Pines A, Wang S, Grant BF, et al. Probability and predictors of remission from life-time nicotine, alcohol, cannabis or cocaine dependence: results from the National Epidemiologic Survey on Alcohol and Related Conditions. Addiction. 2011;106(3):657–69.

45. Ferri M, Amato L, Davoli M. Alcoholics Anonymous and other 12-step programmes for alcohol dependence. Cochrane Database Syst Rev. 2006 Jul 19;(3):CD005032. doi:10.1002/14651858.CD005032.pub2.

46. Canadian Action Network for the Advancement, Dissemination and Adoption of Practice-Informed Tobacco Treatment. Canadian smoking cessation clinical practice guideline. Toronto: Centre for Addiction and Mental Health; 2011.

47. Whitlock EP, Polen MR, Green CA, Orleans T, Klein J; US Preventive Services Task Force. Behavioral counseling interventions in primary care to reduce risky/harmful alcohol use by adults: a summary of the evidence for the U.S. Preventive Services Task Force. Ann Intern Med. 2004;140(7):557–68.

48. Saitz R. Screening and brief intervention for unhealthy drug use: little or no efficacy. Front Psychiatry. 2014;5:121.

49. Glynn TR, van den Berg JJ. A Systematic Review of Interventions to Reduce Problematic Substance Use Among Transgender Individuals: A Call to Action. Transgend Health. 2017;2(1):45–59.

50. Aromin RA. Substance Abuse Prevention, Assessment, and Treatment for Lesbian, Gay, Bisexual, and Transgender Youth. Pediatr Clin North Am. 2016;63(6):1057–77.

51. Reif S, George P, Braude L, Dougherty RH, Daniels AS, Ghose SS, et al. Residential treatment for individuals with substance use disorders: assessing the evidence. Psychiatr Serv. 2014;65(3):301–12.

52. Merkx MJ, Schippers GM, Koeter MW, Vuijk PJ, Poch M, Kronemeijer H, et al. Predictive validity of treatment allocation guidelines on drinking outcome in alcohol-dependent patients. Addict Behav. 2013;38(3):1691–8.

53. Finney JW, Hahn AC, Moos RH. The effectiveness of inpatient and outpatient treatment for alcohol abuse: the need to focus on mediators and moderators of setting effects. Addiction. 1996;91(12):1773–96.

54. McCarty D, Braude L, Lyman DR, Dougherty RH, Daniels AS, Ghose SS, et al. Substance abuse intensive outpatient programs: assessing the evidence. Psychiatr Serv. 2014;65(6):718–26.
55. Smyth BP, Barry J, Keenan E, Ducray K. Lapse and relapse following inpatient treatment of opiate dependence. Ir Med J. 2010;103(6):176–9.
56. Vancouver Coastal Health. Idea: addiction recovery therapeutic community [Internet]. Vancouver: Vancouver Coast Health; 2014 [cited 2021 Oct 3]. Available from: http://vchnews.ca/wp-content/uploads /sites/6/2014/06/Addiction-Recovery-Therapeutic-Community.pdf.
57. Gastfriend DR, Rubin A, Sharon E, Turner WM, Anton RF, Donovan DM, et al. New constructs and assessments for relapse and continued use potential in the ASAM Patient Placement Criteria. J Addict Dis. 2003;22 Suppl 1:95–111.
58. Eliason MJ, Hughes T. Treatment counselor's attitudes about lesbian, gay, bisexual, and transgendered clients: urban vs. rural settings. Subst Use Misuse. 2004;39(4):625–44.
59. Cochran BN, Peavy KM, Robohm JS. Do specialized services exist for LGBT individuals seeking treatment for substance misuse? A study of available treatment programs. Subst Use Misuse. 2007;42(1):161–76.
60. Senreich E. Are specialized LGBT program components helpful for gay and bisexual men in substance abuse treatment? Subst Use Misuse. 2010;45(7–8):1077–96.
61. Centre for Addiction and Mental Health [Internet]. Toronto: CAMH; [cited 2021 Oct 3]. Rainbow services. Available from: https://www.camh .ca/en/your-care/programs-and-services/rainbow-services-lgbtq.
62. Dawson DA, Grant BF, Stinson FS, Chou PS. Estimating the effect of help-seeking on achieving recovery from alcohol dependence. Addiction. 2006;101(6):824–34.
63. Alcholics Anonymous. The AA member – medications and other drugs [Internet]. New York: Alcholics Anonymous World Servies; 2018 [cited 2021 Oct 3]. Available from: https://www.aa.org/assets/en_US/p-11 _aamembersMedDrug.pdf.
64. Kownacki RJ, Shadish WR. Does Alcoholics Anonymous work? The results from a meta-analysis of controlled experiments. Subst Use Misuse. 1999;34(13):1897–916.
65. Moos RH, Moos BS. Participation in treatment and Alcoholics Anonymous: a 16-year follow-up of initially untreated individuals. J Clin Psychol. 2006;62(6):735–50.
66. Owen PL, Slaymaker V, Tonigan JS, McCrady BS, Epstein EE, Kaskutas LA, et al. Participation in alcoholics anonymous: intended and unintended change mechanisms. Alcohol Clin Exp Res. 2003;27(3): 524–32.

67. Mäkelä K. Rates of attrition among the membership of Alcoholics Anonymous in Finland. J Stud Alcohol. 1994;55(1):91–5.

68. Gossop M, Stewart D, Marsden J. Attendance at Narcotics Anonymous and Alcoholics Anonymous meetings, frequency of attendance and substance use outcomes after residential treatment for drug dependence: a 5-year follow-up study. Addiction. 2008;103(1):119–25.

69. Alcoholics Anonymous [Internet]. New York: Alcoholics Anonymous World Services; 1939. Chapter 8, To wives; [cited 2021 Oct 3]. Available from: https://www.aa.org/assets/en_US/en_bigbook_chapt8.pdf.

70. Beck AK, Forbes E, Baker AL, Kelly PJ, Deane FP, Shakeshaft A, et al. Systematic review of SMART Recovery: Outcomes, process variables, and implications for research. Psychol Addict Behav. 2017;31(1):1–20.

71. Kelly PJ, Deane FP, Baker AL. Group cohesion and between session homework activities predict self-reported cognitive-behavioral skill use amongst participants of SMART Recovery groups. J Subst Abuse Treat. 2015;51:53–8.

72. Magill M, Ray LA. Cognitive-behavioral treatment with adult alcohol and illicit drug users: a meta-analysis of randomized controlled trials. J Stud Alcohol Drugs. 2009;70(4):516–27.

73. Reback CJ, Shoptaw S. Development of an evidence-based, gay-specific cognitive behavioral therapy intervention for methamphetamine-abusing gay and bisexual men. Addict Behav. 2014;39(8):1286–91.

74. Rawson RA, Shoptaw SJ, Obert JL, McCann MJ, Hasson AL, Marinelli-Casey PJ, et al. An intensive outpatient approach for cocaine abuse treatment. The Matrix model. J Subst Abuse Treat. 1995;12(2):117–27.

75. Christie D, Channon S. The potential for motivational interviewing to improve outcomes in the management of diabetes and obesity in paediatric and adult populations: a clinical review. Diabetes Obes Metab. 2014;16(5):381–7.

76. Marsden J, Stillwell G, Barlow H, Boys A, Taylor C, Hunt N, et al. An evaluation of a brief motivational intervention among young ecstasy and cocaine users: no effect on substance and alcohol use outcomes. Addiction. 2006;101(7):1014–26.

77. Berg RC, Ross MW, Tikkanen R. The effectiveness of MI4MSM: how useful is motivational interviewing as an HIV risk prevention program for men who have sex with men? A systematic review. AIDS Educ Prev. 2011;23(6):533–49.

78. Katzman MA, Bleau P, Blier P, Chokka P, Kjernisted K, Van Ameringen M; Canadian Anxiety Guidelines Initiative Group on behalf of the Anxiety Disorders Association of Canada/Association Canadienne des troubles anxieux and McGill University. Canadian clinical practice guidelines

for the management of anxiety, posttraumatic stress and obsessive-compulsive disorders. BMC Psychiatry. 2014;14 Suppl 1:S1.

79. Dube SR, Felitti VJ, Dong M, Chapman DP, Giles WH, Anda RF. Childhood abuse, neglect, and household dysfunction and the risk of illicit drug use: the adverse childhood experiences study. Pediatrics. 2003;111(3):564–72.

80. Dube SR, Miller JW, Brown DW, Giles WH, Felitti VJ, Dong M, et al. Adverse childhood experiences and the association with ever using alcohol and initiating alcohol use during adolescence. J Adolesc Health. 2006;38(4):444.e441–10.

81. Söchting I, Corrado R, Cohen I, Ley R, Brasfield C. Traumatic pasts in Canadian Aboriginal people: further support for a complex trauma conceptualization? BCMJ. 2007;49(6):320–6.

82. Brown C. The pervasiveness of trauma among Canadian women in treatment for alcohol use. Paper presented at: Looking Back, Thinking Ahead: Using Research to Improve Policy and Practice in Women's Health Conference; 2009 Mar 15–19; Halifax, NS.

83. Torchalla I, Nosen L, Rostam H, Allen P. Integrated treatment programs for individuals with concurrent substance use disorders and trauma experiences: a systematic review and meta-analysis. J Subst Abuse Treat. 2012;42(1):65–77.

84. Najavits LM, Krinsley K, Waring ME, Gallagher MW, Skidmore C. A Randomized Controlled Trial for Veterans with PTSD and Substance Use Disorder: Creating Change versus Seeking Safety. Subst Use Misuse. 2018 Sep;53(11):1788–800.

85. Empson S, Cuca YP, Cocohoba J, Dawson-Rose C, Davis K, Machtinger EL. Seeking Safety group therapy for co-occurring substance use disorder and PTSD among transgender women living with HIV: a pilot study. J Psychoactive Drugs. 2017;49(4):344–51.

86. Alberta Alcohol and Drug Abuse Commission. Canadian addiction survey 2004: Alberta report [Internet]. Edmonton: Legislative Assembly of Alberta; 2006. Available from: http://www.assembly.ab.ca/lao/library/egovdocs/2006/alad/153968.pdf.

87. Canadian Human Rights Commission. Canadian Human Rights Commission's policy on alcohol and drug testing [Internet]. Ottawa: Government of Canada; 2009 [cited 2021 Oct 3]. Available from: https://publications.gc.ca/collections/collection_2009/ccdp-chrc/HR4-6-2009E.pdf.

88. McLellan AT, Skipper GS, Campbell M, DuPont RL. Five year outcomes in a cohort study of physicians treated for substance use disorders in the United States. BMJ. 2008 Nov 4;337:a2038.

89. Brewster JM, Kaufmann IM, Hutchison S, MacWilliam C. Characteristics and outcomes of doctors in a substance dependence monitoring programme in Canada: prospective descriptive study. BMJ. 2008 Nov 3;337:a2098.

90. Shield KD, Rylett M, Gmel G, Gmel G, Kehoe-Chan TA, Rehm J. Global alcohol exposure estimates by country, territory and region for 2005 – a contribution to the comparative risk assessment for the 2010 global burden of disease study. Addiction. 2013;108(5):912–22.

91. Canadian Centre on Substance Abuse. Canadian drug and slcohol summary, 2017 [Internet]. Ottawa: CCSA; 2017. Available from: http://www.ccsa.ca/Resource%20Library/CCSA-Canadian-Drug-Summary-Alcohol-2017-en.pdf.

92. Butt P, Cesa F, Gliksman L, Paradis C, Stockwell T. Alcohol and health in Canada: A summary of evidence and guidelines for low-risk drinking [Internet]. Ottawa: Canadian Centre on Substance Abuse; 2011 [cited 2021 Oct 3]. Available from: https://www.uvic.ca/research/centres/cisur/assets/docs/report-alcohol-and-health-in-canada.pdf.

93. World Health Organization. Global status report on alcohol and health. Geneva (Switzerland): World Health Organization; 2011.

94. Stockwell T, Zhao J, Panwar S, Roemer A, Naimi T, Chikritzhs T. Do "Moderate" Drinkers Have Reduced Mortality Risk? A Systematic Review and Meta-Analysis of Alcohol Consumption and All-Cause Mortality. J Stud Alcohol Drugs. 2016;77(2):185–98.

95. Stockwell T, Zhao J. Alcohol's contribution to cancer is underestimated for exactly the same reason that its contribution to cardioprotection is overestimated. Addiction. 2017;112(2):230–2.

96. Matching alcoholism treatments to client heterogeneity: project MATCH three-year drinking outcomes. Alcohol Clin Exp Res. 1998;22(6):1300–11.

97. Maisel NC, Blodgett JC, Wilbourne PL, Humphreys K, Finney JW. Meta-analysis of naltrexone and acamprosate for treating alcohol use disorders: when are these medications most helpful? Addiction. 2013;108(2):275–93.

98. King AC, Volpicelli JR, Frazer A, O'Brien CP. Effect of naltrexone on subjective alcohol response in subjects at high and low risk for future alcohol dependence. Psychopharmacology (Berl). 1997;129(1):15–22.

99. Mason BJ, Heyser CJ. Acamprosate: a prototypic neuromodulator in the treatment of alcohol dependence. CNS Neurol Disord Drug Targets. 2010;9(1):23–32.

100. Mason BJ, Quello S, Goodell V, Shadan F, Kyle M, Begovic A. Gabapentin treatment for alcohol dependence: a randomized clinical trial. JAMA Intern Med. 2014;174(1):70–7.

101. Skinner MD, Lahmek P, Pham H, Aubin HJ. Disulfiram efficacy in the treatment of alcohol dependence: a meta-analysis. PLoS One. 2014;9(2):e87366.

102. Diehl A, Ulmer L, Mutschler J, Herre H, Krumm B, Croissant B, et al. Why is disulfiram superior to acamprosate in the routine clinical setting? A retrospective long-term study in 353 alcohol-dependent patients. Alcohol Alcohol. 2010;45(3):271–7.

103. Fuller RK, Branchey L, Brightwell DR, Derman RM, Emrick CD, Iber FL, et al. Disulfiram treatment of alcoholism. A Veterans Administration cooperative study. JAMA. 1986;256(11):1449–55.

104. National Center on Addiction and Substance Abuse at Columbia University. Addiction medicine: closing the gap between science and practice. New York: Columbia University; 2012.

105. Nunes EV. Gabapentin: a new addition to the armamentarium for alcohol dependence? JAMA Intern Med. 2014;174(1):78–9.

106. Jonas DE, Amick HR, Feltner C, Bobashev G, Thomas K, Wines R, et al. Pharmacotherapy for adults with alcohol use disorders in outpatient settings: a systematic review and meta-analysis. JAMA. 2014;311(18):1889–900.

107. Boyle P. Cancer, cigarette smoking and premature death in Europe: a review including the Recommendations of European Cancer Experts Consensus Meeting, Helsinki, October 1996. Lung Cancer. 1997;17(1):1–60.

108. Anthonisen NR, Skeans MA, Wise RA, Manfreda J, Kanner RE, Connett JE; Lung Health Study Research Group. The effects of a smoking cessation intervention on 14.5-year mortality: a randomized clinical trial. Ann Intern Med. 2005;142(4):233–9.

109. US Department of Health and Human Services. The health consequences of smoking: a report of the Surgeon General. Washington (DC): US Department of Health and Human Services; 2004.

110. Reid JL, Hammond D, Rynard VL, Madill CL, Burkhalter R. Tobacco use in Canada: patterns and trends. Waterloo (ON): Propel Centre for Population Health Impact, University of Waterloo; 2017.

111. Hoffman L, Delahanty J, Johnson SE, Zhao X. Sexual and gender minority cigarette smoking disparities: An analysis of 2016 behavioral risk factor surveillance system data. Prev Med. 2018;113:109–15.

112. McCabe SE, Matthews AK, Lee JGL, Veliz P, Hughes TL, Boyd CJ. Tobacco use and sexual orientation in a national cross-sectional study: age, race/ethnicity, and sexual identity-attraction differences. Am J Prev Med. 2018;54(6):736–45.

113. Health Canada [Internet]. Ottawa: Government of Canada; 2017 Mar [cited 2021 Oct 3]. Canadian tobacco alcohol and drug (CTADS): 2015 summary. Available from: https://www.canada.ca/en/health-canada/services/canadian-alcohol-drugs-survey/2015-summary.html

114. Shahab L, Goniewicz ML, Blount BC, Brown J, McNeill A, Alwis KU, et al. Nicotine, carcinogen, and toxin exposure in long-term e-cigarette and

nicotine replacement therapy users: a cross-sectional study. Ann Intern Med. 2017;166(6):390–400.

115. Arrazola RA, Singh T, Corey CG, Husten CG, Neff LJ, Apelberg BJ, Bunnell RE, Choiniere CJ, King BA, Cox S, McAfee T, Caraballo RS; Centers for Disease Control and Prevention (CDC). Tobacco use among middle and high school students – United States, 2011–2014. MMWR Morb Mortal Wkly Rep. 2015 Apr 17;64(14):381–5. https://www.cdc.gov /mmwr/preview/mmwrhtml/mm6414a3.htm.

116. Pacek LR, McClernon FJ. Decline in the perceived risk of cigarette smoking between 2006 and 2015: findings from a U.S. nationally representative sample. Drug Alcohol Depend. 2018 Apr;185:406–10.

117. Vardavas CI, Anagnostopoulos N, Kougias M, Evangelopoulou V, Connolly GN, Behrakis PK. Short-term pulmonary effects of using an electronic cigarette: impact on respiratory flow resistance, impedance, and exhaled nitric oxide. Chest. 2012;141(6):1400–6.

118. Jensen RP, Luo W, Pankow JF, Strongin RM, Peyton DH. Hidden formaldehyde in e-cigarette aerosols. N Engl J Med. 2015;372(4):392–4.

119. Quebec Coalition for the Control of Tobacco [Internet]. Montreal: Quebec Coalition for the Control of Tobacco. Press release, Tobacco and Vaping Products Act: new developments lead some health groups to reconsider their support for Bill S-5; 2018 Feb 12 [cited 2021 Oct 3]. Available from: https://www.newswire.ca/news-releases/tobacco-and-vaping-products -act-new-developments-lead-some-health-groups-to-reconsider-their- support-for-bill-s-5–673813903.html.

120. Chaiton M, Diemert L, Cohen JE, Bondy SJ, Selby P, Philipneri A, et al. Estimating the number of quit attempts it takes to quit smoking successfully in a longitudinal cohort of smokers. BMJ Open. 2016;6(6):e011045.

121. Salgado García FI, Derefinko KJ, Bursac Z, Hand S, Klesges RC. Planning a Change Easily (PACE): A randomized controlled trial for smokers who are not ready to quit. Contemp Clin Trials. 2018;68:14–22.

122. Baskerville NB, Dash D, Shuh A, Wong K, Abramowicz A, Yessis J, et al. Tobacco use cessation interventions for lesbian, gay, bisexual, transgender and queer youth and young adults: A scoping review. Prev Med Rep. 2017;6:53–62.

123. Cahill K, Stevens S, Perera R, Lancaster T. Pharmacological interventions for smoking cessation: an overview and network meta-analysis. Cochrane Database Syst Rev. 2013 May 31;2013(5):CD009329.

124. Mills EJ, Thorlund K, Eapen S, Wu P, Prochaska JJ. Cardiovascular events associated with smoking cessation pharmacotherapies: a network meta- analysis. Circulation. 2014;129(1):28–41.

125. University of Ottawa Heart Institute. Ottawa model for smoking cessation. Ottawa: University of Ottawa Heart Institute; 2016.

126. Collier R. Antismoking drug still recommended to Canadians despite side effects and US advisory. CMAJ. 2009 Feb 17;180(4):381. doi:10.1503/cmaj.090114.

127. Thomas KH, Martin RM, Knipe DW, Higgins JP, Gunnell D. Risk of neuropsychiatric adverse events associated with varenicline: systematic review and meta-analysis. BMJ. 2015 Mar;350 mar12 8:h1109.

128. Anthenelli RM, Benowitz NL, West R, St Aubin L, McRae T, Lawrence D, et al. Neuropsychiatric safety and efficacy of varenicline, bupropion, and nicotine patch in smokers with and without psychiatric disorders (EAGLES): a double-blind, randomised, placebo-controlled clinical trial. Lancet. 2016;387(10037):2507–20.

129. Chang PH, Chiang CH, Ho WC, Wu PZ, Tsai JS, Guo FR. Combination therapy of varenicline with nicotine replacement therapy is better than varenicline alone: a systematic review and meta-analysis of randomized controlled trials. BMC Public Health. 2015;15:689.

130. Becker WJ, Findlay T, Moga C, Scott NA, Harstall C, Taenzer P. Guideline for primary care management of headache in adults. Can Fam Physician. 2015;61(8):670–79.

131. Qaseem A, Wilt TJ, McLean RM, Forciea MA, Denberg TD, Barry MJ, et al.; Clinical Guidelines Committee of the American College of Physicians. Noninvasive treatments for acute, subacute, and chronic low back pain: a clinical practice guideline from the American College of Physicians. Ann Intern Med. 2017;166(7):514–30.

132. Volkow ND, McLellan AT. Opioid abuse in chronic pain – misconceptions and mitigation strategies. N Engl J Med. 2016;374(13):1253–3.

133. Chou R, Turner JA, Devine EB, et al. The effectiveness and risks of long-term opioid therapy for chronic pain: a systematic review for a National Institutes of Health Pathways to Prevention Workshop. Ann Intern Med. 2015;162(4):276–86.

134. Ray WA, Chung CP, Murray KT, Hall K, Stein CM. Prescription of Long-Acting Opioids and Mortality in Patients With Chronic Noncancer Pain. JAMA. 2016;315(22):2415–23.

135. Busse JW, Craigie S, Juurlink DN, Buckley DN, Wang L, Couban RJ, et al. Guideline for opioid therapy and chronic noncancer pain. CMAJ. 2017;189(18):E659–66.

136. Shah A, Hayes CJ, Martin BC. Characteristics of Initial Prescription Episodes and Likelihood of Long-Term Opioid Use - United States, 2006–2015. MMWR Morb Mortal Wkly Rep. 2017;66(10):265–9.

137. Lea T, Mao L, Bath N, Prestage G, Zablotska I, de Wit J, et al. Injecting drug use among gay and bisexual men in Sydney: prevalence and associations with sexual risk practices and HIV and hepatitis C infection. AIDS Behav. 2013;17(4):1344–51.

138. Cochran SD, Ackerman D, Mays VM, Ross MW. Prevalence of non-medical drug use and dependence among homosexually active men and women in the US population. Addiction. 2004;99(8):989–98.

139. Dhalla IA, Mamdani MM, Sivilotti ML, Kopp A, Qureshi O, Juurlink DN. Prescribing of opioid analgesics and related mortality before and after the introduction of long-acting oxycodone. CMAJ. 2009;181(12):891–6.

140. Rudd RA, Aleshire N, Zibbell JE, Gladden RM. Increases in drug and opioid overdose deaths – United States, 2000–2014. MMWR Morb Mortal Wkly Rep. 2016;64(50–51):1378–82.

141. Office of the Chief Coroner. Illicit drug overdose deaths in BC, January 1, 2007–December 31, 2016 [Internet]. Vancouver: British Columbia Coroners Service; 2016 [cited 2017 Oct 26]. Available from: https://www2.gov.bc.ca/assets/gov/public-safety-and-emergency-services/death-investigation/statistical/illicit-drug.pdf.

142. Public Health Agency of Canada [Internet]. Ottawa: Government of Canada; 2018 [cited 2019 Oct 3] National report: Apparent opioid-related deaths in Canada (January 2016 to March 2017). Avaialbe from: https://www.canada.ca/en/public-health/services/publications/healthy-living/apparent-opioid-related-deaths-report-2016.html.

143. Office of the Chief Coroner. Fentanyl-detected illicit drug overdose deaths, January 1, 2012 to December 31, 2017 [Internet]. Vancouver: British Columbia Coroners Service; 2018 [cited 2019 Oct 26]. Available from: https://www2.gov.bc.ca/assets/gov/public-safety-and-emergency-services/death-investigation/statistical/fentanyl-detected-overdose.pdf.

144. Bruneau J, Ahamad K, Goyer MÈ, Poulin G, Selby P, Fischer B, et al.; CIHR Canadian Research Initiative in Substance Misuse. Management of opioid use disorders: a national clinical practice guideline. CMAJ. 2018;190(9):E247–57.

145. Poole R, Kennedy OJ, Roderick P, Fallowfield JA, Hayes PC, Parkes J. Coffee consumption and health: umbrella review of meta-analyses of multiple health outcomes. BMJ. 2017;359:j5024.

146. Romanelli F, Smith KM, Thornton AC, Pomeroy C. Poppers: epidemiology and clinical management of inhaled nitrite abuse. Pharmacotherapy. 2004;24(1):69–78.

147. Farré M, de la Torre R, González ML, Terán MT, Roset PN, Menoyo E, et al. Cocaine and alcohol interactions in humans: neuroendocrine effects and cocaethylene metabolism. J Pharmacol Exp Ther. 1997;283(1):164–76.

148. Shoptaw S, Klausner JD, Reback CJ, Tierney S, Stansell J, Hare CB, et al. A public health response to the methamphetamine epidemic: the

implementation of contingency management to treat methamphetamine dependence. BMC Public Health. 2006;6:214.

149. Menza TW, Jameson DR, Hughes JP, Colfax GN, Shoptaw S, Golden MR. Contingency management to reduce methamphetamine use and sexual risk among men who have sex with men: a randomized controlled trial. BMC Public Health. 2010;10:774.

150. Aaron S, McMahon JM, Milano D, Torres L, Clatts M, Tortu S, et al. Intranasal transmission of hepatitis C virus: virological and clinical evidence. Clin Infect Dis. 2008;47(7):931–4.

151. Pani PP, Trogu E, Vecchi S, Amato L. Antidepressants for cocaine dependence and problematic cocaine use. Cochrane Database Syst Rev. 2011(12):CD002950.

152. Indave BI, Minozzi S, Pani PP, Amato L. Antipsychotic medications for cocaine dependence. Cochrane Database Syst Rev. 2016;3:CD006306.

153. Minozzi S, Cinquini M, Amato L, Davoli M, Farrell MF, Pani PP, Vecchi S. Anticonvulsants for cocaine dependence. Cochrane Database Syst Rev. 2015 Apr 17;(4):CD006754.

154. Amato L, Minozzi S, Pani PP, Solimini R, Vecchi S, Zuccaro P, Davoli M. Dopamine agonists for the treatment of cocaine dependence. Cochrane Database Syst Rev. 2011 Dec 7;(12):CD003352.

155. Castells X, Cunill R, Pérez-Mañá C, Vidal X, Capellà D. Psychostimulant drugs for cocaine dependence. Cochrane Database Syst Rev. 2016 Sep 27;9(9):CD007380.

156. Pérez-Mañá C, Castells X, Torrens M, Capellà D, Farre M. Efficacy of psychostimulant drugs for amphetamine abuse or dependence. Cochrane Database Syst Rev. 2013(9):CD009695.

157. Ling W, Chang L, Hillhouse M, Ang A, Striebel J, Jenkins J, et al. Sustained-release methylphenidate in a randomized trial of treatment of methamphetamine use disorder. Addiction. 2014;109(9):1489–1500.

158. Santos GM, Coffin P, Santos D, Huffaker S, Matheson T, Euren J, et al. Feasibility, Acceptability, and Tolerability of Targeted Naltrexone for Nondependent Methamphetamine-Using and Binge-Drinking Men Who Have Sex with Men. J Acquir Immune Defic Syndr. 2016;72(1):21–30.

159. Schmitz JM, Stotts AL, Rhoades HM, Grabowski J. Naltrexone and relapse prevention treatment for cocaine-dependent patients. Addict Behav. 2001;26(2):167–80.

160. Ray LA, Bujarski S, Courtney KE, Moallem NR, Lunny K, Roche D, et al. The Effects of Naltrexone on Subjective Response to Methamphetamine in a Clinical Sample: a Double-Blind, Placebo-Controlled Laboratory Study. Neuropsychopharmacology. 2015;40(10):2347–56.

161. Weiss RD, Griffin ML, Gallop RJ, Najavits LM, Frank A, Crits-Christoph P, et al. The effect of 12-step self-help group attendance and participation

on drug use outcomes among cocaine-dependent patients. Drug Alcohol Depend. 2005;77(2):177–84.

162. Maude-Griffin PM, Hohenstein JM, Humfleet GL, Reilly PM, Tusel DJ, Hall SM. Superior efficacy of cognitive-behavioral therapy for urban crack cocaine abusers: main and matching effects. J Consult Clin Psychol. 1998;66(5):832–7.

163. Peirce JM, Petry NM, Stitzer ML, Blaine J, Kellogg S, Satterfield F, et al. Effects of lower-cost incentives on stimulant abstinence in methadone maintenance treatment: a National Drug Abuse Treatment Clinical Trials Network study. Arch Gen Psychiatry. 2006;63(2):201–8.

164. Garcia-Rodriguez O, Secades-Villa R, Higgins ST, Fernandez-Hermida JR, Carballo JL, Errasti Perez JM, et al. Effects of voucher-based intervention on abstinence and retention in an outpatient treatment for cocaine addiction: a randomized controlled trial. Exp Clin Psychopharmacol. 2009;17(3):131–8.

165. Schumacher JE, Milby JB, Wallace D, Meehan DC, Kertesz S, Vuchinich R, et al. Meta-analysis of day treatment and contingency-management dismantling research: Birmingham Homeless Cocaine Studies (1990–2006). J Consult Clin Psychol. 2007;75(5):823–8.

166. Iseger TA, Bossong MG. A systematic review of the antipsychotic properties of cannabidiol in humans. Schizophr Res. 2015;162(1–3):153–61.

167. Leweke FM, Piomelli D, Pahlisch F, Muhl D, Gerth CW, Hoyer C, et al. Cannabidiol enhances anandamide signaling and alleviates psychotic symptoms of schizophrenia. Transl Psychiatry. 2012;2:e94.

168. ElSohly MA, Mehmedic Z, Foster S, Gon C, Chandra S, Church JC. Changes in Cannabis Potency Over the Last 2 Decades (1995–2014): Analysis of Current Data in the United States. Biol Psychiatry. 2016;79(7):613–19.

169. Silins E, Horwood LJ, Patton GC, Fergusson DM, Olsson CA, Hutchinson DM, et al.; Cannabis Cohorts Research Consortium. Young adult sequelae of adolescent cannabis use: an integrative analysis. Lancet Psychiatry. 2014;1(4):286–93.

170. Wilson W, Mathew R, Turkington T, Hawk T, Coleman RE, Provenzale J. Brain morphological changes and early marijuana use: a magnetic resonance and positron emission tomography study. J Addict Dis. 2000;19(1):1–22.

171. Allan GM, Finley CR, Ton J, Perry D, Ramji J, Crawford K, et al. Systematic review of systematic reviews for medical cannabinoids: Pain, nausea and vomiting, spasticity, and harms. Can Fam Physician. 2018;64(2):e78-e94.

172. Kermode-Scott B. Canadians authorised to use cannabis for medical purposes to be allowed to grow their own again. BMJ. 2016;354:i4480.

173. Department of Justice [Internet]. Ottawa: Government of Canada; 2017 [cited 2018]. Current cannabis laws, 2017. Available from: http://www .justice.gc.ca/eng/cj-jp/marijuana/law-loi.html.

174. Hasin DS, Wall M, Keyes KM, Cerdá M, Schulenberg J, O'Malley PM, et al. Medical marijuana laws and adolescent marijuana use in the USA from 1991 to 2014: results from annual, repeated cross-sectional surveys. Lancet Psychiatry. 2015;2(7):601–8.

175. Choo EK, Benz M, Zaller N, Warren O, Rising KL, McConnell KJ. The impact of state medical marijuana legislation on adolescent marijuana use. J Adolesc Health. 2014;55(2):160–6.

176. Fischer B, Murphy Y, Kurdyak P, Goldner E, Rehm J. Medical marijuana programs – why might they matter for public health and why should we better understand their impacts? Prev Med Rep. 2015;2:53–6.

177. Allan GM, Ramji J, Perry D, Ton J, Beahm NP, Crisp N, et al. Simplified guideline for prescribing medical cannabinoids in primary care. Can Fam Physician. 2018;64(2):111–20.

178. Canadian College of Family Physicians. The College of Family Physicians of Canada statement on Health: Canada's proposed changes to medical marijuana regulations. Toronto: CCFP; 2013 [cited 2018 Oct 4]. Available from: http://www.cfpc.ca/uploadedFiles/Health_Policy /CFPC_Policy_Papers_and_Endorsements/CFPC_Policy_Papers/ Medical%20Marijuana%20Position%20Statement%20CFPC.pdf.

179. Fischer B, Russell C, Sabioni P, van den Brink W, Le Foll B, Hall W, et al. Lower-Risk cannabis use guidelines: a comprehensive update of evidence and recommendations. Am J Public Health. 2017 Aug;107(8):e1–12.

180. Fisher J, Hirshman E, Henthorn T, Arndt J, Passannante A. Midazolam amnesia and short-term/working memory processes. Conscious Cogn. 2006;15(1):54–63.

181. Anglin D, Spears KL, Hutson HR. Flunitrazepam and its involvement in date or acquaintance rape. Acad Emerg Med. 1997;4(4):323–6.

182. Vermeeren A, Coenen AM. Effects of the use of hypnotics on cognition. Prog Brain Res. 2011;190:89–103.

183. Billioti de Gage S, Pariente A, Bégaud B. Is there really a link between benzodiazepine use and the risk of dementia? Expert Opin Drug Saf. 2015;14(5):733–47.

184. Weich S, Pearce HL, Croft P, et al. Effect of anxiolytic and hypnotic drug prescriptions on mortality hazards: retrospective cohort study. BMJ. 2014;348:g1996.

185. Nielsen S, Lintzeris N, Bruno R, Campbell G, Larance B, Hall W, et al. Benzodiazepine use among chronic pain patients prescribed opioids: associations with pain, physical and mental health, and health service utilization. Pain Med. 2015;16(2):356–66.
186. Ashton H. The treatment of benzodiazepine dependence. Addiction. 1994;89(11):1535–41.
187. Vicens C, Fiol F, Llobera J, Campoamor F, Mateu C, Alegret S, et al. Withdrawal from long-term benzodiazepine use: randomised trial in family practice. Br J Gen Pract. 2006;56(533):958–63.
188. Ashton H. The diagnosis and management of benzodiazepine dependence. Curr Opin Psychiatry. 2005;18(3):249–55.
189. Tupper KW, Wood E, Yensen R, Johnson MW. Psychedelic medicine: a re-emerging therapeutic paradigm. CMAJ. 2015;187(14):1054–9.
190. Krebs TS, Johansen P. Lysergic acid diethylamide (LSD) for alcoholism: meta-analysis of randomized controlled trials. J Psychopharmacol. 2012;26(7):994–1002.
191. Bogenschutz MP, Forcehimes AA, Pommy JA, Wilcox CE, Barbosa PC, Strassman RJ. Psilocybin-assisted treatment for alcohol dependence: a proof-of-concept study. J Psychopharmacol. 2015;29(3):289–99.
192. Johnson MW, Garcia-Romeu A, Cosimano MP, Griffiths RR. Pilot study of the 5-HT2AR agonist psilocybin in the treatment of tobacco addiction. J Psychopharmacol. 2014;28(11):983–92.
193. Thomas G, Lucas P, Capler NR, Tupper KW, Martin G. Ayahuasca-assisted therapy for addiction: results from a preliminary observational study in Canada. Curr Drug Abuse Rev. 2013;6(1):30–42.
194. Grob CS, McKenna DJ, Callaway JC, Brito GS, Neves ES, Oberlaender G, et al. Human psychopharmacology of hoasca, a plant hallucinogen used in ritual context in Brazil. J Nerv Ment Dis. 1996;184(2):86–94.
195. Schep LJ, Knudsen K, Slaughter RJ, Vale JA, Mégarbane B. The clinical toxicology of γ-hydroxybutyrate, γ-butyrolactone and 1,4-butanediol. Clin Toxicol (Phila). 2012;50(6):458–70.
196. Stall R, Paul JP, Greenwood G, Pollack LM, Bein E, Crosby GM, et al. Alcohol use, drug use and alcohol-related problems among men who have sex with men: the Urban Men's Health Study. Addiction. 2001;96(11):1589–601.
197. Rosen RC, Catania JA, Ehrhardt AA, Burnett AL, Lue TF, McKenna K, et al. The Bolger conference on PDE-5 inhibition and HIV risk: implications for health policy and prevention. J Sex Med. 2006;3(6):960–75.
198. Tchaikovski SN, Rosing J. Mechanisms of estrogen-induced venous thromboembolism. Thromb Res. 2010;126(1):5–11.
199. Pomp ER, Rosendaal FR, Doggen CJ. Smoking increases the risk of venous thrombosis and acts synergistically with oral contraceptive use. Am J Hematol. 2008;83(2):97–102.

200. Ip EJ, Yadao MA, Shah BM, Doroudgar S, Perry PJ, Tenerowicz MJ, et al. Polypharmacy, Infectious Diseases, Sexual Behavior, and Psychophysical Health Among Anabolic Steroid-Using Homosexual and Heterosexual Gym Patrons in San Francisco's Castro District. Subst Use Misuse. 2017;52(7):959–68.

201. Krueger RB. Diagnosis of hypersexual or compulsive sexual behavior can be made using ICD-10 and DSM-5 despite rejection of this diagnosis by the American Psychiatric Association. Addiction. 2016;111(12):2110–11.

202. Kelly BC, Bimbi DS, Nanin JE, Izienicki H, Parsons JT. Sexual compulsivity and sexual behaviors among gay and bisexual men and lesbian and bisexual women. J Sex Res. 2009;46(4):301–8.

203. Grov C, Parsons JT, Bimbi DS. Sexual compulsivity and sexual risk in gay and bisexual men. Arch Sex Behav. 2010;39(4):940–9.

204. Kalichman SC, Rompa D. The Sexual Compulsivity Scale: further development and use with HIV-positive persons. J Pers Assess. 2001;76(3):379–95.

205. Sexual Compulsives Anonymous. Secret Shame: sexual compulsion in the lives of gay men and lesbians. New York: SCA International Service Organization; 1991.

206. Leavens E, Marotta J, Weinstock J. Disordered gambling in residential substance use treatment centers: an unmet need. J Addict Dis. 2014;33(2):163–73.

207. Elmquist J, Shorey RC, Anderson S, Stuart GL. Eating disorder symptoms and length of stay in residential treatment for substance use: a brief report. J Dual Diagn. 2015;11(3–4):233–7.

10 Reproductive Health

CARRIE SCHRAM

Introduction

The number of 2SLGBTQ families with children has been steadily increasing in Canada. In 2016, 12.0 per cent of 2SLGBTQ families included children, up from 8.6 per cent in 2001. The majority, 80 per cent, with children were same-sex female couples. As of 2016, about half of all 2SLGBTQ families had parents who were married.[1] It is expected that the number of 2SLGBTQ families with children will continue to grow, and many 2SLGBTQ people will seek assistance and support from their primary care providers.

Historically, the fertility needs of 2SLGBTQ people as a population have been poorly met by the medical community,[2,3] and many gaps in service and care remain today. Some of these challenges are geographical as fertility clinics are almost exclusively located in major cities in Canada, and others are legislative because of some restrictions on services outlined by the Canadian Assisted Human Reproduction Act (AHRA).[4] Those pertaining to the 2SLGBTQ population will be highlighted as needed throughout this chapter. Other challenges remain because of a heteronormative culture that persists within medicine and is especially strong in fertility, where conception has traditionally been perceived as between "male" and "female" and focused on conception in heterosexual relationships. As a result of this history, many 2SLGBTQ people are understandably apprehensive about seeking reproductive care and have valid concerns about the care and treatment they will receive. Thankfully, fertility medicine and legislation are evolving to better meet the needs of our diverse population in a way that is respectful and affirming to all people. Care may not yet be perfect, but primary care providers can help reassure 2SLGBTQ patients that their needs and desires should be respected and help them advocate, when needed, to receive comprehensive and affirming care.

It must be acknowledged that there is incredible diversity among all people, including those in the 2SLGBTQ population, and no assumptions should be made about the needs and desires of anyone from a reproductive perspective. This chapter strives to provide guidance for meeting the reproductive needs of the 2SLGBTQ population, but primary care providers are encouraged to ask about the needs and desires of their patients, to be nonjudgmental, not to make assumptions, and to remain open minded and supportive. For some people in the 2SLGBTQ community, pursuing fertility is particularly emotional or otherwise challenging because of previous negative experiences with the medical community or the reminder of how they do not conform to a heterosexual "norm" that still prevails in society. Primary care providers are encouraged to take the time to explore these aspects of reproductive care, when present, and to give patients a safe space to express their fears and apprehensions, as well as hopes, for their future family.

Part 1: Reproductive Function

2SLBGTQ people not on hormone therapy have typical reproductive function as predicted by their age and personal risk factors. For those on hormone therapy, reproductive function is altered acutely and, at times, permanently, by hormone use. The potential effects of hormone therapy for people born with ovaries and those with sperm is further explored in Part 3 and Part 4, respectively, of this chapter. This section will focus on typical reproductive function for people with ovaries and those with sperm who are not on hormone therapy.

For people with ovaries, a natural fertility study of six different heterosexual Western populations demonstrated a baseline rate of infertility of 5 to 8 per cent when marriage occurred by 25 years of age.[5] The rate of infertility in these populations rose slowly but steadily until age 35, at which point it rose more dramatically, with a mean age of last birth of 40 to 41 years of age.[5] Natural fertility studies have limitations, and caution should be used when applying this data to people of non-Western origins, but these results are consistent with what we see today. At present in Canada, the rate of infertility (lack of conception within 12 months of well-timed attempts) is approximately 16 per cent.[6] This rate has doubled since the 1980s[6] and is due in large part to decreased egg quantity and quality associated with increased age and delayed childbearing.

From a probability of conception perspective, people with ovaries who start trying to conceive have a 90 per cent chance of pregnancy within 12 months at age 30, but this decreases to a 77 per cent chance by age 35 and to a chance of only about 50 per cent by age 40.[6] On a per cycle basis, people with eggs have a probability of conception of about 25 per cent in their 20s, decreasing to 15 per cent by age 36 and to only about 8 per cent by age 40.[7] At the same time, the risk of spontaneous abortion rises with age as does the risk of complications during pregnancy.[7,8] As a result, the Society of Obstetricians and Gynaecologists of Canada (SOGC) has published a clinical practice guideline on advanced reproductive age and fertility[8] and a committee opinion on delayed childbearing,[7] which discuss in detail the effects of age on fertility and make numerous recommendations. Specifically, the SOGC recommends counselling people with ovaries that after 32 years of age, fertility begins to decline significantly.[7]

For people with sperm, although fertility changes with age are less dramatic than for people with eggs, they do occur. Semen quality decreases and the risk of genetic disorders and neurodevelopmental disorders (such as schizophrenia and autism) in offspring increase for individuals older than 40 years of age.[7] Although the relative risk remains small, it does increase more significantly for people with sperm who are over 50 years of age, and it is recommended that people in these age groups who want to conceive be counselled about these risks.[7]

Part 2: Healthy Lifestyles to Optimize Reproductive Health

To optimize reproductive health, all people who want to conceive with their genetic material or carry a pregnancy, should be encouraged to maintain a healthy lifestyle. This includes a healthy diet, regular physical activity, a healthy body mass index (BMI), and the avoidance of smoking, excessive alcohol use, and drug use.

For people with ovaries who want to personally conceive, BMI has a significant impact on conception and risk of spontaneous abortion. Specifically, for every kg/m^2 above 29 kg/m^2, the spontaneous conception rate is 4 per cent less per cycle,[9] and spontaneous abortion rates increase in people with a BMI of more than 25 kg/m^2.[10] Outcomes with fertility treatment, including in vitro fertilization, are similarly negatively impacted by increased BMI.[11] It is also well known that an elevated BMI is a risk factor in pregnancy and places people and their babies at increased risk of gestational diabetes, gestational hypertension, and needing an operative delivery.[7] For people with sperm, BMI is also significant. Sperm count and motility are similarly negatively affected for people with sperm and a BMI of more than 25 kg/m^2.[12] Therefore, for all people who want to conceive with their genetic material and/ or carry a pregnancy, working to maintain a healthy BMI is important. For people with an elevated BMI, weight loss must be addressed with sensitivity, and even small reductions will improve the probability of a healthy ongoing pregnancy and delivery.

Although many people recognize the need to abstain from habits such as smoking, alcohol use, and drug use in pregnancy, many people do not recognize the significance of these habits on conception. For people with eggs, smoking has an increased relative risk of infertility and increases the risk of spontaneous abortion.[13,14] For people with sperm, smoking decreases sperm count and motility.[15] Although alcohol in moderation does not appear to have a negative impact on conception, use beyond the low-risk guidelines decreases pregnancy rates, increases risk of spontaneous abortion,[14] and reduces sperm count and motility.[15] Similarly, there are THC receptors throughout the reproductive tracts of all people, and cannabis use has been associated with cycle abnormalities in people with eggs, lower conception rates, and decreased sperm motility for those with sperm.[16] Other recreational drugs also have significant negative effects on conception and pregnancy and, while explored here in detail, should be avoided for a variety of health reasons.

Lastly, reproductive health for all people may be impacted by exposure to sexually transmitted infections (STIs). Bacterial infections, such as chlamydia, can have a negative impact on tubal function for people with fallopian tubes and a negative impact on sperm production for people with testicles, making conception more difficult. Refer to chapter 6 for more information on STIs.

Part 3: Reproductive Options for Prospective Parents with Ovaries Only

When discussing fertility with people with ovaries, it is important to ask them first if they want to have a family and, if so, how they envision it happening. Do they personally want to conceive? Would they prefer to use their eggs but have a partner or someone else carry the pregnancy? Do they see themselves using an anonymous sperm donor or a known donor? It cannot be assumed that a person will want a child with their genetic material, to carry a pregnancy or not carry a pregnancy, regardless of gender identity or sexual orientation.

For people who want to conceive with their eggs and carry that pregnancy, the options are to conceive with a known sperm donor or an anonymous sperm donor. Known sperm donors are people, usually a family member of a partner or a close friend, who have agreed to provide sperm to the prospective parent with eggs. Often, conception occurs with minimal to no medical involvement. The prospective parent with eggs will monitor for ovulation, and insemination will occur on one or more occasions at that time. People with regular cycles will usually use phone applications alone or together with home cervical mucous monitoring, home urinary luteinizing hormone (LH) monitoring, or basal body temperature monitoring to help with timing.

Insemination is often performed with a needleless syringe purchased from a pharmacy or by placing sperm in a menstrual cup and placing it up by the cervix. With well-timed inseminations, pregnancy rates are the same as those in the general population. Some patients will seek guidance around timing and the number of inseminations to perform. Timing is the same as for any person trying to conceive and can be estimated based on cycle length. For example, for someone with a regular 28-day cycle, it is reasonable to inseminate on days 12 and 14. Those with irregular cycles or who are unsuccessful may benefit from fertility specialist consultation.

Special caution needs to be taken with using known sperm donors. There is an obvious risk of STIs given that body fluids are being inserted into the recipient. STI screening can help reassure the recipient of a reduced risk, but it is well known that not all STIs are immediately detectable (e.g., HIV seroconversion can occur weeks to months after exposure) and a negative screen does not guarantee the donor is not actively infected at the time of donation. There are also social and legal risks. Although desires for contact with offspring may be clear at the time of donation, desires by both parties may change over time, which can affect personal relationships. In extreme cases, people have taken legal action to obtain access to a child and/or financial support for a child conceived with a known donor. For this reason, it is recommended people using known donors strongly consider legal counsel for themselves and the donor and have a document in writing to ensure all parties' rights are respected.

Use of an anonymous sperm donor is much safer for the prospective parent(s) from infection, social, and legal perspectives but has other disadvantages including cost, need for medical involvement and lack of a childhood relationship with the donor, which some people desire. At present, the AHRA[4] prohibits payment for gamete donation, resulting in very few Canadian sperm donors. The result is most sperm used in Canada is imported from sperm donation centres in the United States and, to a lesser degree, Europe. Some Canadian companies specialize in importing this sperm in accordance with Health Canada requirements. The Canadian companies are readily accessible on the Internet and provide detailed instructions for the process of sperm purchase and access to donor profiles and information. At present, sperm can be released only to medical professionals and given the improved pregnancy rates with intrauterine insemination (IUI) versus intracervical or vaginal insemination,[17] especially with sperm that has previously been frozen, it is recommended patients do IUI for anonymous donor sperm. In addition, given the costs (which for insemination includes not only the cost of the sperm sample itself but also the shipping and possible thawing/washing/preparation fees), most people will use a single sperm sample per cycle, along with cycle monitoring at a fertility centre and IUI to optimize chances.

This means that people choosing this path will usually attend a fertility centre several times during their cycle to perform insemination. Conception rates are slightly lower with sperm that has been frozen versus fresh sperm, with people less than 35 years of age having a pregnancy rate of approximately 20 per cent per cycle, decreasing to approximately 5 per cent by age 40.[18]

The AHRA[4] outlines necessary processes and limitations that govern the use of known donor sperm. The intention of these are to maximize safety while accommodating a need for access to known donor sperm. The regulations are updated periodically, and it is best to refer patients to experienced fertility specialists for up-to-date information if they want to use medical assistance with a known donor.

For people with ovaries who want to conceive with their genetic material but not carry that pregnancy, there is the option of in vitro fertilization (IVF) with a partner or surrogate to carry the pregnancy. This is much more medicalized and expensive than home insemination or IUI, but for some people it is necessary for medical reasons or preferable for social reasons. The process of having a partner carry a pregnancy for the couple, where the other individual's egg is used, known as reciprocal IVF, is becoming increasingly popular. Those who choose this route often do so to allow both partners who will co-parent the child to be physically involved in the pregnancy.[19] Use of a gestational carrier or surrogate is distinct from this as there is no romantic relationship between the egg donor and surrogate and no intention for the surrogate to co-parent the child as there is in reciprocal IVF.

People with ovaries considering hormone therapy with testosterone should consider their reproductive plans before initiating treatment, if possible. Presently, little is known about the effects, if any, of testosterone on long-term ovarian function. Case studies, however, are encouraging as trans men have been found to have normal age-related responses to ovarian stimulation even after years of testosterone therapy.[20,21] People with ovaries considering hormone therapy with testosterone should discuss reproductive concerns with their hormone prescriber or fertility specialist. With time, more research should help clarify what effect, if any, testosterone has on the ovaries long term, but in the meantime a discussion can be had and consideration can be given to egg harvesting and freezing.

For people who are considering hormone therapy, considering having their ovaries removed, or are aging and do not have plans for conception in the near future, it is very reasonable to consider egg or embryo freezing. With both egg freezing and embryo freezing, the individual with ovaries is required to do basic fertility testing and then work with a specialist to create a plan to produce a large number of eggs, ideally 15 to 20. This requires gonadotropic hormone injections and close medical monitoring, plus an egg retrieval procedure, which is performed transvaginally, usually under conscious sedation. When egg freezing is the goal, the eggs are then retrieved and frozen for future use. When there is a partner with sperm or a sperm donor, instead of freezing the eggs, the eggs can be fertilized and embryos grown to the blastocyst stage. Not all eggs retrieved will be mature, not all will fertilize, not all that fertilize will become blastocysts, and not all blastocysts will be euploid. Hence the goal is to retrieve a large number of eggs to optimize the chances of having at least one child. The cost of egg and embryo freezing varies based on medical protocols but is usually upwards of $10,000 plus yearly banking fees. More specific details on prognosis, the procedure, and costs is best had in discussion with a fertility specialist who can provide patient-specific information based on individual circumstances.

Part 4: Reproductive Options for Prospective Parents with Sperm Only

People with sperm who want to have a family with their genetic material need to have both an egg donor and surrogate to carry the pregnancy. Both the egg donor and surrogate may be known to the prospective parent(s) or be anonymous. As with known sperm donors, it is advised that anyone using known egg donors or surrogates obtain legal counsel and contracts to clearly state intentions and protect the parenting rights and responsibilities of all parties involved.

The AHRA[4] currently prohibits payment for gametes, including eggs, in Canada beyond reimbursement of medical and direct expenses with receipts (such as parking). As a result, obtaining eggs can be challenging as relatively few people will donate altruistically, without direct financial gain. Similarly, at present the AHRA also prohibits payment for surrogate pregnancy services beyond reimbursement of medical and direct receiptable expenses.

Many people with sperm who need eggs and a surrogate will therefore ask family or friends for help or seek care from abroad, most commonly the United States, where additional payment is legal and there is easier access to eggs and surrogates. For people with sperm who need both an egg donor and a surrogate, the costs for medical and associated expenses in Canada can be significant, and these are often amplified if they seek them in another country.

For people with sperm who want to begin hormone therapy with estrogen, there is a significant risk of reduced sperm count sufficient to cause infertility, which may not return if hormone therapy is discontinued. Experts recommend that anyone with sperm who is starting hormone therapy with estrogen and who may want to have a biological child in the future bank their sperm.[22,23] Sperm banking is less invasive and costly than egg and embryo freezing but does have an upfront fee and yearly storage fees. Interested patients should meet with a fertility specialist to discuss their individual needs and desires.

Part 5: When to Refer to a Fertility Specialist

There are many circumstances in which patients may want to seek fertility consultation or in which you may feel that the care of a fertility specialist is indicated. Referral can occur at any stage: fertility planning with no active plans for conception, fertility preservation before hormonal or surgical intervention, active conception planning and initiation, or after trying to conceive in the community without success.

Fertility Planning

Primary care providers are well equipped to talk to their patients about fertility in general and expected changes with age. For most 2SLGBTQ patients, there is no need for specialist consultation well in advance of trying to conceive. However, for patients at increased risk of infertility, including those of advanced age, those who have more complex fertility desires (such as reciprocal IVF or the need for a surrogate), or those with personal fertility risk factors, referral in the planning stage can help optimize fertility when conception is more actively desired. It is also valuable for people considering gamete or embryo freezing as freezing at a younger age, particularly for eggs, is advantageous and results in greater probability of success in the future.

Before Hormone Therapy or Transition-Related Surgery

As previously discussed, it is recommended that individuals planning to begin hormone therapy who may want to someday have children with their genetic material meet with a fertility specialist before starting therapy. The purpose of this visit is to discuss what is currently known about hormone therapy and fertility, an area of medicine in which there is ongoing research, and to discuss fertility preservation options. People considering or planning permanent fertility-altering surgery, such as oophorectomy or orchiectomy, should be counselled and offered referral. Certainly, people can choose to not have consultation or preserve their fertility, but it is important that they have the opportunity to make an informed decision.

If your patient has already been on hormone therapy and has questions or concerns from a fertility perspective, it is valuable to refer them for consultation, discussion, and consideration of testing. There is individual variability in response to hormone therapy from a fertility perspective, and it should not be assumed that a person is infertile even after years of treatment.

Conception Initiation

For people who want to start trying to conceive but require assistance, particularly with donor gametes, it is advisable to seek consultation three to six months before they want to start trying. This allows for time to meet with the fertility specialist, discuss options, make informed choices, and complete any agreed upon testing before initiation. Of note, the Canadian Fertility and Andrology Society recommends that all people involved in third-party reproduction (including heterosexual people, single parents by choice, 2SLGBTQ people, donors, recipients, and their partners, if present) receive counselling prior to treatment.[24] This can also take time to arrange and complete but rarely more than a few months. The cost, however, does fall to the individuals involved.

After Trying to Conceive

The SOGC recommends referral for further fertility evaluation after six months of well-timed attempts at conception for people with ovaries who are 35–37 years of age and earlier for people with ovaries who are over 37 years of age.[7] For people not yet 35 years of age, it is reasonable to try up to 12 months, although referring sooner, especially if there are any risk factors for reduced fertility (such as cycle irregularity, suspicion of endometriosis, history of chlamydia or gonorrhea, family history of difficulty conceiving, or others) or if patients are expressing concerns about tracking their cycles or insemination timing, or are becoming frustrated or burnt out by the trying process. For all people, trying to conceive can be stressful, and seeking help and support from fertility specialists or counsellors when appropriate can help people navigate this important journey.

Part 6: What Patients Can Expect from a Fertility Clinic

Most importantly, when patients are seen by fertility specialists, they should expect non-discriminatory and respectful care. This is consistent with the Canadian AHRA, which states that "persons who seek to undergo assisted reproduction procedures must not be discriminated against, including on the basis of their sexual orientation or marital status."[4] Patients should also expect to be heard and have their needs and desires discussed and addressed in a professional manner.

With respect to testing, what is offered and recommended will vary according to patient needs and desires, as well as conception plans. At a minimum, fertility clinics will often require screening for HIV, hepatitis B, hepatitis C, and syphilis within 12 months of a proposed treatment date, in keeping with the standards of care within the fertility profession. Beyond this, recommended testing will vary according to patient plans and risk factors.

For people with ovaries, additional testing beyond the screening mentioned above may include blood work for rubella and varicella immunity status, additional blood work based on risk factors (i.e., ovarian reserve testing for people more than 35 years of age to help triage escalation of care), a sonohysterogram for uterine anatomy and tubal patency, and cycle monitoring. For patients who do not have risk factors for subfertility, it is very reasonable to discuss the risks and benefits of this additional testing and make an informed choice about what to pursue. For example, it is reasonable to decline a sonohysterogram if there are no risk factors for uterine or tubal pathology, but it would also be reasonable to do a sonohysterogram before undergoing insemination if the patient wishes, to ensure there are no unidentified issues, given the cost of donor sperm. Historically, 2SLGBTQ people have been required, or felt pressured, to do testing they did not desire. Primary care providers can help by supporting and advocating for their 2SLGBTQ patients when it comes to testing to ensure they are being offered comprehensive care aligned with their choices and values.

For people with sperm, additional testing may include hormonal profile testing and a semen analysis. If any concerns are identified, more specialized semen analysis testing or a scrotal ultrasound may be recommended.

In terms of costs, medical consultation and the majority of tests are covered by provincial and territorial funding programs, and some treatments including insemination are also covered. At the time of writing, Ontario is the only province or territory to fund in vitro fertilization (with some restrictions). It is important to be aware that some more specialized tests, medications and biological materials (donor sperm and eggs) are not covered by provincial health plans. Some private insurers will cover some fertility medications and costs, but this varies widely. As coverage changes over time and varies by province and territories, it is prudent to have patients call fertility centres or have a consultation (which is covered) to learn more about costs related to their specific goals and situation.

Conclusion

Increasingly, more 2SLGBTQ people and couples are having children and will seek the advice and support of their primary care providers to create their families. Being informed about the options available to help 2SLGBTQ people conceive is an important part of comprehensive care. Primary care providers are also uniquely positioned to counsel 2SLGBTQ patients early in their journeys to help preserve fertility when appropriate and to advocate for informed and sensitive care, when needed.

References

1. Statistics Canada [Internet]. Ottawa: Government of Canada; 2017 Aug 2 [cited 2018 Mar 15]. Same sex couples in Canada in 2016. Available from: http://www12.statcan.gc.ca/census-recensement/2016/as-sa/98-200 -x/2016007/98-200-x2016007-eng.cfm.
2. Corbett SL, Frecker HM, Shapiro HM, Yudin MH. Access to fertility services for lesbian women in Canada. Fertil Steril. 2013 Oct;100(4):1077–80.
3. Ross LE, Steele LS, Epstein R. Service use and gaps in services for lesbian and bisexual women during donor insemination, pregnancy, and the postpartum period. J Obstet Gynaecol Can. 2006 Jun;28(6):505–11.

4. Assisted Human Reproductive Act, S.C. 2004, C.2.
5. Eijkemans MJ, van Poppel F, Habbema DF, Smith KR, Leridon H, te Velde ER. Too old to have children? Lessons from natural fertility populations. Hum Reprod. 2014 Jun;29(6):1304–12.
6. Public Health Agency of Canada [Internet]. Ottawa: Government of Canada; 2017 [cited 2018 Mar 18]. Fertility. Available from: https://www.canada.ca/en/public-health/services/fertility/fertility.html.
7. Johnson JA, Tough S, Wilson RD, Audibert F, Blight C, Brock S JA, et al.; SOGC Genetics Committee. Delayed child-bearing. J Obstet Gynaecol Can. 2012 Jan;34(1):80–93.
8. Liu K, Case A, Cheung AP, Sierra S, AlAsiri S, Carranza-Mamane B, et al.; Reproductive Endocrinology and Infertility Committee. Advanced reproductive age and fertility. J Obstet Gynaecol Can. 2011 Nov;33(11):1165–75.
9. van der Steeg JW, Steures P, Eijkemans MJ, Habbema JD, Hompes PG, Burggraaff JM, et al. Obesity affects spontaneous pregnancy chances in subfertile, ovulatory women. Hum Reprod. 2008 Feb;23(2):324–8.
10. Rittenberg V, Seshadri S, Sunkara SK, Sobaleva S, Oteng-Ntim E, El-Toukhy T. Effect of body mass index on IVF treatment outcome: an updated systematic review and meta-analysis. Reprod Biomed Online. 2011 Oct;23(4):421–39.
11. Koning AM, Mutsaerts MA, Kuchenbecker WK, Broekmans FJ, Land JA, Mol BW, et al. Complications and outcome of assisted reproduction technologies in overweight and obese women. Hum Reprod. 2012 Feb;27(2):457–67.
12. Oliveira JB, Petersen CG, Mauri AL, Vagnini LD, Renzi A, Petersen B, et al. Association between body mass index and sperm quality and sperm DNA integrity. A large population study. Andrologia. 2018 Apr;50(3):e12889.
13. Augood C, Duckitt K, Templeton AA. Smoking and female infertility: a systematic review and meta-analysis. Hum Reprod. 1998 Jun;13(6):1532–9.
14. Homan GF, Davies M, Norman R. The impact of lifestyle factors on reproductive performance in the general population and those undergoing infertility treatment: a review. Hum Reprod Update. 2007 May-Jun;13(3):209–23.
15. Anifandis G, Bounartzi T, Messini CI, Dafopoulos K, Sotiriou S, Messinis IE. The impact of cigarette smoking and alcohol consumption on sperm parameters and sperm DNA fragmentation (SDF) measured by Halosperm(®). Arch Gynecol Obstet. 2014 Oct;290(4):777–82.
16. Park B, McPartland JM, Glass M. Cannabis, cannabinoids and reproduction. Prostaglandins Leukot Essent Fatty Acids. 2004 Feb;70(2):189–97.

17. Guzick DS, Carson SA, Coutifaris C, Overstreet JW, Factor-Litvak P, Steinkampf MP, et al.; National Cooperative Reproductive Medicine Network. Efficacy of superovulation and intrauterine insemination in the treatment of infertility. N Engl J Med. 1999 Jan;340(3):177–83.

18. Ferrara I, Balet R, Grudzinskas JG. Intrauterine insemination with frozen donor sperm. Pregnancy outcome in relation to age and ovarian stimulation regime. Hum Reprod. 2002 Sep;17(9):2320–4.

19. Klatsky P [Internet]. New York: Huffington Post; 2017 Jun 22 [cited 2018 Mar 15]. Co-maternity and reciprocal IVF: empowering lesbian parents with options. Available from: https://www.huffingtonpost.com /entry/co-maternity-and-reciprocal-ivf-empowering-lesbian _us_594b0f7be4b062254f3a5b69

20. Gidoni YS, Raziel A, Strassburger D, Kasterstein E, Ben-Ami I, Ron-El R. Can we preserve fertility in female to male transgender after long term testosterone treatment – case report. Fertil Steril. 2013;100(3):S169–70.

21. Rodriguez-Wallberg KA, Dhejne C, Stefenson M, Degerblad M, Olofsson JI. Preserving eggs for men's fertility. A pilot experience with fertility preservation for female-to-male transsexuals in Sweden. Fertil Steril. 2014;102(3 Supp):e160–1.

22. Bourns A [Internet]. Toronto: Sherbourne Health Centre; 2015 [cited 2018 Apr 3]. Guidelines and protocols for hormone therapy and primary health care for trans clients. Available from: http://sherbourne.on.ca/wp -content/uploads/2014/02/Guidelines-and-Protocols-for-Comprehensive -Primary-Care-for-Trans-Clients-2015.pdf.

23. Deutsch M [Internet]. San Francisco: University of California, San Francisco, Transgender Care 2015; [cited 2018 Apr 3]. Information on estrogen hormone therapy. Available from: https://transcare.ucsf.edu /article/information-estrogen-hormone-therapy.

24. Havelock J, Liu K, Levitan S, Petropanagos A, Lawrence K. Guidelines for third-party reproduction: Clinical practice guidelines. Dorval (QC): Canadian Fertility and Andrology Society; 2016.

11 Trans and Non-binary Health: Gender-Affirming Hormone Therapy and Primary Care

AMY BOURNS

The content of this chapter has been adapted from the 2019 Sherbourne Health *Guidelines for Gender-Affirming Primary Care with Trans and Non-binary Patients*, published by Rainbow Health Ontario.[1] These recommendations are based on 15 years of experience providing gender-affirming services in a primary care setting and a growing body of evidence to guide clinical decision making. They are meant to be applied with flexibility – adaptations may be considered in relation to an individual patient's anatomic, social, or psychological situation or according to patient or systemic resource limitations. Sherbourne Health's guidelines are updated periodically to incorporate new research and to reflect an evolution of the understanding and values of trans and non-binary communities. The guidelines also include several tools that can be used to assist providers at the point of care and have been adapted into an online interactive educational tool, "The Trans Primary Care Guide," which can be found at https://www.rainbowhealthontario.ca/TransHealthGuide/.

An Introduction to Trans and Non-binary Communities and Their Health Care

Trans and Non-binary Communities: Size, Diversity, and Language

A recent compilation of population-based surveys in the United States suggests that the number of self-identified trans people is growing and currently represents approximately 0.6 per cent of the population (as a conservative estimate), with a higher prevalence among youth.[2] The Trans PULSE Project,* which studied trans people in Ontario, Canada,

---

* Trans PULSE was a multi-year community-based research initiative that used mixed methods to better understand the health of trans communities in Ontario. The core

showed that although urban centres are often sought out by trans people wanting to access health care, approximately 70 per cent of trans Ontarians were living outside the Greater Toronto Area.[3]

Trans PULSE also revealed a very diverse patient population with respect to age, ethnicity, sexuality, income, and education. While many trans individuals were highly educated, income security was a common concern. The study also included many findings related to experiences of transphobia and violence, as well as challenges with finding a provider willing to provide gender-affirming care.[4,5] Taken as a whole, mental health and suicidality were marked concerns. Of particular significance was the finding that these problems became much less prominent for trans patients who had undergone medical (i.e., hormonal or surgical) interventions to affirm their gender identity (when medical transition was part of how an individual wanted to transition).[6]

As discussed in the chapter 1 of this text, the use of language regarding gender identity and gender expression is constantly evolving and providing concrete definitions is bound to be imperfect. With this caveat in mind, this chapter will use the term *transmasculine* to refer to patients who were assigned female at birth (or *AFAB*) but whose sense of self is of being a man or on the masculine spectrum. Similarly, the term *transfeminine* will be used to refer to patients who were assigned male at birth (or *AMAB*) but whose sense of self is of being a woman or on the feminine spectrum. Fundamental to this work is using respectful and affirming language that aligns with a patient's self-identification whenever possible. Readers are directed to the glossary of terms, as well as recommendations for improving provider-patient communication in chapters 2 and 3.

The Role of the Primary Care Provider (PCP)

Health care professionals are increasingly in consensus that trans and non-binary communities are an underserved population – one whose health care needs can be effectively addressed in the context of primary care. Accordingly, primary care providers (PCPs) have taken an increasingly important role in providing gender-affirming care to trans patients. Since PCPs usually have familiarity and a longitudinal relationship with

researchers have more recently acquired Canadian Institutes of Health Research (CIHR) funding to conduct a national study – an unparalleled opportunity to gather large-scale, robust data about the health of trans people across Canada. Preliminary findings can be found on the Trans PULSE Canada website: https://transpulsecanada.ca.

patients, they are ideally situated to facilitate and support a patient's transition process. *The Lancet*[7] identified Toronto, along with Vancouver, Boston, and Sydney, as cities where effective, comprehensive care is provided to trans patients in the context of primary care.

One of the historical barriers to providing gender-affirming care has been the absence of education about trans health in medical, nursing, and other health professional education.[8] Individual efforts are being made to incorporate gender diversity and trans-related health topics into the curriculum at a number of Canadian medical and nursing schools, but there remains no standardized curriculum or learning objectives for these programs. The historical lack of education and available resources – as well as lingering perceptions that transition-related care falls exclusively under the domain of specialists – has limited the number of PCPs working with trans patients.

While the situation is improving, the historical shortage of clinicians available to provide gender-affirming primary care has often led to trans patients experiencing protracted searches, long waitlists, or distant travel to find providers able to assist with their transition goals. Providing timely transition-related care can have a substantial positive effect on mental health, including a significant decrease in suicidality and suicide attempts.[6] Research to this effect resonates with the experience of clinicians involved in the provision of trans care and underscores the importance of timely access to gender-affirming care.

Referral to an endocrinologist may be appropriate and helpful for patients seeking gender-affirming hormone therapy, particularly in the case of a medically complex patient, but it is not required as a matter-of-course. Furthermore, outside major urban areas, an endocrinologist with experience treating trans patients may not be available, thus requiring a consultation may result in an unduly long and painful wait. If consultation is sought, it may be helpful to initiate low/initial doses of a hormone regimen until consultation can be obtained. E-consult services, if available, can be a useful source of timely input and support.

An Individualized Approach

Given the spectrum of gender identity and the variation in each person's expression, there is no single pathway for a trans person to follow to actualize the presentation of their authentic self. While hormones or surgeries are medically necessary for many trans people to create alignment with their experienced gender, for others it may be sufficient to modify their presentation through changes in legal identification and modifications to features such as dress, gait, voice, and hair.

When hormones are required as part of a transition, some patients may seek maximum feminization/masculinization, while others may seek a more androgynous appearance. Hormone therapy may also be helpful for patients who do not want to make a social transition or who are unable to do so.[9] Both the dose and route of hormone treatments may be individualized to meet a patient's specific treatment goals. The duration of therapy may also be personalized: patients who have not undergone gonadectomy, for example, may opt to discontinue hormone therapy if the irreversible changes (see discussion below) are adequate to maintain the needed presentation.

While hormone therapy is generally required before genital surgery or gonadectomy (unless contraindicated), it is not considered a requirement before breast, chest, or other gender-affirming procedures.[10] The decision to undergo surgical interventions is also highly individual.

Considerations for Non-binary Patients

Research suggests that at least 20 per cent of trans-identified people do not have a binary gender identity (see chapter 1).[11] Like other trans patients, non-binary patients may seek medical assistance with modification of primary and secondary sex characteristics. Unfortunately, lack of familiarity with non-binary identities and normative assumptions on the part of health care providers may lead to additional barriers to accessing gender-affirming treatments.[12]

Individuals who identify as non-binary have the same range of needs for and entitlement to gender-affirming hormone therapy and surgeries as binary-identified trans people. It is important to discuss with non-binary patients the desired configuration of primary and secondary sex characteristics and expectations regarding outcomes. While dose, duration, route, and type of hormone therapy can be individualized, it may not be possible to achieve certain combinations of effects (for example, a deeper voice without facial hair growth). Some non-binary people may express the need for contrasting masculine and feminine characteristics, such as breasts and facial hair to align with their experienced gender.[13]

HORMONE PLANNING AND INITIATION

The traditional model of hormone provision, which emphasizes the provider's role in assessing a patient's eligibility and readiness for hormone therapy, has been criticized for compromising patient autonomy and positioning the provider as a "gatekeeper" to treatment.[14] In response, a number of health centres in the United States* implemented in the 1990s and early 2000s what has become known as the "informed consent model" for hormone provision.

This model focuses on obtaining informed consent as the threshold for the initiation of hormone therapy, without requiring an in-depth mental health assessment or referral, unless significant mental health concerns are identified. The current version of the World Professional Association for Transgender Health (WPATH) Standards of Care (SOC-7), recognizes the validity of both the traditional and informed consent approaches to the initiation of gender-affirming hormone therapy.[10] The informed consent model should be differentiated from "hormones on demand," which implies that anyone who asks for hormones will receive a prescription in all cases, giving no scope to the expertise or judgment of the prescribing clinician.[15,16]

The approach described here is rooted in the informed consent model and considers the decision to initiate hormone therapy as a collaborative, patient-centred process that supports psychosocial preparedness. The PCP (with or without the support of a multidisciplinary team) can facilitate a decision-making process that informs, educates, and supports patients. The provider or care team takes an active role in assisting a patient in meeting their transition-related goals and addressing any existing barriers to the safe administration of hormone therapy.

Some providers may be concerned about the possibility of regret: treating a patient with hormone therapy who later realizes a preference for the gender role typically associated with the sex assigned at birth. Regardless, this is a very rare occurrence. A survey of 12 clinics in the United States (representing 1944 patients treated) operating under the informed consent model revealed a prevalence of cases of regret of 0.8 per cent, with just 0.1 per cent leading to a reversal of gender transition. No cases of malpractice claims, settlements, or judgments relating to regret were reported or found following a thorough literature review conducted as part of the same study.[17]

Providers may additionally have concerns regarding the impact of hormone therapy on a patient's physical health. There is a lack of high-quality long-term prospective studies for most trans-specific health concerns, but a number of retrospective studies from the Netherlands present some reassuring safety data.[18-21] Emerging evidence suggests

---

* Examples include Tom Waddell Health Center in San Francisco, Callen Lorde Community Health Center in New York City, and Fenway Health in Boston.

that modern hormone regimens do not have a significant negative impact on morbidity and mortality. Following a recent systematic review for the Endocrine Society, Weinand and Safer conclude "current literature suggests that hormone therapy is safe when followed carefully for certain risks," though they acknowledge the limitations associated with the lack of high-quality studies.[22]

Known risks (explored below) should be considered and mitigated when possible. For each patient seeking hormone therapy, it is important to consider not only the possible risks of treatment but the often-substantial risks of withholding treatment. In addition to experiencing adverse effects on mental health, those who are not able to access hormone therapy through a provider may opt to take hormones without a prescription (in the case of feminizing hormones, this may include less safe forms of estrogen) without monitoring, potentially putting themselves at risk.[23] Two studies pointedly illustrate that the bulk of morbidity and mortality suffered by transgender patients is related to the challenges of being trans in our society, rather than any risks of hormone therapy.[18,24]

The Hormone Planning Period

Typically, new patients are seen for a number of visits before the initiation of hormone therapy. This period allows the provider to become acquainted with the patient, provide education regarding the anticipated effects and the potential risks of hormone therapy, determine the need for services such as fertility preservation, and offer additional support if needed. The number of visits needed to complete these tasks can vary depending on the length of time available for each visit, the experience of the provider, and clinical factors. The tasks for the planning period are listed in box 11.1 and expanded upon below.

Box 11.1. Tasks for the Planning Period

- Do a general medical intake and take medical history.
- Orient to the process and explain the rationale for the planning period and follow up/monitoring.
- Obtain/review previous medical records (if the patient is new to the practice).
- Explore gender identity and expression.
- Confirm gender dysphoria/gender incongruence and exclude rare differential diagnoses.

- Discuss gender-affirming goals.
- Review expected effects (reversible versus irreversible), potential side effects, risks, and contraindications to hormone therapy.
- Explore social supports and plans for work/school, and discuss available ancillary supports as needed (counselling, peer support, etc.).
- Review lifestyle and mental health considerations.
- Perform a focused physical exam, baseline investigations, and routine health promotion/disease prevention/screening commensurate with age.
- Discuss fertility, contraception, and sexual health (fertility preservation, if a priority for the patient, should be considered before hormone initiation).
- Ensure capacity to consent.
- Discuss funding of medications and other possible transition-related costs; submit request for public funding of medication if available.
- Discuss/initiate risk mitigation if conditions exist that increase risks or side effects associated with hormone therapy.
- Discuss options and choose an initial hormone regimen.
- Provide a prescription and review follow-up plan.

Provision of hormone therapy in some cases may be undertaken without completing the usual tasks of the planning period. This is primarily under the rubric of harm reduction in situations where the delay of treatment could cause significant harm to the patient. Examples include a patient who is already using hormones without a prescription or someone who is experiencing extreme distress regarding their gender presentation.

Exploration of Gender Identity and Expression

Health care providers are not typically taught how to speak with patients about their history and experience with gender. However, it is an important part of understanding trans patients' needs and informing the discussion around the development of an individualized care plan.

Box 11.2 provides an example of questions that may be used to guide the conversation about a patient's experience of gender. Additionally, it may be helpful to explain the rationale for obtaining this history and to reassure the patient that there are no "wrong answers" nor any specific narrative that the provider is looking to hear.

Box 11.2. Possible Questions to Explore Gender Identity and Expression

- How would you describe your gender identity? *If prompting is needed:* For example, some people identify as a man, a trans man, gender-queer, etc.
- Do you remember the time when you realized that your gender was different from the one you were assigned at birth? *Or:* Do you remember when you first started to see your gender as _____?
- Can you tell me a bit about what's happened since realizing this? *If prompting is needed:* Some people find this to be a difficult realization and may not feel comfortable discussing it, while other people are fortunate to have people in their life they feel safe talking with – what was it like for you?
- Have you taken any steps to express your gender differently/to feel more comfortable in your gender? *If prompting is needed:* Some people ask others to use a different name and pronoun or make changes to their hair or clothing styles.
- *If they have taken steps to express their gender differently:* What was that like for you? How did that feel?

Source: Adapted from *Trans Care BC: Primary Care Toolkit*, October 2018.[25]

Diagnosis

The provision of hormone therapy has generally been preceded by a diagnosis of gender dysphoria (or previously gender identity disorder), as outlined in the *Diagnostic and Statistical Manual of Mental Disorders, Volume 5 (DSM-5)*.[26] Both the medical and trans communities have widely debated the appropriateness of using a psychiatric diagnosis (or a diagnosis at all) for trans individuals. The aim to destigmatize gender diversity while securing access to care has been a central dilemma in this debate.[27]

Since "transvestism" first appeared in the World Health Organization's (WHO) 8th edition of the *International Statistical Classification of Diseases and Related Health Problems (ICD-8)* in 1965, (and "transexualism" in the *DSM-III* in 1980) there has been continuous evolution of the name, criteria, and categorical placement for diagnoses describing trans experiences.[28] The revision of the diagnosis and its criteria in 2013 in the *DSM-5*[26] represented a step towards depathologizing gender difference and validating the spectrum of gender identities (see box 11.3 for criteria).

Box 11.3. The Criteria for the *DSM-5* Diagnosis of Gender Dysphoria[26]

A. A marked incongruence between one's experienced/expressed gender and assigned gender, of at least six months duration, as manifested by at least two of the following:
   1. A marked incongruence between one's experienced/expressed
      gender and primary and/or secondary sex characteristics (or in
      young adolescents, the anticipated secondary sex characteristics).
   2. A strong desire to be rid of one's primary and/or secondary sex char-
      acteristics because of a marked incongruence with one's experienced/
      expressed gender (or in young adolescents, a desire to prevent the
      development of the anticipated secondary sex characteristics).
   3. A strong desire for the primary and/or secondary sex characteris-
      tics of the other gender.
   4. A strong desire to be of the other gender (or some alternative gen-
      der different from one's assigned gender).
   5. A strong desire to be treated as the other gender (or some alterna-
      tive gender different from one's assigned gender).
   6. A strong conviction that one has the typical feelings and reactions
      of the other gender (or some alternative gender different from
      one's assigned gender).
B. The condition is associated with clinically significant distress or impairment in social, occupational or other important areas of functioning.

The WHO has taken a further step in depathologizing trans identities in its *ICD-11*, which was released in May 2019. It has renamed
the diagnosis *gender incongruence* and removed the diagnosis from the
category of mental health disorders, placing it instead in a category of
"Conditions Related to Sexual Health." Additionally, in contrast to the
DSM-5 diagnosis, there is no criteria for significant distress or impairment[29] (see box 11.4).

This change represents a concerted effort to abandon the psycho-
pathological model of trans experiences and supports the provision of
gender-affirming treatments to a wider population of trans and non-
binary people. As societal acceptance and access to supportive communities and care increases, the distress experienced by some trans people
is likely to decrease.[30] Eliminating the criteria for significant distress
or impairment as a prerequisite for treatment allows for the timely

provision of gender-affirming therapies as a preventive measure, rather than waiting for distress and impairment to manifest through the withholding of these treatments.

We advocate for the provision of gender-affirming hormone therapy to those who meet the diagnostic criteria for gender dysphoria or the description of gender incongruence. Thus, the terminology *gender dysphoria/gender incongruence* will be used in this chapter when referring to diagnoses for which hormone therapy is indicated. The term *gender dysphoria* will be used on its own when referring specifically to the discomfort/distress experienced by some trans people because of incongruence of gender.

Box 11.4. Description of Gender Incongruence in the ICD-11[29]

Gender incongruence of adolescence and adulthood is characterized by a marked and persistent incongruence between an individual's experienced gender and the assigned sex, which often leads to a desire to "transition" in order to live and be accepted as a person of the experienced gender, through hormonal treatment, surgery or other healthcare services to make the individual's body align, as much as desired and to the extent possible, with the experienced gender. The diagnosis cannot be assigned prior to the onset of puberty. Gender variant behaviour and preferences alone are not a basis for assigning the diagnosis.

In addition to establishing a diagnosis of gender dysphoria or incongruence, it is recommended that the provider work to rule out other diagnoses that may explain the presentation. Possible differential diagnoses include schizophrenia and other psychotic disorders, dissociative disorders, and body dysmorphic disorder. These diagnoses are rarely found to underlie the desire for gender-affirming treatment, but can occur and thus should be ruled out. If the presentation is unclear, obtaining the opinion of a psychiatrist is appropriate. The provider should take care to refer to a psychiatrist who has experience working with trans people whenever possible. If the presentation is clear, then consultation with psychiatry is not necessary.

Patient Expectations

One of the prescribing provider's roles is to help the patient develop reasonable expectations about treatment before it is initiated. Changes associated with hormones can be slow, and the underlying body structure will not change. Transfeminine patients will maintain shoulder and hip width and existing facial bone structure. Transmasculine patients will also maintain existing facial and body structure. Hormonal treatment of adults does not impact a person's height. Additionally, feminizing hormone therapy does not affect voice pitch in transfeminine individuals (see "Limitations to Feminizing Hormone Therapy" below). Despite a desire to, people may not easily "pass" as the gender to which they are transitioning. This can be stressful and disheartening for some people, and the possibility should be tactfully discussed by the provider.

It may be helpful to provide the patient with a copy of the estimated timelines for hormonal effects (see tables 11.2 and 11.7 later in the chapter), while emphasizing that physiologic responses to hormone therapy are highly individual. While some resources available on the Internet espouse a "more is better" approach to hormone administration, there is no evidence to support this approach.

Psychosocial Preparation and Support

Gender transition can be a phase of significant adjustment in an individual's life. Like any major life change, the aim is to enable patients with supports that facilitate healthy adjustment. Mental health counselling is not required before hormone therapy, but some patients may benefit from extra support. Support in a peer group setting (such as Gender Journeys)* can be immensely beneficial for some patients. Some patients may benefit from individual therapy with a trans-positive therapist with whom they can discuss concerns about the transition process and receive additional psychological support. Removing any requirement for the therapist to provide an "approval letter" before hormone initiation can enhance effectiveness of this support by allowing the therapeutic relationship to evolve in a more trusting and open manner.[15]

It is encouraged that patients discuss their transition with family members (including chosen family) and friends, as they too will have

---

*   Gender Journeys is an 11-week program in which individuals can explore their gender identity, learn about different aspects of social and medical transitioning, and build communities. Developed at Sherbourne Health and running since 2005, Gender Journeys groups are now offered in several cities throughout the country. Copies of the manual for this program can be downloaded free of charge from https://www.rainbowhealthontario.ca/lgbt2sq-health/resource-library/

their own reactions and be affected by the patient's transition. Asking about how transitioning might influence the vocational or educational situation of the patient is important (see box 11.5). Providers can help patients develop positive strategies for dealing with gender change in school or the workplace.[31] Unfortunately, it is not uncommon for transition to result in the loss of a job or struggle in the academic setting.[32]

In the past, WPATH advocated for a three-month period of life experience in the congruent gender role before hormone therapy. The rationale for this step was to enable the establishment of coping mechanisms for the above-mentioned social stressors. This requirement for a "real-life experience" has been shown to be both stressful and potentially dangerous, since it requires the adoption of a gender role before acquiring any physical changes commensurate with that gender. As of 2011 in WPATH SOC-7, there is no longer a requirement for a gender role experience of any duration before the provision of hormone therapy or surgical interventions, with the exception of external genital surgery.[10]

Box 11.5. Asking about Psychosocial Preparation and Supports

Questions such as these can be used to open the conversation about psychosocial preparation and supports:

- Have you thought about how you will manage the changes in your appearance and gender expression at work or school?
- Who has supported you along the way? *If they have not spoken with anyone else yet:* Who do you think might be supportive if you bring this up with them?
- Have you done anything to prepare yourself for this step? *If prompting is needed:* Have you talked with any peers or asked friends or family for support? Have you done any reading or research?
- Do you anticipate any challenges?
- Some people find it helpful to have the support of a counsellor for either decision making or ongoing support after beginning hormone therapy – would you be interested in a referral to a trans-competent counsellor?

Adapted from: Trans Care BC: Primary Care Toolkit, October 2018.[25]

Mental Health and Lifestyle Considerations

Trans patients invariably experience some degree of minority stress. Adapting Meyer's definition of this in relation to lesbian, gay, and bisexual populations,[33] minority stress in the trans population may be thought of as the chronic psychological strain resulting from stigma and expectations of rejection and discrimination, decisions about disclosure of gender identity, and the internalization of transphobia that trans people face in a cissexist society.

In addition to minority stress, many trans people are exposed to gender-based interpersonal violence, including during the formative years of childhood and adolescence.[34] Negative experiences in health care settings can further exacerbate the effects of this trauma. As a result, in addition to ensuring that they take a gender-affirming approach, it is to the benefit of trans and non-binary patients for providers to be familiar with and practise trauma-informed care. A 2018 review in *Canadian Family Physician* describes the principles of trauma-informed care and their application in primary care.[35]

Minority stress and trauma are often associated with the adoption of behaviours such as smoking and excessive substance use (see chapter 9). In addition, gender dysphoria may impact a person's relationship with their body and contribute to the risk for these behaviours. Such behaviours, particularly tobacco use, may increase the risks associated with hormone therapy. It is worthwhile for the provider and patient to work to decrease modifiable risks as much as possible, with the understanding that this is not always feasible before starting treatment, and a harm-reduction approach may be necessary.

The initiation of hormone therapy and the expectation of aligning one's body with an internal sense of gender may create an opportunity for a patient to begin to develop a new relationship with their body and initiate lifestyle changes that positively impact health. It is not uncommon for this time of transition to provide the impetus and inspiration for lasting positive lifestyle changes.

In the past, the presence of active suicidal thoughts or plans has been considered an absolute contraindication to hormone administration, particularly testosterone. However, as discussed above, Trans PULSE demonstrated higher rates of suicidality before hormone administration, with decreasing rates following access to transitional treatments.[6] Additionally, a prospective study of transmasculine participants initiating testosterone demonstrated a significant improvement in psychological functioning in multiple domains, including depressive symptoms, following three months of treatment.[36]

These findings suggest the need for a reconsideration of best practice. If a patient is in acute crisis and unable to provide informed consent, this would certainly constitute an absolute contraindication. If an acute safety issue exists, hospitalization may be necessary, and this would become the immediate priority for the PCP. However, a patient who is at risk of suicide but able to provide informed consent may benefit greatly from the initiation of hormone therapy. This can be particularly true when gender dysphoria/gender incongruence is the main source of the patient's psychological distress.

It is suggested that these types of situations are best approached on a case-by-case basis, with an assessment of the risks and benefits of hormone provision in relation to the individual patient's mental health. The best course of action may be to start the patient on low-dose therapy while strategizing around suicide risk reduction (for example, by establishing a crisis plan and connecting the patient with additional mental health supports and treatment). Providers may also consider using an ethical decision-making framework (if their organization has one) or consulting with an ethicist.

Capacity to Consent

As with any other medical intervention, patients must demonstrate an understanding of the risks and benefits of hormone treatment. Obtaining informed consent is a process that PCPs engage in daily, and when prescribing hormones to trans patients, the same basic principles apply.

Questions may arise around capacity to consent in individuals with cognitive or developmental disabilities, in those with significant mental health challenges, or in younger patients. Since there is no specific age determining when an individual is eligible to provide consent for medical interventions in Canada, it is determined on a case-by-case basis and at the discretion of the provider.[37] If there are persistent concerns regarding a patient's capacity to consent, a referral to a psychiatrist with experience working with trans people may be helpful.

Physical Exam and Baseline Investigations

A focused physical exam is recommended before the initiation of hormone therapy. The exam should include screening for conditions such as hypertension, obesity, and active liver disease, which may increase the risks of hormone therapy. Physical examination, particularly of the breast/chest and genitalia, may be uncomfortable for trans patients.

Fortunately, with the exception of STI and Pap testing (when indicated per provincial and territorial guidelines), examination of these areas is no longer recommended for routine screening.

Previously, genital examination was recommended before hormone initiation to rule out the possibility of an intersex condition; however, it is suggested that inquiry into any history suggestive of an intersex condition (i.e., ambiguous genitalia, unexpected or absence of pubertal changes), along with baseline hormone levels within expected ranges, may be sufficient. Findings suggestive of an intersex condition merit consultation with an endocrinologist before treatment.

For adolescent patients who may not have completed puberty, examination of the breast/chest and genitals is useful to establish the pubertal Tanner stage. Initial treatment options for youth who have not reached Tanner stage 5 include pubertal suppression with a GnRH analogue. If puberty is not yet complete, providing care under the guidance of an expert, or referral to a specialized clinic or another provider with expertise in supporting trans children and youth is recommended.

Inspection and measurement of the breasts to document a baseline may be helpful in the future determination of eligibility for publicly covered breast augmentation in some provinces (e.g., to be eligible for funding in Ontario, patients must have no breast growth following 12 months of estrogen therapy, unless contraindicated). Aside from interest in surgery, some patients may simply like to track changes to these measurements; however, others may find such measurements uncomfortable or intrusive.

Chapter 2 provides recommendations and discussion on minimizing potential discomfort with physical examination.

Laboratory tests are performed to identify any existing health problems such as liver dysfunction, high cholesterol, or diabetes (see tables 11.3, 11.6, and 11.10 later in the chapter). If present, these conditions should ideally be managed before or concurrently with the initiation of hormones. The values will also provide a useful baseline to help with future monitoring for endocrine changes. Measurement of hormone levels may reveal whether any exogenous hormones are being taken. Any major irregularities could also indicate an intersex condition.

Fertility and Contraception

Trans people have the same range of reproductive interests as cis people, and many are at childbearing age at the time of transition. Masculinizing and feminizing hormone therapy regimens have variable temporary and long-term impacts on fertility. Though there are numerous ways that people may create families without the use of their own gametes, many people have a wish for genetically related children. Accordingly, there is a need for discussion regarding both birth control and fertility preservation before the initiation of hormone therapy.

Patients should be counselled on options for fertility preservation before hormone initiation. If indicated, referral for fertility preservation should be initiated as soon as possible as the process may take several months. Alternatively, patients who want to conceive in the near future may opt to delay medical transition to minimize the potential need for harvesting and storing or advanced reproductive technologies (ARTs), which can be costly and involve procedures that can intensify feelings of gender dysphoria.

Trans Patients with Ova

In most cases, testosterone therapy leads to reversible amenorrhea without depletion of ovarian follicles.[38] Despite reduced fertility during testosterone administration, it should not be considered an adequate method of contraception. Given the teratogenic potential of testosterone, transmasculine patients on testosterone should be counselled on the risk of pregnancy, and those who are sexually active with people with sperm should be offered contraceptive options, such as progesterone-only contraception or an intrauterine system/device (IUS/IUD). Anecdotally, it may be easier to insert an IUS/IUD before initiating testosterone due to the subsequent atrophic changes of the vaginal and cervical tissues.

After testosterone is initiated, the provider should check with the patient periodically regarding their sexual behaviour and reiterate the necessary precautions if the patient becomes sexually active with people who produce sperm. If accidental pregnancy does occur, testosterone therapy should be discontinued immediately if maintaining the pregnancy is desired or under consideration. Counselling regarding all options, including pregnancy termination, should be provided. If termination is chosen, it may be helpful for the provider to directly contact a local abortion clinic to ensure that the patient will be received appropriately.

Little is known about the long-term effects of testosterone on ovarian function. Reassuringly, many transmasculine people have successfully conceived after discontinuing testosterone to pursue pregnancy,[39] and case studies have demonstrated a normal age-related response to ovarian stimulation following several years of testosterone therapy.[40,41] Still, given the possibility of permanent effects on fertility, patients with ova should be counselled regarding options for fertility preservation before testosterone initiation, as well as the option to delay hormone therapy. While ideally completed before starting hormones, fertility preservation can also be performed following (temporary or permanent) discontinuation of testosterone.

For additional information regarding fertility and fertility preservation in patients with ova, see chapter 10.

Trans Patients with Sperm

The administration of feminizing hormone therapy results in a reduction of testicular volume and has a suppressive effect on sperm motility and density in a cumulative, dose-dependent manner.[42] Hamada et al.[43] noted poor sperm quality in transfeminine individuals even before the initiation of hormone therapy, an effect that may be related to factors such as the practice of "tucking,"* psychological stress, undisclosed hormone use, or unidentified genetic polymorphisms.

Nonetheless, it is important to counsel transfeminine patients regarding the need for birth control if they are sexually active with partners who may become pregnant and check in periodically regarding sexual behaviour to reiterate precautions if necessary.

Patients should also be counselled regarding options for fertility preservation before starting hormones. Sperm cryopreservation following ejaculation is the simplest and most reliable form of preservation. STI screening (i.e., chlamydia, gonorrhea, HIV, syphilis, and hepatitis serologies) is required before banking, and PCPs can expedite the process for patients by completing these tests before referral. In a variety of scenarios, semen analysis can be helpful in assessing current fertility and informing options.

Testicular sperm extraction (TESE) involves the percutaneous removal of sperm from the testes or epididymis under local anaesthetic.[44] This procedure may be considered when ejaculation is overly burdensome or difficult. Resulting sperm counts are often low and thus multiple samples and/or the use of in vitro fertilization or intracytoplasmic sperm injection may be required.[38] Patients with sperm may also attempt conception or undergo fertility preservation following the suspension of hormone therapy for three to six months since testicular function may recover to a variable degree.[45] TESE and ART

---

* Tucking refers to the process of concealing the penis and scrotum so that they are not conspicuous through clothing. One common method involves "tucking" the genitalia back between the legs and binding along the perineum and/or between the buttocks.

can be useful in overcoming reduced fertility secondary to hormone therapy.

See chapter 10 for additional information regarding fertility and fertility preservation in patients with sperm.

Feminizing Hormone Therapy

The goal of hormone therapy in transfeminine patients is to reduce the endogenous effects of testosterone and to induce feminine secondary sex characteristics in keeping with the patient's individual goals. Most commonly, this requires the suppression of endogenous androgens and the addition of estrogen.

This treatment results in both reversible and irreversible feminization. General effects such as reduction in muscle mass, reduction of body and (to a lesser extent) facial hair, and changes in skin, as well as sweat and odour patterns, are reversible. Changes in facial and body subcutaneous fat distribution are generally considered reversible effects but to some degree may not be. Sexual and gonadal effects, including changes in libido and reduction in erectile function, are generally considered reversible, while reduced testicular and prostatic size, sperm count reduction, and the resulting impact on fertility may be irreversible.[45] Breast development is considered irreversible and would require surgical intervention to reverse.

Anti-androgens

Treatment with physiologic doses of estrogen alone is not usually sufficient to suppress testosterone levels into the physiologic female range in transfeminine patients who have not undergone gonadectomy.[19] Because of the potential for adverse effects with higher doses of estrogen (discussed below), androgen-suppressing agents are used as part of a feminizing regimen in transfeminine patients with gonads.

The anti-androgens most commonly used in Canada are spironolactone and cyproterone. Spironolactone is a potassium-sparing diuretic, which acts as an anti-androgen at higher doses through direct blockade of peripheral androgen receptors. It also exerts secondary suppressive effects on androgen synthesis and has weak estrogenic and progestational activity. Given that its primary mechanism of action is at the receptor level, it will not always cause a significant change in blood testosterone levels. As a result, effectiveness should be evaluated by a patient's reported response (i.e., absence of spontaneous arousal, slowing of facial and body hair growth, skin changes) rather than serum levels.

Cyproterone is a synthetic steroid with progestin-like activity. Like spironolactone, it exerts anti-androgenic effects by binding to androgen receptors. In addition, its progestational activity exerts negative feedback on testosterone production through a reduction in gonadotropins. Anecdotally, cyproterone has been shown to be a more potent anti-androgen than spironolactone, with more rapid effects and a more marked suppression of libido and erectile function.

In the absence of sufficient data to guide a preferential choice of one anti-androgen over another, the decision can be made individually with each patient based on medical history and preference regarding risk and side effect profiles (see table 11.1).

Table 11.2 shows the starting/low, customary, and maximum doses for spironolactone and cyproterone. Generally, spironolactone can be started at 50 mg once daily, and increased every two to four weeks or more barring negative effects. Doses can be divided twice daily, or given once daily in the morning (for those who experience problematic nocturia) or at night (for those who have concerns around daytime bathroom safety). Total daily doses up to 300 mg/day have been used but are rarely required.

Cyproterone can be initiated at 12.5 mg and increased by 12.5 mg every two to four or more weeks (to a rare maximum of 50 mg) if required. Lower doses or less frequent dosing (e.g., one-quarter of a 25 mg tablet twice weekly, one-eighth of a 25 mg tablet every other day) have been used with success for patients who wish to maintain sexual function or minimize other side effects. Time intervals for dose titration should take into consideration existing medical conditions, blood work results, and individual transition-related goals.

If an adequate response is not achieved with maximum doses of the initially chosen agent, or side effects prohibit titration to adequate effect, a trial of the alternative agent is indicated (in the absence of contraindications). When discontinuing spironolactone, consider a taper in patients with hypertension or renal dysfunction, with monitoring of blood pressure and volume status.

Table 11.3 displays the monitoring parameters for both spironolactone and cyproterone. Note that additional parameters are required after estrogen is initiated (see table 11.6 later in the chapter).

If contraindications exist or if intolerance is a concern for both spironolactone and cyproterone, GnRH analogues (leuprolide or busrelin) may be considered. GnRH analogues flood the pituitary gland's GnRH receptors, leading to a downregulation of the response to endogenous GnRH and sustained suppression of luteinizing hormone (LH) and follicle-stimulating hormone (FSH) release. In the absence

Table 11.1. Effects, Side Effects, and Contraindications of Anti-androgens

	Spironolactone	Cyproterone
Drug Effects	Breast growth* Reduced erectile function[†] Decreased fertility[†] Reduced prostatic and testicular volume[†] Slowed growth of facial/body hair Decreased androgenic alopecia	Breast growth* Reduced erectile function[†] Decreased fertility[†] Reduced prostatic and testicular volume[†] Slowed growth of facial/body hair Decreased androgenic alopecia
Side Effects	Hyperkalemia Renal impairment Polyuria, polydipsia, risk of dehydration Hypotension, orthostasis, dizziness Somnolence Gastrointestinal side effects Rash	Liver enzyme elevation Hepatotoxicity (acute liver failure, rare) Depression, especially in first 6–8 weeks Possible increased risk of VTE CBC changes: anemia, thrombocytosis, myelosuppression (rare) Prolactinemia (esp. with estrogen), possible increased risk of prolactinoma
Contraindications	Renal insufficiency Addison's disease or other conditions associated with hyperkalemia (type IV tubular acidosis) Hyperkalemia Avoid concomitant use of ACE inhibitors, ARBs, other potassium-sparing diuretics (if concomitant use is not avoidable, use with caution; consider low dose, slow titration and frequent monitoring because of the high risk of hyperkalemia) trimethoprim-sulfamethoxazole potassium supplements eplerenone, heparin, low molecular weight heparin	Active liver disease and hepatic dysfunction Severe renal insufficiency Severe chronic depression (caution in all patients with a history of depression) Previous or existing liver tumours Presence or history of meningioma Existing thromboembolic process Avoid concomitant use of hepatotoxic medications

ACE = angiotensin converting enzyme, ARB = angiotensin II receptor blocker, CBC = complete blood count, VTE = venous thromboembolism

* Irreversible

[†] May be irreversible

Table 11.2. Options and Recommended Doses of Anti-androgens in Feminizing Therapy

	Starting/Low Dose	Usual Dose	Maximum Dose
Spironolactone (oral)	50 mg daily to 2x/day	100 mg 2x/day	150 mg 2x/day*
Cyproterone (oral)	12.5 mg (¼ 50 mg tab) every second day or daily	12.5 mg (¼ 50 mg tab) to 25 mg (½ 50 mg tab) daily	50 mg daily*

* Rarely required or used. Maximal effect does not necessarily require maximal dosing. Use clinical judgment in selecting optimal individual dosing.

Table 11.3. Recommended Parameters for Monitoring Anti-androgen Therapy

		Baseline*	3–6 Months	12 Months
Spironolactone	History	Screen for contraindications/ potential drug interactions	Side effects (polyuria, orthostasis), desired effects	
	PE	I _____BP _____ I +/– Breast inspection[†] (baseline)		
	Key labs	Cr, lytes, total testosterone	Cr, lytes, total testosterone	Cr, lytes, total testosterone
Cyproterone	History	Screen for contraindications/ potential drug interactions	Side effects (depression, low energy), desired effects	
	PE	Wt, BP, +/– breast inspection[†]	Wt, BP, abdominal exam	
	Key labs	CBC, AST/ALT, Cr, lytes, total testosterone	CBC,[‡] AST/ ALT, total testosterone, Cr, lytes	CBC,[‡] AST/ALT, total testosterone, fasting glucose or HbA1c, lipid profile, +/– Cr, lytes[§]

Note. Additional parameters required with estrogen as per table 11.6; pre-existing conditions or risk factors may require earlier/more frequent monitoring of specific parameters.

AST = aspartate sminotransferase, ALT = alanine aminotransferase, BP = blood pressure, CBC = complete blood count , Cr = creatinine, HbA1c = glycosylated hemoglobin

* If not done in the preceding 3 months

[†] Inspection and measurement of the breasts to document a baseline may be helpful in the future determination of eligibility for publicly covered breast augmentation (available in some provinces).

[‡] Red blood cell parameters can be expected to decrease with androgen blockade, female reference ranges for lower limits of normal should be used.

[§] Necessary only if risks/concerns identified

of stimulation by these gonadotropins, endogenous sex hormone production by the gonads ceases. GnRH analogues are commonly used for pubertal suppression in trans youth and have also been used in adults (in some European regimens) undergoing gender-affirming hormone therapy.[46,47]

Drawbacks include high cost, repeat (often painful) injections or frequent nasal spray dosing, and possible side effects, including headache, mood changes, and weight gain. If providers lack experience with the use of GnRH analogues, consultation or communication with an endocrinologist or another experienced provider before initiation is recommended.

Finasteride is a less effective anti-androgen and is generally not recommended for this purpose,[48] although it may be considered for those who desire very mild anti-androgenic effects (dose range 1–5 mg daily). Finasteride is commonly added to a feminizing regimen for those who continue to exhibit scalp hair loss on a standard feminizing hormone regimen (usually 1 mg daily or one-quarter of a 5 mg tab daily), though its benefit in this setting of already suppressed androgenic activity has not been firmly established. It should also be noted that there are reports of permanent sexual dysfunction with the use of finasteride for scalp hair loss in cis men.

If the administration of anti-androgens is problematic, another option is the removal of the major source of endogenous testosterone, that is, orchiectomy. For transfeminine patients who are unable to access or are not seeking vaginoplasty (as a part of which orchiectomy is routinely performed), orchiectomy alone is a choice that may be considered. For the vast majority of transfeminine patients who have undergone gonadectomy, androgen suppression will no longer be required. The androgen-blocker can be stopped immediately after surgery or tapered over four to six weeks or more post-operatively.

In some cases, the effects of anti-androgens may be sought without the additional feminizing effects of estrogen, or when estrogen is contraindicated. In addition to potential hot flashes, low mood, and fatigue, there may be a loss of bone mineral density, akin to that demonstrated in cis men who have undergone long-term androgen blockade without hormone replacement for the treatment of prostate cancer.[49] This treatment may, however, be considered in some circumstances, following detailed discussion with the patient, and with preventive measures and monitoring for bone loss in place. Periodic bone mineral density testing for those on prolonged monotherapy with an anti-androgen can be used to identify any concerning loss of bone density.

Estrogen

Estrogens act directly on estrogen receptors to initiate feminization. The effects and expected time course of a standard regimen consisting of an anti-androgen and estrogen are shown in table 11.4. The degree and rate of physical effects are largely dependent on patient-specific factors such as age, genetics, and body habitus, and to some extent the dose and route used, selected according to a patient's specific goals and risk profile.[50]

There is a lack of consensus among providers on the preferred timing of the initiation of estrogens in relation to an anti-androgen. Common approaches have included both the initiation of an anti-androgen prior (usually one to three months) to the addition of estrogen, or alternatively, the simultaneous introduction and subsequent titration of both components.

Several forms and routes of estrogen have been used for feminization. Current formulations, along with recommended doses, can be found in table 11.5. The most common form used is oral 17-β estradiol (Estrace).[46] While conjugated estrogens (e.g., Premarin) have historically been used because of their accessibility and affordability, they are no longer recommended. Disadvantages include ethical concerns (in obtaining equine estrogens), inability to readily measure levels in the bloodstream, and implications for increased cardiovascular and thromboembolic risk.[13]

Oral formulations are subject to first-pass gastrointestinal (GI) and liver metabolism which, according to the "first-pass hypothesis," contribute to negative hepatic and prothrombotic effects.[54] Sublingual, transdermal, and injectable routes all bypass this stage during which much estradiol is oxidized to the less potent estrone.

The administration of estrogen via the sublingual route has gained interest in recent years given its accessibility (oral formulations of micronized estradiol can be dissolved under the tongue), affordability (compared to the transdermal route), and the proposed benefits of bypassing first-pass metabolism.

A study comparing oral and sublingual single-dose pharmacokinetics of micronized 17-β estradiol in postmenopausal cis women demonstrated rapid absorption with sublingual dosing, followed by a rapid fall in serum levels over the first six hours.[55] It has been noted that this may more closely mimic natural ovarian estrogen secretion.[13] Sublingual dosing also demonstrated lower circulating ratios of estrone to estradiol, higher peak estradiol levels (up to 13-fold over corresponding oral at a 1 mg dose), and higher 24-hour area under the curve for

Table 11.4. Effects and Expected Time Course of Feminizing Hormones

Effect	Expected Onset*	Expected Maximum Effect*
Body fat redistribution	3–6 months	2–3 years
Decreased muscle mass/strength	3–6 months	1–2 years[†]
Softening of skin/decreased oiliness	3–6 months	Unknown
Decreased libido	1–3 months	3–6 months
Decreased spontaneous erections	1–3 months	3–6 months
Erectile dysfunction	Variable	Variable
Breast growth	3–6 months	1–2 years
Decreased testicular volume	3–6 months	2–3 years
Decreased sperm production	Unknown	>3 years
Thinned/slowed growth of body/facial hair	6–12 months	>3 years[‡]
Scalp hair loss stops, no regrowth	1–3 months	Variable

* Estimates represent unpublished clinical and published observations[51–53]

[†] Significantly dependent on amount of exercise

[‡] Complete removal of male facial and body hair requires electrolysis, laser treatment, or both

Source: Adapted from Hembree et al. 2017, *The Endocrine Treatment of Gender Dysphoric/Gender Incongruent Persons: An Endocrine Society Guideline.*[48]

estradiol, which the authors postulate may translate into greater physiologic action.[55] The rapid peaks and increased periodicity may make monitoring serum levels more difficult.

While it is theoretically plausible that higher peak levels and increased periodicity may lead to increased risks (and unwanted side effects), there are no data yet that demonstrate any harm[48] or establish how potential harms may be offset by possible benefits. Thus, while further studies are needed, sublingual dosing may have benefits over oral dosing, and could be considered as an alternative to switching to injections or the addition of a progestin when patients are dissatisfied with their degree of feminization and are seeking to explore alternative strategies.

Similar to the sublingual route, injectable estrogens bypass first-pass metabolism and result in higher peaks and increased periodicity over oral forms.

Injectable estrogen (in the form of estradiol valerate compounded for intramuscular (IM) injection) is available through some compounding pharmacies. A single-dose pharmacokinetic study of IM estradiol valerate demonstrated peak levels at three to five days with an average half-life of four to five days.[56] Similar pharmacokinetics were demonstrated in a single study of subcutaneously injected estradiol.[57] Physiologic levels are attained through weekly or biweekly administration, which some patients prefer over daily oral dosing. There have been anecdotal reports of an acceleration in breast development following a switch to injectable from oral estradiol, but no outcome studies have been done. Challenging this observation, a recent study found no association between serum estradiol levels and breast development (though only oral and transdermal forms were used).[58]

If patients want to self-inject, it is important to instruct them on the technique for safe injection and sharps disposal. Directly observing a patient self-inject makes it possible to correct any issues with technique. A written step-by-step guide on self-injection for patients is available from Fenway Health.[59]

Transdermal estradiol bypasses first-pass metabolism, results in relatively steady serum levels, and seems to have the best overall safety profile. Notably, studies of transdermal estradiol in menopausal cis women suggest no increased risk of venous thromboembolism (VTE),[60] and the improved safety profile is also reflected in studies in transfeminine patients.[18,61] Because of this, transdermal estradiol is recommended preferentially for transfeminine patients who are over 40 or who have risk factors for cardiovascular (CV) or thromboembolic disease. It is most commonly administered in the form of the estradiol patch (Estradot), which is available from most pharmacies but is unfortunately more expensive than oral forms.

Other transdermal options include creams and gels. Estradiol creams are only available via compounding. Gel is available in a product formulated for the treatment of menopausal cis women (Estragel), however the area of skin needed for absorption of the gel is quite large, even for low/starting doses, so it is not a first choice for most trans patients. Cream and gel formulations may be effective for some transfeminine patients, but physiologic estrogen levels may be difficult to achieve in others. Again, these transdermal forms are expensive. Note that specific details and dosing of compounded formulations should be discussed with the compounding pharmacist.

Reducing estrogen dosing is not required post-operatively,[13] but some patients may find that a lower dose suffices to maintain desired feminization in the absence of any endogenous testosterone. Consideration should be given to bone mineral density in agonadal patients on low dose estrogen (see "Osteoporosis and BMD Screening").

Table 11.5. Formulations and Recommended Doses of Estrogen for Feminizing Hormone Therapy

	Starting Dose	Usual Dose	Maximum Dose
Estradiol (oral)	1–2 mg daily	4 mg daily or 2 mg 2x/day	6 mg daily or 3 mg 2x/day
Estradiol (transdermal, patch)*	50 mcg daily/apply patch 2x/week	Variable	200 mcg daily/apply patches 2x/week†
Estradiol (transdermal, gel)‡	2.5 g daily (2 pumps, contains 150 mcg estradiol)	Variable	6.25 g daily (5 pumps, contains 375 mcg estradiol), may be limited by surface area requirements for gel application
Estradiol valerate injectable§	3–4 mg weekly or 6–8 mg every 2 weeks	Variable	10 mg every week‖

* Estradot brand

† 200 mcg daily given as two 100 mcg patches applied twice weekly (4 patches/week)

‡ Estragel brand

§ Estradiol valerate IM must be prepared by a compounding pharmacy, opened multi-use vials should be discarded after 28 days

‖ Given as 1 mL of 10 mg/mL estradiol valerate

Progestins

With the exception of cyproterone, the use of progestins in transfeminine patients continues to be controversial.[48] Progestins have a suppressive effect on LH, and therefore on testosterone production, and have at times been used as part of feminizing regimens for transfeminine patients. There have also been anecdotal reports of improved breast and/or areolar development, mood, sleep, and libido with the use of progestins.[62,63] However, a clear impact has yet to be demonstrated.

Progestins have a role in histologic differentiation during breast development and lactation in cis women; however, it is uncertain whether progestins add to breast volume in this population. A 2014 review of the literature regarding the effects of cross-sex hormone therapy on breast development in transfeminine patients identified a small number of low-quality studies that addressed the topic. The authors concluded that there was no evidence to suggest that progestins enhanced breast development. However, the absence of such an effect was not able to be definitively confirmed.[62]

In addition to weight gain and edema, depression is an often-cited side effect of progestins. Anecdotally, some patients may experience a favourable impact on mood, while others may experience negative effects.[54,61] Some protocols have suggested the adjunctive use of progestins when traditional treatments don't achieve adequate androgen suppression, while others suggest a trial of a progestin as an option for transfeminine patients with low libido.[25]

The use of progestins in feminizing hormone therapy has traditionally been avoided by many centres based on harms demonstrated in the Women's Health Initiative study.[64] However, the University of California San Francisco (UCSF) Center for Excellence in Transgender Health cautions against the direct application of these data to transfeminine patients.[13] Thus, while not routinely recommended, a trial may be considered in certain circumstances following a frank discussion of expectations, side effects, and potential risks.

Micronized bio-identical progesterone, Prometrium (100–200 mg daily), is chosen preferentially over medroxyprogesterone acetate Provera (5–20 mg daily), because of a preferable safety profile. Injected depo-medroxyprogesterone acetate, Depo-Provera, is seldom used in transfeminine patients. If a progestin is prescribed, some clinicians advise limiting the treatment duration to a maximum of two to three years, or the use of cyclical dosing (i.e., administered 10 days per month).[65]

Special Considerations for Older Transfeminine Patients

There is little information in the literature to guide recommendations for the initiation or maintenance of feminizing hormone regimens in older transfeminine patients. Unique considerations in older populations include changes in endogenous hormone levels, physiologic changes that may affect response to medications, a higher burden of existing medical conditions, and multiple pre-existing medications leading to the increased potential for drug interactions.

It is not uncommon for transfeminine patients to seek to initiate hormone therapy at older ages.[66] Feminizing effects may be slower and more subtle for those initiating therapy at an advanced age. Despite this, a large number of transfeminine patients have initiated hormone therapy at advanced ages with an acceptable degree of safety and satisfaction. There is no reason to withhold hormone therapy from elderly patients simply because of age.[67] For some older transfeminine patients who have had to delay transition until later in life, maximizing feminization may take precedence over concerns about risk. For such patients, an "active period" of treatment with doses used for younger patients may be considered following a thorough discussion of risks and benefits.

For transfeminine patients over 50, it is reasonable to mimic physiologic hormone levels in menopausal cis women, which can usually be attained with estrogen doses typically administered to post-menopausal cis women (e.g., starting/low-dose topical formulations). For those with gonads, required anti-androgen doses may also be lower because of age-related decreases in serum testosterone. The preferential use of spironolactone in older transfeminine patients (with healthy renal function) has been suggested given the possible increased thromboembolic risk associated with cyproterone.[67]

For those over age 50 who have been on feminizing hormone therapy for some time, some guidelines suggest considering complete discontinuation of hormone therapy. However, those without gonads will likely experience symptoms akin to menopause along with potential loss of bone mineral density, and those with gonads may experience a return of virilization.[13]

As with all trans patients, decisions about hormone therapy should be individualized following a thorough discussion of risks and benefits.

Monitoring and Dose Adjustments

Standard monitoring of a feminizing regimen should be employed at 3, 6, and 12 months (additionally, creatinine and electrolytes should be checked between four- and six-weeks following initiation of spironolactone and change in dosage). Some providers prefer to see patients monthly until an effective dose is established. Follow-up visits should include a functional inquiry, targeted physical exam, blood work, and health promotion and disease prevention counselling, as indicated.

Functional inquiry should include subjective positive or negative impacts on mental health, as well as any noted physiologic changes. It may be helpful to remind patients that changes related to androgen blockade and estrogen administration may take months to years for full effect.

The first changes will likely be loss of spontaneous and morning arousal. Breast development, skin and hair changes, and fat redistribution take longer. Some patients may experience a small amount of physiologic galactorrhea early in the course of treatment. If galactorrhea is from more than one duct or bilateral, and non-bloody, no further workup is warranted.

Generally, physical changes are considered to be complete after two to three years on hormone therapy (see table 11.4). Periodically, the clinician should counsel around monitoring for signs and symptoms of VTE, particularly in those at increased risk. Patients should also be reminded about the importance of adequate calcium and vitamin D intake. Examination should be focused and minimally include blood pressure and weight. Inspection and measurement of the breasts following 12 months of a feminizing regimen (and comparison to baseline) is indicated in those seeking publicly funded breast augmentation to determine whether eligibility criteria have been met (available only in some provinces; criteria vary by province). Blood work should be completed according to table 11.6, with more frequent monitoring as deemed necessary if concerns are identified.

Dose titration of anti-androgen and estrogen may be performed over three to six months or more and will depend on patient goals, physical response, measured serum hormone levels, and other lab results. Titration schedules vary between clinicians and can be tailored to individual patient needs and variables.

Hormone levels for those seeking a more androgynous appearance may intentionally be mid-range between male and female norms. For many transfeminine patients, the goal will be to achieve the suppression of testosterone into the female range. Be mindful that patients may experience clinically relevant results without total suppression of testosterone because of the peripheral androgen blockade, which is not measured.

In the vast majority of cases, the measurement of total testosterone (rather than both total and free) is adequate to assess the degree of androgen suppression. Measurements and calculated estimates of free testosterone are imprecise and generally don't add value. In rare cases, the calculation of free or bioavailable testosterone may be helpful for fine-tuning hormone regimens – for example where there is persistent virilization despite a total testosterone in the female range.[13]

Serum estradiol levels should also be monitored. The Endocrine Society guidelines recommend serum estradiol levels be maintained "at the level for premenopausal females (100 to 200 pg/mL),"[48] which corresponds approximately to 370 to 735 pmol/L. Again, it is important to keep in mind that clinical effects are the goal of therapy, not specific lab values. Anecdotally, we have found that most patients

Table 11.6. Recommended Blood Work for Monitoring Feminizing Hormone Therapy

Test	Baseline	4–6 Weeks	3 Months	6 Months	12 Months‖	Yearly	According to Guidelines for Cis Patients or Provider Discretion
CBC*	X		x	x	X	x	
ALT/AST†	X		x	x	X	x	X
Creatinine/lytes‡	X	X	x	x	x	x	
Hba1c or fasting glucose	X				X		X
Lipid profile	X				X		X
Total testosterone	X		X	X	X	X	
Estradiol	X		X	X	X	X	
Prolactin§	X				x	x	X
Other	Hep B, C						
	Consider: HIV, syphilis, and other STI screening as indicated, frequency depending on risk						

Notes. In this table, smaller and lighter grey x's indicate parameters that are measured under particular circumstances. Individual parameters should be considered more frequently if concerns are identified or existing risk factors are present.

AST = aspartate sminotransferase, ALT = alanine aminotransferase, CBC = complete blood count, HbA1c = glycosylated hemoglobin

* At baseline for all, and regularly with cyproterone; for Hb/Hct use female reference for lower limit of normal and male reference for upper limit of normal

† At baseline for all and regularly with cyproterone; otherwise repeat once at 6–12 months then as needed

‡ Cr, lytes should be monitored at each visit with spironolactone, but is only required at baseline and then once between 6–12 months with cyproterone unless risk factors or concerns re: renal disease are present, use male reference range for upper limit of normal for Cr

§ Prolactin should be monitored at least yearly with the use of cyproterone and more frequently if elevation is noted

‖ During first year of treatment only

reach considerable feminization at estradiol levels between 200 and 500 pmol/L.

For those on injectable (or sublingual) estrogen, levels taken at peak may be expected to exceed recommended targets. For monitoring injectable estrogen, most guidelines recommend checking serum levels at mid-cycle, while some clinicians prefer to measure at trough (i.e., just before the next injection is due). The latter adds convenience for patients who prefer to come into clinic for their injections. There may also be utility in varying the timing of blood work to gather information regarding serum levels throughout the cycle (peak, mid-cycle and trough), especially if a patient is reporting cyclic symptoms (e.g., hot flashes, headaches, fatigue). In such cases, wide fluctuations should prompt consideration of increased frequency of injections or a route with less periodicity.[13]

If the sex marker associated with the patient's health card has not been changed, the reported reference ranges will refer to the sex assigned at birth. As reference ranges vary between laboratories, it is important to be able to refer to reference ranges for the affirmed gender from the specific laboratory. These can often be found on laboratory websites or can be obtained by request from the lab.

Limitations to Feminizing Hormone Therapy

In the vast majority of cases, hormone levels in the female range can be achieved fairly readily if that is the goal. Yet the physiologic results in transfeminine patients may not meet a patient's hopes and expectations for feminization, and some may experience ongoing dysphoria or dissatisfaction. These limitations to feminizing hormone therapy should be reviewed with patients before initiation to minimize disappointment from unachievable expectations.

Feminizing therapy does not affect the pitch of the voice in transfeminine patients. Some patients may benefit from voice therapy with a qualified and supportive speech and language therapist who can work with the patient to modify their vocal characteristics. Obtaining publicly covered services can be challenging, though many private drug plans will cover voice therapy with a note from the PCP. A variety of surgical techniques have also been used to feminize the voice by altering the vocal cords. These procedures are also not publicly covered and carry risks for vocal and other complications, though some patients may benefit from these procedures if vocal therapy has not produced satisfactory changes.

Although feminizing therapy slows the rate of growth of hair on the face and neck, it does not eliminate it. Plucking, waxing, or depilatory chemicals are temporary measures, therefore many patients will seek permanent hair reduction by laser hair removal or electrolysis. Both of these techniques can be painful, require multiple sessions and may require lifelong treatment for sustained effect. Unfortunately, these procedures can be costly and are not publicly covered.

Additionally, feminizing hormone therapy does not affect the underlying bony structure of the face. Some softening of the facial features (possibly through fat redistribution) has been anecdotally reported by patients. Some transfeminine individuals may desire facial feminization surgery; however, this procedure is not publicly covered.

Breast growth is an aspect of feminization that is very important to many transfeminine patients. Unfortunately, many women will be dissatisfied with their degree of breast development. Though likely dependant on many factors such as genetics, body habitus and age, a 2014 review of the literature by Wierckx et al. found that most transfeminine patients experienced modest breast development (average cup size less than A, or developmental Tanner stage 2 to 3).[62] A recent multicentre prospective cohort study of transfeminine patients on various hormone regimens found that the majority of breast development occurred during the first six months of treatment, and by the end of the one-year study period most women had AAA cup size or smaller, while only 3.6 per cent obtained a cup size greater than A.[58]

Both Wierckx's review[62] and the cohort study[58] found that neither type nor dosage of estrogen had an effect on final breast size, with the latter study further establishing no relationship between serum estradiol levels and breast development after one year. As discussed above, there is no evidence to support that progestins confer any benefit.[62] The extent to which the degree of testosterone suppression may affect breast development is unknown. Research to date examining factors impacting breast development in transfeminine patients is scarce and of low quality. More research is needed to guide recommendations in regards to this aspect of feminizing therapy.

Precautions and Risk Mitigation with Estrogen Therapy

Many providers new to trans care have concerns about the safety of estrogen, particularly with respect to CV/VTE events and malignancies. As more evidence emerges on modern feminizing regimens, fears of a significant negative impact on morbidity and mortality are being set aside. Following a recent comprehensive review of the literature, Weinand and Safer concluded that the compiled evidence suggests feminizing therapy for transgender individuals is "safe without a large risk of adverse events when followed carefully for a few well-documented medical concerns,"[22] which will be reviewed in more detail below.

Pre-existing medical conditions and risk factors may increase risks with estrogen administration and should be considered to enable individualized discussions with patients regarding their unique risks and benefits of treatment. Available measures to reduce associated risks (see table 11.7 and expanded discussion below) should be considered and discussed with patients, and, if possible, undertaken before or concurrently with the initiation of hormone therapy. In some cases, patients may want to begin hormone therapy in the setting of ongoing increased risk, that is, immitigable risk or having declined measures for risk mitigation. In these situations, a careful informed consent process should be undertaken, considering individual capacity to make an informed decision, the severity of potential harms from treatment, and the harms that may result from not pursuing treatment.

The initiation of feminizing hormone therapy should ideally be done in collaboration with relevant specialists who may already be involved in a patient's care. In some cases, a new referral may be helpful in informing decisions about risks and their mitigation. However, efforts should be taken to ensure that this does not cause undue delay. If accessibility to a specialist is limited, an e-consult can be both timely and beneficial.

There are a small number of contraindications to estrogen:

- unstable ischemic CV disease
- estrogen-dependent cancer
- end-stage chronic liver disease
- psychiatric conditions that limit the ability to provide informed consent
- hypersensitivity to one of the components of the formulation

Specific Conditions: Risk Mitigation and Long-Term Preventive Care

VENOUS THROMBOEMBOLISM (VTE)
Historically, studies on transfeminine patients have revealed a significant increase in thromboembolic events with estrogen administration, with the highest risk during the first year of treatment. Potential variables affecting the risk of VTE in transfeminine patients include type, route, and dose of estrogen; selection of anti-androgen; the use of progestin; and pre-existing risk factors.

Many of the patients in the original studies evaluating thromboembolic risk were taking ethinyl estradiol, which is now known to be significantly more thrombogenic than estradiol.[18] Studies on menopausal

Table 11.7. Precautions with Estrogen Therapy and Considerations in Minimizing Associated Risks

Precaution to Estrogen Therapy	Considerations in Minimizing Associated Risks
Strong family history of abnormal clotting	Rule out genetic clotting disorder, if affected see "hypercoagulable state," consider transdermal route of administration, consider spironolactone as preferred anti-androgen
Metabolic syndrome	Dietary and medical management of component disorders, consider cardiac stress test, consider transdermal route of administration
Severe, refractory, or focal migraine*	Consider referral to neurology, consider daily migraine prophylaxis, ensure all other cerebrovascular risk factors are optimized, consider transdermal route of administration, consider spironolactone as preferred anti-androgen
Seizure disorder	Consider referral to neurology, consult with a pharmacist re: possible estrogen interaction with anticonvulsant medication
Other cardiac disease	Consider referral to cardiology
Hyperprolactinemia	Determine etiology and manage as indicated, if prolactin > 80 mcg/L or symptomatic: rule out prolactinoma, refer to endocrinology as needed, consider spironolactone as preferred anti-androgen
History of benign intracranial hypertension	Consider referral to neurology/neurosurgery
Hepatic dysfunction	Dependent on etiology, e.g., minimize alcohol consumption, weight loss in NAFLD, consider referral to hepatology/gastroenterology, use transdermal, sublingual, or injectable route of administration, consider spironolactone as preferred anti-androgen
Strong family history of breast cancer	Refer to genetics/familial breast cancer program for further risk stratification and genetic testing as indicated
Prior history of estrogen-sensitive cancer	Refer to oncology
Autoimmune conditions (e.g., RA, MS, IBD)	Start low dose, titrate slowly in collaboration with any involved specialists
Personal or family history of porphyria (rare)	Consider referral to porphyria clinic or internist with experience in porphyria
Stable ischemic cardiovascular disease*	Consider referral to cardiology, ensure optimal medical (including prophylactic antiplatelet agent(s) if indicated per national guidelines) and/or surgical management as indicated, risk factor optimization, use transdermal route of administration +/− lower dose, consider spironolactone as preferred anti-androgen

Precaution to Estrogen Therapy	Considerations in Minimizing Associated Risks
Cerebrovascular disease*	Consider referral to neurology, ensure optimal medical management (including prophylactic antiplatelet agent(s) if indicated per current national guidelines) and risk factor optimization, use transdermal route of administration +/– lower dose
Hypercoagulable state or personal history of DVT or PE	Identify and minimize existent risk factors, prophylactic anti-coagulation if indicated per current national guidelines, consider referral to hematology/thrombosis clinic, use transdermal route of administration +/– lower dose, consider spironolactone as preferred anti-androgen
Marked hypertriglyceridemia	Identify and address barriers to optimal lipid control, refer to dietitian, minimize alcohol consumption, consider antilipemic pharmacologic therapy, consider endocrinology referral, use transdermal route of administration
Uncontrolled high blood pressure	Identify and address barriers to optimal BP control, use spironolactone as preferred anti-androgen, add additional antihypertensives as needed (avoid ACEs/ARBs with spironolactone), consider cardiac stress test, consider transdermal route of administration, consider referral to cardiology
Uncontrolled diabetes	Identify and address barriers to optimal glycemic control, refer to dietitian, encourage lifestyle modification, initiate antiglycemic agent(s) per national guidelines, consider cardiac stress test, consider transdermal route of administration
Smoker	Encourage and support smoking cessation, consider referral to smoking cessation program/offer NRT and/or bupropion/varenicline, or negotiate a decrease in smoking, consider cardiac stress test, use transdermal route of administration +/– lower dose, consider spironolactone as preferred anti-androgen, consider low-dose ASA prophylaxis

ACEs = angiotensin converting enzyme inhibitors, ARBs = angiotensin receptor blockers, ASA = acetylsalicylic acid, BP = blood pressure, DVT = deep vein thrombosis, GI = gastroenterology, IBD = inflammatory bowel disease, MS = multiple sclerosis, NAFLD = non-alcoholic fatty liver disease, NRT = nicotine replacement therapy, PE = pulmonary embolus, RA = rheumatoid arthritis, VTE = venous thromboembolism

* Imparts moderate to high risk of an adverse outcome without risk mitigation

cis women have suggested increased thrombogenicity and CVD risk with the use of conjugated estrogens (Premarin) over estradiol.[68,69]

Studies on the risk of VTE associated with oral estradiol use in menopausal cis women have yielded variable results, with some suggesting no increased risk and others suggesting a 2.5- to 4-fold increased risk. Risk in this setting may also have been impacted by choice of co-administered progestin.[60,70] A recent retrospective study involving transfeminine individuals taking a regimen of spironolactone and oral estradiol (4–8 mg/day) showed no increased risk of VTE over baseline in the general population.[71] A comparison of their results with those of Wierckx et al.,[72] which demonstrated a 5.1 per cent increase in lifetime risk of VTE in transfeminine patients taking largely transdermal or oral estradiol in combination with cyproterone, prompted the authors to speculate on the potential role of cyproterone in conferring increased thrombogenic risk. Most recently, a large cohort study of 2842 transfeminine patients in the United States demonstrated an increased incidence of VTE, with two- and eight-year risk differences of 4.1 and 16.7 per 1000 persons compared to cis men, and 3.4 and 13.7 risk differences compared to cis women. Despite the relatively large cohort size, detailed analysis by specific hormone regimens was precluded.[73]

Transdermal forms have been shown to have minimal effects on hemostatic variables and to confer minimal or no thrombotic risk in menopausal cis women, even in those with a prior history of thrombosis.[70] As discussed above, sublingual and injectable formulations may also be associated with decreased VTE risk by bypassing first-pass metabolism and the associated hepatic production of clotting factors, but how this balances with the potential impact of high-serum values observed shortly after administration is unknown.

Risk increases in patients who are over age 40, highly sedentary or obese, and particularly in smokers or those who have underlying thrombophilic disorders. Transdermal formulations should be used whenever possible in patients with risk factors. Routine screening for thrombophilic disorders before estrogen initiation is not recommended and should be restricted to those with a personal or strong family history of thromboembolic events.[74] The UCSF Center for Excellence in Transgender Health presents helpful algorithms to address various scenarios of VTE history or risk factors and estrogen use.[13] The routine use of prophylactic ASA or anticoagulation is not recommended in transfeminine patients without another indication per national thrombosis guidelines.[41]

It is currently common practice to discontinue estrogen therapy two to four weeks before surgical procedures, including vaginoplasty, because of the assumed increased risk of VTE. The necessity of this practice has come into question by some experts who cite a lack of supportive evidence, in addition to suspecting a strong association between hormone cessation and post-operative depression.[13] More research is needed to address this question. In the meantime, we encourage our patients to discuss hormone cessation recommendations with their surgeon. In general, estrogen can be restarted post-operatively once a patient is ambulatory.

CARDIOVASCULAR DISEASE AND RELATED METABOLIC RISK FACTORS

Studies in cis women demonstrating an increased risk of CV events with the use of estrogen gave rise to concerns about the extent to which estrogen preparations could cause harmful CV events in transgender women.[64,75] A 2010 Cochrane review of hormone replacement therapy in menopausal cis women found no increased all-cause mortality, CV-related mortality, non-fatal myocardial infarction (MI), angina, or need for angioplasty or bypass surgery. The same review demonstrated a small increase in stroke, limited to a subgroup of women who started hormone replacement therapy more than 10 years following menopause.[76]

The extrapolation from the use of estrogen in cis populations to trans populations is problematic for a number of reasons, including significant differences in the average age of initiation and associated risk factors at baseline, different hormone regimens and doses, as well as differences in genetic makeup and natal hormonal milieu.

Studies in trans populations, however, have been limited to small prospective studies and some larger retrospective cohort studies that did not account for significant risk factors, including tobacco use.[18,24,72,77] Furthermore, many of the studies on transfeminine patients do not distinguish between the dosage or form of oral estradiol used (ethinyl estradiol, conjugated equine estrogens, or 17-β estradiol), the concomitant use of progesterone, or the type of anti-androgen, which further complicates interpreting their data. Though also hampered by these limitations, it is noteworthy that the US cohort demonstrated rates of MI in transfeminine participants similar to those observed in cis men, with a very small increase noted in the rate of ischemic stroke.[73]

A large 2010 meta-analysis of transfeminine patients using feminizing hormones demonstrated an increase in triglyceride concentrations of 0.26 mmol/L, with no changes in any other lipid parameters or in blood pressure. Very few CV events were reported, and the authors concluded that data were insufficient to allow meaningful assessment of clinically important CV-related outcomes.[78]

A systematic review of 29 studies commissioned by the Endocrine Society in 2017 arrived at similar conclusions, reporting a statistically significant increase in triglycerides without changes in other lipid parameters, and very few cases of MI, stroke, and CV-related mortality. Again, the evidence was noted to be of poor quality.[48]

The effect of feminizing hormones on blood sugar and diabetes type II (DMII) risk is also unclear. Some studies suggest an increase in insulin resistance and fasting glucose.[79-81] Higher rates of DMII have been observed in transfeminine patients compared to age-matched cisgender men and women,[72] but the degree to which hormone therapy is implicated versus other factors is unknown. The Endocrine Society guidelines state that there is limited evidence to determine whether estrogen has a beneficial or detrimental effect on blood sugar or DMII risk in transfeminine patients.[48]

Most experts and organizations take a similar approach regarding risk mitigation with estrogen: CV risk factors in transfeminine patients should be optimally managed, according to existing national guidelines, and a transdermal route of estrogen should be used preferentially in those with existing risk factors or high triglycerides.[13,48,65,82] Optimal management of CV parameters can be reached before, or concurrently with, the administration of feminizing hormone therapy and can be managed according to guidelines if concerns arise during treatment.

While the assessment of baseline risk before the initiation of hormone therapy can be estimated by sex-based risk calculators using sex assigned at birth (e.g., Framingham),[83] risk calculations become more challenging after changes in the hormonal milieu. Depending on the age of hormone initiation and duration of hormone exposure, providers may choose to use the risk calculator for sex assigned at birth, affirmed gender, or an average of both.[76] Prophylactic antiplatelet agent(s) for CVD are not routinely recommended for primary prevention.

OSTEOPOROSIS AND BONE MINERAL DENSITY SCREENING

Sex hormones affect bone mineral density (BMD) and the subsequent risk of osteoporosis. A hypogonadal state induces loss of bone in both cis men and cis women. In studies of older cis men, serum estradiol levels show a stronger association with the maintenance of BMD than testosterone levels.[83,84]

Although multiple studies have found a lower BMD in transfeminine individuals before estrogen therapy when compared to age-matched cis men,[85-87] bone support appears to be adequate in transfeminine patients who are maintained on estrogen. Previous evidence has been conflicting; however, a recent systematic review commissioned by the Endocrine Society found a statistically significant increase in BMD values at 12 and 24 months compared with baseline values before feminizing hormone therapy.[48]

In accordance with national recommendations for cis people, BMD testing should be offered to all transfeminine patients over age 65, and screening to identify people at higher risk of osteoporosis (including those who smoke, are HIV positive, have a high alcohol intake, or have a body weight less than 60 kg) can begin at age 50. As in cis populations, the presence of certain high-risk conditions such as hyperparathyroidism or malabsorption syndrome warrant screening before age 50.[86]

High-risk scenarios unique to trans populations that should prompt earlier screening include patients who have undergone orchiectomy and have been on low-dose or no hormones for any significant length of time (i.e., >2 years). Screening may also be considered for those who have been on anti-androgens or a GnRH analogue for a significant length of time without the co-administration of exogenous estrogen.

There are no studies to guide the interpretation of BMD results and fracture risk in trans people. Current tools (e.g., FRAX, CAROC) are age- and sex-based, and it is unclear whether better approximations are obtained using sex assigned at birth or affirmed gender. Some guidelines suggest that this decision may be made on an individual basis, depending on the age at which hormones are initiated. Alternatively, in some cases it may be reasonable to assess fracture risk using both sex calculators and using an intermediate value.[48]

Despite reassuring data regarding risks, all transfeminine patients should ensure a daily intake of 1000 IU vitamin D and 1200 mg of calcium (total of diet + supplements). Weight-bearing exercise should also be encouraged.

HYPERPROLACTINEMIA/PROLACTINOMA
There is a theoretical increased risk of hyperprolactinemia and prolactinoma in transfeminine patients on feminizing hormone therapy. Elevations in serum prolactin are common and, while typically benign, there have been multiple case reports of prolactinoma in transfeminine patients following long-term hormone therapy.[88-91] There remains no clear evidence, however, to suggest an increased risk compared to cis women.[13]

Some point out concerns regarding the potential for estrogen to mask the symptoms of a prolactinoma given they are similar to the desired effects of estrogen.[19,62,92] Thus, some guidelines recommend checking prolactin at baseline and monitoring every one to two years during treatment.[48] The recommended response to elevations includes decreasing the estrogen dose and, if elevations are persistent or above a certain threshold, imaging of the sella turcica.

Various arguments are emerging that these routine practices may be unnecessary. While the elevations in prolactin seen in transfeminine patients have historically been attributed to estrogen, recent studies implicate cyproterone as having a major role.[93,94] These findings have prompted some to suggest that monitoring of prolactin is unnecessary if cyproterone is not being used.[94] Second, Deutsch's group points out that given the recommendation for expectant management of asymptomatic prolactinoma, such routine monitoring for hyperprolactinemia (and associated prolactinoma) would not have an impact on management[94] and could lead to needless harm and cost. As such, they recommend checking prolactin only in the presence of symptoms, that is, visual disturbances, excessive galactorrhea, or new onset of headaches.[13]

A reasonable approach may be to monitor prolactin at baseline, particularly in those with a history of hyperprolactinemia or those who use medications that may increase prolactin (e.g., antipsychotics), and then yearly if cyproterone is being used. If significant elevation (>60–70 mcg/L) is noted on cyproterone, a trial switch to spironolactone can be considered before decreasing the estrogen dose. Levels can be checked six to eight weeks after any medication adjustments. Imaging can be considered in the setting of persistent elevations of more than 80 mcg/L and should always be ordered if symptoms are present.

BREAST CANCER

Estrogens stimulate epithelial growth and the development of acini and lobules in the breasts of transfeminine people. How the risk of breast cancer in transfeminine individuals compares with that of cis women or cis men has been a matter of debate. Evidence to date suggests that the risk of breast cancer in transfeminine patients is not higher and may potentially be lower than in cisgender women.[62,72,95–97]

Longer duration of feminizing hormone exposure (i.e., number of years taking estrogen), family history of breast cancer, obesity (BMI > 35), and the use of progestins likely increase the level of risk.[50] Those with a strong family history of breast and/or ovarian cancer who are considering estrogen should be referred to a familial breast cancer program and undergo genetic screening, as indicated. It is unfortunately not known to what extent BRCA mutations influence the risk of developing breast cancer in transfeminine patients on estrogen, but the reasonable expectation of increased risk is important to take into account. A 2014 case report discusses the treatment of a BRCA1 positive trans woman who declined prophylactic mastectomy and continued on estrogen therapy under informed consent.[98]

Transfeminine patients should receive counselling around breast self-awareness as is recommended for cis women. In general, annual clinical breast examination (as well as breast self-exam) as a part of routine breast cancer screening is of questionable utility, but may be useful in transfeminine patients to assess the degree of breast development or to assess for implant complications if the patient has undergone breast augmentation.

A 2009 study that assessed the feasibility and acceptability of screening mammography in transfeminine participants found that screening was technically possible, nearly painless, and of high personal importance.[99] However, the finding that transfeminine patients have a high prevalence of dense breasts – 60 per cent dense or very dense on mammography[99] – raises questions about the sensitivity and specificity of mammography in trans women compared to cis women.[13]

Recommendations for initiation and frequency of screening mammography in transfeminine patients vary between organizations. A reasonable approach is to perform mammography in transfeminine patients every two years if older than 50 years old AND on estrogen for more than five years total (i.e., years do not have to be consecutive), and to consider initiating screening at a younger age if additional risk factors are present.

When implants are present, the technical approach of a diagnostic mammogram rather than a screening mammogram is necessary.[99] In addition, routine imaging to screen for implant rupture may be recommended depending on the implant type. In the case of saline implants, rupture causes a visible deflation and thus diagnosis is clinical and routine imaging is not indicated. In the case of silicone implants, "silent" (non-visible) rupture can occur. Recommendations for screening vary between surgeons and implant manufacturers. Currently Gender Reassignment Surgery (GRS) Montreal recommends an annual ultrasound for silicone implants from the fifth year onward.[100] If a rupture is suspected but not confirmed by ultrasound, an MRI can be performed.

PROSTATE CANCER

It is reasonable to assume that the risk of both benign prostatic hypertrophy and prostate cancer is significantly decreased by the androgen deprivation associated with feminizing hormone therapy or gonadectomy. Although rare, there have been cases of prostate cancer reported in transfeminine patients, generally occurring in those who started hormone therapy after the age of 50.[101] It is important to note that feminizing therapy will lower prostate-specific antigen (PSA) values even in the presence of prostate cancer, thus impacting its utility in this population. Some recommend a reduction in the upper limit of normal for PSA to 1 ng/L in transfeminine patients with suppressed testosterone.[102]

As with cis men, routine PSA screening is not recommended in transfeminine patients in the absence of significant risk factors. There is little evidence to support a role for annual digital rectal exam in prostate cancer screening; however, it may be considered according to a provider's routine practice with cis men or if symptoms arise. Keep in mind that prostate volume is expected to decrease in the presence of feminizing therapy. In patients who have undergone vaginoplasty, the prostate remains in situ and may be palpated anteriorly via digital vaginal exam in a gender-affirming lithotomy position.

LIVER/GALLBLADDER

Estrogen may be associated with transient liver enzyme elevations and, rarely, clinical hepatotoxicity.[50] Baseline elevation in liver enzymes should be investigated and any existing hepatic disease optimized before or concurrently with the initiation of estrogen therapy. Spironolactone should be selected preferentially over cyproterone in those with hepatic disease or concomitant use of hepatotoxic medication and healthy renal function. Injectable, transdermal, or sublingual routes are preferable in those with pre-existing liver disease or use of hepatotoxic medication, given that they bypass first-pass metabolism.

Chronic hepatitis C should not be considered a contraindication to feminizing hormone therapy, nor hormone therapy a contraindication to hepatitis C treatment. There is theoretical potential for interactions between estradiol and some interferon-free direct acting agent treatment regimens for hepatitis C, which could increase serum concentrations of estrogen. Co-administration has not been studied and the clinical significance (if any) is not known. It is recommended that providers check for potential drug interactions using the University of Liverpool's *HEP Drug Interactions Checker*[103] and choose treatment regimens and monitoring parameters in consultation with a pharmacist.

Estrogen use has been shown to increase the risk of cholelithiasis and subsequent cholecystectomy.[50]

HUMAN IMMUNODEFICIENCY VIRUS (HIV) AND
ANTI-RETROVIRAL (ARV) DRUGS

See chapter 7 for information on HIV and its treatment in trans and non-binary populations.

SEIZURE DISORDERS AND ANTICONVULSANT THERAPY

Hormones appear to influence seizure occurrence by multiple mechanisms. Higher estrogen levels in particular are associated with an increased frequency of seizures in cisgender women.[104] Consultation with a neurologist can be considered in those with pre-existing seizure disorders. In addition, some anticonvulsant drugs impact estrogen metabolism through induction of the CYP450 isoenzyme, resulting in the accelerated conversion of estrogen to inactive metabolites. Of the common anticonvulsants used in Canada, phenobarbital, phenytoin, carbamazepine, and topiramate are all CYP450 inducers, whereas valproic acid, gabapentin, and lamotrigine do not appear to interact with estrogen.[105] If a patient is on a CYP450-inducing anticonvulsant for a seizure disorder, neuropathic pain, or mood stabilization, it is reasonable to consult a specialist or pharmacist to inquire about switching to a non-inducer or considering adjustments to estrogen dosage before initiation.

SEXUAL FUNCTION AND FATIGUE

Some transfeminine patients undergoing feminizing hormone therapy may experience loss of libido or sexual function. Though sexual desire and function are multifaceted, having hormonal, anatomical, and psychologic components, it is likely that androgen blockade and suppression play a significant role.

Should a patient report problematic sexual desire or function, all contributing aspects should be explored and considered. When appropriate, a trial of a decreased dose of anti-androgen or, if cyproterone is being used, a switch to spironolactone can be considered. The addition of a progestin may also be trialed for low libido, following a discussion of potential risks/side effects and the lack of clear evidence for benefit. Loss of erectile function is common, and although it may be welcome for some, others may wish to retain sexual function. Phosphodiesterase-5 (PDE-5) inhibitors (e.g., sildenafil or tadalafil) can be helpful for transfeminine patients wanting to maintain erectile function.

Gonadectomy (+/– vaginoplasty) has a variable impact on libido. As summarized by Wierckx et al., some studies found no change or a decrease in sexual desire following surgery, while others observed an increase.[106] Nonetheless, it appears relatively consistent across studies that approximately one-third of post-operative transfeminine patients experienced significant distress as a result of low libido and met the criteria for hypoactive sexual desire disorder.[106–108]

Those who have undergone gonadectomy often have free and total testosterone levels that are below the normal range for ovulating cis women. Though studies investigating the relationship between libido and testosterone levels in both cis and transfeminine patients are limited, inconsistent, and sometimes contradictory, weak evidence exists to suggest a potential benefit for low-dose transdermal testosterone supplementation to bring serum levels into the female range.[107,109]

A low-dose testosterone patch or low-concentration gel can be used. Dose ranges used in the treatment of sexual dysfunction in cis women may be used as a guide (typically 0.2–1 mg of topical testosterone daily). This should be done carefully, with close monitoring for any unwanted masculinizing effects. Serum levels should also be monitored closely until a therapeutic dose is established. Serum levels within the female range are unlikely to have significant metabolic implications. This supplementation is contraindicated in the presence of prostate or other androgen-sensitive cancer.

Similarly, this intervention can be considered for post-op transfeminine patients experiencing significant fatigue, assuming a workup for other causes is negative or any contributing factors such as iron deficiency, hypothyroidism, sleep apnea, or depression are optimally managed.

Long-Term Follow-Up

The long-term follow-up of transfeminine patients on feminizing hormone therapy should involve (at least) annual preventive care visits. Preventive care checklists endorsed by the College of Family Physicians of Canada exist for cisgender patients,[110] but use of these forms for trans patients is awkward and can lead to missed elements important in their comprehensive primary care. An adapted preventive care checklist for transfeminine patients designed for access at the point of care is available as part of Sherbourne Health's *Guidelines for Gender-Affirming Primary Care with Trans and Non-binary Patients*, published by Rainbow Health Ontario and available for download from https://www.rainbowhealthontario .ca/guidelines.

Masculinizing Hormone Therapy

Testosterone

The cornerstone of hormone therapy for transmasculine patients is testosterone. The goal of treatment is virilization – the development of masculine secondary sexual characteristics. Generally, the desired androgenic effects of testosterone therapy include deepened voice, cessation of menses, clitoral growth, increased muscle mass, fat redistribution, and hair growth in androgen-dependent areas, including facial hair. Breast tissue may lose glandularity but generally does not lose mass or hemi-circumference.[111]

Voice changes and clitoral growth are irreversible changes. Fat redistribution and increased muscle mass are generally considered reversible effects, but some degree of redistribution may be irreversible. The cessation of menses is generally achievable within the first three to six months of therapy.

Fertility is decreased during testosterone administration but should not be relied upon as contraception. While there may be an irreversible reduction in fertility, many transmasculine people have conceived healthy pregnancies following the discontinuation of testosterone.

The effects of testosterone and their expected time courses are shown in table 11.8. Typically, patients taking testosterone will experience masculinizing changes over a period of months to years. The timeframe of physiologic changes may be slightly slower with the use of transdermal preparations. The degree and rate of physical effects are also dependent on the dose of administration,[50] as well as patient-specific factors such as age, ethnicity, genetics, body habitus, and lifestyle. Coarsening of body hair, as well as facial hair growth, begin soon after initiation of testosterone but take a number of years to reach full expression. Clitoral growth usually begins in the first few months of therapy and may be accompanied by mild clitoral discomfort and increased spontaneous arousal.

If cessation of menses is not achieved within the first 6 months of therapy, the testosterone dosage may need to be increased if not already at a maximum dose. In patients who prefer low-dose testosterone, or occasionally in patients using transdermal preparations, a progestin may be used, either in the form of a levonorgestrel-releasing IUS (e.g., Mirena), or an injectable medroxyprogesterone acetate (MPA) (Depo-Provera).

Some patients may want to have cessation of menses without virilization. For these individuals, the levonorgestrel-releasing IUS or injectable MPA can be used independently, without adding testosterone.

Table 11.8. Effects and Expected Time Course of Masculinizing Hormones

Effect	Expected Onset*	Expected Maximum Effect*
Skin oiliness/acne	1–6 months	1–2 years
Facial/body hair growth	3–6 months	4–5 years
Scalp hair loss	6–12 months[†]	Variable
Increased muscle mass/strength[‡]	6–12 months	2–5 years
Body fat redistribution	1–6 months	2–5 years
Cessation of menses	1–6 months	n/a
Clitoral enlargement	3–6 months	1–2 years
Vaginal atrophy	1–6 months	1–2 years
Deepened voice	6–12 months	1–2 years

* Estimates represent published and unpublished clinical observations[4–7]

[†] Highly dependent on age and inheritance; may be minimal

[‡] Significantly dependent on amount of exercise

Source: Adapted from Hembree et al., *The Endocrine Treatment of Gender-Dysphoric/ Gender Incongruent Persons: An Endocrine Society Guideline*[48]

While the use of MPA has been shown to affect bone accretion in adolescents, there is evidence to suggest that peak bone mass and future osteoporotic fracture risk are not affected.[112]

Alternatively, a GnRH analogue (leuprolide, Lupron; or busrelin, Suprefact) can be used to suppress menses *and* the expression of endogenous female hormones. Drawbacks include high cost, repeat (often painful) injections or frequent nasal spray dosing, and possible side effects including headache, mood changes, and weight gain. It should also be noted that the administration of a GnRH analogue in the absence of exogenous hormone use, for a significant amount of time (i.e., >2 years), can decrease bone mineral density. If providers lack experience with the use of GnRH analogues, consultation or communication with an endocrinologist or another experienced provider before initiation is recommended.

All patients with childbearing potential (i.e., uterus and ova) who are considering testosterone should be counselled regarding its teratogenic impact (specifically hyper-androgenization of the fetus), regardless of current sexual practices. Patients should be aware of their ongoing risk of pregnancy, despite testosterone therapy or amenorrhea (see "Fertility and Contraception" above).

Table 11.9. Formulations and Recommended Doses of Testosterone for Masculinizing Hormone Therapy

	Starting/Low Dose	Maximum Dose
Testosterone enanthate (IM/SC)*	20–50 mg each week or 40–100 mg every 2 weeks	100 mg each week or 200 mg every 2 weeks
Testosterone cypionate (IM/SC)*	20–50 mg each week or 40–100 mg every 2 weeks	100 mg each week or 200 mg every 2 weeks
Testosterone patch (transdermal)†	2.5–5 mg daily	5–10 mg daily
Testosterone gel 1% (transdermal)‡	2.5–5 g daily (2–4 pumps, equivalent to 25–50 mg testosterone)	5–10 g daily (4–8 pumps, equivalent to 50–100 mg testosterone)

Note. Testosterone (in all forms) is a controlled substance in Canada; prescriptions should be written in accordance with provincial or territorial requirements for controlled substances.

IM = intramuscular, SC = subcutaneous

* Testosterone enanthate is compounded in sesame oil, and testosterone cypionate is compounded in cottonseed oil; patients with allergy to either of these compounds should use the alternative agent.

† Androderm brand; per drug monograph, the 12.2 mg patch delivers 2.5 mg/day while the 24.3 mg patch delivers 5 mg per day.

‡ Each pump bottle provides 60 doses, 1 dose = 1.25 g of gel, equivalent to 12.5 mg of testosterone.

In Canada, currently available options for testosterone administration are limited to injectable and transdermal preparations (patch or gel). Injectable formulations are most commonly used because of superior efficacy and affordability. Table 11.9 outlines the formulations and recommended doses of testosterone therapy currently available.

The advantage of transdermal preparations is the relatively steady state of testosterone delivery, as opposed to the periodicity associated with injectables. Some reported drawbacks include local reactions, higher cost, fear of skin-to-skin transmission, problems with the adhesion of patches, and an unpleasant odour with gel.[113]

Patches should be applied to a flat, clean, dry, and undamaged area of skin on the back, stomach, upper arm, or thigh. Gel should be applied to the upper arms, shoulders, or abdomen. If a gel formulation is used, patients should be counselled regarding the risk of inadvertent exposure to others who come into contact with the patient's skin. This is of particular importance for patients who care for young children and/or have intimate partners who are pregnant or considering pregnancy. Testosterone gel should be allowed to dry before getting dressed, and the site of application should remain dry for at least two hours (to allow for absorption into the dermis). Thorough handwashing should be performed following application, and gloves worn if the gel is applied by someone else.

While IM injection is the most common means of administering parenteral testosterone, subcutaneous (SC) delivery has also been used with clinical efficacy and is very well tolerated. Proponents describe less discomfort for patients, a decreased rate of injection site complications, and an increased capacity for self-injection. A study of adult transmasculine individuals demonstrated achievement of amenorrhea in 51 of 53 pre-menopausal participants with careful dose adjustment of SC testosterone cypionate. Of 63 total participants, 61 had testosterone levels within the male range on a dose of 100 mg weekly or less (median dose 75–80 mg). The same study reported that all 22 patients who had switched from IM to SC injections had a mild ($n = 2$) or marked ($n = 22$) preference for the SC route.[113]

Pharmacokinetic studies to date, though small, suggest that the SC route of testosterone is associated with a greater half-life compared to IM, with a comparable trough level and total drug exposure (area under the curve).[114,115] Based on these studies' findings, some suggest a 10 to 15 per cent dose reduction in testosterone when switching from IM to SC. A subsequent testosterone level can be obtained to ensure that desired levels are maintained.

While the IM route remains better studied and often more familiar to both patients and providers, enough evidence exists suggesting reasonable safety and efficacy to offer the SC route as an option for patients.

If patients want to self-inject, it is important to instruct them on technique for safe injection and sharps disposal. Directly observing a patient self-inject is helpful for the correction of any problems with technique and to reassure patients that they are injecting correctly. A written step-by-step guide on self-injection for patients is available from Fenway Health.[52]

Some surgeons have advocated for the topical application of testosterone to the clitoris as an adjunct to growth before metoidioplasty (surgical reconstruction of the hypertrophied clitoris to create a phallus). There is no definitive evidence for this practice, and it is not routinely recommended; however, if undertaken, the applied dose should be subtracted from the patient's total testosterone dosage.[51]

No reduction in testosterone dosing is required following bilateral or unilateral oophorectomy with hysterectomy;[53] however, some patients may choose to lower their dose due to the absence of concerns regarding the return of menses. Consideration should be given to bone mineral density in agonadal patients on low-dose testosterone (see "Osteoporosis and Bone Mineral Density Screening").

Considerations in Older Transmasculine Patients

There is little information in the literature to guide recommendations for the initiation or maintenance of masculinizing hormone regimens in older transmasculine patients. Unique considerations in older populations include changes in endogenous hormone levels; physiologic changes that may affect response to medications; a higher burden of existing medical conditions; and multiple concurrent medications, leading to the increased potential for drug interactions.

It is not uncommon for trans patients to seek to initiate hormone therapy at older ages,[66] though there is evidence to suggest that transmasculine patients may generally seek treatment at an earlier age on average than transfeminine patients.[116] In one centre, 71 of 74 patients over 50 seeking gender-affirming hormone therapy during a period of 30 months identified as trans women versus only 3 who identified as trans men.[66]

Testosterone treatment in hypogonadal cis men is often continued into old age, and there is no upper age limit to this treatment.[117] Adverse outcomes in cis populations have largely highlighted issues with prostate cancer risk, which is not a concern in transmasculine patients. Increases in hematocrit and overt polycythemia are more common in older cis men than younger cis men,[118] and can be expected to also be the case for older transmasculine patients. As discussed further below, the impact of testosterone on CV outcomes is minimal and is likely highly dependent on pre-existing risk factors. Modifiable risk factors that may be present in older transmasculine patients should be managed according to existing national guidelines.

With appropriate monitoring and risk management, there is no reason not to initiate testosterone therapy in a patient simply because of older age, and no compelling argument to require discontinuation at any age.[67] Several studies have shown that testosterone levels in many cis men fall gradually and to a modest degree between the ages of 40 and 79 (an average of 0.4 per cent per year in one study)[119] and may fall more markedly after the age of 80.[120] However, because of the variability of this decline,[121] the upper limit of normal total testosterone (<28.8 nmol/L at LifeLabs) is not stratified by age in adults, and there is no normal "andropausal range" akin to the menopausal range for estrogen in cis women.

Therefore, as transmasculine patients age, dose reductions can be discussed and considered in accordance with patients' goals. Some guidelines suggest considering complete discontinuation for patients over 50; however, those without gonads may experience symptoms of hypogonadism, along with potential BMD loss. Those with or without gonads may be expected to experience reduced muscle mass, body hair and libido,[53] though in some cases the irreversible changes induced by testosterone may be sufficient to maintain a presentation that is consistent with a patient's needs.

As with all trans patients, decisions about hormone therapy at an advanced age should be individualized, following a thorough discussion of risks and benefits.

Monitoring and Dose Adjustments

As with treatment for transfeminine patients, monitoring should be done at 3, 6, and 12 months after starting therapy. Some clinicians prefer to see patients monthly until an effective dose is established. Follow-up visits should include a functional inquiry, a targeted physical exam, blood work, and health promotion and disease prevention counselling.

Functional inquiry should include noted positive or negative impacts on overall well-being, mood/mental health, and energy levels (including fluctuation). It is useful to inquire about changes in libido and how the patient is managing any change. Inquiry regarding physiological changes should include discussing menstruation. There may be some irregular bleeding or spotting in the first few months of treatment. However, once sustained cessation is achieved, any vaginal bleeding without explanation (e.g., missed dose(s) or lowered dose of testosterone) warrants a workup for endometrial hyperplasia or cancer.

Patients should be reminded about the importance of adequate calcium and vitamin D intake and encouraged to participate in regular, moderate physical activity. With regular exercise, lean muscle mass tends to begin to increase soon after treatment begins. Patients should be advised to increase resistance in weightlifting slowly, since there has been evidence of tendon rupture with testosterone administration. This is likely a result of the rapid increase of muscle mass without the ability for compensatory changes in the tendons.

Examination should be focused and minimally include blood pressure and weight. Blood work should be completed according to table 11.10, with more frequent monitoring as needed if concerns are identified. Hemoglobin (Hb) and hematocrit (Hct) – via complete blood count, (CBC) – should be undertaken because of the risk for polycythemia

Table 11.10. Recommended Blood Work for Monitoring Masculinizing Hormone Therapy

Test	Baseline	3 Months	6 Months	12 Months‡	Yearly	According to Guidelines for Cis Patients or Provider Discretion
CBC*	X	X	X	X	X	
ALT/AST	X		X§			X
Fasting glucose/ HbA1c	X		X§			X
Lipid profile	X		X§			X
Total testosterone	X	X	X	X	X	
LH†	x			x	X	
Other	Hep B/C, pregnancy test					
	Consider: HIV, syphilis and other STI screening as indicated, frequency depending on risk					

Notes. In this table, smaller and lighter grey x's indicate parameters that are measured under particular circumstances. Individual parameters should be considered more frequently if concerns are identified or existing risk factors are present.

AST = aspartate sminotransferase, ALT = alanine aminotransferase, CBC = complete blood count, LH = luteinizing hormone, HbA1c = glycosylated hemoglobin

* Male reference ranges should be used for Hb/Hct (lower limit of female range can be used if menstruating).

† Post-gonadectomy only: elevated LH may have implications regarding bone mineral density (see "Osteoporosis and Bone Mineral Density Screening").

‡ During first year of treatment only

§ Once at either the 6- or 12-month mark

(male reference ranges should be used for the upper limit of normal). Liver enzymes, fasting glucose or glycosylated hemoglobin (HbA1c), and lipids, should be checked at least once between 6 and 12 months or potentially earlier if concerns were identified before initiation. The need for ongoing monitoring of liver enzymes should be guided by individual risk.

Titration of doses will generally occur in the early phases of treatment. For example, with injectable testosterone, a starting dose of 30 mg injected weekly could be increased by 10 to 20 mg every four to six weeks. Speed of titration will depend on lab results, patient goals, response, and side effects.

Some patients will intentionally seek testosterone levels midway between the male and female range. For patients seeking maximum masculinization, the target dose will bring the testosterone level into the physiologic male range. It is important to keep in mind, however, that clinical effects are the goal of therapy, not specific lab values. If a patient is happy with the rate and degree of masculinization, there is no need to increase the dose to achieve a certain range.

If levels are at the lower end of the male range and patients are concerned about slow progress, or low energy, libido, mood, or breakthrough bleeding, the dose can be slowly increased with close monitoring. Once the midpoint of the male reference range is attained, additional benefit is questionable. After the first year of treatment, hormone levels can be monitored yearly in the absence of metabolic shifts such as substantial weight gain, concerns regarding regression of virilization, or the emergence of symptoms potentially related to hormone levels (e.g., cyclic symptoms such as migraines or pelvic cramping/bleeding).[13]

When monitoring injectable testosterone, some clinicians prefer to check serum levels at trough (i.e., just before the next injection is due) while others prefer mid-cycle. There may be utility in varying the timing of blood work to gather information regarding serum levels throughout the cycle (peak, mid-cycle, and trough), especially if a patient is reporting cyclic symptoms or breakthrough bleeding. In such cases, wide fluctuations should prompt consideration of increasing the frequency of injections or switching to a route with less periodicity.[13]

Supraphysiologic levels should be avoided because of the increased risk of adverse events and side effects, as well as the potential for the aromatization of excess testosterone into estrogen. Dose adjustment is warranted if supraphysiologic doses are measured at mid-cycle or trough. Since changes to the integument occur with testosterone administration, patients on a transdermal formulation may require ongoing titration to maintain or obtain physiologic changes. Some transmasculine patients may require titration of topical testosterone to the extent that they need to apply upwards of 6 or more pumps of gel daily. If patients find this cumbersome or are "running out" of surface area, some compounding pharmacies can create a higher concentration of gel (e.g., 5 per cent rather than the standard 1 per cent) so that the volume applied is less. Note that specific details and dosing of compounded formulations should be discussed with the compounding pharmacist.

If the sex marker associated with the patient's health card has not been changed, the reference ranges reported from the laboratory will refer to the sex assigned at birth. Reference ranges vary between laboratories, so it is important to refer to reference ranges for the affirmed gender from the specific laboratory. These can often be found on laboratory websites or obtained by request from the lab.

Precautions and Risk Mitigation with Testosterone Therapy

Providers may have concerns about the safety of testosterone, particularly with respect to metabolic impacts, CV events, and malignancies. As more evidence emerges in transgender populations, fears of a significant impact on morbidity and mortality in transmasculine patients are being set aside. Following a recent comprehensive review of the literature, Weinand and Safer concluded that the compiled evidence suggests that masculinizing therapy for transgender individuals is safe without a large risk of adverse events when followed carefully for a few well-documented medical concerns,[22] which will be reviewed in more detail below.

Pre-existing medical conditions and risk factors may impart increased risks with testosterone administration and should be considered to enable individualized discussions with patients regarding the risks and benefits of treatment. Measures available to reduce associated risks (see table 11.11 and expanded discussion below) should be considered and discussed with patients and, if possible, undertaken before or concurrently with the initiation of hormone therapy. In some cases, patients may want to begin hormone therapy in the setting of ongoing increased risk, that is, immitigable risk or having declined measures for risk mitigation. In such situations, a careful informed consent process should be undertaken, considering individual capacity to make an informed decision, the severity of potential harms from treatment, and the harms that may result from not treating.

Initiating testosterone should ideally be done in collaboration with relevant specialists who may already be involved in a patient's care. In some cases, a new referral may be helpful in informing decisions about risks and their mitigation. However, efforts should be taken to ensure that this does not cause undue delay. If access to a specialist is limited, an e-consult can be both timely and beneficial.

There are a small number of contraindications to testosterone therapy:

Table 11.11. Precautions with Testosterone Therapy and Considerations in Minimizing Associated Risks

Precautions with Testosterone Therapy	Considerations in Minimizing Associated Risks
Stable ischemic cardiovascular disease	Consider referral to cardiology, ensure optimal medical (including prophylactic antiplatelet agent(s) if indicated, per national guidelines) and surgical management as indicated, optimize risk factors, consider transdermal route of administration, and/or low dose/slow titration with monitoring
Uncontrolled high blood pressure	Identify and address barriers to optimal BP control, initiate antihypertensive(s) as needed, consider cardiac stress test, consider low dose/slow titration with monitoring, consider referral to cardiology
Uncontrolled diabetes	Identify and address barriers to optimal glycemic control, refer to dietitian, encourage lifestyle modification, initiate antiglycemic agent(s) per national guidelines, consider endocrinology referral, consider cardiac stress test, consider low dose/slow titration with monitoring
Uncontrolled dyslipidemia	Identify and address barriers to optimal lipid control, refer to dietitian, initiate antilipemic pharmacologic therapy per national guidelines, consider endocrinology referral, consider cardiac stress test, consider low dose/slow titration with monitoring
Hepatic dysfunction	Dependent on etiology, e.g., minimize alcohol consumption, weight loss in NAFLD, consider referral to hepatology/gastroenterology, consider low dose/slow titration with monitoring
Polycythemia	Identify etiology and address contributing factors, consider referral to hematology, consider transdermal route of administration and/or low dose/slow titration with monitoring
History of DVT/PE or hypercoagulable state	Identify and minimize existent risk factors, use prophylactic anti-coagulation if indicated per current national guidelines, consider referral to hematology/thrombosis clinic, consider transdermal route of administration, and/or low dose/slow titration with monitoring for polycythemia
Chronic respiratory disease that may be worsened by erythrocytosis/polycythemia	Consider transdermal route of administration and/or low dose/slow titration with monitoring, consider referral to respirology
Severe/uncontrolled sleep apnea	Initiate CPAP or oral device, refer to dietitian and encourage lifestyle changes if overweight, monitor for changes in CPAP pressure requirements

Precautions with Testosterone Therapy	Considerations in Minimizing Associated Risks
Androgen-sensitive epilepsy	Refer to neurology
Smoker	Encourage and support smoking cessation, consider referral to smoking cessation program/offer NRT and/or bupropion/varenicline, or negotiate a decrease in smoking, consider cardiac stress test; consider transdermal route of administration
Migraines	Consider daily migraine prophylaxis, consider transdermal route of administration
Inter-menstrual bleeding/ menorrhagia	Workup per national guidelines,[122] gynecology referral as needed
Oligo-/amenorrhea	Identify etiology (i.e., PCOS, rule out pregnancy), consider pelvic ultrasound (transvaginal if possible), consider progesterone-induced menstrual bleed before testosterone initiation
Autoimmune conditions (e.g., RA, MS, IBD)	consider low dose/slow titration with monitoring in collaboration with any involved specialists

- pregnancy or breastfeeding
- active, known, androgen-sensitive cancer
- unstable ischemic CV disease
- active endometrial cancer
- poorly controlled psychosis or acute homicidality
- psychiatric conditions that limit the ability to provide informed consent
- hypersensitivity to one of the components of the formulation

Specific Conditions: Risk Mitigation and Long-Term Preventive Care

CARDIOVASCULAR DISEASE AND RELATED METABOLIC RISK FACTORS
There are well-known differences in CV risk between cis men and cis women. In addition, increased risk is suggested in women with poly-cystic ovarian syndrome (a hyper-androgenic state). Overall, studies of testosterone therapy for hypogonadal cis men remain conflicting and inconclusive: while multiple large studies have suggested no increased risk, others have suggested an increased risk in CV events and/or

subclinical atherosclerosis. Together, these findings have contributed to concerns about the impact of testosterone on CV risk in transmasculine patients.

However, multiple studies in transmasculine patients have been reassuring. For example, a large long-term cohort study out of the Netherlands found no increased risk for CV mortality in transmasculine participants.[18] A meta-analysis conducted by Elamin et al. in 2010 and the Endocrine Society's systematic review in 2016 both demonstrated a statistically significant rise in triglycerides and low-density lipoprotein levels, as well as a decrease in high-density lipoprotein levels, with testosterone administration in trans men. However, the clinical significance of these changes was debatable, and the overall evidence regarding CV outcomes was insufficient to allow meaningful conclusions.[48,78]

Studies regarding the effect of testosterone on insulin resistance have shown mixed results, with some studies reporting an increase in insulin resistance[81] while others have suggested no impact.[80,123] A 2013 case-control study demonstrated an increased prevalence of DMII in transmasculine individuals at baseline compared with control cisgender men and women, as well as a small increase in incidence over a seven-year period, however the number of cases was low. The authors suggest that the discrepancy may have been related to lifestyle differences rather than testosterone administration.[72]

The risk of hypertension among transmasculine patients using testosterone is also unclear, as data have been inconclusive. It appears that testosterone therapy likely leads to a small increase in blood pressure that is statistically significant but may not be clinically significant. For example, Elamin et al.'s meta-analysis revealed an average increase in systolic blood pressure of 1.74 mmHg.[78]

Overall, the data seem to suggest that the CV and metabolic risks associated with testosterone in transmasculine patients are at most minimal, and have likely been overestimated in the past. However, patients with risk factors such as PCOS or existing dyslipidemia may be at increased risk of further abnormalities with testosterone administration.

Most experts and organizations take a similar approach regarding CV risk mitigation with testosterone: CV risk factors in transmasculine patients should be optimally managed according to existing national guidelines. Optimal management of CV parameters can be attained before or concurrently with the administration of masculinizing hormone therapy and managed per guidelines if concerns emerge during treatment.

While the assessment of baseline risk before the initiation of hormone therapy can be estimated by sex-based risk calculators (e.g., Framingham)[83] using sex assigned at birth, risk calculations become more challenging following alterations in the hormonal milieu. Depending on the age of hormone initiation and duration of hormone exposure, providers may choose to use the risk calculator for sex assigned at birth, affirmed gender, or an average of both.[53] Prophylactic antiplatelet agents are not generally recommended for primary prevention, and a decision to prescribe should be made in accordance with national guidelines.[124]

OBSTRUCTIVE SLEEP APNEA

Sleep apnea may be worsened or unmasked by testosterone therapy.[117] Those with risk factors and/or suggestive signs or symptoms of sleep apnea should be screened via sleep study. As continuous positive airway pressure (CPAP) requirements may change with masculinizing therapy, they should be reassessed periodically via sleep study following testosterone initiation.

HEPATIC DYSFUNCTION

Transient elevation of liver enzymes may occasionally occur with testosterone initiation and generally spontaneously resolves unless another cause of hepatic dysfunction is present.

According to the Endocrine Society,[48] past concerns regarding liver toxicity with testosterone have been alleviated with more recent reports that indicate minimal risk of serious liver disease. Liver enzymes should be checked at baseline and again at 6 or 12 months, with more frequent and ongoing monitoring depending on individual risk factors, concomitant medications, and previous results.

Chronic liver disease, including chronic hepatitis C, does not constitute a contraindication to testosterone.[13] No known drug interactions exist between testosterone and treatment regimens for hepatitis C.[103]

POLYCYTHEMIA

Testosterone increases renal erythropoietin production, which in turn induces increased marrow production of red blood cells. Associated amenorrhea also impacts Hb/Hct levels, so an increase in red cell mass and concentration are expected with testosterone therapy. No action is required unless Hb/Hct results exceed the male range (as mentioned above, if the sex marker has not been changed, reported reference ranges may not be applicable).

If levels exceed the male range, adjustments are recommended given that the associated higher blood viscosity may lead to an increased risk of adverse vascular events – particularly in those with other risk factors such as smoking or sleep apnea. This may necessitate a dose reduction, but adjustments to minimize periodicity may also resolve the problem. This can be achieved by increasing the injection frequency (for example 100 mg once weekly, rather than 200 mg every two weeks), or by switching to a transdermal formulation. Transdermal formulations can be used preferentially in those with a history of or major risk factors for polycythemia.[125]

PSYCHIATRIC EFFECTS

The peaks and troughs of serum testosterone associated with the injectable route may lead to fluctuations in energy and mood. Some transmasculine patients may report significant fatigue and lower mood as serum levels fall leading up to the next injection. In such cases, it may be useful to vary the timing of blood work to gather information about serum levels throughout the cycle (peak, mid-cycle, and trough). If this is a problem, increasing the frequency of injections or changing to a transdermal route of administration to attain a more steady serum level is often helpful.

There have been some concerns regarding negative psychiatric effects with testosterone use. A small number of case reports note an increase in psychiatric symptoms including mania in cis men, particularly in those with a history of bipolar disorder. Observational data in trans populations have noted increased aggression, hypersexuality and occasionally psychotic symptoms. Adverse effects were often associated with higher doses or supraphysiologic serum levels of testosterone.[50]

The first prospective study of the impact of testosterone on mental health in transmasculine patients demonstrated no increase in hypomania or psychotic symptoms three months after testosterone initiation.[36] Several studies demonstrate improved psychological functioning in multiple domains with testosterone initiation in transmasculine people.[36,126,127]

Overall, there is no convincing evidence that testosterone administration is associated with the onset or worsening of mental health conditions.[53] Nonetheless, it is prudent to exercise some caution in patients with bipolar disorder or psychotic disorders, particularly when suboptimally managed. Transdermal preparations result in a steady serum testosterone level and are preferred in patients prone to mood or other psychiatric disturbances.

VAGINAL BLEEDING AND ENDOMETRIAL CANCER

There has been some debate regarding the impact of testosterone on the endometrium and risk of endometrial cancer. PCOS, which is associated with higher levels of circulating endogenous androgens, has been associated with an increased risk of endometrial cancer.[128] The local aromatization of testosterone to estrogen, thereby creating a uterine environment of unopposed estrogen, has been postulated to be a mechanism by which an increased risk might occur.[129]

There is one case report of endometrial cancer in a transgender man reported in the literature,[130] and we have had one case at our centre (unpublished). Retrospective long-term studies have revealed no cases.[18,116,131] Histopathologic studies have had variable findings, with some showing a tendency towards an atrophic endometrium,[132–134] some showing no change,[135,136] and two small studies suggesting a tendency towards a proliferative endometrium and hyperplasia.[137,138] Taken in sum, the evidence to date does not suggest an increased risk of endometrial cancer with testosterone administration.

Nonetheless, when initiating testosterone, unexplained frequent, irregular, or heavy bleeding may indicate existing pathology and should be investigated before or concurrently with testosterone, especially in the presence of other risk factors for endometrial hyperplasia and cancer. Unaddressed pathology (including benign causes) may at the very least complicate the attainment of cessation of menses with testosterone.

For patients who are experiencing oligo- or amenorrhea at baseline, workup is suggested before testosterone administration, including a pregnancy test when indicated by sexual history. Alternatives to traditional workup in those who may experience transvaginal imaging or procedures as overly invasive include watchful waiting for amenorrhea at six months following testosterone initiation, transabdominal ultrasonography, or progesterone challenge[13] – though the last may also be emotionally difficult. In some cases, a referral to a culturally competent gynecologist may be helpful.

A pelvic or transabdominal ultrasound may reveal previously unknown PCOS or a thickened endometrium. Some have suggested a potential benefit with the induction of a menstrual period for such patients before starting testosterone, with the rationale that it is preferable to start out with a thinner lining and may hasten the cessation of menses. However, once again, this may be emotionally difficult for some.

Routine screening for endometrial cancer in transmasculine patients on testosterone is not recommended. However, once sustained menstrual cessation is achieved, any vaginal bleeding without explanation (e.g., missed dose(s) or lowered dose of testosterone) warrants workup including endometrial biopsy for endometrial hyperplasia or cancer.

PELVIC PAIN

The differential diagnosis for chronic pelvic pain (>6 months) in transmasculine patients is broad. Causes to consider in transmasculine patients include vaginitis, cystitis, STIs, post-surgical sequelae, and musculoskeletal and psychological causes. Obedin-Maliver explores the approach to chronic pelvic pain in transmasculine patients in depth as part of the UCSF Center for Excellence in Transgender Care's primary care guidelines.[13]

Some transmasculine patients may report pelvic pain secondary to uterine cramping associated with cyclic testosterone dosing or following orgasm. The mechanism of this pain is poorly understood. Non-steroidal anti-inflammatories (NSAIDs) are often effective. Prevention or reduction of post-orgasmic pain may be attained through the administration of an NSAID approximately one hour before sexual activity. Patients may also obtain some relief by adjusting testosterone route or frequency to minimize serum peaks and troughs. Definitive management with hysterectomy may also be an option, especially if other motivating factors for this procedure are present.

ATROPHIC CHANGES

Testosterone therapy may result in atrophy and dryness of vaginal tissues, particularly following oophorectomy. This may lead to discomfort or dyspareunia in patients who want to have receptive frontal (vaginal) sex. This may sometimes be improved with topical estrogen therapy as in postmenopausal cis women. Some systemic absorption does occur but is not likely sufficient to interfere with physiologic masculinization if testosterone is maintained. Lubricants and moisturizers may also be helpful.

OSTEOPOROSIS AND BONE MINERAL DENSITY SCREENING

Sex hormones are well known to impact BMD, and the subsequent risk of osteoporosis. A hypogonadal state induces loss of bone in both cis men and cis women. Serum estradiol levels show a stronger association with maintenance of BMD than do testosterone levels. It is likely that the aromatization of testosterone to estrogen contributes significantly to bone density in cis men.[67]

Baseline BMD before testosterone administration in transmasculine individuals has been found in one study to be in the expected range for sex assigned at birth.[139] Some studies to date show no change in BMD with testosterone over time,[54,140] while others have shown an increase.[141,142] A recent systematic review commissioned by the Endocrine Society found no statistically significant change at 12 and 24 months compared with baseline values before initiating masculinizing hormone therapy.[48]

In accordance with national recommendations for cis individuals, BMD testing should be offered to all transmasculine patients over age 65, and screening to identify people at higher risk of osteoporosis (including those who smoke, are HIV positive, have a high alcohol intake or have a body weight of less than 60 kg) can begin at age 50. As in cis populations, the presence of certain high-risk conditions such as hyperparathyroidism or malabsorption syndrome warrant screening before age 50.[143] Patients who have undergone oophorectomy and have been on low-dose or no exogenous testosterone for any significant length of time (i.e., > 2 years) are also considered to be at high risk.

One small study suggested that LH levels may be associated with BMD in patients who have undergone gonadectomy – that is, if LH is elevated, the patient may not be achieving adequate hormonal support for bone maintenance.[144] Thus in transmasculine patients, BMD testing may additionally be considered in agonadal patients with elevated LH.

There are no studies to guide the interpretation of BMD results and fracture risk in trans people. Current tools (e.g., FRAX, CAROC) are age- and sex-based, and it is unclear whether better approximations are obtained using sex assigned at birth or affirmed gender. The Endocrine Society guidelines suggest that this decision may be made on an individual basis, depending on the age at which hormones are initiated. Alternatively, in some cases it may be reasonable to assess fracture risk using both sex calculators and using an intermediate value.[48]

Despite reassuring data regarding risks, all transmasculine patients should ensure a daily intake of 1000 IU vitamin D and 1200 mg of calcium (total of diet and supplements). Moderate and gradual weight-bearing exercise should also be encouraged.

BREAST CANCER

Testosterone therapy is not thought to significantly increase the risk of breast cancer in transmasculine patients.[48] Transmasculine patients who have undergone chest reconstruction likely have a significantly lower risk than cis women since there is much less tissue present in which malignancy could develop, though there is residual breast tissue, particularly in the axillary regions. There are, however, several reports of transmasculine patients developing breast cancer on testosterone, even after chest reconstruction.[95–97,145]

For those who have undergone chest reconstruction and are presenting with physical concerns, chest and axillary lymph node examination should be performed to assess for abnormalities in the remaining tissue. If an abnormality is detected post-surgically by the patient or by physical exam, ultrasound is recommended as an initial investigation, given that mammography would be technically very difficult. Focused MRI may also be useful to investigate chest abnormalities in transmasculine patients who have undergone chest reconstruction.

In the absence of other significant risk factors, no routine screening investigations are needed post-chest reconstruction. Transmasculine patients who have not undergone chest reconstruction should follow the same guidelines for screening mammography as cis women. Breast/chest self-awareness can be encouraged for all transmasculine patients.

CERVICAL CANCER AND PAP TESTS

Testosterone does not appear to increase the risk of cervical cancer; however, transmasculine patients are at risk and are often underscreened.[146] Transmasculine patients with a cervix should be screened with Papanicolaou (Pap) tests following the guidelines for cis women. Human papillomavirus (HPV) vaccination should be offered to patients under age 45.

Pap testing may be emotionally difficult or painful for transmasculine patients. Several strategies may be employed to minimize the discomfort that may be associated with this examination (see chapter 3, as well as the excellent resources *Tips for Providing Paps to Trans Men*,[147] and *Cervical Cancer Screening for Patients on the Female-to-Male Spectrum: A Narrative Review and Guide for Clinicians*[148])

Barring contraindications, topical 2% lidocaine jelly may be applied vaginally 5 to 10 minutes before the procedure in those who find speculum examination painful because of atrophic changes. The use of vaginal estrogens for one week before the exam may also be helpful. To minimize histological misinterpretation, it is important to note on the cytology requisition that a patient is on testosterone, as well as their menstrual status. Inadequate samples are more common in patients on testosterone and repeat may be required.[146] The use of both brush and broom may increase yield in patients with atrophic changes.[149]

OVARIAN CANCER

Analogous to concerns of an increased risk for ovarian cancer in cis women with elevated androgen levels, it has been postulated that testosterone therapy in transmasculine patients may increase risk. There have been a small number of case reports of ovarian cancer in transmasculine individuals.[150,151] Small histologic studies have shown hyperplasia of the ovarian stroma and an increase in fibrous collagen content with testosterone administration, but no evidence of polycystic ovary morphology,[133,152] whereas one recent study did report multifollicular ovaries.[136] Overall, there is no evidence to suggest an increased risk of ovarian cancer in transmasculine patients on testosterone,[22] and thus no cause to perform oophorectomy in transmasculine patients solely for primary prevention.

HUMAN IMMUNODEFICIENCY VIRUS (HIV) AND ANTI-RETROVIRAL (ARV) DRUGS

See chapter 7 for information on HIV and its treatment in trans and non-binary populations.

ACNE

Many transmasculine patients will experience a significant increase or worsening of acne upon initiation of testosterone. This may be limited to the face or may also involve the chest and back; in a minority of patients the acne may be severe. Acne is generally worse in the first year of hormone therapy, peaking in severity at six months.[153] Acne may be managed as for cisgender patients. Severe acne may also improve by changing the formulation, route, and/or frequency of testosterone. Dose reductions need only be considered after all treatments and alternatives have been exhausted.[51]

HAIR LOSS

Androgenic alopecia may occur as a result of testosterone therapy and, as in cis men, is often genetically determined. Thinning is also related to the duration of therapy.[153] Finasteride may be effectively used to treat male pattern hair loss in transmasculine patients by blocking the conversion of testosterone to dihydroydrotestosterone.* Patients considering this option should be counselled that this may impact facial hair growth, and the potential negative impact on other aspects of

---

* The typical dose of Finasteride for alopecia is 1 mg per day. For those paying out of pocket, it is much more affordable to prescribe the 5 mg tablet and have the patient carefully split the tablet and take 1/4 tab daily

masculinization early in transition are unknown. Minoxidil may alternatively be used as a topical agent applied to the scalp.[51]

Long-Term Follow-Up

The long-term follow-up of transmasculine patients on masculinizing hormone therapy should involve (at least) annual preventive care visits. Preventive care checklists endorsed by the College of Family Physicians of Canada exist for cisgender patients,[154] but use of these forms for trans patients is awkward and can lead to missed elements important in their comprehensive primary care. An adapted preventive care checklist for transmasculine patients designed for access at the point of care is available as part of Sherbourne Health's *Guidelines for Gender-Affirming Primary Care with Trans and Non-binary Patients*, published by Rainbow Health Ontario and available for download from https://www.rainbowhealthontario.ca/guidelines.

Conclusion

PCPs across Canada play an essential role in ensuring that the health care needs of trans and non-binary patients are met and gender-affirming treatments are delivered in a timely way. Transition pathways can vary widely between individuals; however, for many trans people, hormone therapy is an essential part of transition. This chapter has presented a guideline for gender-affirming hormone provision and primary care as a resource for PCPs that is based on extensive experience, emerging evidence, and standards of care from several national and international medical associations. E-consults and mentorship programs are also available to support PCPs when needed and play an important role in building our collective capacity to serve trans and non-binary patients.

References

1. Bourns A. Guidelines for gender-affirming primary care with trans and non-binary patients. 4th ed. Toronto: Rainbow Health Ontario; 2019 [cited 2019 Sep 30]. Available from: https://www.rainbowhealthontario.ca/guidelines.
2. Flores A, Herman J, Gates G, Brown T. How many adults identify as transgender in the United States? [Internet]. California: The Williams Institute; 2016 [cited 2019 Feb 4]. Available from: https://williamsinstitute.law.ucla.edu/wp-content/uploads/How-Many-Adults-Identify-as-Transgender-in-the-United-States.pdf.

3. Scheim AI, Bauer GR. Sex and gender diversity among transgender persons in Ontario, Canada: results from a respondent-driven sampling survey. J Sex Res. 2015;52(1):1–14.

4. Giblon R, Bauer GR. Health care availability, quality, and unmet need: a comparison of transgender and cisgender residents of Ontario, Canada. BMC Health Serv Res. 2017;17(1):283.

5. Bauer G, Zong X, Scheim A, Hammond R, Thind A. Factors impacting transgender patients' discomfort with their family physicians: A respondent-driven sampling survey. PLoS One. 2015 Dec;10(12):e0145046.

6. Bauer G, Pyne J, Francino M, Hammond R. La Suicidabilité parmi les personnes trans en Ontario: implications en travail social et en justice sociale. Serv Soc. 2013; 59(1):35–62.

7. Wylie K, Knudson G, Khan SI, Bonierbale M, Watanyusakul S, Baral S. Serving transgender people: clinical care considerations and service delivery models in transgender health. Lancet. 2016 Jul;388(10042):401–11.

8. MacKinnon K, Tarasoff LA, Kia H. Predisposing, reinforcing, and enabling factors of trans-positive clinical behaviour change: A summary of the literature. Int J Transgenderism. 2016;17(2):83–92.

9. Meyer W 3rd. World Professional Association for Transgender Health's Standards of Care requirements of hormone therapy for adults with gender identity disorder. Int J Transgenderism. 2009;11(2):127–32.

10. Coleman E, Bockting W, Botzer M, Cohen-Kettenis P, DeCuypere G, Feldman J, et al. Standards of care for the health of transsexual, transgender, and gender-nonconforming people, version 7. Int J Transgenderism. 2012;13(4):165–232.

11. Grant J, Mottet L, Tanis J. Injustice at every turn: A report of the National Transgender Discrimination Survey. Washington (DC): National Centre for Transgender Equality; 2011.

12. Koehler A, Eyssel J, Nieder T. Genders and individual treatment progress in (non-)binary trans individuals. J Sex Med. 2018;15(1):102–13.

13. Deutsch M [Internet]. San Francisco: University of California, San Francisco; 2016 [cited 2019 Feb 4]. Guidelines for the primary and gender-affirming care of transgender and gender nonbinary people. Available from: http://transhealth.ucsf.edu/protocols.

14. Grimstad F. Connect the dots: Informed consent in the medical care of transgender and gender-nonconforming patients. Obstet Gynecol 2017;129(3):579.

15. Cavanaugh T, Hopwood R, Lambert C. Informed consent in the medical care of transgender and gender non-conforming patients. AMA J Ethics. 2016 Nov;18(11):1147–55.

16. Catherine White Holman Wellness Centre [Internet]. Vancouver: Catherine White Holman Wellness Society; 2012 Aug 4 [cited 2018 July

18]. Informed consent FAQs. Available from: http://www.cwhwc.com/about-us/informed-consent-faqs/.

17. Deutsch M. Use of the informed consent model in the provision of cross-sex hormone therapy: a survey of the practices of selected clinics. Int J Transgenderism. 2012;13(3):140–6.

18. van Kesteren P, Asscheman H, Megens J, Gooren L. Mortality and morbidity in transsexual subjects treated with cross-sex hormones. Clin Endocrinol (Oxf). 1997;47(3):337–42.

19. Gooren LJ, Giltay EJ, Bunck MC. Long-term treatment of transsexuals with cross-sex hormones: extensive personal experience. J Clin Endocrinol Metab. 2008 Jan;93(1):19–25.

20. Wierckx K, Van Caenegem E, Schreiner T, Haraldsen I, Fisher AD, Toye K, et al. Cross-sex hormone therapy in trans persons is safe and effective at short-time follow-up: results from the European network for the investigation of gender incongruence. J Sex Med. 2014 Aug;11(8):1999–2011.

21. Martin dH, Bakker A, Gooren L. Long term hormonal treatment for transgender people. BMJ Br Med J Online. 2017;359.

22. Weinand J, Safer J. Hormone therapy in transgender adults is safe with provider supervision; A review of hormone therapy sequelae for transgender individuals. J Clin Transl Endocrinol. 2015;2(2):55–60.

23. Rotondi N, Bauer G, Scanlon K, Kaay M, Travers R, Travers A. Nonprescribed hormone use and self-performed surgeries: "do-it-yourself" transitions in transgender communities in Ontario, Canada. Am J Public Health. 2013;103(10):1830–6.

24. Asscheman H, Giltay E, Megens J, de Ronde W, van Trotsenburg M, Gooren L. A long-term follow-up study of mortality in transsexuals receiving treatment with cross-sex hormones. Eur J Endocrinol. 2011;164(4):635–42.

25. Trans Care BC. Gender-affirming care for trans, Two-Spirit, and gender diverse patients in BC: a primary care toolkit [Internet]. Vancouver: Provincial Health Services Authority; 2017 Oct [cited 2019 July 16]. Available from: http://www.phsa.ca/transgender/Documents/Primary%20Care%20Toolkit.pdf.

26. American Psychiatric Association. Diagnostic and statistical manual of mental disorders. 5th ed [Internet]. New York: American Psychiatric Association Publishing; 2013 [cited 2019 July 16]. Available from: https://dsm.psychiatryonline.org/doi/book/10.1176/appi.books.9780890425596.

27. Beek T, Cohen-Kettenis P, Bouman W, de Vries A, Steensma T, Witcomb G. Gender incongruence of adolescence and adulthood: acceptability

and clinical utility of the World Health Organization's proposed ICD-11 criteria. PLoS One. 2016;11(10):e0160066.

28. Kreukels B, Steensma T, de Vries A. Gender dysphoriaand disorders of sex development: progress in care and knowledge. New York: Springer; 2014.

29. World Health Organization. International classification of diseases. 11th ed. [Internet]. Geneva (Switzerland): WHO; 2019 May 25 [cited 2019 July 16]. Available from: https://icd.who.int/en

30. Drescher J, Cohen-Kettenis P, Winter S. Minding the body: situating gender identity diagnoses in the ICD-11. Int Rev of Psychiatry. 2012;24(6):568–77.

31. Mizock L, Woodrum T, Riley J, Sotilleo E, Yuen N, Ormerod A. Coping with transphobia in employment: strategies used by transgender and gender-diverse people in the United States. Int J Transgenderism. 2017;18(3):282–94.

32. Bauer G, Nussbaum N, Travers R, Munro L, Pyne J, Redman N. We've got work to do: workplace discrimination and employment challenges for trans people in Ontario. Trans PULSE E-Bulletin. 2011 May;2(1). Available from: https://transpulseproject.ca/research/workplace-discrimination -and-employment-challenges-for-trans-people-in-ontario/

33. Testa R, Habarth J, Peta J, Balsalm K, Bockting W. Development of the gender minority stress and resilience measure. Psychol Sex Orientat Gend Divers. 2015;2(1):65–77.

34. Richmond K, Burnes T, Carroll K. Lost in trans-lation: interpreting systems of trauma for transgender patients. Traumatology. 2012;18(1):45–57.

35. Purkey E, Patel R, Phillips S. Trauma-informed care: better care for everyone. Can Fam Physician. 2018;64(3):170–2.

36. Keo-Meier C, Herman L, Reisner S, Pardo S, Sharp C, Babcock J. Testosterone treatment and MMPI-2 improvement in transgender men: a prospective controlled study. J Consult Clin Psychol. 2015;83(1):143–56.

37. College of Physicians and Surgeons of Ontario [Internet]. Toronto: CPSO; 2015 [cited 2019 Feb 4]. Policy statement #3-15, consent to treatment. Available from: https://www.cpso.on.ca/CPSO/media/documents /Policies/Policy- Items/Consent-To-Treatment.pdf?ext=.pdf.

38. De Roo C, Tilleman K, T'Sjoen G, De Sutter P. Fertility options in transgender people. Int Rev Psychiatry. 2016;28(1):112–19.

39. Light A, Obedin-Maliver J, Sevelius J, Kerns J. Transgender men who experienced pregnancy after female-to-male gender transitioning. Obstet Gynecol. 2014;124(6):1120–7.

40. Rodriguez-Wallberg K, Dhejne C, Stefenson M, Degerblad M, Olofsson JI. Preserving eggs for men's fertility. a pilot experience with fertility

preservation for female-to-male transsexuals in Sweden. Fertil Steril 2014;102(3):e160–1.

41. Gidoni YS, Raziel A, Strassburger D, Kasterstein E, Ben-Ami I, Ron-El R. Can we preserve fertility in a female to male trangender after a long term testosterone treatment- case report. Fertil Steril 2013;100(3 suppl):S169–70.

42. Payer A, Meyer WJ 3rd, Walker P. The ultrastructural response of human Leydig cells to exogenous estrogens. Andrologia. 1979;11(6):423–36.

43. Hamada A, Kingsberg S, Wierckx K, T'Sjoen G, De Sutter P, Knudson G, et al. Semen characteristics of transwomen referred for sperm banking before sex transition: A case series. Andrologia. 2015;47(7):832–8.

44. Wallace S, Blough K, Kondapalli L. Fertility preservation in the transgender patient: expanding oncofertility care beyond cancer. Gynecol Endocrinol. 2014;30(12):868–71.

45. De Sutter P. Reproductive options for transpeople: Recommendations for revision of the WPATH's Standards of Care. Int J Transgenderism. 2009;11(3):183–5.

46. Dittrich R, Binder H, Cupisti S, Hoffmann I, Beckmann MW, Mueller A. Endocrine treatment of male-to-female transsexuals using gonadotropin-releasing hormone agonist. Exp Clin Endocrinol Diabetes. 2005 Dec;113(10):586–92.

47. Gava G, Cerpolini S, Martelli V, Battista G, Seracchioli R, Meriggiola MC. Cyproterone acetate vs leuprolide acetate in combination with transdermal oestradiol in transwomen: a comparison of safety and effectiveness. Clin Endocrinol (Oxf). 2016;85(2):239–46.

48. Hembree WC, Cohen-Kettenis PT, Gooren L, Hannema SE, Meyer WJ, Murad MH, et al. Endocrine treatment of gender-dysphoric/gender-incongruent persons: an Endocrine Society clinical practice guideline. J Clin Endocrinol Metab. 2017 Nov 1;102(11):3869–903.

49. Bienz M, Saad F. Androgen-deprivation therapy and bone loss in prostate cancer patients: a clinical review. Bonekey Rep. 2015;4:716.

50. Feldman J, Safer J. Hormone therapy in adults: suggested revisions to the sixth version of the Standards of Care. Int J Transgenderism. 2009 Aug;11(3):146–82.

51. Gorton N, Buth J, Spade D. Medical therapy and health maintenance for transgender men: a guide for healthcare providers [Internet]. San Francisco (CA): Lyon Martin Women's Health Services; 2005 [cited 2019 Feb 4]. Available from: https://www.nickgorton.org/Medical%20 Therapy%20and%20HM%20for%20Transgender%20Men_2005.pdf.

52. Fenway Health. Transgender health injection guide [Internet]. Boston (MA): Fenway Health; 2015 [cited 2019 Feb 4]. p. 29. Available from: https://fenwayhealth.org/wp-content/uploads/2015/07/COM-1880-trans -health_injection-guide_small_v2.pdf.

53. Center of Excellence for Transgender Health [Internet]. [cited 2019 Feb 4]. Available from: http://www.transhealth.ucsf.edu.

54. Levy A, Crown A, Reid R. Endocrine intervention for transsexuals. Clin Endocrinol (Oxf). 2003 Oct;59(4):409–18.

55. Price TM, Blauer KL, Hansen M, Stanczyk F, Lobo R, Bates GW. Single-dose pharmacokinetics of sublingual versus oral administration of micronized 17 beta-estradiol. Obstet Gynecol. 1997 Mar;89(3):340–5.

56. Düsterberg B, Nishino Y. Pharmacokinetic and pharmacological features of oestradiol valerate. Maturitas. 1982 Dec;4(4):315–24.

57. Sierra-Ramírez JA, Lara-Ricalde R, Lujan M, Velázquez-Ramírez N, Godínez-Victoria M, Hernádez-Munguía IA, et al. Comparative pharmacokinetics and pharmacodynamics after subcutaneous and intramuscular administration of medroxyprogesterone acetate (25 mg) and estradiol cypionate (5 mg). Contraception. 2011 Dec;84(6):565–70.

58. de Blok CJM, Klaver M, Wiepjes CM, Nota NM, Heijboer AC, Fisher AD, et al. Breast development in transwomen after 1 year of cross-sex hormone therapy: Results of a prospective multicenter study. J Clin Endocrinol Metab. 2018 01;103(2):532–8.

59. Fenway Health. Transgender health injection guide [Internet]. Boston (MA): Fenway Health; 2015. Available from: https://fenway health.org/wp-content/uploads/2015/07/COM-1880-trans-health _injection-guide_small_v2.pdf.

60. Canonico M, Plu-Bureau G, Lowe GD, Scarabin PY. Hormone replacement therapy and risk of venous thromboembolism in postmenopausal women: systematic review and meta-analysis. BMJ. 2008 May;336(7655): 1227–31.

61. Toorians AWFT, Thomassen MCLGD, Zweegman S, Magdeleyns EJP, Tans G, Gooren LJG, et al. Venous thrombosis and changes of hemostatic variables during cross-sex hormone treatment in transsexual people. J Clin Endocrinol Metab. 2003 Dec;88(12):5723–9.

62. Wierckx K, Gooren L, T'Sjoen G. Clinical review: breast development in trans women receiving cross-sex hormones. J Sex Med. 2014 May;11(5):1240–7.

63. Orentreich N, Durr NP. Proceedings: mammogenesis in transsexuals. J Invest Dermatol. 1974 Jul;63(1):142–6.

64. Rossouw JE, Anderson GL, Prentice RL, LaCroix AZ, Kooperberg C, Stefanick ML, et al.; Writing Group for the Women's Health Initiative Investigators. Risks and benefits of estrogen plus progestin in healthy postmenopausal women: principal results From the Women's Health Initiative randomized controlled trial. JAMA. 2002 Jul 17;288(3):321–33.

65. Cavanaugh T, Hopwood R, Gonzalez A, Thompson J [Internet]. Boston, MA: Fenway Health; 2015 Oct [cited 2019 Feb 4]. The medical care of

transgender persons. Available from: https://www.lgbthealtheducation
.org/publication/transgender-sod/.

66. Bouman WP, Claes L, Marshall E, Pinner GT, Longworth J, Maddox V, et al.
Sociodemographic variables, clinical features, and the role of preassessment
cross-sex hormones in older trans people. J Sex Med. 2016 Apr;13(4):711–9.

67. Gooren L, Lips P. Conjectures concerning cross-sex hormone treatment of
aging transsexual persons. J Sex Med. 2014 Aug;11(8):2012–19.

68. Shifren JL, Rifai N, Desindes S, McIlwain M, Doros G, Mazer NA. A
comparison of the short-term effects of oral conjugated equine estrogens
versus transdermal estradiol on C-reactive protein, other serum markers
of inflammation, and other hepatic proteins in naturally menopausal
women. J Clin Endocrinol Metab. 2008 May;93(5):1702–10.

69. Ho JYP, Chen MJ, Sheu WHH, Yi YC, Tsai ACW, Guu HF, et al. Differential
effects of oral conjugated equine estrogen and transdermal estrogen
on atherosclerotic vascular disease risk markers and endothelial
function in healthy postmenopausal women. Hum Reprod. 2006
Oct;21(10):2715–20.

70. Canonico M, Oger E, Plu-Bureau G, Conard J, Meyer G, Lévesque H, et al.;
Estrogen and Thromboembolism Risk (ESTHER) Study Group. Hormone
therapy and venous thromboembolism among postmenopausal women:
impact of the route of estrogen administration and progestogens: the
ESTHER study. Circulation. 2007 Feb 20;115(7):840–5.

71. Arnold JD, Sarkodie EP, Coleman ME, Goldstein DA. Incidence of venous
thromboembolism in transgender women receiving oral Estradiol. J Sex
Med. 2016;13(11):1773–7.

72. Wierckx K, Elaut E, Declercq E, Heylens G, De Cuypere G, Taes Y, et
al. Prevalence of cardiovascular disease and cancer during cross-sex
hormone therapy in a large cohort of trans persons: a case-control study.
Eur J Endocrinol. 2013 Oct;169(4):471–8.

73. Getahun D, Nash R, Flanders WD, Baird TC, Becerra-Culqui TA,
Cromwell L, et al. Cross-sex hormones and acute cardiovascular
events in transgender persons: A cohort study. Ann Intern Med. 2018
Aug;169(4):205–13.

74. Ott J, Aust S, Promberger R, Huber JC, Kaufmann U. Cross-sex hormone
therapy alters the serum lipid profile: a retrospective cohort study in 169
transsexuals. J Sex Med. 2011 Aug;8(8):2361–9.

75. Simon JA, Lin F, Vittinghoff E, Bittner V, Res Grp HE; Heart and Estrogen-
Progestin Replacement Study (HERS) Research Group. The relation
of postmenopausal hormone therapy to serum uric acid and the risk
of coronary heart disease events: the Heart and Estrogen-Progestin
Replacement Study (HERS). Ann Epidemiol. 2006;16(2):138–45.

76. Main C, Knight B, Moxham T, Gabriel Sanchez R, Sanchez Gomez LM,
Roqué i Figuls M, et al. Hormone therapy for preventing cardiovascular

disease in post-menopausal women. Cochrane Database Syst Rev. 2013 Apr;(4):CD002229.

77. Dhejne C, Öberg K, Arver S, Landén M. An analysis of all applications for sex reassignment surgery in Sweden, 1960–2010: prevalence, incidence, and regrets. Arch Sex Behav. 2014 Nov;43(8):1535–45.

78. Elamin MB, Garcia MZ, Murad MH, Erwin PJ, Montori VM. Effect of sex steroid use on cardiovascular risk in transsexual individuals: a systematic review and meta-analyses. Clin Endocrinol (Oxf). 2010 Jan;72(1):1–10.

79. Fung R, Hellstern-Layefsky M, Lega I. Is a lower dose of cyproterone acetate as effective at testosterone suppression in transgender women as higher doses? Int J Transgenderism. 2017 Apr;18(2):123–8.

80. Elbers JMH, Giltay EJ, Teerlink T, Scheffer PG, Asscheman H, Seidell JC, et al. Effects of sex steroids on components of the insulin resistance syndrome in transsexual subjects. Clin Endocrinol (Oxf). 2003 May;58(5):562–71.

81. Polderman KH, Gooren LJ, Asscheman H, Bakker A, Heine RJ. Induction of insulin resistance by androgens and estrogens. J Clin Endocrinol Metab. 1994 Jul;79(1):265–71.

82. Bourns A. Guidelines and protocols for hormone therapy and primary health care for trans clients [Internet]. Toronto: Sherbourne Health; 2015 [cited 2019 Feb 4].Available from: http://sherbourne.on.ca/wp-content /uploads/2014/02/Guidelines-and-Protocols-for-Comprehensive -Primary-Care-for-Trans-Clients-2015.pdf.

83. Amin S, Zhang Y, Sawin CT, Evans SR, Hannan MT, Kiel DP, et al. Association of hypogonadism and estradiol levels with bone mineral density in elderly men from the Framingham study. Ann Intern Med. 2000 Dec;133(12):951–63.

84. Gennari L, Khosla S, Bilezikian JP. Estrogen and fracture risk in men. J Bone Miner Res. 2008 Oct;23(10):1548–51.

85. Van Caenegem E, Wierckx K, Taes Y, Schreiner T, Vandewalle S, Toye K, et al. Preservation of volumetric bone density and geometry in trans women during cross-sex hormonal therapy: a prospective observational study. Osteoporos Int. 2015 Jan;26(1):35–47.

86. Van Caenegem E, Taes Y, Wierckx K, Vandewalle S, Toye K, Kaufman JM, et al. Low bone mass is prevalent in male-to-female transsexual persons before the start of cross-sex hormonal therapy and gonadectomy. Bone. 2013 May;54(1):92–7.

87. Increase in lumbar spine Z-score after 10 years of cross-sex hormonal treatment in transwomen and transmen [Internet]. Endocrine Society; [cited 2019 Feb 4]. Available from: https://www.endocrine.org/meetings /endo-annual-meetings/abstract-details

88. Gooren LJ, Assies J, Asscheman H, de Slegte R, van Kessel H. Estrogen-induced prolactinoma in a man. J Clin Endocrinol Metab. 1988 Feb;66(2):444–6.

89. Cunha FS, Domenice S, Câmara VL, Sircili MHP, Gooren LJG, Mendonça BB, et al. Diagnosis of prolactinoma in two male-to-female transsexual subjects following high-dose cross-sex hormone therapy. Andrologia. 2015 Aug;47(6):680–4.

90. Kovacs K, Stefaneanu L, Ezzat S, Smyth HS. Prolactin-producing pituitary adenoma in a male-to-female transsexual patient with protracted estrogen administration. A morphologic study. Arch Pathol Lab Med. 1994 May;118(5):562–5.

91. Serri O, Noiseux D, Robert F, Hardy J. Lactotroph hyperplasia in an estrogen treated male-to-female transsexual patient. J Clin Endocrinol Metab. 1996 Sep;81(9):3177–9.

92. Mueller A, Gooren L. Hormone-related tumors in transsexuals receiving treatment with cross-sex hormones. Eur J Endocrinol. 2008;159(3): 197–202.

93. Bisson JR, Chan KJ, Safer JD. Prolactin levels do not rise among transgender women treated with Estradiol and Spironolactone. Endocr Pract. 2018 Jul;24(7):646–51.

94. Freda PU, Beckers AM, Katznelson L, Molitch ME, Montori VM, Post KD, et al; Endocrine Society. Pituitary incidentaloma: an endocrine society clinical practice guideline. J Clin Endocrinol Metab. 2011 Apr;96(4):894–904.

95. Brown GR, Jones KT. Incidence of breast cancer in a cohort of 5,135 transgender veterans. Breast Cancer Res Treat. 2015 Jan;149(1):191–8.

96. Gooren LJ, van Trotsenburg MAA, Giltay EJ, van Diest PJ. Breast cancer development in transsexual subjects receiving cross-sex hormone treatment. J Sex Med. 2013 Dec;10(12):3129–34.

97. de Blok CJM, Wiepjes CM, Nota NM, van Engelen K, Adank MA, Dreijerink KMA, Barbé E, Konings IRHM, den Heijer M. Breast cancer risk in transgender people receiving hormone treatment: nationwide cohort study in the Netherlands. BMJ. 2019 May 14;365:l1652.

98. Colebunders B, T'Sjoen G, Weyers S, Monstrey S. Hormonal and surgical treatment in trans-women with BRCA1 mutations: a controversial topic. J Sex Med. 2014 Oct;11(10):2496–9.

99. Weyers S, Villeirs G, Vanherreweghe E, Verstraelen H, Monstrey S, Van den Broecke R, et al. Mammography and breast sonography in transsexual women. Eur J Radiol. 2010 Jun;74(3):508–13.

100. GRS Montreal. Screening recommendations for implant rupture. Email to Amy Bourns; 2018.

101. Gooren L, Morgentaler A. Prostate cancer incidence in orchidectomised male-to-female transsexual persons treated with oestrogens. Andrologia. 2014 Dec;46(10):1156–60.
102. Trum HW, Hoebeke P, Gooren LJ. Sex reassignment of transsexual people from a gynecologist's and urologist's perspective. Acta Obstet Gynecol Scand. 2015 Jun;94(6):563–7.
103. HEP Interactions [Internet]. Liverpool (England): University of Liverpool; [cited 2019 Feb 4]. Available from: https://www.hep-druginteractions.org/checker
104. Foldvary-Schaefer N, Falcone T. Catamenial epilepsy: pathophysiology, diagnosis, and management. Neurology 2003;61(6 Suppl 2):S2–S15
105. Carl JS, Weaver SP, Tweed E, Edgerton L. Effect of antiepileptic drugs on oral contraceptives. Am Fam Physician. 2008 Sep 1;78(5):634–5.
106. Wierckx K, Elaut E, Van Hoorde B, Heylens G, De Cuypere G, Monstrey S, et al. Sexual desire in trans persons: associations with sex reassignment treatment. J Sex Med. 2014 Jan;11(1):107–18.
107. Kronawitter D, Gooren LJ, Zollver H, Oppelt PG, Beckmann MW, Dittrich R, et al. Effects of transdermal testosterone or oral dydrogesterone on hypoactive sexual desire disorder in transsexual women: results of a pilot study. Eur J Endocrinol. 2009 Aug;161(2):363–8.
108. Elaut E, De Cuypere G, De Sutter P, Gijs L, Van Trotsenburg M, Heylens G, et al. Hypoactive sexual desire in transsexual women: prevalence and association with testosterone levels. Eur J Endocrinol. 2008 Mar;158(3):393–9.
109. A retrospective study on the use of androgen therapy in trans feminine patients to treat HSSD. Paper presented at: EPATH conference; 2015 Mar 13; Ghent, Belgium.
110. Ridley J, Ischayek A, Dubey V, Iglar K. Adult health checkup: Update on the Preventive Care Checklist Form©. Can Fam Physician. 2016; 62(4):307–13.
111. Futterweit W, Schwartz IS. Histopathology of the breasts of 12 women receiving long-term exogenous androgen therapy. Mt Sinai J Med. 1988 Sep;55(4):309–12.
112. Kaunitz AM [Internet]. Netherlands: Wolters Kluwer; 2018 [cited 2019 Feb 4]. Depot medroxyprogesterone acetate for contraception: efficacy, side effects, metabolic impact, and benefits. UpToDate. Available from: https://www.uptodate.com/contents/depot-medroxyprogesterone-acetate-for-contraception-efficacy-side-effects-metabolic-impact-and-benefits.
113. Spratt DI, Stewart II, Savage C, Craig W, Spack NP, Chandler DW, et al. Subcutaneous injection of Testosterone is an effective and preferred

alternative to intramuscular injection: Demonstration in female-to-male transgender patients. J Clin Endocrinol Metab. 2017 01;102(7):2349–55.

114. Wilson DM, Kiang TKL, Ensom MHH. Pharmacokinetics, safety, and patient acceptability of subcutaneous versus intramuscular testosterone injection for gender-affirming therapy: A pilot study. Am J Health Syst Pharm 2018;75(6):351–8.

115. McFarland J, Craig W, Clarke NJ, Spratt DI. Serum testosterone concentrations remain stable between injections in patients receiving subcutaneous testosterone. J Endocr Soc. 2017;1(8):1095–103.

116. Gooren LJG, Giltay EJ. Review of studies of androgen treatment of female-to-male transsexuals: effects and risks of administration of androgens to females. J Sex Med 2008;5(4):765–76.

117. Bhasin S, Brito JP, Cunningham GR, Hayes FJ, Hodis HN, Matsumoto AM, et al. Testosterone therapy in men with hypogonadism: an Endocrine Society clinical practice guideline. J Clin Endocrinol Metab. 2018 May;103(5):1715–44.

118. Haddad RM, Kennedy CC, Caples SM, Tracz MJ, Boloña ER, Sideras K, et al. Testosterone and cardiovascular risk in men: a systematic review and meta-analysis of randomized placebo-controlled trials. Mayo Clin Proc. 2007 Jan;82(1):29–39.

119. Wu FC, Tajar A, Pye SR, Silman AJ, Finn JD, O'Neill TW, et al.; European Male Aging Study Group. Hypothalamic-pituitary-testicular axis disruptions in older men are differentially linked to age and modifiable risk factors: the European Male Aging Study. J Clin Endocrinol Metab. 2008 Jul;93(7):2737–45.

120. Handelsman DJ, Yeap B, Flicker L, Martin S, Wittert GA, Ly LP. Age-specific population centiles for androgen status in men. Eur J Endocrinol. 2015 Dec;173(6):809–17.

121. Travison TG, Vesper HW, Orwoll E, Wu F, Kaufman JM, Wang Y, et al. Harmonized reference ranges for circulating testosterone levels in men of four cohort studies in the United States and Europe. J Clin Endocrinol Metab. 2017 01;102(4):1161–73.

122. Singh S, Best C, Dunn S, Leyland N, Wolfman WL, Leyland N, et al.; CLINICAL PRACTICE – GYNAECOLOGY COMMITTEE. Abnormal uterine bleeding in pre-menopausal women. J Obstet Gynaecol Can. 2013 May;35(5):473–5.

123. Meriggiola MC, Armillotta F, Costantino A, Altieri P, Saad F, Kalhorn T, et al. Effects of testosterone undecanoate administered alone or in combination with letrozole or dutasteride in female to male transsexuals. J Sex Med. 2008 Oct;5(10):2442–53.

124. Bell AD, Roussin A, Cartier R, Chan WS, Douketis JD, Gupta A, et al. The use of antiplatelet therapy in the outpatient setting: Canadian

Cardiovascular Society Guidelines Executive Summary. Can J Cardiol. 2011;27(2):208–21.

125. Dobs AS, Meikle AW, Arver S, Sanders SW, Caramelli KE, Mazer NA. Pharmacokinetics, efficacy, and safety of a permeation-enhanced testosterone transdermal system in comparison with bi-weekly injections of testosterone enanthate for the treatment of hypogonadal men. J Clin Endocrinol Metab. 1999 Oct;84(10):3469–78.

126. Colton Meier S, Fitzgerald K, Pardo S, Babcock J. The effects of hormonal gender affirmation treatment on mental health in female-to-male transsexuals. J Gay Lesbian Ment Health. 2011 Jul 1;15(3):281–99.

127. Gómez-Gil E, Zubiaurre-Elorza L, Esteva I, Guillamon A, Godás T, Cruz Almaraz M, et al. Hormone-treated transsexuals report less social distress, anxiety and depression. Psychoneuroendocrinology. 2012 May;37(5):662–70.

128. Cattrall FR, Healy DL. Long-term metabolic, cardiovascular and neoplastic risks with polycystic ovary syndrome. Best Pract Res Clin Obstet Gynaecol. 2004 Oct;18(5):803–12.

129. Futterweit W. Endocrine therapy of transsexualism and potential complications of long-term treatment. Arch Sex Behav. 1998 Apr;27(2):209–26.

130. Urban RR, Teng NNH, Kapp DS. Gynecologic malignancies in female-to-male transgender patients: the need of original gender surveillance. Am J Obstet Gynecol. 2011 May;204(5):e9–12.

131. Schlatterer K, Yassouridis A, von Werder K, Poland D, Kemper J, Stalla GK. A follow-up study for estimating the effectiveness of a cross-gender hormone substitution therapy on transsexual patients. Arch Sex Behav. 1998 Oct;27(5):475–92.

132. Miller N, Bédard YC, Cooter NB, Shaul DL. Histological changes in the genital tract in transsexual women following androgen therapy. Histopathology. 1986 Jul;10(7):661–9.

133. Grynberg M, Fanchin R, Dubost G, Colau J, Brémont-Weil C, Frydman R, et al. Histology of genital tract and breast tissue after long-term testosterone administration in a female-to-male transsexual population. Reprod Biomed Online. 2010;20(4):553–8.

134. Perrone AM, Cerpolini S, Maria Salfi NC, Ceccarelli C, De Giorgi LB, Formelli G, et al. Effect of long-term testosterone administration on the endometrium of female-to-male (FtM) transsexuals. J Sex Med. 2009 Nov;6(11):3193–200.

135. Mueller A, Kiesewetter F, Binder H, Beckmann MW, Dittrich R. Long-term administration of testosterone undecanoate every 3 months for testosterone supplementation in female-to-male transsexuals. J Clin Endocrinol Metab. 2007 Sep;92(9):3470–5.

136. Loverro G, Resta L, Dellino M, Edoardo DN, Cascarano MA, Loverro M, et al. Uterine and ovarian changes during testosterone administration in young female-to-male transsexuals. Taiwan J Obstet Gynecol. 2016 Oct;55(5):686–91.
137. Futterweit W, Deligdisch L. Histopathological effects of exogenously administered testosterone in 19 female to male transsexuals. J Clin Endocrinol Metab. 1986 Jan;62(1):16–21.
138. Mikhaïlichenko VV, Fesenko VN, Khmelnitskiï NV, Ozhiganova IN, Novikov AI, Korolev VV, et al. [Morphological and functional changes of organs of female and male reproductive systems at change of sex.] Urologiia. 2013;(3):18–23.
139. Van Caenegem E, Wierckx K, Taes Y, Schreiner T, Vandewalle S, Toye K, et al. Body composition, bone turnover, and bone mass in trans men during testosterone treatment: 1-year follow-up data from a prospective case-controlled study (ENIGI). Eur J Endocrinol. 2015 Feb;172(2):163–71.
140. Mueller A, Haeberle L, Zollver H, Claassen T, Kronawitter D, Oppelt PG, et al. Effects of intramuscular testosterone undecanoate on body composition and bone mineral density in female-to-male transsexuals. J Sex Med. 2010 Sep;7(9):3190–8.
141. Nota NM, Dekker MJHJ, Klaver M, Wiepjes CM, van Trotsenburg MA, Heijboer AC, et al. Prolactin levels during short- and long-term cross-sex hormone treatment: an observational study in transgender persons. Andrologia. 2017 Aug;49(6):e12666.
142. Turner A, Chen TC, Barber TW, Malabanan AO, Holick MF, Tangpricha V. Testosterone increases bone mineral density in female-to-male transsexuals: a case series of 15 subjects. Clin Endocrinol (Oxf). 2004 Nov;61(5):560–6.
143. Papaioannou A, Morin S, Cheung AM, Atkinson S, Brown JP, Feldman S, et al.; Scientific Advisory Council of Osteoporosis Canada. 2010 clinical practice guidelines for the diagnosis and management of osteoporosis in Canada: summary. CMAJ. 2010 Nov 23;182(17):1864–73.
144. van Kesteren P, Lips P, Gooren L, Asscheman H, Megens J. Long-term follow-up of bone mineral density and bone metabolism in transsexuals treated with cross-sex hormones. Clin Endocrinol (Oxf). 1998;48(3):347–54.
145. Gooren L, Bowers M, Lips P, Konings IR. Five new cases of breast cancer in transsexual persons. Andrologia. 2015 Dec;47(10):1202–5.
146. Peitzmeier SM, Khullar K, Reisner SL, Potter J. Pap test use is lower among female-to-male patients than non-transgender women. Am J Prev Med. 2014 Dec;47(6):808–12.
147. Potter M. Tips for providing paps to trans men [Internet]. Toronto: Rainbow Health Ontario; updated 2018 [cited 2018 Jun 1]. Available

from: https://www.rainbowhealthontario.ca/wp-content/uploads
/2020/04/Tips_Paps_TransMen.pdf.

148. Potter J, Peitzmeier SM, Bernstein I, Reisner SL, Alizaga NM, Agénor
M, et al. Cervical Cancer Screening for Patients on the Female-to-Male
Spectrum: a Narrative Review and Guide for Clinicians. J Gen Intern
Med. 2015 Dec;30(12):1857–64. doi:10.1007/s11606-015-3462-8.

149. Davis-Devine S, Day SJ, Anderson A, French A, Madison-Henness D,
Mohar N, et al. Collection of the BD SurePath Pap Test with a broom
device plus endocervical brush improves disease detection when
compared to the broom device alone or the spatula plus endocervical
brush combination. Cytojournal. 2008 Feb;6:4.

150. Dizon DS, Tejada-Berges T, Koelliker S, Steinhoff M, Granai CO. Ovarian
cancer associated with testosterone supplementation in a female-to-male
transsexual patient. Gynecol Obstet Invest. 2006;62(4):226–8.

151. Hage JJ, Dekker JJ, Karim RB, Verheijen RH, Bloemena E. Ovarian cancer
in female-to-male transsexuals: report of two cases. Gynecol Oncol. 2000
Mar;76(3):413–15.

152. Ikeda K, Baba T, Noguchi H, Nagasawa K, Endo T, Kiya T, et al.
Excessive androgen exposure in female-to-male transsexual persons of
reproductive age induces hyperplasia of the ovarian cortex and stroma
but not polycystic ovary morphology. Hum Reprod. 2013;28(2):453–61.

153. Wierckx K, Van de Peer F, Verhaeghe E, Dedecker D, Van Caenegem E,
Toye K, et al. Short- and long-term clinical skin effects of testosterone
treatment in trans men. J Sex Med 2014;11(1):222–9.

154. Dubey V, Matthew R, Iglar K, Duerksen A. Preventive care checklist
forms [Internet]. 2018 Jun 29 [cited 2019 Dec 30]. Available at: https://
portal.cfpc.ca/CFPC/Resources/EN/Periodic_Health_Examination
/content_id_1184.aspx.

12 Indigenous LGBTQ and Two-Spirit Health

ZONGWE BINESIKWE CRYSTAL HARDY

Introduction

My name is Zongwe Binesikwe Crystal Hardy, Sounding Thunderbird Woman, Bear Clan, from Rocky Bay First Nation in northern Ontario. I live and work out of Thunder Bay, Ontario, as an Anishinaabe Two-Spirit storyteller and nurse practitioner. My pronouns are *they/them/she/her*. I am a PhD candidate in nursing at Queen's University, with an area of study focused on decolonizing trauma work. My thesis, "Storytelling as Medicine: Autoethnography of a Two-Spirit Anishinaabe Nurse Practitioner," explores the use of ceremonial self-reflective practice using expressive arts to promote resilience and address compassion fatigue in nurses.

The term *Two-Spirit* is used by some First Nations, Métis, and Inuit peoples on Turtle Island (Canada) to describe their sexual, gender, or spiritual identity as having both a masculine and a feminine spirit. In this chapter, I use the term *Indigenous* when discussing First Nations (Status or non-Status), Inuit, and Métis peoples. Another term you may have heard is *Aboriginal*; this term comes from the 1982 Constitution, meaning "from the Origins." Because of the colonial history of Canada, Indigenous 2SLGBTQ people face increased risks of bias and social isolation related to the intersectionality of race, gender, and sexual orientation. Many of the programs available to Indigenous patients have been created from a non-Indigenous perspective and may not be considered culturally safe. For health care providers to better understand the needs of Indigenous 2SLGBTQ individuals, it is necessary to consider the historical and contemporary impacts of colonization. While resources exist for both Indigenous patients and LGBTQ patients separately, there are currently limited resources available for Indigenous patients who are 2SLGBTQ. This chapter will direct readers to available resources, as well as outline the history of Indigenous peoples in Canada and contemporary issues facing Indigenous 2SLGBTQ individuals.

Storytelling

Throughout this chapter, I will tell the stories of historical and current events that affect the health and well-being of Indigenous peoples in Canada, particularly those that affect people who are 2SLGBTQ. It is important to note that much of the historical writing about Indigenous peoples was done by European settlers who typically were not academics;[1] thus, observations were made through a Eurocentric lens and impacted by colonial biases. Although research continues to provide more information, there has been limited inquiry focused on the unique cultural and health care needs of Indigenous 2SLGBTQ people.[2]

Within North America, the transmission of knowledge has historically been through storytelling. Storytelling is a holistic and experiential teaching method to pass on cultural beliefs, values, rituals, and ways of life. Some Indigenous peoples may have lost their voice (the ability to speak their truths) because of historical attempts at assimilation and cultural genocide. This loss is felt by Indigenous 2SLGBTQ individuals, and the reclamation of their voices is paramount to promote good health. A powerful example of this reclamation can be seen in Elder Ma-Nee Chacaby's autobiography:[3]

> My name is Ma-Nee Chacaby. I am an Ojibwe-Cree elder, and I have both a male and a female spirit inside of me. I have experienced a long, complicated, and sometimes challenging journey over the course of my life. My earliest memories are of gathering kindling, making snowshoes, and hunting and trapping in my isolated Canadian community, where alcoholism was widespread in the 1950s. In 2013, more than a half a century later, I performed a healing ceremony and then helped lead the first gay pride parade in my city, Thunder Bay, Ontario.

Our patients also utilise storytelling techniques by sharing their knowledge and experience of their health journeys through illness narratives. Illness narratives often occur as oral stories outlining how lives have been impacted by a health issue.[4] Contemporary Western health care very often focuses on viewing patients primarily by their symptoms or diagnosis; however, it is important for health care providers to seek out stories from patients.

Indigenous Peoples in Canada

Three groups of Indigenous peoples in Canada were distinctly recognized in the 1982 Constitution: First Nation, Inuit, and Métis. More than one million people in Canada identify as Indigenous people.[5] The terms *Indigenous* and *Aboriginal* are used to include First Nations, Inuit, and Métis peoples[6] – these terms will be used interchangeably throughout this chapter. There are hundreds of distinct Indigenous cultures, languages, and societies in Canada.

The First Nations peoples in Canada used to be called *Indians*, since early European explorers thought they had landed in India.[1] The term *Indian*, although now considered derogatory, continues to be used as a legal definition under Canadian Law, such as the Indian Act. The Indian Act of 1876, which evolved from the Gradual Civilization Act of 1857, is a federal law defining relations between the Canadian government and First Nations peoples. These laws and policies predate the confederation of Canada and were designed to benefit the British Empire through the establishment of Canada as a colony and part of the British Commonwealth. Under the Gradual Civilization Act, Indian peoples could have rights if they "pledged to live as White."[7] The Indian Act went on to control and define in absolute the citizenship of First Nations peoples, including their language, cultural, social, political, and economic rights. An Indian Registry was created to keep the names of all Indian peoples in Canada. Status First Nation individuals are listed in the Indian Register and are issued identification cards (known as Status or treaty cards) that contain information regarding band and registration number.[8] In contrast, non-Status First Nation individuals are not registered with the federal government and their names do not appear in the Indian Registry. Indians were considered "wards of the State." *Enfranchisement* is the term used for losing one's "Indian Status." Enfranchisement could happen in many circumstances, from serving in the military to owning land to obtaining a university degree: these accomplishments could not happen without losing "Indian Status" and all protected rights that come with Status. Enfranchisement had a significant impact on Indigenous women. For example, under the Indian Act, if an Indigenous woman married a non-Indigenous man, she would lose her Status.[8] In April 1985, a Bill to Amend the Indian Act (Bill C-31) was passed into law to address gender discrimination and restore Status to those who had been forcibly enfranchised.[9] These individuals may identify with Bill C-31 status. The Inquiry into Missing and Murdered Indigenous Women and Girls (MMIWG) identified sex and gender discrimination in the Indian Act as a fundamental institutionalized policy that contributes to the tragic violence against Indigenous Women, Girls and 2SLGBTQ peoples.[10]

The Indigenous peoples of the Arctic are known as Inuit; however, there is also a large population in Ottawa. The word *Inuit* means "the people" in the Inuit language of Inuktut.[11] Some Inuit do not identify with the term *Indigenous*. Métis are a people of mixed ancestry (Indigenous and European)[12] whose cultural origins trace back to the late eighteenth century near the Red River in Manitoba. Métis culture is unique and distinct from both First Nations and European culture.

There is not one way to be Indigenous, just as there is not one way to be LGBTQ or Two-Spirit. The experiences of LGBTQ and Two-Spirit individuals may overlap, but they are distinct identities.[2] Therefore, many services focused on only LGBTQ care or Indigenous patient populations may not meet the individual needs of the patient. For example, Indigenous Two-Spirit people have stated that some Aboriginal health care centres were not welcoming of their expressions of Two-Spirit identity.[2] They also reported that LGBTQ-specific services often have limited knowledge of the Two-Spirit identity or the unique concerns of Indigenous communities.[2] Health care providers can ask patients how they identify their ethnicity and to share relevant stories to help the provider understand patients' backgrounds.

Indigenous History

Indigenous peoples have a historical legacy with the Canadian government. To understand the health and wellbeing of Indigenous 2SLGBTQ individuals, we must consider the historical impacts of colonization as well as its contemporary effects.[13] To provide historical and current context, providers can familiarize themselves with the following important documents and inquiries that impact the Indigenous peoples of Canada.

Royal Proclamation of 1763

The Royal Proclamation of 1763 is a document that set out guidelines for European settlement of Aboriginal territories in North America. It recognizes Indigenous peoples as independent Nations and owners of the land they occupied.[14] Some Indigenous academics consider the Royal Proclamation as an important step towards self-determination as it is powerful evidence of the recognition of Aboriginal rights in Canadian law.

The Indian Act of 1876

The Indian Act of 1876 is the principal statute through which the federal government manages Indigenous issues. The focus of this legislation was to "civilize" Indigenous peoples through coercion and control by prohibiting them from speaking their languages, practising their traditional religion, and outlawing cultural ceremonies. The Indian Act denied women Status, introduced the Indian residential school system (IRSS), created reservations, renamed individuals with European names, and restricted First Nations people from leaving reserves without permission from an Indian Agent. The Indian Act imposed the band council system – a system that did not take into account traditional governance structures – and denied First Nations people the right to vote.[15]

First Nations people were also prohibited from owning property, attending university, lobbying the government, hiring legal counsel, seeking legal claims, or starting political organizations. Indigenous peoples in Canada were not granted the unfettered right to vote until 1960. Indigenous peoples were forced to live on segregated lands (reserves), which were not adequately resourced with basic services and did not correspond to traditional lands. Permission from an Indian Agent was required to leave the reserve, to produce or sell goods outside the reserve, and even for sustenance hunting and fishing on-reserve. Cultural and traditional practices were outlawed on- and off-reserve, and Indigenous languages were prohibited.

Métis Road Allowance

As Canada expanded into the prairies in the late 1800s, the Dominion Land Survey divided the territory into homesteads, without taking into account land on which Métis and First Nations peoples lived. Within the homesteads, space was left for roads and railways, and on each side of these thoroughfares was 10 feet of Crown land. As farmers claimed homesteads, Métis peoples were forced to live, hunt, trap, and survive on these thin strips of land in conditions of imposed poverty. Between 1900 and 1960, regulations shaped an increasingly difficult time for Metis peoples as the government enforced stricter laws – for example, declaring it illegal to hunt or trap without a licence – leading to the arrest and jailing of Métis peoples. Métis children were not allowed to go to school as their families did not pay property taxes; the land they lived on was defined as Crown land on which they were "squatting." Generations of Métis peoples were denied access to education in this manner.[16]

High Arctic Relocation

In the 1950s, the Canadian government relocated Inuit, who they declared were citizens of Canada, to the High Arctic. This enabled the Canadian government to exert sovereignty, or land claim, over this highly disputed territory during the Cold War, making the Arctic a part of Canada. This relocation is highly controversial, with the government initially insisting the move was voluntary, while Inuit maintained it was a forced migration so that Canada could colonize the High Arctic. Relocation to this unknown territory caused untold hardship for Inuit peoples, as basic infrastructure and services were not provided and continue to be extremely limited.[17] In 2010, the Canadian government apologized for this "tragic chapter" in Canadian history.[18]

Royal Commission on Aboriginal Peoples of 1996

The Royal Commission on Aboriginal Peoples was mandated to review the challenges affecting the relationship between Aboriginal peoples, the Canadian government, and Canadian society and proposed effective solutions to these challenges.[19] The *Report of the Royal Commission on Aboriginal Peoples* contains five volumes that concern governmental policies related to original Indigenous nations.[19] Some of the major recommendations included legislation committing to a new relationship with Aboriginal peoples; recognition of an Aboriginal order of government; expansion of the Aboriginal land and resource base; and initiatives to address social, education, and health needs.[19]

United Nations Declaration of the Rights of Indigenous Peoples

In September 2007, the United Nations Declaration of the Rights of Indigenous Peoples (UNDRIP) was adopted by the United Nations General Assembly as a standard of achievement to be pursued in a spirit of partnership and mutual respect.[20] The Declaration establishes a universal framework of standards for the survival, dignity, and well-being of the Indigenous peoples of the world.[20] The UNDRIP received near unanimous approval, with only four countries in opposition: the United States, New Zealand, Australia, and Canada. Canada has since reversed its position.[20]

Truth and Reconciliation Commission of Canada, 2015

The Truth and Reconciliation Commission of Canada (TRC) aimed to acknowledge the legacy of residential schools and further the process of reconciliation with Indigenous peoples[21]. The TRC was a result of the Indian Residential School Settlement Agreement of 2007: the largest class action lawsuit in Canadian history – and it does not even include Metis, Inuit, or day school survivors. Indigenous children were forced to attend government-funded, church-run residential schools that had the express goal of assimilation into Euro-Canadian culture. The last residential school closed in 1996.

In 2008, Prime Minister Stephen Harper gave a historic apology to the Indigenous peoples of Canada, saying, "The two primary objectives of the IRSS were to remove and isolate children from their families, homes, traditions and cultures, and to assimilate them into the dominant culture. These objectives were based on the belief that Aboriginal cultures and spiritual beliefs were inferior and unequal. Indeed, some sought, as infamously said, to 'kill the Indian in the child'. Today, we recognize this was wrong and it caused great harm, and has no place in our country." Survivors came forward to expose the horrific cruelty, abuse, and trauma inflicted on generations of Indigenous families through these school systems, and the TRC came to the conclusion that the IRSS was a system of cultural genocide.[22]

The Indian Residential School Settlement agreement gave compensation to some survivors, established the Aboriginal Healing Foundation, and established the Truth and Reconciliation Commission, which explored the impact of the IRSS. The Inquiry lasted from 2008 to 2015, during which time thousands of testimonies were heard across the country and more than 6000 people with lived experience of the IRSS were interviewed. There are 94 Calls to Action centred on the themes of legacy, education, language and culture, health, justice, and reconciliation.[21] Some of the recommendations include reducing the number of Indigenous children in the child welfare system; addressing the educational and employment gaps; and closing the gaps in health outcomes, well-being, quality of life, and life expectancy between Indigenous and non-Indigenous peoples in Canada.[23]

The National Inquiry into Missing and Murdered
Indigenous Women and Girls

The MMIWG Inquiry was launched in 2015 to examine the systemic causes of violence against Indigenous women, girls, and members of the 2SLGBTQ community.[24] Indigenous women, girls, and 2SLGBTQ peoples face an astonishing amount of violence in Canada, where they are 12 to 19 times as likely to be missing or murdered than any other group. Not only are they victims of violence at these alarming rates, but they are also massively overrepresented in the criminal justice and child apprehension systems. In some provinces, 85 per cent of incarcerated women are Indigenous.[25] They are 5 to 12 times as likely to lose their children to care,[26] where 90 per cent of apprehended children are Indigenous in some provinces.[21] The MMIWG Inquiry collected data through a decolonizing, culturally specific, and rights-based approach that highlighted the resilience, resistance, and cultural resurgence of Indigenous women, girls, and 2SLGBTQ people. The final report on MMIWG was released in June 2019.[24]

Colonization

Colonization is the action of settling among and establishing control over the Indigenous peoples of an area. Colonization and assimilation of Indigenous peoples into Euro-Canadian society has impacted health, traditional roles, connection to culture, socioeconomic conditions, and access to services.[27] The impact of colonization can be viewed as one of the most influential factors affecting the health of Indigenous peoples today.[28]

During colonization, Indigenous peoples living outside of typical European gender and sexual norms faced discrimination, oppression, violence, and murder.[29] Colonial patriarchy marginalized Indigenous women and Two-Spirit people through the Indian Act and its governance systems, which in turn inform the barriers which Indigenous women and Two Spirit people continue to face today.[6] The colonial system affected not only Indigenous women and Two-Spirit people but Indigenous men and Indigenous LGBTQ people as well,[30] while trans people fail to be recognized at all because of the colonial notion of the gender binary.[28]

The root causes of health inequalities should be considered within historical, economic, and sociopolitical contexts to promote equity in health care.[27] The impacts of colonialism on Indigenous communities intentionally resulted in vast disparities in social determinants of health, including poverty, housing insecurity, high rates of substance use, unemployment, and violence.[31] The intersectionality of ethnicity, gender, and social exclusion places Indigenous 2SLGBTQ people at risk for harassment and physical and sexual assault.[32] Patterns of discrimination including violence, isolation, health care bias, self-denial, and internalized homo/bi/transphobia produce negative health effects such as increased rates of alcohol and drug use, greater risks for sexually transmitted infections, and high rates of depression and suicide.[33]

True decolonization will involve reshaping Indigenous governance and honouring self-determination, gender variance, and the contributions of Indigenous women, Two-Spirit, and LGBTQ individuals.[28]

Christianity

Colonization introduced Christianity and moralistic teachings regarding gender and sexuality into Indigenous communities, implementing a colonial sex/gender binary and effectively a cultural genocide.[30] Children in schools were separated into two gendered groups defined by colonizers and expected to conform to strongly contrasting behaviours.[30] Within this religious belief system, sex for the exclusive purpose of reproduction and the immorality of homosexuality are core teachings.[29] This European gender binary was violently imposed on Indigenous communities through Christianity and the IRSS.[2] Those individuals who did not conform to the gender binary were seen as "unclean" or "unwell" and placed into mental health institutions. Similarly, any same sex relationships were viewed as immoral. This history has been passed through generations of Indigenous peoples, causing lack of trust of both the education and the health care systems.

Indian Residential School System

From 1857 to 1996, more than 150,000 children ages 6 to 15 years old were forcibly taken from their homes and placed into the IRSS. Children were traumatized when they were taken from their parents and placed into government-funded, church-controlled, residential learning institutions. Many children suffered significant physical, emotional, and sexual abuse perpetrated by teachers and moral authorities, as well as prolonged hunger and other experiments. Those who were lucky enough to make it home often were disconnected from their families and communities by mental health issues. The residential schools were created to separate Aboriginal children from their families to minimize family ties and cultural linkages,[21] and the trauma these children experienced has had lasting effects on their ability to parent their own children. As Sir John A. MacDonald, Canada's first prime minister, told the House of Commons in 1883:[21]

> When the school is on the reserve the child lives with its parents, who are savages; he is surrounded by savages, and though he may learn to read and write his habits, and training and mode of thought are Indian. He is simply a savage who can read and write. It has been strongly

pressed on myself, as the head of the Department, that the Indian children should be withdrawn as much as possible from the parental influence, and the only way to do that would be to put them in central training industrial schools where they will acquire the habits and modes of thought of white men.

The Government of Canada pursued this cultural genocide as a means to separate itself from financial obligations to Aboriginal peoples and gain control over the land and resources.[21]

The Sixties Scoop and the Child Welfare System

The practice of removing children from their families was not done only through the residential school system. During the 1960s, Indigenous children were placed into the child welfare system,[34] and the term *Sixties Scoop* is used to describe the placement of "neglected" or disadvantaged Indigenous children with non-Indigenous families.[35]

There continues to be an overrepresentation of Indigenous children in out-of-home care due to multiple disadvantages, including systemic racism.[36] These disadvantages relate to social determinants of health facing their families – for example poverty, poor housing conditions imposed on Indigenous communities, and substance use related to unresolved intergenerational trauma.

Currently, the number of Indigenous children in the child welfare system exceeds that at the height of the residential school movement.[36] Severing the parent-child relationship was a fundamental tenet of the IRSS, and children who survived the IRSS were denied healthy parental role models; as adults, they face increased structural and personal challenges in caring for their own families.[36]

Intergenerational Trauma

Stressful and traumatic events have immediate effects on health and well-being but can also be passed down through generations.[37] Survivors transmit the trauma they experienced to later generations when they don't recognize or have the opportunity to address their issues.[38] Over time, these behaviours become normalized within the family and community, leading to the next generation suffering the same or related problems.[38] Some of the consequences of unresolved trauma include depression, anxiety, family violence, suicidal and homicidal thoughts, and addictions. High-risk-taking behaviours can exist when a patient is having difficulty coping with past or current experiences.

Trauma-Informed Care

In addition to the intergenerational trauma of forced relocation and cultural genocide, Indigenous peoples tend to experience higher rates of personal traumas including assault, abuse, and systemic racism.[2] Studies have shown that Two-Spirit individuals and gay and bisexual Indigenous men are more likely than their non-Indigenous counterparts to report being physically or sexually assaulted, which may include childhood sexual abuse.[2] Trans-identified Indigenous people report being subjected to physical or sexual violence motivated by transphobia[2] within their home communities as well as urban settings. This violence is often endorsed against those who defy binary gender identities.

Trauma-informed care involves the holistic treatment of a patient by taking into account past traumatic events and subsequent coping mechanisms.[39] Indigenous peoples are exposed to single and cumulative traumatic incidents over the course of their lives,[13] through exposure to or witnessing actual or threatened physical injury or death. These incidents can cause post-traumatic stress disorder (PTSD), which affects Indigenous women and gender diverse people more often than their non-Indigenous counterparts. A history of childhood abuse and violence may increase the risk of PTSD, which is further compounded by poverty and low educational attainment.

Some patients may speak about their traumas factually without visible emotion.[39] Often this is the patient's attempt to cope with the traumatic event through detachment.[39] Trauma-informed care can involve listening to the patient's narrative to broaden the provider's understanding of the patient's past. When Indigenous peoples interact with the health care system, it would be beneficial for health care providers to use a trauma-informed lens: recognizing the prevalence of trauma and how it affects all individuals involved.

Environments

On-Reserve

Indian reservations were created through the Indian Act as fixed geographical areas that imposed restrictions on the people forced to live within them. Throughout Canada, many Indigenous peoples are currently living in conditions similar to those in developing countries,[39] and those on reserves face significant jurisdictional issues. The First Nations and Inuit Health Branch, now called Indigenous Services Canada, supports the delivery of public health and health promotion services on-reserve and within Inuit communities. For those communities that are remote and isolated, Indigenous Services Canada offers primary health care services.

Indigenous 2SLGBTQ peoples have delayed accessing care when they feel unsafe because of biases.[2] Furthermore, the quality and access to these services are below the average standard, particularly for services related to 2SLGBTQ care. Confidentiality can be difficult to maintain in smaller communities, especially if family members or close community contacts work at the nursing station or health clinic. Individuals may fear being ostracised if they disclose their sexual orientation or gender identity. There are also significant concerns because of the lack of stable health care or qualified providers on-reserve. Health care providers can address issues of visibility and acceptance by creating welcoming environments through gender diverse posters, intake forms, and clinician language and behaviour. Countless Indigenous 2SLGBTQ individuals leave their homes to seek out gender-diverse communities and services.[40] Unfortunately, moving away from their communities may lead to social isolation and disconnection from family.

Urban Life

Indigenous peoples move to urban centres for many reasons, including access to health care, education, employment, and housing.[41] Similarly, 2SLGBTQ individuals may move to urban areas because of a lack of family or community acceptance of their sexual orientation and gender identity.[42] The experience of Indigenous 2SLGBTQ individuals varies. This variability of acceptance depends on the individual, their family, and their community. Some communities have a very strong Christian or Catholic faith that remained in place after colonization and may not be as accepting as other communities that are not Christian or Catholic.

After relocating to an urban centre, some Indigenous 2SLBGTQ people continue to face many of the same challenges as people moving to Canada from other countries[13] (see chapter 15 on newcomers and refugees). They have left their home communities only to face racism within 2SLGBTQ-specific services.[2] This marginalization can have significant effects on the well-being of Indigenous sexual- and gender-minority individuals[2] and is a key factor in creating the gap in health outcomes.[39] However, on a positive note, Indigenous 2SLGBTQ people have come together to create communities based on empowerment and Indigenous teaching to reduce marginalization.[43]

Health Access and Equity

Access to primary health care can be a problem for many Indigenous 2SLGBTQ people. The compartmentalized care offered doesn't achieve a holistic picture of health and fails to account for the reality of homophobia and heterosexism.[13] It can be helpful for health care providers to be aware of and collaborate with the 2SLGBTQ services and resources available in their area.

The health disparities and inequities that Indigenous peoples face in Canada can be directly and indirectly linked to social, economic, cultural, and political inequities. Indigenous 2SLGBTQ individuals' experiences cannot be simply understood from knowledge of broader Indigenous or gender-diverse populations.[40] Compounded marginalization can be understood in the theory of intersectionality.[44] Health care providers can help mitigate this marginalization through the provision of culturally safe care.

Cultural Safety Continuum

Cultural safety in health care involves empowerment of the health care provider and the patient – which is determined by the patient. The adoption of culturally safe principles can lead to more equitable health outcomes in Indigenous communities.[2]

Cultural safety follows on a continuum (see figure 12.1). It begins with cultural awareness, which is recognizing our own cultural values, beliefs, and perceptions and how they are the same or different from other cultures. The next stage is cultural sensitivity, which is being aware of and understanding a deeper level of emotions that attach to your own culture and how your culture may be perceived by others. Then comes cultural competency, which focuses on the skills, knowledge, and attitudes of the health care provider. Finally, cultural safety, which goes beyond awareness and helps us to understand the limitations of competence. Some recommendations[2] to promote cultural safety in health care include the following:

- Learning about the colonization of Indigenous communities in Canada
- Examining one's own biases
- Recognizing one's own social location
- Being mindful of the power imbalance between provider and patient
- Addressing the root causes of health disparities

Figure 12.1. Cultural Safety Continuum

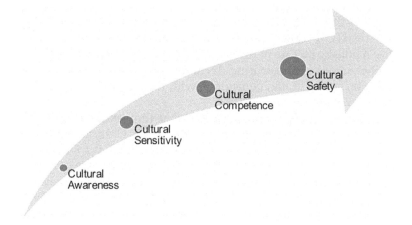

Gender Identity

Before European contact, Indigenous peoples respected alternative gender identities as a part of the sacred web of life and society.[29] There have been 150 documented Indigenous nations that counted third genders among their members.[45] Indigenous identity had little to do with biological sex or associated roles and was more concerned with a holistic understanding of being, which may be incorporated into ceremonies.[30] There was respect for gender equality and gender fluidity.[46] Individual uniqueness was embraced, and diversity was viewed as an asset, unlike traditional European ideals of dichotomous gender roles.[29]

Many Indigenous communities had their own terms that demonstrated LGBTQ or Two-Spirit identities [47] such as:

- Crow: *boté, bate, bade* ("split testicles")
- Cree: *ayekkwe, a:yahkwew* ("split testicles")
- Lakota: *winkte* ("would be woman," "dreams of double woman")
- Navajo: *nutlys, natli, nadleehi* ("he changes," "being transformed")

Two-Spirit

Two-Spirit can be defined as a self-descriptor increasingly used by Aboriginal gay, lesbian, bisexual, and transgender people who live within a traditional Aboriginal worldview. It asserts that all aspects of identity are interconnected, where sexuality is inseparable from experiences of culture and communities.[43] Self-identifying as Two-Spirit is an act of decolonization as it allows individuals to separate from essentialist and sometimes derogatory Euro-colonial terms.[29]

The term *Two-Spirit* affirms the interrelatedness of all aspects of identity including gender, sexuality, community, culture, and spirituality.[43] Two-Spirit individuals occupy distinct gender roles and cultural expectations for those roles.[47] Many of the shamans, visionaries, dreamers, and medicine givers in pre-colonized Indigenous communities were Two-Spirits.[48]

Not all Indigenous LGBTQ individuals will identify with the term *Two-Spirit*[2] and many Indigenous individuals don't label themselves as LGBTQ or Two-Spirit. Some may identify with a nation-specific term that best represents the gender diversity traditionally found in their community.[2] When addressing patients, health care providers could offer their own name and pronoun to provide an opportunity for the patient to share – or ask the patient if they identify with a particular term.

Holistic Care

Within an Indigenous perspective, wellness is viewed as a whole and healthy person through a sense of balance of spirit, emotion, mind, and body.[49] Negative health outcomes are largely caused by life stressors.[50] We can use a life course perspective that focuses on exposure to a variety of health determinants throughout different life stages, from gestation through childhood and early adulthood to older adulthood.[51] The social determinants of health have a differential impact on health across the life course. Health issues such as chronic illnesses may create conditions that influence health[52] through perceived disability. The idea of holistic care and interconnectedness can be found throughout Indigenous cultures.

Seven Sacred Grandfather Teachings

The Anishinabek (Ojibway) story of the seven grandfather teachings has been shared through the generations.[53] The teachings offer ways in which to love and respect each other and nature:[53]

- Wisdom: To cherish knowledge is to know wisdom
- Love: To know love is to know peace
- Respect: To honour all of creation is to have respect

Figure 12.2. Medicine Wheel

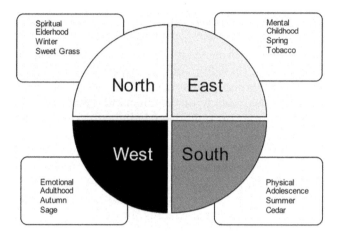

- Bravery: Bravery is to face the foe with integrity
- Honesty: Honesty in facing a situation is to be brave
- Humility: Humility is to know yourself as a sacred part of creation
- Truth: Truth is to know all of these things

Medicine Wheel Teachings

The medicine wheel emphasizes a holistic approach to maintain balance in life (see figure 12.2). It is a circular symbol representing the wholeness of traditional Indigenous life. It represents not only spirituality but also the emotional and physical aspects of people's beliefs.[54] It would be useful for providers to have familiarity with Indigenous beliefs of health and well-being. It may also be helpful to have a medicine wheel or some Indigenous artwork visible in a clinical space to promote a sense of cultural awareness for patients.

Mental Health

Within the medicine wheel, mental health is represented by direction of East (see figure 12.2). The sacred medicine of tobacco sits in the Eastern direction as it was the first medicine gifted to Ojibway people by the Creator. Tobacco is used to communicate with the Spirit world and is used as an offering or a gift. Everything begins in the East – childhood, spring, and mental health.

Mental well-being is the intelligent and conscious drive to know and activate one's being and becoming.[49] Indigenous peoples, including those who are 2SLGBTQ, are more likely to report mental health problems (including anxiety, depression, and PTSD) than their non-Indigenous counterparts.[13] Generations of Indigenous children continue to be born into circumstances of hopelessness, poverty, discrimination, racism, and violence. These adverse childhood events negatively impact health outcomes. There can be issues with management of emotions and the lack of positive coping skills. Low self-esteem has been noted as a risk factor for substance use and other risky behaviours for Indigenous 2SLGBTQ people.[2]

As discussed, mental health service usage rates are reportedly high among Indigenous 2SLGBTQ individuals.[4] Negative mental and physical health outcomes have been attributed to the effects of racist, sexist, cissexist, and heterosexist discrimination and violence.[2]

High rates of alcoholism, addictions, and attempted and completed suicides of Indigenous 2SLGBTQ people can be attributed to colonialism, structures of anti-Indigenous racism, social isolation, and inadequate support.[29] As previously mentioned, sexual- and gender-minority Indigenous individuals in rural and on-reserve environments can face significant barriers to accessing culturally safe services.[2]

Mood Disorders

Social isolation and exclusion can prevent individuals from pursuing education and training, promoting lack of income and potential for poverty.[52] Poverty creates lack of control and can result in anxiety, insecurity, low self-esteem, and feelings of hopelessness.[52] These types of psychological stressors have been linked to violence, addictions, poor parenting skills, social isolation, and lack of social support.[52] Research has shown that Two-Spirit people reported their first drink at an earlier age than their non-Indigenous counterparts and report drinking to manage their moods, relax, make friends, and deal with feelings of inferiority.[13] Two-Spirit people are more likely to experience depression and anxiety related to intersections of racism, homophobia, transphobia, heteronormativity, and intergenerational trauma.[32] Indigenous 2SLGBTQ individuals may continue to feel the stigma of other people viewing homosexuality and transsexuality as mental health disorders.[32] Unfortunately, the lack of access to culturally safe care continues to impact the mental health status of Indigenous 2SLGBTQ people in Canada.[52]

Suicide

Suicide was the leading cause of death among Indigenous youth ages 10 to 19 years old in the year 2000.[55] Many statistics underestimate these rates given that approximately 25 per cent of deaths are recorded as accidental by coroners.[56] Furthermore, these statistics are not classified by sexual orientation or gender identity.[57] Intergenerational trauma and removal from family ties may play a large role in suicidal ideation and action among Indigenous 2SLGBTQ people.[2]

Research has shown that Indigenous peoples identifying as trans experience high levels of suicide risk, with nearly half of sample populations reporting at least one attempt.[2] Indigenous people who identify as Two-Spirit have a greater suicide risk than the Indigenous heterosexual population.[32]

Physical Health

Within the medicine wheel, physical health is represented by the direction of South (see figure 12.2). The sacred medicine of cedar sits in the Southern direction. Cedar is used for purification of the home and body and is often used in sweat lodge and fasting ceremonies for protection of the individuals involved. Adolescence, summer, and physical health are located in the Southern door of the medicine wheel.

Physical well-being is behaving in a way to actualize the intention and desire of the spirit in the world[2] by treating your physical body as a sacred vessel. Biomedicine has a large focus on physical wellness, but health care providers may consider viewing physical ailments as a lack of balance within the holistic self. Physical issues that may impact the health of Indigenous 2SLGBTQ people are non-ceremonial tobacco use, alcohol and substance use, and sexual health conditions.

Non-ceremonial Tobacco Use

Tobacco is a sacred medicine that is used as a prayer vessel to the Creator and all things spiritual.[54] During ceremonies, tobacco is often used along-side the other three medicines (cedar, sweetgrass, and sage).[33] When praying to the Creator, tobacco is held in the left hand because it is the hand that sits closest to the heart.[33] When an individual needs guidance from an Elder or a spiritual leader, tobacco is offered.[33] If the tobacco is accepted by the Elder or spiritual leader, they are bound to honour the request for guidance.[33]

The forceful removal of the connection to culture sees Indigenous peoples using tobacco in a non-ceremonious way. Indigenous adults have been found twice as likely to smoke cigarettes as other adults in Canada,[52] and its use among Indigenous 2SLGBTQ individuals has been strongly correlated with experiences of racial discrimination.[2]

Sexual Health

Within the health care system, many approaches to sexual education and health screening occur within a heteronormative model.[32] Indigenous youth have high levels of early sexual activity onset, unprotected sex, and history of abuse, which exposes them to greater risk of sexually transmitted infections and HIV.[13] Research suggests that Indigenous 2SLGBTQ peoples experience higher rates of HIV infection than their non-Indigenous peers,[2] particularly in the Prairie provinces. Programs targeted at educating Indigenous 2SLGBTQ communities about HIV/AIDS have already seen positive outcomes.[32] It is helpful for health care providers to be aware of HIV/AIDS service organizations in their area, as well as other Indigenous agencies providing sexual and reproductive health services, such as Indigenous midwifery programs.

One often overlooked aspect of Indigenous Two-Spirit care is reproductive health care and fertility support. Indigenous peoples report having extremely limited access to Indigenous sperm, eggs, and surrogates in main-stream fertility services. This is also a result of colonial biases in the development of health care services and is experienced as a form of medical violence by Indigenous peoples.

Emotional and Social Health

Within the medicine wheel, emotional health is represented by the direction of West (see figure 12.2). The sacred medicine of sage sits in the West. Sage is used for releasing what is troubling the mind and for removing negative energy. It is also used for cleansing homes and sacred bundles are carried by Indigenous peoples. Adulthood, autumn, and emotional health are located in the Western door of the medicine wheel.

In general, emotional health can be tied to social interactions. Emotional well-being and relationships with others are at the heart level of one's being.[4] It may be beneficial to ask the patient about any experiences that might affect their emotional or social health. Indigenous people may have been impacted by living on-reserve, attending a residential school, and disconnection from community through adoption or fostering. While community building and promoting self-expression can be used to improve emotional and social health, it can also combat systemic homophobia and transphobia.[32]

Connection to Community

The connection to community influences the health of an individual and their family.[52] The degree of social and cultural cohesion within a community can be considered cultural continuity.[52] Cultural continuity involves traditional intergenerational connectedness that can only be maintained through intact families and the engagement of elders passing on traditions to subsequent generations.[52]

Spiritual Health

Within the medicine wheel, spiritual health is represented by the direction of North (see figure 12.2). The sacred medicine of sweetgrass sits in the Northern direction. Sweetgrass is viewed as the sacred hair of Mother Earth. It has a sweet aroma that reminds us of the gentleness, kindness, and love she has for us. Sweetgrass can be used in healing or sharing circles to calm the participants. It can also be used for smudging and purification. Elderhood, winter, and spiritual health are located in the Northern door of the medicine wheel.

Spiritual wellbeing is central to the primary vision of one's life.[49] Christianity introduced through colonization impacted traditional Aboriginal worldviews by outlawing traditional ceremony, language, and ways of life, and silencing Indigenous gender and sexual diversity.[29]

Traditional Healing

While there is no succinct definition of traditional healing, it can be viewed as practices that date back to before the spread of Western biomedicine that are designed to promote mental, physical, emotional, and spiritual well-being.[51] Elders and Traditional Knowledge Keepers use spiritual ceremonies and share oral histories that reveal how their ancestors restored harmony to families and communities through Indigenous wisdom.[21] Each Indigenous nation has its own traditions, culture, and language.[21] Indigenous cultural resources, like traditional health practices, ceremonies, and spirituality, can help combat the impact of life stressors.[50] The use of stories, songs, and sacred items, like the wampum belt, peace pipe, eagle feather, cedar boughs, drums, and regalia, can be used to restore harmony and balance.[21]

For Indigenous 2SLGBTQ people, claiming traditional cultural roles and responsibilities can promote positive self-identities.[32] This process of reclamation and self-acceptance has been expressed as "coming in" – as opposed to "coming out."[32] An individual is considered to be coming in when they can embrace the identity that fits with who they are, rather than trying to conform to pre-existing identities or labels.[32]

Conclusion

Services must be responsive to the needs of Indigenous LGBTQ and Two-Spirit patients, and be consciously aware of the colonial root of oppression.[23,58] The colonial legacy has had lasting impacts on the health of Indigenous communities.[2] Although pre-colonial Indigenous ways of life cannot be restored, positive identities and healthy self-concepts can be, through the knowledge of traditional cultural roles.[29]

Self-determination may be one of the most important determinants of health for Indigenous people as it influences all the other determinants, including education, housing, and health services. Indigenous control over health care does not mean a complete rejection of the biomedical model, but rather the provision of culturally safe health care with the inclusion of traditional healing practices.[51]

Health care providers must be kind and considerate to all patients, especially those who identify as Indigenous LGBTQ and Two-Spirit. It is important to build the therapeutic relationship by fostering trust and respect, and ensure you are meeting the needs of the patient.

To better provide support for Indigenous 2SLGBTQ patients, health care providers can implement any of the following recommendations:

- Create safe spaces for Indigenous 2SLGBTQ.
- Seek out stories from your patients to understand their backgrounds, particularly their childhood events.
- Ask patients how they identify their ethnicity and gender.
- Review important documents affecting Indigenous peoples of Canada.
- Participate in cultural safety training, as well as self-reflection.
- Provide care using a trauma-informed lens that recognizes the prevalence of trauma and how it affects all individuals involved.
- Address issues of visibility and acceptance by providing welcoming environments through gender-diverse posters, intake forms, and clinician language and behaviour.
- Promote a sense of cultural awareness through visible Indigenous artwork in the clinical space.

- Offer your own name and pronoun to provide an opportunity for patients to share their names and pronouns.
- Be aware of Indigenous-specific and 2SLGBTQ resources available in your area.

For further resources in supporting Indigenous 2SLGBTQ patients, you can find valuable information in Fraser Health Authority's *Providing Diversity Competent Care to Two-Spirit Patients – A Handbook for Health Care Providers,* https://www.fraserhealth.ca/-/media/Project/FraserHealth/FraserHealth/Health-Professionals/Professionals-Resources/Diversity-Services/201609Providing DiverseCareto2SClients.pdf; *An Introduction to the Health of Two Spirit People* by Sarah Hunt, https://www.ccnsa-nccah.ca/docs/emerging/RPT-HealthTwoSpirit-Hunt-EN.pdf, and *A Wise Practices Guide: Voices of Aboriginal Trans People,* https://www.rainbowhealthontario.ca/wp-content/uploads/2008/11/OurRelativesSaid.pdf.

References

1. Magocsi PR. Aboriginal Peoples of Canada: a short introduction. Toronto: University of Toronto Press; 2002.
2. Rainbow Health Ontario. Two-Spirit and LGBTQ Indigenous health [Internet]. Toronto: Rainbow Health Ontario; 2016 Jul [cited 2018 Mar 31 2018]. Available from: https://www.rainbowhealthontario.ca/wp-content/uploads/2016/07/2SLGBTQINDIGENOUSHEALTHFactH eet.pdf.
3. Chacaby MN. A Two-Spirit journey: the autobiography of a lesbian Ojibwe-Cree Elder. Winnipeg: University of Winnipeg Press; 2016. p. 3.
4. Hyden LC. Illness narrative. In: Ritzer G, editor. The Blackwell encyclopedia of sociology. Hoboken (NJ): Wiley; 2007. Available from: https://doi.org/10.1002/9781405165518.wbeosi016.
5. Government of Canada [Internet]. Ottawa: Government of Canada; 2018 [cited 2021 Jan 3]. Available from: https://www.canada.ca/en/services/culture/canadian-identity-society/indigenous-peoples-cultures.html.
6. Vowel C. Indigenous writes: a guide to First Nations, Metis and Inuit issues in Canada. Winnipeg: High Water Press; 2016.
7. Robinson A. Gradual civilization act. In: The Canadian Encyclopedia. Toronto: Historica Canada; 2016 Mar 3 [cited 2021 Jan 21]. Available from https://www.thecanadianencyclopedia.ca/en/article/gradual-civilization-act.

8. Justice Canada [Internet]. Ottwa: Government of Canada; 1985 [cited 2021 Jan 31]. Indian act. Available from; https://laws.justice.gc.ca/eng /acts/I-5/.

9. Henderson WB. Indian act. In: The Canadian Encylopedia. Toronto: Historica Canada; 2006 Feb 7 [updated 2020 Dec 16; cited 2021 Jan 21]. Available from: https://www.thecanadianencyclopedia.ca/en/article/ indian-act.

10. National Inquiry into Missing and Murdered Indigenous Women and Girls. Reclaiming power and peace: final report [Internet]. Vancouver: MMIWG; 2019 [cited 2021 Jan 31]. Available from: https://www.mmiwg -ffada.ca/final-report/.

11. Crown-Indigenous Relations and Northern Affairs Canada [Internet]. Ottawa: Government of Canada; 2018 [cited 2018 Mar 31]. Inuit. Available from: https://www.rcaanc-cirnac.gc.ca/eng/1100100014187/1534785248701.

12. Gaudry A. Métis. In: The Canadian Encyclopedia. Toronto: Historica Canada; 2009 [cited 2018 Mar 31]. Available from: https:// thecanadianencyclopedia.ca/en/article/metis.

13. Ristock J, Zoccole A, Passante L. Aboriginal Two-Spirit and LGBTQ migration, mobility and health research project: Winnipeg final report [Internet]. Winnipeg: University of Manitoba; 2010 Nov [cited 2018 Mar 31]. Available from: http://www.2spirits.com/PDFolder/MMH Report.pdf.

14. Crown-Indigenous Relations and Northern Affairs Canada [Internet]. Ottawa: Government of Canada; 2013 Nov 27 [cited 2018 Mar 31]. Royal Proclamation of 1763: relationships, rights and treaties. Available from https://www.rcaanc-cirnac.gc.ca/eng/1379594359150/1607905375821.

15. Joseph B [Internet]. Toronto: CBC News; 2016 Apr 13 [cited 2018 Mar 31]. Things you may not know about the Indian Act. Available from: http://www.cbc.ca/news/indigenous/21-things-you-may -not-know-about-the-indian-act-1.3533613.

16. Royal Canadian Geographical Society. Canadian geographic Indigenous People's atlas of Canada. Ottawa: Royal Canadian Geographical Society; 2018. Metis; Road Allowance People.

17. Madwar, S. Inuit High Arctic relocations in Canada. In: The Canadian Encyclopedia. Toronto: Historica Canada; 2018 [cited 2021 Jan 31]. Available from: https://www.thecanadianencyclopedia.ca/en/article /inuit-high-arctic-relocations.

18. Crown-Indigenous Relations and Northern Affairs Canada [Internet]. Ottawa: Government of Canada; 2010 Sep 15 [cited 2021 Jan 31]. Apology for the Inuit High Arctic relocation. Available from https://www.rcaanc -cirnac.gc.ca/eng/1100100016115/1534786491628.

19. Royal Commission on Aboriginal Peoples. Final report [Internet]. Ottawa: Government of Canada; 1996 [modified 2016 Nov 2; cited 2018 Mar 31]. Available from: https://www.bac-lac.gc.ca/eng/discover/aboriginal -heritage/royal-commission-aboriginal-peoples/Pages/final-report.aspx.

20. United Nations. United Nations declaration on the rights of Indigenous Peoples [Internet]. New York: United Nations; 2007 [cited 2018 Mar 31]. Available from: http://www.un.org/esa/socdev/unpfii/documents /DRIPS_en.pdf.

21. Truth and Reconciliation Commission of Canada. Honouring the truth, reconciling the future [Internet]. Winnipeg: TRC; 2015 [cited 2021 Jan 31]. Available from: http://nctr.ca/assets/reports/Final%20Reports /Executive_Summary_English_Web.pdf. p. 8.

22. Crown-Indigenous Relations and Northern Affairs Canada [Internet]. Ottawa: Government of Canada; 2008 Jun 11 [modified 2010 Sep 15; cited 2021 Jan 31]. Statement of apology to former students of Indian residential schools. Available from: https://www.rcaanc-cirnac.gc.ca/eng/110010001 5644/1571589171655.

23. Truth and Reconciliation Commission of Canada. Calls to Action. 2012. [cited 2021 Jan 31]. Available from http://nctr.ca/assets/reports/Calls_to _Action_English2.pdf.

24. National Inquiry into Missing and Murdered Indigenous Women and Girls [Internet]. Vancouver: MMIWG; 2018 [cited 2018 Mar 31]. National Inquiry into Missing and Murdered Indigenous Women and Girls. Available from http://www.mmiwg-ffada.ca.

25. Mahony TH. Women and the criminal justice system [Internet]. Ottawa: Statistics Canada; 2011 Apr [cited 2021 Jan 31]. Available from: https:// www150.statcan.gc.ca/n1/en/pub/89-503-x/2010001/article/11416 -eng.pdf.

26. Hyslop K [Internet]. How poverty and underfunding land Indigenous kids in care. Vancouver: The Tyee; 2018 May 14 [cited 2021 Jan 31]. Available from: https://thetyee.ca/News/2018/05/14/Indigenous -Kids-Poverty-Care/.

27. MacDonald C, Steenbeek A. The impact of colonization and Western assimilation on health and wellbeing of Canadian Aboriginal People. Int J Reg Local Hist. 2015;10(1):32–46. doi:10.1179/2051453015Z.00000000023.

28. Greenwood M, de Leeuw S, Lindsay NM, Reading C. Determinants of Indigenous Peoples' health in Canada: beyond the social. Toronto: Canadian Scholars' Press; 2015.

29. Alaers J. Two-Spirited people and social work practice: exploring the history of Aboriginal gender and sexual diversity. Crit Soc Work. 2010;11(1). doi:10.22329/csw.v11i1.5817.

30. Innes RA, Anderson K. Indigenous men and masculinities: legacies, identities, regeneration. Winnipeg: University of Manitoba Press; 2015.
31. Brotman S, Ryan B, Jalbert Y, Rowe B. Reclaiming space-regaining health. J Gay Lesbian Soc Serv. 2002;14(1):67–87.
32. Hunt S. An introduction to the health of Two-Spirit people: historical, contemporary and emergent issues. Prince George (BC): National Collaborating Centre for Aboriginal Health; 2016.
33. Mulé NJ, Ross LE, Deeprose B, Jackson BE, Daley A, Travers A, et al. Promoting LGBT health and wellbeing through inclusive policy development. Int J Equity Health. 2009 May;8(1):18.
34. Hanson E [Internet]. Vancouver: University of British Columbia; 2009 [cited 2018 Mar 31]. The Sixties Scoop. Available from: http:// indigenousfoundations.arts.ubc.ca/sixties_scoop/.
35. Dickason OP. A concise history of Canada's First Nations. Toronto: Oxford University Press; 2006.
36. Trocmé N, Knoke D, Blackstock C. Pathways to the overrepresentation of Aboriginal children in Canada's child welfare system. Soc Serv Rev. 2004;78(4):577–600.
37. Bombay A, Matheson K, Anishman H. Intergenerational Trauma: Convergence of Multiple Processes among First Nations Peoples in Canada. J Aborig Health. 2009;5(3):6–47.
38. Berube K. The intergenerational trauma of First Nations still runs deep. The Globe and Mail [Internet]; 2015 Feb 16 [cited 2018 Mar 31]. Available from https://www.theglobeandmail.com/life/health-and-fitness/health-advisor/the-intergenerational-trauma-of-first-nations-still-runs-deep/article23013789/.
39. Daschuk J. Clearing the plans: disease, politics of starvation and the loss of Aboriginal life. Regina: University of Regina Press; 2013.
40. Scheim A, Jackson R, James L, Dopler TS, Pyne J, Bauer GR. Barriers to well-being for Aboriginal gender-diverse people: results from the Trans PULSE Project in Ontario, Canada. Ethn Inequal Health Soc Care. 2013;6(4):108–20.
41. Crown-Indigenous Relations and Northern Affairs Canada [Internet]. Ottawa: Government of Canada; 2010 [cited 2018 Mar 31]. Fact sheet: urban Aboriginal population in Canada. Available from http://www.aadnc-aandc.gc.ca/eng/1100100014298/1100100014302.
42. Abramovich IA. No Safe place to go – LGBTQ youth homelessness in Canada: reviewing the literature. Can J Fam Youth. 2012;4(1):29–51.
43. Wilson A. N'tacimowin inna nah': Our coming in stories. Can Womens Stud. 2008;26(3/4):193–9.

44. Hancock AM. When multiplication doesn't equal quick addition: examining intersectionality as a research paradigm. Perspect Polit. 2007;5(1):63–79.

45. Egan L. Two-Spirit people of Aboriginal tribes of North America. 2013 Apr 18 [cited 2018 Mar 31]. In: Ega L. WordPress blog [Internet]. Available from http://leighannaega_wordpress.com/2013/04/18/28/.

46. Suzack C, Huhndorf AM, Perreault J, Barman J. Indigenous women and feminism: politics, activism, culture. Vancouver: University of British Columbia Press; 2011.

47. Roscoe W. Changing ones: third and fourth genders in Native North America. New York: St. Martin's Press; 1998.

48. Pullin Z [Internet]. Media (PA): Kosmos; 2014 [cited 2018 Mar 31]. Two Spirit: the story of a movement unfolds. Available from: http://www.kosmosjournal.org/news/two-spirit-the-story-of-a-movement-unfolds/.

49. Dumont J. Definition of wellness: honouring our strengths. Saskatoon: University of Saskatchewan; 2014.

50. Walters KL, Simoni JM. Reconceptualizing native women's health: an "indigenist" stress-coping model. Am J Public Health. 2002 Apr;92(4):520–4.

51. Waldram J, Herring DA, Young TK. Aboriginal health in Canada: historical, cultural, and epidemiological perspectives. Toronto: University of Toronto Press; 2006.

52. Reading C, Wien F. Health inequalities and social determinants of Aboriginal Peoples' health. Prince George (BC): National Collaborating Centre for Aboriginal Health; 2013.

53. O'Brien M [Internet]. Seven Grandfather Teachings Document. c2000 – [cited 2018 Mar 31]. Available from http://ojibweresources.weebly.com/ojibwe-teachings--the-7-grandfathers.html.

54. Georgian College Resources Centre [Internet]. Barrie (ON): Georgian College; 2000 [cited 2018 Mar 31]. Medicine wheel. Available from http://ojibweresources.weebly.com/medicine-wheel.html.

55. Health Canada. A statistical profile on the health of First Nations in Canada: for the year 2000. Ottawa: Government of Canada; 2005.

56. White J, Jodoin N. Aboriginal youth: a manual of promising suicide prevention strategies. Calgary: Centre for Suicide Prevention; 2007.

57. First Nations Centre. Suicide prevention and Two-Spirited people. Ottawa: National Aboriginal Health Organization; 2012.

58. Robinson M. Two-Spirit and bisexual people: different umbrella, same rain. J Bisex. 2017;17(1):7–29.

13 Older 2SLGBTQ Adults and End-of-Life Decision Making

JACQUELINE GAHAGAN, EMILY HUGHES,
AND ELISE JACKSON

Introduction

Aging is a process we all must face, but how we experience aging and end of life can vary greatly. Two-Spirit, lesbian, gay, bisexual, transgender, and queer (2SLGBTQ)* seniors, in particular, face unique challenges as they age and navigate end-of-life care.

Although there has been a trend of increasing acceptance of younger 2SLGBTQ individuals within broader society, such as the introduction of gender-neutral bathrooms in schools, the same trend has not been observed for 2SLGBTQ seniors.[1] For older 2SLGBTQ populations, locating culturally sensitive and appropriate health care services is often made challenging by lingering negative perceptions and biases about homosexuality and transgender identities that are reflected in health and social care policies and programs.[2-4] This can be compounded by a lack of knowledge and training among health and social care providers regarding the unique needs of older 2SLGBTQ adults.

The negative impacts of these issues can be seen across all 2SLGBTQ populations and throughout the life course.[5,6] Older 2SLGBTQ populations experience health disparities and poor health outcomes at higher rates than their age-matched heterosexual peers, including a higher prevalence of hypertension, substance abuse, mental health issues, and

---

* The use of the term *queer* may be experienced negatively or positively among older 2SLGBTQ adults. Given the historical use of the term as derogatory, its use may be offensive and traumatizing to some, while others have reclaimed the term in an act of empowerment. Thus, when communicating with older adults, it is of particular importance to reflect back the language that they themselves use to describe their identities.

HIV.[7] A lifetime of stigma, bias, and discrimination not only imparts higher rates of poor health outcomes but can also result in higher rates of social isolation and neglect.[1,6] The dearth of 2SLGBTQ-specific health and social resources, programs, and policies can further contribute to these health inequities.[8,9]

In addition, the health and social issues faced by older 2SLGBTQ populations can be exacerbated by the variety of modifiable and non-modifiable determinants of health, such as income, age, and education, among others.[10–12] The result, for many older 2SLGBTQ individuals, is that fear of discrimination or bias within health care systems and among health and social care providers decreases the likelihood of active engagement in many facets of care, including end-of-life (EOL) discussions and decision making. Previous research has indicated that many older 2SLGBTQ adults will "go back into the closet" as they age and as they are required to interact more frequently with health and social care systems.[2,13–15]

In some instances, the choice to not identify as 2SLGBTQ is made to buffer themselves against the perceived or actual stigma and discrimination within what are often experienced as both complex and hetero-normative and cisnormative systems. This has translated into a lack of visibility for these populations and their specific needs. For example, a study conducted in White Rock, British Columbia, in 2013 showed that front-line staff from every residential care facility in the city and surrounding area believed none of their residents to be 2SLGBTQ-identified despite statistics showing 2SLGBTQ seniors make up at least 6 per cent of the population.[16] Misconceptions like these perpetuate the invisibility, at best, and neglect, at worst, of 2SLGBTQ populations within older adult care environments.

Recognizing and reconciling the negative impacts of the long history of discrimination against 2SLGBTQ populations is crucial in relation to both healthy aging and EOL care for these populations – particularly among older generations who may have been subjected to unwanted medical interventions (e.g., reparative therapy) or experienced legal sanctions in their younger years. The inclusion of 2SLGBTQ needs is an important component in ensuring culturally competent and safe care, particularly in relation to EOL decision making, when reliance on health care systems and health care providers becomes more acute. This chapter offers an overview of some of the key issues faced by older 2SLGBTQ populations as they age and make decisions about their EOL needs and concludes with some suggestions on how health and social care providers can help address these challenges.

2SLGBTQ Aging and End of Life in the Shadow of AIDS

Aging and 2SLGBTQ community norms and expectations about health and social care are often intertwined with the long history of the AIDS epidemic, particularly in North America. In the early days of the epidemic, many gay men were told by their health care providers not to expect to live into older adulthood and to prepare for end of life while in their 20s and 30s. With the advent of highly active antiretroviral therapy in the mid-1990s, gay men living with HIV increasingly aged into the older adult population. The long history of loss associated with AIDS, including the loss of friends, lovers, and families of choice, necessitated a rethinking of how to address the aging and EOL needs of older 2SLGBTQ populations.[17-19] Although living into old age is now possible for those with HIV, the challenges of navigating health and social care systems because of homophobia, transphobia and the stigma associated with HIV have remained.

Shifting Towards a 2SLGBTQ Understanding of Healthy Aging

The concept of *healthy aging* has appeared in the published literature for many years.[9,20-22] However, while often implied when discussing aging in the 2SLGBTQ population, it is neither well understood nor studied. Current research suggests the need for a more nuanced examination of how, for example, a variety of intersecting determinants of health can impact on the health outcomes of older 2SLGBTQ populations. Issues of sexual orientation and gender identity, as well as other determinants of health – such as education, socioeconomic status, marital status, race, and ethnicity – can collectively and synergistically impact the healthy aging and EOL processes.[23] These issues may make incorporating EOL conversations in clinical care settings particularly challenging.

The ways in which healthy aging is understood vary widely. For example, the Public Health Agency of Canada,[24] in its "new vision on healthy aging," supports a vision that "values and supports the contributions of older people; celebrates diversity, refutes ageism and reduces inequities; and provides age-friendly environments and opportunities for older Canadians to make healthy choices, which will enhance their independence and quality of life."[24] What is absent from that definition, as well as many other recent definitions of "healthy aging," is the recognition that 2SLGBTQ and other minority populations face different challenges as they age and therefore require different strategies in developing EOL approaches within health and social care sectors.

For example, older 2SLGBTQ adults are more likely to live alone, less likely to have children or other biological relatives in their lives, and more likely to turn to their "chosen families" for help with health and social care issues. While the issue of resilience is an important concept in understanding healthy aging, we do not have a strong understanding of how this applies to older 2SLGBTQ adults since most of the work in this area refers to heterosexual, cisgender adults. However, the key mechanisms associated with resilience, such as the ability to withstand and "bounce back" from adversity, generally evolve over the life course in all individuals, 2SLGBTQ people included.[25]

Aging in Place and Aging in Care

To be truly effective, aging and EOL care strategies need to be thought of as a community conversation – one that requires a patient-centred approach free from hetero- and cisnormative assumptions about sexual orientation, a male–female binary, marital status, or families of origin. These conversations also need to take place in open and accepting health and social care environments. It is critically important for health care providers to incorporate discussions of and with patients' *family of choice* when making EOL decisions or when providing EOL care.[15]

For some older 2SLGBTQ adults, the desire to age in place by remaining in their home for as long as possible is driven by the desire to avoid having to come out to health and social care providers (as well as fellow residents and their families). This may result in what is referred to as *forgone health care*, resulting in poorer health outcomes and worse EOL experiences.[26,27] While cost is traditionally considered the key variable in forgone health care, older 2SLGBTQ populations in Canada may not avail themselves of health care to continue to bypass a system they have purposefully avoided for much of their lives. Further, this is a system that many have paid into for much of their lives and will not benefit from.

So far, this chapter has discussed several aspects of what makes healthy aging and EOL planning challenging for older 2SLGBTQ adults. What follows covers the ways in which health care providers can support older 2SLGBTQ populations with inclusive clinical practices.

A Practical Approach to Older 2SLGBTQ-Inclusive Clinical Care

Advance Care Planning and End of Life

Before an individual becomes unable to make their own health care decisions, it is important that an advance care plan (ACP) is in place.

The plan consists of a competent individual providing guidance regarding their wishes for care and assigning someone to make decisions on their behalf should they become unable – for example, either a power of attorney (POA) or substitute decision maker (SDM).

If a POA is not assigned, and the individual is not married or in a common-law relationship, a parent or sibling could legally be designated as an SDM, regardless of the individual's relationship with this person. If no family member (as usually defined by legislation, legal or biological family) is available, decisions about health care could end up being made by another unfamiliar party, such as a public guardian and trustee or a court, who may not have insight into that individual's preferences and values.

These issues are of particular importance to 2SLGBTQ populations because of the historic and systemic invalidation of their lived identities.[28] Some common barriers to EOL planning for all seniors include a lack of access to the necessary information, an absence of perceived need, and the desire to avoid thinking about end of life. Social isolation, which is more common in 2SLGBTQ populations, may make it difficult to identify POAs. Furthermore, fear of disclosing sexual orientation, gender identity, or gender expression to care providers may be exacerbated by previous negative experiences with the health care system.

Health care providers should encourage all their patients, including their 2SLGBTQ patients, to create an ACP at any age. For more information, people can access advancecareplanning.ca, where patients, providers, and friends/families can use region-specific tools to create an ACP.

For transgender and gender-diverse patients, it is important to use specific language in the ACP, wherever possible, that respects their gender identity and expression.

2SLGBTQ-specific considerations for post-death include the following:

- Specify in the ACP whether the individual consents to an autopsy after death. Post-mortem autopsies can present problems if the coroner's office insists on recording an individual's sex assigned at birth on the death certificate, or if the autopsy "outs" the trans identity of the individual.
- In the case of casket ceremonies, open casket should reflect the deceased's preferences regarding gender identity and gender expression. Similarly, memorials and gravestones should be chosen to reflect the deceased's gender identity. These details should be specified through the ACP.[29]

- Inconsistencies between the deceased's legal documents and lived identity can cause numerous problems. Some funeral homes may refuse to bury trans-identified individuals according to their lived identity. Seek out a funeral home that is 2SLGBTQ inclusive and specify the use of this home in the ACP.
- Ensure that the insurance company is 2SLGBTQ inclusive. Some individuals experience issues with insurance companies, including an unwillingness to pay on the policy because of the trans identity or gender nonconformity of the policyholder.[29]

Completing an ACP, however, is not enough; other stakeholders need to know it exists and need to be able to access it.[28] To achieve this, health care providers should do the following:

- Have a copy of the ACP.
- Encourage patients to have conversations with partners, family members, and friends about ACPs and ensure they also have copies.
- Advise patients to have detailed discussions with their POA(s) and potential SDMs.
- Recommend that individuals carry a note in their wallet (or in their phone emergency health section) stating that they have an ACP, along with instructions on where to find it and who to contact in case of an emergency.
- Inform patients that advancecareplanning.ca gives the individual the option of emailing an ACP to anyone they choose, including themselves.

Psychosocial Well-Being

Psychosocial well-being is an essential part of healthy living at all stages of life and promotes healthy aging in older populations. The involvement of affirming family members (biological or chosen), other relationships, spirituality, and mental health all contribute to an individual's psychosocial well-being, which may be experienced differently by 2SLGBTQ communities.

Family and Community

When working with aging 2SLGBTQ communities, there are unique considerations with respect to social and cultural context. Many 2SLGBTQ individuals have experienced rejection by their families, including

parents, siblings, and partners. Additionally, children of transgender individuals may feel abandoned or betrayed by a parent's transition and thus
may not be willing to provide elder care.[29] Furthermore, while 2SLGBTQ
individuals may have developed strong community networks throughout their lives, these support systems may be weakened or diminished as
they age because of mortality, illness (including higher rates of HIV and
AIDS), disability, and social isolation. This degradation of support networks is reflected in statistics that show that older trans adults are two to
three times as likely to age alone as the general population. When asked
who would take care of them in the event that they needed assistance,
over 30 per cent of trans respondents were unable to provide an answer.[30]

For a care provider, some ways to help include the following:

- Facilitate referral to a community service agency to improve social
  and community connection, if desired by the individual.
- When possible, refer to professionals and organizations who are
  known to be competent and sensitive, or follow-up to ensure that
  the unique needs of the individual are being met.
- Place less emphasis on family of origin and acknowledging that
  many 2SLGBTQ people have created families of choice.[30] 2SLGBTQ
  families of choice are extremely important but have historically
  been denied visitation in health care facilities and excluded from
  medical and EOL decisions.[1] Ask your patient who they want to
  have present for these conversations.
- Frankly discuss loneliness with patients and how it impacts their
  health. Providers may consider partnering with other agencies to
  develop programing, home-visit programs, and opportunities to
  reduce isolation (for example, a drop-in day health program with a
  meal).

Violence and Abuse

2SLGBTQ individuals experience higher rates of violence and abuse
than the general population.[31] This violence can occur in interpersonal
and institutional contexts – including experiences of being denied
access to services and health care because of sexual orientation or gender identity and expression.[32] For older 2SLGBTQ adults, violence may
manifest in unique ways that care providers should be cognizant of,
such as the following:

- People may threaten to "out" their sexual orientation or gender
  identity and expression. This is particularly concerning for

people who experienced a time when their identity was illegal or
pathologized.
- They may be blackmailed or financially exploited by caregivers.
- They can be denied care, abused, or neglected by a caregiver.
- Caregivers or facilities may deny their lived identity (for example,
  by dressing them in ways that do not correspond to their gender
  identity or expression, or by preventing 2SLGBTQ partners from
  sharing rooms in long-term-care facilities).

When screening for elder abuse in 2SLGBTQ patients, consider asking about these aspects, and support the individual in addressing any
issues – whether by legal recourse, or by finding new housing or new
care providers. It is also important to be aware that the likelihood of
experiencing violence is even higher for 2SLGBTQ individuals who
also have other marginalized identities, such as being racialized, disabled, Indigenous, and so on. Please see chapters 14 and 15 for more
information on intersectionality.

Spirituality and Attitudes Towards Death and Dying

Spiritual and religious beliefs about death are important to address
with all individuals at the end of life. Historically, many faith-based
institutions have been unsupportive of, have intentionally mistreated,
and have excluded 2SLGBTQ populations, even those actively seeking
spiritual care. Although 2SLGBTQ individuals may identify as spiritual, this ostracization from religious communities can be an important
consideration and may impact logistics, such as burial.[29]

Additionally, recent media reports have brought medical assistance
in dying to wider community attention. 2SLGBTQ communities tend to
report higher support for medical assistance in dying than the general
population.[33] With the recent Canadian legalization of medical assistance in dying, it is important to know how to address this topic with
2SLGBTQ seniors, who may show interest in accessing these services.

Aging within a community with a high prevalence of HIV may also
affect a person's attitudes towards death and dying.[34] A diminished
support network, because of acquaintances dying from AIDS and
related complications, may contribute to isolation and loneliness and
leave a person with less support. For some individuals, EOL planning
may have begun many years ago, when fewer people lived with HIV
for a time. Individuals may have been living HIV-positive for decades,
leading to significant psychological and financial impacts, such as
difficulty in obtaining employment, and they may not have planned

financially for the future given their short life expectancy at the time of diagnosis. In these cases, EOL arrangements and advanced care planning may need to be updated. However, there remain many AIDS service organizations that provide support to PHAs (people living with HIV/AIDS). In particular, specialized HIV hospice and hospital care is available to PHAs in many large centres (for example, the Dr. Peter Centre in Vancouver and Casey House in Toronto).

Mental Health and Isolation

Mental illness affects people of all gender identities and sexual orientations but is particularly prevalent in 2SLGBTQ communities. Almost half (48 per cent) of trans and 30 per cent of older LGB adults suffer from depression compared to 5 per cent of heterosexual and cisgender older adults.[29] Furthermore, older 2SLGBTQ adults report lower self-acceptance and more feelings of isolation. In a 2011 US study, 40 per cent of transgender adults aged over 55 reported their gender identity as a reason their children no longer had contact with them, while over half stated they had lost close friends as a result of their gender identity.[35] Other factors contributing to this include but are not limited to higher likelihood of aging alone, long-term effects of experiencing violence, historical and continued stigma and marginalization, and rejection by religious or spiritual institutions.[36] Individuals who are HIV-positive may experience additional stress, financial concerns, and stigma. Being mindful of these challenges can be helpful when assessing mental health concerns and care planning. Addressing the isolation that these populations experience is often more effective than treating their symptoms with medication.[28]

Long-Term and Palliative Care Settings

Health care providers are often responsible for initiating conversations about long-term and palliative care with patients and their family members. Sexuality, gender identity, and gender expression remain important considerations in these settings; however, most long-term and palliative care environments are currently neither 2SLGBTQ-inclusive nor have estimates of the number of 2SLGBTQ-identified residents. A lack of reliable estimates and knowledge around the needs of 2SLGBTQ seniors means that facilities often cannot justify the associated cost of undertaking education or leadership to support communities that they do not believe exist in their facilities. As discussed earlier, this perpetuates a lack of visibility and erases the identities of 2SLGBTQ seniors.

Furthermore, there is an absence of anti-discrimination policies specific to 2SLGBTQ populations in the context of long-term care.[15] There is evidence to suggest that 2SLGBTQ-identified individuals would benefit immensely from policy initiatives that name homophobia, biphobia, and transphobia as grounds for elder abuse.[1]

It is a common desire among older 2SLGBTQ individuals not to be cared for in a long-term-care facility.[27] Many express concerns about how they would be treated in an institutional setting; fear they would be ridiculed by staff, other residents, and residents' families; and worry they would not be able to be safely "out" in a facility.[36]

The following are a few practical considerations for clinicians when thinking about long-term and palliative care settings for 2SLGBTQ patients:

- Sexuality and intimacy are significant human needs across the life course, and they remain important within the context of long-term and palliative care.
- It is important for health care providers to avoid heteronormative assumptions and to recognize that 2SLGBTQ-identified individuals may have unique needs and challenges regarding care.
- Staff, clinicians, and allied health care providers should work together to create and maintain an affirming and inclusive environment for all residents of care facilities. Many intake forms do not include any questions or data on sexual orientation or gender identity and expression.[15] This prevents individuals from being matched to a care environment with 2SLGBTQ-inclusive training and resources, non-gendered washrooms, and so on.
- It is important to include loved ones, as identified by the individual, in the decision-making and planning process for long-term and palliative care.

Physical Health

In addition to facing unique health concerns, such as high rates of HIV, post-surgical complications from gender-affirming surgery, and the effects of hormone replacement therapy, 2SLGBTQ adults are at risk for overall lower levels of health and higher levels of disability and disease as they age. Reasons for these disparities have already been described, such as lower use of health care services, denial of health care or insurance, and higher stress from external and internalized stigma. Additionally, 2SLGBTQ populations have lower rates of protective health behaviours (regular physical activity, for example) combined with higher rates of smoking, as well as fewer protective factors, such as social support, community involvement, or social engagement.[29,8]

HIV

Gay male communities and trans communities experience dispropor-tionately high rates of HIV compared to the general population.[37] Older people are generally more likely to delay HIV testing, and health care providers are less likely to suggest testing. However, HIV screening is important to discuss with older patients seeking care.

When treating seniors with HIV, there are unique considerations (please see chapter 7 for further information on HIV and aging):

- HIV progresses more quickly in older people and impacts the aging process.[37]
- Older people are generally more likely to adhere to drug regimens, but cognitive decline may impact their ability to remember to take medications.
- Elderly populations have higher rates of AIDS-related cancer, osteoporosis, kidney disease, liver disease, and HIV-related dementia and other neurodegenerative disorders.[37]
- HIV medications may cause side effects or drug–drug interactions. This should particularly be considered in the treatment of elderly patients who have more comorbidities and of trans individuals who have been prescribed gender-affirming hormone therapies.
- Patients should be offered information about safer sexual health practices and provided with appropriate protection and disclosure of HIV status. These needs are often overlooked in older adult populations.

Cognitive Decline

While the onset of cognitive impairment is distressing for any indi-vidual and their loved ones, there are additional aspects to take into account for an 2SLGBTQ patient diagnosed with cognitive decline. Some individuals may experience confusion around their gender iden-tity and gender expression as their cognitive abilities change and their memory is impacted.[34] This can be extremely distressing, and caregiv-ers should be counselled on how to address this issue. Some actions that caregivers can take to ameliorate this distress and help individuals maintain their identity include the following:

- Dressing individuals in a way that is congruent with their gender identity and expression. As cognitive impairment increases the dependency of individuals on caregivers, it is essential that caregivers understand the wishes of the person they are caring for regarding their physical gender expression.[38]
- Displaying of photos and other memorabilia of a person's life and loved ones (including their chosen family) in their home environment. Reminiscence therapy interventions, such as creating photo albums and narrated videos, and listening to favorite music, have been shown to increase well-being, reduce depression and apathy, and improve cognition in individuals with cognitive decline.[39]
- Use of blister packs, supervised medication administration, and regular medication reviews by family doctors and pharmacists as cognitive decline can lead to reduced adherence with medication regimens, including hormones required for physical transition.[34] Such interventions can help individuals continue to live according to their true identity.
- Creating a 2SLGBTQ friendly care environment, whether in a nursing/retirement home with inclusive staff and policies, including specific training in caring for 2SLGBTQ seniors, or through promoting the presence of chosen family and loved ones who affirm the individual's identity.[34]
- Recognizing that the fluctuating nature of cognitive decline may result in inconsistencies in an individual's understanding or expression of their identity. This does not negate the validity of their 2SLGBTQ identity, and caregivers should provide support and care that aligns with the individual's previously expressed wishes regarding their sexual orientation or gender identity whenever possible.
- Try to ensure that discussions surrounding EOL care and advanced care planning occur with a SDM while the individual is still able to express their wishes. It is important to designate a POA who respects the person's wishes and lived identity.

Recommendations for Health and Social Care

As stated earlier, various intersecting determinants of health, including sexual orientation and gender identity, can impact the stigma and discrimination faced by older 2SLGBTQ adults. When we consider these issues, as well as the longstanding minority stress experienced by 2SLGBTQ populations across the life course, it is clear that additional support is needed to ensure that health and social care providers and programs are meeting the unique needs of these often marginalized populations. The key takeaway message for health and social care providers is the importance of ensuring that hetero- and cisnormative assumptions are not part of the clinical care discussions about EOL. Informed decision making based on an understanding of the unique needs of the patient is crucial. An important step in providing culturally competent and safe care for older 2SLGBTQ populations is to collectively move towards informed EOL conversations.

Conclusion

Building on a foundation of patient-centred care and patient-informed decision making allows a shift away from the silencing of older 2SLGBTQ populations towards open conversations about aging and EOL issues. This is particularly relevant to informing health and social care in that it allows for bidirectional conversations about how to address specific health and social care needs leading up to and including end of life. In this regard, aging and EOL decision making are key processes for 2SLGBTQ patients and health and social care providers to explore collectively and collaboratively.

References

1. Brotman S, Ryan B, Cormier R. The health and social service needs of gay and lesbian elders and their families in Canada. Gerontologist. 2003 Apr;43(2):192–202.
2. de Vries B. Stigma and LGBT aging: Negative and positive marginality. In: Orel NA, Fruhauf CA, editors. The lives of LGBT older adults: Understanding challenges and resilience. Washington, DC, US: American Psychological Association; 2015. pp. 55–71.
3. Griebling TL. Sexuality and aging: a focus on lesbian, gay, bisexual, and transgender (LGBT) needs in palliative and end of life care. Curr Opin Support Palliat Care. 2016 Mar;10(1):95–101.
4. Mulé NJ, Ross LE, Deeprose B, Jackson BE, Daley A, Travers A, et al. Promoting LGBT health and wellbeing through inclusive policy development. Int J Equity Health. 2009 May;8(18):18.
5. Aldredge PA, Conlon A. Reflections: gay men and lesbians at end-of-life. J Soc Work End Life Palliat Care. 2012;8(2):113–18.
6. de Vries B. LG(BT) persons in the second half of life: the intersectional influences of stigma and cohort. LGBT Health. 2014 Mar;1(1):18–23.

7. Averett P, Yoon I, Jenkins CL. Older lesbians: experiences of aging, discrimination and resilience. J Women Aging. 2011;23(3):216–32.
8. Fredriksen-Goldsen KI, Cook-Daniels L, Kim HJ, Erosheva EA, Emlet CA, Hoy-Ellis CP, et al. Physical and mental health of transgender older adults: an at-risk and underserved population. Gerontologist. 2014 Jun;54(3):488–500.
9. Gahagan J, Colpitts E. Understanding and measuring LGBTQ pathways to health: a scoping review of strengths-based health promotion approaches in LGBTQ health research. J Homosex. 2017;64(1):95–121.
10. Brotman S, Ryan B, Collins S, Chamberland L, Cormier R, Julien D, et al. Coming out to care: caregivers of gay and lesbian seniors in Canada. Gerontologist. 2007 Aug;47(4):490–503.
11. Murray E, Numer M, Merritt B, Gahagan J, Comber S. Healthy-aging among LGBT seniors in Canada: A review of the literature. Int J Health Wellness Soc. 2012;1(4):179–92.
12. Fredriksen-Goldsen KI, Bryan AE, Jen S, Goldsen J, Kim HJ, Muraco A. The Unfolding of LGBT lives: key events associated with health and well-being in later life. Gerontologist. 2017 Feb;57 suppl 1:S15–29.
13. Stinchcombe A, Smallbone J, Wilson K, Kortes-Miller K. Healthcare and end-of-life needs of lesbian, gay, bisexual, and transgender (LGBT) older adults: A scoping review. Geriatrics (Basel). 2017 Mar;2(1):13.
14. Wilson K, Kortes-Miller K, Stinchcombe A. Staying out of the closet: LGBT Older adults' hopes and fears in considering end-of-life. Can J Aging. 2018 Mar;37(1):22–31.
15. QMUNITY. Ageing out: moving towards queer and trans competent care for seniors [Internet]. Vancouver: QMUNITY; 2015 Mar [cited 2021 Oct 3]. Available from: http://qmunity.ca/wp-content/uploads/2015/03/AgingOut.pdf.
16. Emlet CA, Fredriksen-Goldsen KI, Kim HJ, Hoy-Ellis C. The relationship between sexual minority stigma and sexual health risk behaviors among HIV-positive older gay and bisexual men. J Appl Gerontol. 2017 Aug;36(8):931–52.
17. Lyons A, Pitts M, Grierson J, Thorpe R, Power J. Ageing with HIV: health and psychosocial well-being of older gay men. AIDS Care. 2010 Oct;22(10):1236–44.
18. Masten J. "A shrinking kind of life": gay men's experience of aging with HIV. J Gerontol Soc Work. 2015;58(4):319–37.
19. Daley A, MacDonnell J, Brotman S, St Pierre M, Aronson J, Gillis L. Providing health and social services to older LGBT adults. Annu Rev Gerontol Geriatr. 2017;37:143–60.
20. Herrick AL, Lim SH, Wei C, Smith H, Guadamuz T, Friedman MS, et al. Resilience as an untapped resource in behavioral intervention design for gay men. AIDS Behav. 2011 Apr;15(S1 Suppl 1):S25–9.

21. Lachowsky N, Gahagan J, Anderson K. Pathways to health equity for LGBTQ populations. In: Arya N, Piggott T, editors. Under-served: health determinants of indigenous, inner-city, and migrant populations in Canada. Toronto: Canadian Scholars; 2018.
22. Mikkonen J, Raphael D. Social determinants of health: the Canadian facts. Toronto: York University School of Health Policy and Management; 2010.
23. Colpitts E, Gahagan J. The utility of resilience as a conceptual framework for understanding and measuring LGBTQ health. Int J Equity Health. 2016 Apr;15(1):60.
24. Public Health Agency of Canada. Healthy aging in Canada: a new vision, a vital investment from evidence to action [Internet]. Ottawa: Governement of Canada; 2006 Jul [cited 2021 Oct 3]. p. 12. https://www.health.gov.bc.ca/library/publications/year/2006/Healthy_Aging_A_Vital_latest_copy_October_2006.pdf.
25. Kalousova L, Burgard SA. Debt and foregone medical care. J Health Soc Behav. 2013 Jun;54(2):204–20.
26. Towne SD Jr. Socioeconomic, geospatial, and geopolitical disparities in access to health care in the US 2011–2015. Int J Environ Res Public Health. 2017 May;14(6):573.
27. Services and Advocacy for LGBT Elders [Internet]. Washington (DC): US Department of Health and Human Services, Administration on Aging; 2016 [cited 2021 Oct 3]. Welcome to the National Resource Center on LGBT Aging. Available from: http://www.lgbtagingcenter.org/index.cfm.
28. Witten TM. Graceful exits: intersection of aging, transgender identities, and the family/community. J GLBT Fam Stud. 2009;5(1–2):35–61.
29. Witten TM. End of life, chronic illness, and trans-identities. J Soc Work End Life Palliat Care. 2014;10(1):34–58.
30. Hash KM, Netting FE. Long-term planning and decision-making among midlife and older gay men and lesbians. J Soc Work End Life Palliat Care. 2007;3(2):59–77.
31. Witten TM. Transgender bodies, identities, and healthcare: effects of perceived and actual violence and abuse. Res Sociol Health Care. 2008;25:225–49. doi:10.1016/S0275-4959(07)00010-5.
32. Frazer S. LGBT health and human services needs in New York State. Albany (NY): Empire State Pride Agenda Foundation; 2009.
33. Stein GL, Bonuck KA. Attitudes on end-of-life care and advance care planning in the lesbian and gay community. J Palliat Med. 2001 Summer;4(2):173–90.
34. Byrne, M., Rodriguez, M. Massaquoi, N, Murzin, K. What's so queer about dying? Panel discussion at: 519 Church Street Community Centre; 2016 Apr 30; Toronto, ON.

35. Grant JM, Lisa A. Mottet Justin, Tanis Jack, Harrison Jody, Herman L,
    Keisling M. Injustice at every turn: A report of the National Transgender
    Discrimination Survey. Washington (DC): National Center for
    Transgender Equality and National Gay and Lesbian Task Force; 2011.
36. Cartwright C, Hughes M, Lienert T. End-of-life care for gay, lesbian,
    bisexual and transgender people. Cult Health Sex. 2012;14(5):537–48.
37. Canadian Working Group on HIV and Rehabilitation [Internet]. Toronto:
    Realize Canada; 2013 [cited 2021 Oct 3]. HIV and aging. Available from:
    http://www.realizecanada.org/en/our-work/hiv-and-aging/.
38. Twigg J, Buse CE. Dress, dementia and the embodiment of identity.
    Dementia. 2013 May;12(3):326–36.
39. Caddell LS, Clare L. Interventions supporting self and identity in
    people with dementia: A systematic review. Aging Ment Health. 2011
    Sep;15(7):797–810.

14 Caring for 2SLGBTQ Disabled People

A.J. WITHERS, LAURA MACDONALD,
AND ELIZABETH HARRISON

Introduction

2SLGBTQ people are disabled people,* have disabled lovers, have disabled kids, and care for disabled people in their chosen families and families of origin. Attending to 2SLGBTQ issues, therefore, requires attending to disability issues. This chapter provides a brief overview of the social-historical context of the relationship between health care providers and disabled 2SLGBTQ people. It examines some of the issues that impact disabled 2SLGBTQ people's health and offers health care providers recommendations for the provision of safe and effective care.

There is very little research on disabled 2SLGBTQ people and even less that is specific to health and health care. This is, we would argue, a symptom of broader social injustices resulting in the erasures of disabled people and 2SLGBTQ people, making the intersection of these two groups virtually invisible. The evidence for this chapter, therefore, is largely extrapolated from applying broader disability research to existing knowledge about 2SLGBTQ populations and vice versa. Further, the synthesis of knowledge from these discrete bodies of research is informed by the authors' undivided identities as queer disabled people and experiences as care providers or scholars.

---

* While *people with disabilities* may be a more familiar term to some readers, we use the term *disabled people* in alignment with the social and radical models of disability.[6,13,18] We use *disability* as an umbrella term to describe those people who are typically defined or define themselves as disabled. We want to note that not everyone who is typically classified as disabled considers themselves disabled. In particular, the Deaf community generally considers itself a linguistic minority rather than a disability group.

The disability community is very diverse. 2SLGBTQ people and other marginalized groups experience disproportionate rates of disability. One study demonstrated that 55 per cent of trans people in Ontario are disabled or chronically ill.[1] A US study found that lesbians were 1.9 times as likely and bisexual women were 2.7 times as likely to be disabled than heterosexual women after adjustment for sociodemographic characteristics; rates for gay and bisexual men were also higher.[2] Racialized people,[3,4] Indigenous people,[4] poor people[4,5] and women[4,5] are all more likely to be disabled than their counterparts. The explanations for this are likely complex. However, social determinants of health research shows that groups that experience discrimination[3] or poverty[4] growing up will have long-term health disparities.

What Is Disability?

Understandings of disability have shifted over time and are culturally specific, including within medicine itself.[6] As a result, there can be fissures between how the medical community views disabled people and how disabled people view themselves. In this section, we will begin by discussing the historical implications of the medical definition of disability for the 2SLGBTQ community and then explore how disabled people relate to their own identities.

As a group, 2SLGBTQ people were pathologized by the medical community for decades. The first edition of the *Diagnostic and Statistical Manual of Mental Disorders (DSM)* pathologized "transvestism" and homosexuality.[7] Classification as a "mental disorder" led to 2SLGBTQ people being forcibly subjected to electroconvulsive therapy,[8,9] lobotomy,[9] or institutionalization.[8] The American Psychiatric Association replaced "homosexuality" with "egodystonic homosexuality" in the *DSM*-III in 1973, and it was not removed completely until 1986.[10] This removal was a response to changes in cultural views of homosexuality and organizing by 2SLGBTQ people.[9,11]

The demedicalization of homosexuality was declared a major victory by 2SLGBTQ activists, many of whom had worked to have it delisted as a mental disorder – as a disability.[*,11-13]

The classification of *gender dysphoria* is viewed more ambiguously in the trans community than the classification of homosexuality was. Some trans people support the inclusion of gender dysphoria in the

---

* *Disability*, while used, has no definition in the *DSM*-II. Because there are a variety of definitions of disability, some definitions do not consider simple inclusion in the *DSM* a disability while others do.

DSM because it provides a route to medical treatments while others oppose it, arguing that it devalues the legitimacy of their identities.[13] Some trans people argue for continued medicalization but as a physical disorder.[13,14]

Although some patients will be unaware of or unconcerned about it, it is important for health providers to understand this history and context as it can inform the relationship between their patients and themselves. It has been argued that the classification of various 2SLGBTQ identities are examples of how psychiatric diagnoses can be socially constructed.[9,13,15] Consequently, disabled 2SLGBTQ people may be particularly sensitive about or resistant to being labelled with a psychiatric diagnosis. As a result, professional relationships with disabled 2SLGBTQ people may be negatively impacted, or disabled 2SLGBTQ people may try to minimize the frequency of health care interactions, which can contribute to the delay or avoidance of care.

It can be argued that the way in which some trans people frame the debate about the classification of gender dysphoria in the *DSM* also erases (otherwise) disabled trans people.[13] Thus, some of these people may feel alienated from the trans/2SLGBTQ community, making some community and health resources inaccessible to, or anxiety provoking for, them.

Medical and Community Understandings of Disability

There is a gap between medical understandings of disability and how many disabled people understand themselves. This may be true even for disabled people who engage actively in the medical system for treatment related to their disabilities. We submit that it is essential for health care providers to understand this disjuncture to provide complete and appropriate care for disabled people, including those who identify as 2SLGBTQ.

Disabilities, according to *Stedman's Medical Dictionary*, "represent disturbances at the individual level."[16] The medical model of disability is a "find it and fix it" approach.[17] Here, all or part of a person is understood as pathological, as improperly functioning and in need of a cure. Where that isn't possible, disability is treated or, if necessary, accommodated.[6] From this perspective, medical practitioners are the experts on disability and disabled people.[6,18] As the medical model is the dominant way of understanding disability in Canada,[6,19] it seems like the obvious way to view disability for many health care providers. Consequently, this perspective largely goes unquestioned by front-line practitioners interacting with disabled people.

While there is a great deal of diversity within this community, for most disabled people, the medical model does not define or explain our experiences or understandings of disability. Diagnoses can be informative for many; however, they are not comprehensive of our identities. Typically, disabled people do not conceptualize their experiences of disability in medical terms. Someone walking slowly because they are in pain generally isn't understanding their body through a medical lens; rather, they are understanding it as walking slowly – as being in pain. While this pain can be awful, it also gives them something that goes unrecognized in the medical model. Being in chronic pain, living in chronic pain, gives people a different sense of being in their bodies, a perspective difficult to articulate to those without pain in their lives. Walking slowly provides a non-normative perspective of the world; it allows for observations and understandings that wouldn't be possible by walking quickly.

The electric wheelchair user, on the other hand, can, at times, move far more quickly than someone on foot. The Deaf person has access to an entire language and linguistic community that is incredibly difficult for the hearing person to access.

Our experiences help create who we are as people: 2SLGBTQ disabled people become who we are as human beings *in* and *through* our disabilities. Within the medical model, however, all of these things are defined only in negative terms: as inherent impairments. But this is not *our* experience – at least not our *entire* experience.

Disability, for many disabled people, is viewed as an identity, not as a quantifiable checklist of deficits. Engaging with 2SLGBTQ disabled people, therefore, means engaging with complex identities. "Madness," for example, is a reclaimed identity that is a plurality of experiences and emotional ways of being. It is shaped by perceptions, thought processes and understandings of one's self and others that do not fall within the defined standards of the present dominant psychiatric construction of "normal."[20] Neurodivergent people are those whose brains function outside of the "normal" range (e.g., people along the autism spectrum, people with brain injuries).

People who are part of the neurodiversity movement reject the pathologization of neurodivergence and argue that it is a meaningful way of life and that neurodiversity is a natural and valuable human variation.[21] There are also a number of disability and Deaf cultural events, and activist groups that fight for social justice for disability communities across North America and around the world. Many disabled people do not want to be cured – they view themselves as fine just as they are.[6,22]

At the same time, disabled people may be misperceived by health care providers. Doctors typically rate the quality of life of disabled people lower than disabled people rate their own quality of life.[23,24] Discrimination against disabled people accessing health care is also well documented.[6,25–27]

The Disjuncture

The disjuncture between how many disabled people see themselves and how many health care providers see disabled people can be profound. In the authors' experience, it can lead to a lack of common understanding of what disabled people's health care needs are, which can result in deficits in care for disabled people.

While disabled people may seek the assistance of medical professionals for help managing our minds and bodies, and we may express dismay and frustration, it is important to appreciate that the medical model allows for a very limited perspective of disability. This limited perspective may constrain what disabled people deem to be acceptable conversations to have with their medical practitioners about their disabilities, entrenching practitioner's negative understandings of disability.

Disability and Sexuality

Disabled people are often depicted as nonsexual or hypersexual.[28] The desexualization of disabled people is harmful as it undermines important parts of their lives and identities. Both of these constructions have the same result: the denial of disabled people's sexuality and sexual agency. As 2SLGBTQ social spaces are often hypersexual spaces, the desexualization of 2SLGBTQ disabled people can be especially harmful as it can cut off access to these spaces and these communities.[29] Conversely, hypersexuality constructs disabled people, especially people of colour[29] and people with intellectual disabilities,[28] as potential threats. Consequently, many disabled people, especially those labelled as intellectually or developmentally disabled, are not given adequate sex education.[28–30] It is important for health care providers to understand disabled people as having or being capable of having rich and rewarding sexualities, sexual or romantic lives, and fantasies. Practitioners should answer questions, offer information, and not make assumptions about their disabled patients' sexualities, sexual health, and sexual curiosities. Disabled people of all sexual identities should be screened for sexually transmitted infections based on frank, non-judgmental assessment of their sexual practices and risk factors.

Benefits and Accommodations

There are a number of disability related benefits that some 2SLGBTQ people may qualify for. A diagnosis is almost never sufficient to qualify for a benefit; rather, benefits typically require an application and additional medical documentation, at a minimum. Disability accommodations are thought of as ways of levelling the playing field, while disability benefits are understood as a supplement or replacement for something that cannot be attained because of a disability or systemic discrimination. Examples of accommodations include disability transit services, extra time on exams, access to specialized equipment or software for work or school, and provision of a communication assistant or interpreter. Benefits might include additional funds for transportation, dietary allowances, or tax exemptions for the purchase of specialized equipment.

Poverty is a serious but reversible threat to health that 2SLGBTQ disabled people are disproportionately affected by. Health care providers are often in the role of gatekeepers to many income supports and have a responsibility to know what accommodations and supports are available to the communities they care for. For health providers to provide comprehensive care, they need to be aware of these benefits, inform patients, and, like those in a growing movement of providers, prescribe income support as part of routine medical care.[31] In response to the growing recognition of the importance of this issue, the College of Family Physicians of Canada has developed a clinical tool to help providers more adequately assess and prescribe income.[32]

Disability benefits often involve cash payments or tax refunds. Examples of disability benefits include disability social assistance (like the Ontario Disability Support Program or Disability Assistance in BC), the Disability Tax Credit, Canada Pension Plan – Disability, short- and long-term disability insurance, and workers' compensation. They are often accessed by people living in poverty or people who would be living in poverty without the benefit.

There can be tensions between health care providers, the de facto gatekeepers of resources essential for living, and their patients who are applying for these benefits and who may be in urgent need of the additional financial resources. Frazee, Gilmour, and Mykitiuk argue that the disability benefit system repositions the "physician-patient relationship [which] is built on trust" as a potentially adversarial one.[33]

Tensions can sometimes arise because of hesitancy to complete forms on the part of the health care provider, for which there may be a number of reasons. Some disability benefit forms do not define "disability,"[33] which may confuse those tasked to fill them out. Practitioners may be unaware that their own understandings of disability and the legal threshold for disability are different. In addition, the lack of a definition may contribute to uncertainty in how to represent situations that involve health conditions that fluctuate from day to day or over periods of time with compounding conditions.[19] Lack of knowledge about people's disabilities and about benefit programs have also been documented as reasons that health care providers may be reluctant to fill out patients' forms.[20] Frazee, Gilmour, and Mykitiuk also describe how "providers' general lack of knowledge about the lives of people experiencing disability can lead them to seriously underestimate the extent to which their patients are precluded from carrying out activities of daily living or to dismiss what their patients tell them."[33] Where hesitancy results from a lack of information, knowledge, or experience, the onus is on the health care provider to obtain the necessary skills and education.* Providers are not expected to be adjudicators or legal experts; rather, their responsibility is to accurately document a patient's condition(s) and experiences.

Providers may also be concerned that their patients are exaggerating their claims in the hopes of obtaining benefits. A US study found self-reported levels of disability for social assistance were "surprisingly accurate" and can be used as "a valid measure" for social assistance eligibility.[34] Contrary to popular opinion, social assistance fraud is very uncommon in Canada.[35,36] While it is important to exercise clinical judgment, distrusting the accounts of disabled people is unwarranted. Some trans patients may be particularly sensitive to actual or perceived scrutiny because of the gender identity probing they may have been subjected to. Having to explain, justify, and describe in detail another core aspect of their identity can be especially emotionally difficult for trans patients.

Disability benefits can also be granted for gender dysphoria and for the symptoms of depression and anxiety that frequently accompany it.[37] Some health care providers may be hesitant to label trans as a disability as many trans people have fought against being categorized as disabled.

However, there is far from consensus in the trans community regarding the classification of disability.[13] Prince notes the potential good intentions behind the hesitance to "medicalize symptoms";[38] however,

---

* There are significant gaps in medical education curricula (to varying degrees, depending on discipline and institution) with respect to the treatment and care for disabled people. In the absence of robust curricula, providers are encouraged to become informed through continuing education and collaboration.

the harms of poverty are well documented.[4] We would argue that if the individual reports having a disability that interferes with the activities of daily living or meets the other criteria for disability benefits, the health care practitioner should assist the individual in completing the benefit application. Delaying, refusing, or poorly completing an application of a disabled 2SLGBTQ individual who would qualify for disability benefits, we suggest, represents a failure of meeting the duty to care for patients.

We would also suggest that one of the best ways to resolve the tensions around benefits and accommodations between 2SLGBTQ patient and provider is for health providers to demonstrate a non-judgmental attitude towards people on social assistance and those needing disability accommodations early on. For example, providers can suggest school or workplace accommodations that the person could need and benefit from; ask if the individual is getting the accommodations they need; and tell their patients that they can bring in social assistance forms for completion, including directing them to any organizational policies related to this service (e.g., timelines, supplementary fees). These simple things can help to make patients more comfortable discussing disability-related needs.

Barriers to Health Care

As evidenced throughout this text, the 2SLGBTQ community experiences systemic barriers to health care. Discrimination and providers' lack of knowledge about 2SLGBTQ issues contribute to people's negative health care experiences and their putting off getting medical treatment.[39,40] We suggest that this is compounded for disabled 2SLGBTQ people as they face multiple barriers to accessing health care.

The typical discussion about access for disabled people is about physical access: ramps, elevators, and so on. These things are important, but they aren't the only considerations when it comes to access for disabled people. Disabled people often face other, less visible barriers to accessing health care. For instance, someone who has pain or is neurodivergent may have difficulty getting to an appointment and sitting in a waiting room because of a combination of factors, including the health care environment. There are numerous other barriers, including financial and social, which are discussed below.

An awareness on the part of health care practitioners of the barriers faced by 2SLGBTQ disabled people is key to work to eliminate or, where that is not possible, mitigate those barriers. The measures that enable accessibility for disabled people should be considered alongside those that make care spaces inclusive of sexually diverse communities as disabled people are important parts of these communities. Creating accessible spaces for disabled patients will not only assist practitioners in providing care for more diverse and marginalized communities but also help them continue to care for their patient base throughout the life cycle (as well as meet human rights or legislated disability access requirements).

Barriers

PHYSICAL SPACE

The physical space where care practitioners meet and interact with patients impacts the accessibility of care for disabled people. Access to the building and onto exam tables have been reported as the two most significant physical barriers for disabled people.[41] Consider factors such as the presence of stairs, narrow doorways, heavy doors, lack of wheelchair accessible washrooms, poor lighting, fragrances, and uniformed security guards (which can be anxiety provoking for some patients) in terms of additional barriers.

LANGUAGE AND COMMUNICATION BARRIERS

Communication is fundamental to providing safe, ethical health care. People can face a multitude of communication barriers, from a practitioner not knowing American Sign Language (ASL) to a patient having a condition affecting their ability to process and recall information. One third of autistic people reported not being able to process information in health care appointments quickly enough for the appointment to be accessible to them, and nearly as many said they faced communication barriers with health providers and staff.[42] Many disabled people reported appointments were too short to meet their communication needs.[42] Many Deaf patients are anxious and fearful of going to the doctor because they are afraid they will be misunderstood.[43] Any or all of these experiences can be frustrating and discourage patients from further interactions with health care providers.

PAST NEGATIVE EXPERIENCES

The prior experiences of 2SLGBTQ disabled people will likely inform how they relate to health providers in the present and future. Morris found that disabled patients were "less likely to rate their provider's bedside manner favorably (74% vs. 59% ...) and to have positive perceptions of their provider's work (46% vs. 32% ...) than patients without disabilities."[44]

In addition to the barriers discussed above, medical abuse against disabled people, especially disabled people of colour[45] has been well documented.[6,45,46] We define *medical abuse* as mistreatment or harm caused by medical practitioners affecting a person or persons under their care. Medical abuse of disabled people is experienced by individuals, but pre-existing power relations and institutional mechanisms allow these abuses to take place. There are some notorious contemporary examples of medical abuse, such as the Huronia Regional Centre, an Ontario psychiatric hospital that closed in 2009,[47] and Ontario nurse Elizabeth Wettlaufer, who murdered eight nursing home residents under her care.[48] We submit that medical abuses often happen in more subtle ways to disabled people, including over- or under-medication[49], refusal to provide treatment because of a pre-existing disability or diagnosis,[6] or a failure to obtain informed consent for medical procedures presumed to be in the patients' best interest.

OTHER BARRIERS

Financial barriers also keep people from seeking care from medical providers; these can include transportation costs; child care; time away from work; or payment for attendant care, interpreters, or other kinds of accompaniment. Additionally, health services that may be indicated for a patient may not be publicly funded. Although Canada has "universal" health care (excluding many migrants), medications, physical therapies, dental care, alternative therapies, counselling, and other forms of treatment must often be paid for out of pocket, rendering them effectively inaccessible to lower-income patients. Studies have demonstrated that this is specifically the case for people with traumatic spinal cord injury,[50] Deaf people,[51] disabled perinatal women,[52] and homeless disabled people.[53] Cost, or even the fear of it, can still be a significant barrier.

The burden of coordinating care between multiple health practitioners, collating results, and scheduling appointments can also be a health care barrier.[54]

Not having attendant care available can also result in the inability to access health care. Likewise, lack of transportation can be a barrier.[54] Even when available, adaptive modes of public transit such as wheel trans (accessible vans) often require riders to book trips in advance with unpredictable availability and little room for flexibility in terms of arrival and departure times. This may result in patients being late to appointments, having to rush through meetings with providers to catch return rides, or being forced to wait for extended time before or after appointments. These issues are often compounded by lack of financial resources and other accessibility issues.

Health care practitioners may also not be knowledgeable about a disabled person's condition(s).[54] Already a barrier for disabled people, this could be particularly problematic for people seeking 2SLGBTQ-specific services like gender affirming treatments or sexual health services.

Reducing and Removing Barriers

Accessibility and Accommodations

Accommodations can be sizable, like building renovations, or they can be small, like writing down instructions at the end of an appointment or having large print copies on hand. Some accommodations, like having accessible parking, ramps, and accessible washrooms will be in place (or, too often, not) regardless of the particular patient, while others could be specific to an individual. Practitioners should have conversations about what accommodations 2SLGBTQ disabled patients need rather than make assumptions. Having a discussion about accessibility takes time; be sure to allow as much time as needed and ensure all members of the health care team are made party to the results of that discussion so the patient doesn't have to continually educate people in your workplace.

Physical Space

Putting in ramps, accessible washrooms, and so on, may seem like a major undertaking, but it is necessary to make spaces accessible. Grants are sometimes available to make services more accessible. Further, accessibility benefits the whole community. Installing a single-stall wheelchair-accessible washroom, for example, can make the entire space more trans friendly as it can be a gender-neutral washroom that non-binary and some trans people will feel more comfortable using. Providing scent-free spaces can also make the space more accessible to everyone. Installing ramps can make the space accessible to patients throughout the lifecycle (as they age, when they have kids in strollers, etc.). Increasingly, jurisdictions are passing legislation (like the Access for Ontarians with Disabilities Act in Ontario[53]) that sets specific accessibility standards for health providers.

There are many different ways to accommodate someone within the confines of a set physical space. An individual may require an alternative space to wait in or be examined in. For example, while far from ideal, one could use a conference room for physical examination of a patient who uses a motorized wheelchair. If this is the case, consider patient privacy and comfort. Some people can become agitated or overwhelmed in public waiting rooms; providing a quiet room to wait for an appointment can be a necessary accommodation. Advance planning can reduce stress and facilitate care for a patient who needs to, for example, be lifted from a wheelchair to an exam table. Home visits or, when an exam isn't required, video or phone calls may also be options for discussions between the patient and the health care provider if the patient has difficulty getting into the office.

No matter how accessibly designed a space is, it is irrelevant if the space is used for another purpose. For example, ramps used for bike locks or hallways and bathrooms used for storage can make a space inaccessible and a disabled person feel unwelcome.

Third-Party Support People

A disabled person may require assistance in their interactions with health care providers for various reasons. Third-party support people may include but are not limited to attendant care providers, communication assistants, and interpreters. Below are some suggestions for working with support people you may encounter in providing care to disabled patients and some important considerations in your approach to care with disabled 2SLGBTQ patients.

INTERPRETERS

People who communicate with ASL (usually members of the Deaf community) may use the services of an interpreter to communicate with health professionals. ASL–English interpreters will have varying levels of exposure to, and familiarity with, terminology and subject matter related to both medical and 2SLGBTQ issues; some may be well-versed in one or both, while others may not. Depending on the length and type of appointment, interpreters may work in groups of two or more.[49] Whenever possible, communicate with the Deaf patient in advance of a meeting, and try to ensure that a preferred interpreter or interpreter service is arranged. Depending on your agency or institution's policies, this may require working around existing procedures to meet an individual's needs.

Deaf interpreters (DIs) are members of the Deaf community who work alongside an ASL interpreter to assist with advocacy and cultural bridging for the Deaf patient. Because of systemic discrimination and lack of access to information, some Deaf people will lack literacy skills or foundational health information. DIs also work with disabled people who require additional communication assistance.[55]

It is the provider's responsibility to book and pay for ASL interpreters,[56] which usually need to be booked well in advance.

COMMUNICATION ASSISTANTS

Some disabled people have physical difficulties producing speech; there are various reasons that this might be the case, from presence of a tracheostomy to neuromotor conditions. Strategies for communicating for these people fall under the umbrella term of *alternative and augmentative communication* (AAC). AAC modalities tend to be highly specific to an individual and may be self-designed or created in collaboration with a speech language pathologist, friends or family members, or other professionals.

Communication assistant (CA) is a broad term that is not specific to any one method or style of facilitating communication. CAs may have formal training or none at all, provide other support (i.e. attendant care), and be an employee (of the patient or an institution) or unpaid (family, friend, volunteer). The choice of CA should be based on the needs and preferences of the disabled person, rather than those of the health care provider(s). Be aware that some people's communication tools, or the assistants using them, may not provide a vocabulary for discussing sexuality or some 2SLGBTQ issues.

ATTENDANT CARE AND SUPPORT PEOPLE

Attendant care and support people can also be paid or unpaid and are present to assist the patient to meet disability related needs. Their role may be to lift the patient onto the exam table or be present to watch for triggers or warning signs of mental health crisis, for example. Depending on the role of this third party, they may or may not need to be present for an exam or a consultation.

CONSIDERATIONS FOR WORKING WITH PATIENTS
WITH SUPPORT PEOPLE

Practitioners may find themselves torn between patient confidentiality and meeting health care needs. While some third parties will have confidentiality agreements, others could be friends, partners, or family members, which can make conversations about sexuality and sexual health difficult. Further, sometimes the interpersonal relationship or dynamic between the support person and the patient can have a bearing on the resulting interaction with health care professionals.

Health care providers can ask to be alone with the patient during the appointment; they can also try to come to an understanding in advance of the appointment regarding sexual health matters. These options may or may not be possible or may be more or less successful depending on the individual's circumstances. If the patient has a friend or family member acting as an ASL interpreter, you can make it clear to the patient that they are entitled to a professional interpreter.

Whenever possible, establish what the patient is comfortable discussing in front of the third party before discussing it. Never "out" someone or reveal other sensitive information without checking in advance. A provider should not assume that because a patient is out to one third party that they are out to another. If sexual health issues need to be discussed and the patient doesn't feel comfortable doing so because of a particular third-party support person, interpreter or CA, someone from their health care team should work with them to find appropriate supports of their choosing to assist them at appointments.

Always speak directly to the patient about their own health care and not to the third party; this communicates respect for the patient and their agency. Speaking to the disabled person directly affirms the provider understands the patient is responsible for decisions related to their health care.

Some ways to avoid miscommunication and increase the likelihood of understanding are asking patients to repeat information back, asking open ended questions, and using pictorial aids.[43] You might also repeat to a person what you believe they meant and ask for confirmation.

A larger space, additional seating, and extra time are required for meetings with more people present.

Referrals

Creatively meeting people's access needs will only go so far. If a space isn't physically accessible, it is important to be able to refer patients to physically accessible options. However, it is notable that physically accessible equipment does not guarantee accessibility of care.[44] There may be reasons that a patient wants to see a specific practitioner and/or doesn't want to go to the physically accessible place you refer them to; reasons can include proximity, 2SLGBTQ friendliness, need for transition support, continuity of care, and so on. If possible, practitioners should communicate with a provider or organization before referring a patient with accessibility needs to see if their particular needs will be met.

When a patient reports a barrier that made an appointment with another provider difficult or impossible, especially when this was a provider you referred them to, we recommend that you work to re-establish trust with the patient. Based on the authors' anecdotal experience, we would argue this is best done by listening to the patient, acknowledging that you understand what the barrier was, apologizing for not being aware that the patient would have a negative experience and, where appropriate, explaining formal complaints processes or telling the patient you will have a conversation with the provider. Where appropriate, ask them for their opinion about future referrals.

Conclusion

As health care providers, attending to 2SLGBTQ issues requires attending to disability issues. Disabled 2SLGBTQ patients, like all people, have multifaceted identities and experiences of oppression that intersect and interlock.

While challenges for health care providers working across these issues can be multifold, the opportunities for dismantling particular sites of oppression are exciting and real. Building robust health care practices grounded in principles of social justice can start with modest actions.

Connecting with a disability advocacy group for information about available resources can be useful for health care providers and their patients alike. Many disability groups welcome support from non-disabled people and do important disability community work. It is essential that providers look to groups *of* disabled people not groups *for* disabled people. Online and real-world sites of grassroots 2SLGBTQ and disability communities or movements can also be sources of history and alternative perspectives for health care providers and may point to meaningful ways engage with these communities.[57–62]

Writing, art pieces, and performances by 2SLGBTQ disabled people can offer health care providers insight into patients' experiences and offer the opportunity to support artists and communities financially as a patron or consumer.[62–69]

The history of medicine and medicalization of disabled 2SLGBTQ bodies is layered and complex. It is our belief that, in beginning to understand and acknowledge these issues, health care providers can work with disabled 2SLGBTQ patients to reduce barriers and enhance the quality and accessibility of health care for all.

References

1. Pyne J, Bauer G, Redman N, Travers R. Improving the health of trans communities: findings from the TRANS Pulse project [Internet]. London (ON): Trans PULSE; 2012 [cited 2018 Feb 15]. Available from: http://transpulseproject.ca/research/improving-the-health -of-trans-communities/.
2. Fredriksen-Goldsen KI, Kim H-J, Barkan SE. Disability among lesbian, gay, and bisexual adults: disparities in prevalence and risk. Am J Public Health. 2012 Jan;102(1):e16–21. Available from: http://www.ncbi.nlm.nih .gov/pubmed/22095356.
3. Nestel S. Colour coded health care: the impact of race and racism on Canadian's health [Internet]. Toronto: Wellesley Institute; 2012 [cited 2018 Feb 15]. Available from: http://www.wellesleyinstitute.com/wp-content /uploads/2012/02/Colour-Coded-Health-Care-Sheryl-Nestel.pdf.
4. Raphael D. Poverty and policy in Canada: implications for health and quality of life. 2nd ed. Toronto: Canadian Scholars' Press; 2011.
5. Arim R. Canadian survey on disability, 2012: a profile of persons with disabilities among canadians aged 15 years or older, 2012 [Internet]. Ottawa: Statistics Canada; 2015 [cited 2018 Feb 15]. Available from: http:// www.statcan.gc.ca/pub/89-654-x/89-654-x2015001-eng.pdf.
6. Withers AJ. Disability politics and theory. Black Point: Fernwood; 2012.
7. American Psychiatric Association. Diagnostic and statistical manual of mental disorders. Washington (DC): American Psychiatric Association; 1952.
8. Frank LR. The history of shock treatment. In: Frank LR, editor. The history of shock treatment. San Francisco (CA): Leonard Roy Frank; 1978.
9. Perone AK. The social construction of mental illness for lesbian, gay, bisexual, and transgender persons in the United States. Qual Soc Work. 2014;13(6):766–71.
10. American Psychiatric Association [Internet]. Arlington (VA): American Psychiatric Association; 1973 [cited 2018 Feb 15]. Homosexuality and sexual orientation disturbance: proposed change in DSM-II, 6th printing, page 44 position statement (retired). Available from: psychiatryonline.org.
11. Silverstein C. Are you saying homosexuality is normal? J Gay Lesbian Ment Health. 2008;12(3):277–87.
12. Stryker S. Transgender history. Berkeley (CA): Seal Press; 2008.
13. Withers A. Disabling trans: political implications and possibilities of constructions of trans as a disability [Internet]. Toronto: York University; 2013 [cited 2018 Feb 16]]. Available from: https://stillmyrevolution.files .wordpress.com/2015/05/withers-fully-completed-doccument.pdf.

14. Gapka S, Raj R. Trans health project: a position paper and resolution adopted by the Ontario Public Health Association (OPHA). Toronto: Ontario Public Health Association; 2003.
15. Withers AJ. Disability, divisions, definitions and disablism: when resisting psychiatry is oppressive. In: Burstow B, LeFrançois BA, Diamond S, editors. Crafting the (r)evolution against psychiatry: theorizing resistance. Montreal: McGill-Queen's University Press; 2014. p. 150–71.
16. Stedman TL. Stedman's medical dictionary 28th ed. Philadelphia (PA): Lippincott Williams & Wilkins; 2006. Disability; p. 547–8.
17. Elliott TR, Dreer L. Disability. In: Ayers S, Baum A, McManus C, Newman S, Wallston K, Weinman J, et al., editors. Cambridge Handbook of Psychology, Health and Medicine. Cambridge: Cambridge University Press; 2007. p. 80–4.
18. Barnes C, Mercer G, Shakespeare T. Exploring disability: a sociological introduction. Cambridge: Polity Press; 1999.
19. Vellacott JW. Walking the talk? models of disability and discourse in employment policy for Canadians with disabilities [dissertation]. [Vancouver (BC)]: University of British Columbia; 2011. Available from: http://hdl.handle.net/2429/36758.
20. Menzies R, Lefrançois BA, Reaume G. Introducing mad studies. In: LeFrançois BA, Menzies R, Reaume G, editors. Mad matters: a critical reader in Canadian mad studies. Toronto: Canadian Scholars' Press; 2013. p. 1–22.
21. Walker N [Internet]. Berkeley (CA): NeuroQueer; 2014 [cited 2018 Feb 16]. Neurodiversity: some basic terms and definitions. Available from: https://neuroqueer.com/neurodiversity-terms-and-definitions/.
22. Cooper C. The road I have taken: Christopher Reeve and the cure. ABILITY magazine [Internet]. [cited 2018 Feb 16]. Available from: https://www.abilitymagazine.com/reeve_interview.html.
23. Gerhart KA, Koziol-McLain J, Lowenstein SR, Whiteneck GG. Quality of life following spinal cord injury: knowledge and attitudes of emergency care providers. Ann Emerg Med. 1994 Nov 29;23(4):807–12. doi:10.1016/s0196-0644(94)70318-3.
24. Saigal S. In their own words: life at adulthood after very premature birth. Semin Perinatol. 2016 Dec;40(8):578–83. doi:10.1053/j.semperi.2016.09.010.
25. Ali A, Scior K, Ratti V, Strydom A, King M, Hassiotis A. Discrimination and other barriers to accessing health care: perspectives of patients with mild and moderate intellectual disability and their carers. PLoS One. 2013 Jan 7;8(8):e70855. doi:10.1371/journal.pone.0070855.
26. Marrocco A, Krouse HJ. Obstacles to preventive care for individuals with disability: implications for nurse practitioner. J Am Assoc Nurse Pract. 2017 May;29(5):282–93. doi:10.1002/2327-6924.12449.

27. Sirch L, Salvador L, Palese A. Communication difficulties experienced by deaf male patients during their in-hospital stay: findings from a qualitative descriptive study. Scand J Caring Sci. 2017 Jun;31(2):368–77. doi:10.1111/scs.12356.
28. Perlin ML, Lynch AJ. Sexuality, disability, and the law: beyond the last frontier? Basingstoke (England): Palgrave Macmillan; 2016.
29. Erickson L. Unbreaking our hearts: cultures of un/desirability and the transformative potential of queer crip porn. Toronto: York Universtiy; 2015.
30. Anderson S. Sex education programs focused on "protection" and "prevention" with little attention given to supporting people to develop healthy, positive sexual relationships. Res Pract Intellect Dev Disabil. 2015 Jan 2;2(1):98–100.
31. Porter C. Taser stun gun figures incomplete. Toronto Star. 2004;B2.
32. College of Family Physicians Canada [Internet]. Toronto: CFPC; 2016 Nov [cited 2018 Nov 18]. Poverty: a clinical tool for primary care providers. Available from: https://web.archive.org/web/20180705131919/http://www.cfpc.ca/poverty_tools/.
33. Frazee C, Gilmour J, Mykitiuk R [Internet]. Rochester (NY): Social Science Research Network; 2011 Jan [cited 2018 Feb18]. The legal regulation and construction of the gendered body and of disability in Canadian health law and policy. Available from: https://papers.ssrn.com/abstract=1775204. p. 78, 79.
34. Benítez-Silva H, Buchinsky M, Man Chan H, Cheidvasser S, Rust J. How large is the bias in self-reported disability? J Appl Econom. 2004 Jan 14;19(6):649–70. doi:10.1002/jae.797.
35. Maki K. Neoliberal deviants and surveillance: welfare recipients under the watchful eye of Ontario works. Surveill Soc. 2011;9(1/2):47–63.
36. Mosher JE. Welfare fraud: the constitution of social assistance as crime [Internet]. Comm Rep Stud Public Policy Doc; 2005 Mar [cited 2018 Feb18]. Available from: http://digitalcommons.osgoode.yorku.ca/reports/161/.
37. 1405–05006 (re), 2015 ONSBT 73 (CanLII). p. 73. Available from: http://canlii.ca/t/gjkzg.
38. Prince MJ. Struggling for social citizenship: disabled Canadians, income security, and prime ministerial eras. Montreal: McGill-Queen's Press; 2016.
39. Maragh-Bass AC, Torain M, Adler R, Ranjit A, Schneider E, Shields RY, et al. Is it okay to ask: transgender patient perspectives on sexual orientation and gender identity collection in healthcare. Acad Emerg Med. 2017;24(6):655–67.
40. Giblon R, Bauer GR. Health care availability, quality, and unmet need: a comparison of transgender and cisgender residents of Ontario, Canada. BMC Health Serv Res. 2017 Apr 18;17(1):283. doi:10.1186/s12913-017-2226-z.

41. Bauer G, Nussbaum N, Travers R, Munro L, Pyne J, Redman N. We've got work to do: workplace discrimination and employment challenges for trans people in Ontario. Trans PULSE E-Bulletin. 2011;2(1):1–3. Available from: http://transpulseproject.ca/wp-content/uploads/2011/05/E3English.pdf.

42. Raymaker DM, McDonald KE, Ashkenazy E, Gerrity M, Baggs AM, Kripke C, et al. Barriers to healthcare: instrument development and comparison between autistic adults and adults with and without other disabilities. Autism. 2017 Nov 22;21(8):972–84. doi:10.1177/1362361316661261.

43. Scheier DB. Barriers to health care for people with hearing loss: a review of the literature. J New York State Nurses Assoc. 2009 Mar 22;40(1):4–11.

44. Morris MA, Maragh-Bass AC, Griffin JM, Finney Rutten LJ, Lagu T, Phelan S. Use of accessible examination tables in the primary care setting: a survey of physical evaluations and patient attitudes. J Gen Intern Med. 2017 Dec 18;32(12):1342–8. doi:10.1007/s11606-017-4155-2. p. 1345.

45. Mingus M. Leaving Evidence [blog on the Internet]. [place unknown]: Mia Mingus. Medical industrial complex visual; 2015 [cited 2018 Jan 26]. Available from: https://leavingevidence.wordpress.com/2015/02/06/medical-industrial-complex-visual/.

46. Higgins M, Swain J. Disability and child sexual abuse: lessons from survivors' narratives for effective protection, prevention and treatment. London: Jessica Kingsley Publishers; 2009.

47. Goar C. Ugly secret of Ontario psychiatric hospitals won't stay hidden. Toronto Star [Internet]. 2013 Jun 7 [updated 2016 Jan 7; cited 2018 Jan 26]; Available from: https://www.thestar.com/opinion/commentary/2013/06/07/ugly_secret_of_ontario_psychiatric_hospitals_wont_stay_hidden_goar.html.

48. Dubinski K. Ex-nurse who killed 8 seniors in her care sentenced to 8 concurrent life terms [Internet]. CBC News. 2017 Jun 23 [cited 2018 Jan 26]; Available from: https://www.cbc.ca/news/canada/london/killer-nurse-wettlaufer-sentencing-1.4175164.

49. Ontario Association of Sign Language Interpreters. ASL-english interpreters: quick tips [Internet]. Toronto: Ontario Association of Sign Language Interpreters; [cited 2018 Feb 25]. Available from: http://www.oasli.on.ca/images/quickcards/OASLI_Quick_Card_Quick_Tips.pdf.

50. Goodridge D, Rogers M, Klassen L, Jeffery B, Knox K, Rohatinsky N, et al. Access to health and support services: perspectives of people living with a long-term traumatic spinal cord injury in rural and urban areas. Disabil Rehabil. 2015 Jul 31;37(16):1401–10. doi:10.3109/09638288.2014.972593.

51. Canadian Association of the Deaf. Communicating accessibility: a project report on federal accessibility legislation [Internet]. Ottawa: CAD.

Available from: https://sci-can.ca/sites/spinalcordinjurycanada.ca/files
/attach/Communicating Accessibility CAD EN.pdf.

52. Tarasoff LA. Experiences of women with physical disabilities during
the perinatal period: a review of the literature and recommendations to
improve care. Health Care Women Int. 2015 Jan 2;36(1):88–107. doi:10.1080
/07399332.2013.815756.

53. Accessibility for Ontarians with Disabilities Act, 2005, SO 2005, c 11.

54. Bauer SE, Schumacher JR, Hall A, Marlow NM, Friedel C, Scheer D, et al.
Disability and physical and communication-related barriers to health care
related services among Florida residents: a brief report. Disabil Health J.
2016 Jul;9(3):552–6.

55. Ontario Association of Sign Language Interpreters [Internet]. Toronto:
Ontario Association of Sign Language Interpreters; [cited 2021 Jan 15].
What is an interpreter?Available from: http://oasli.on.ca/index.php
/interpreters/what-is-an-interpreter.

56. Ontario Association of Sign Language Interpreters. You've been asked to
pay for an interpreter ... [Internet]. Toronto: Ontario Association of Sign
Language Interpreters; [cited 2018 Feb 25]. Available from: http://www
.oasli.on.ca/images/quickcards/OASLI_Quick_Card_Paying_for
_Interpreters.pdf.

57. British Columbia Rainbow Alliance of the Deaf [Internet]. Vancouver:
British Columbia Rainbow Alliance of the Deaf; [cited 2018 Dec 28].
Available from: https://www.facebook.com/BCRAD.YVR.

58. Deaf Queer Resource Center [Internet]. About us; 2009 [cited 2018 Dec 28].
Available from: http://www.deafqueer.org/411/about/.

59. Ontario Rainbow Alliance of the Deaf [Internet]. Toronto: Ontario
Rainbow Alliance of the Deaf; [cited 2018 Dec 28]. Available from:
https://www.facebook.com/oradeaf/.

60. Toronto Disability Pride [Internet]. Toronto: Toronto Disability Pride;
[cited 2018 Dec 29]. Toronto Disability Pride march. Available from:
https://torontodisabilitypride.wordpress.com.

61. Toronto Mad Pride [Internet]. Toronto: Toronto Mad Pride; [cited 2018 Dec
29]. Available from: http://www.torontomadpride.com.

62. Withers AJ. Still my revolution [blog on the Internet]. Toronto: AJ Withers.
c2008– [cited 2018 Dec 28]. Available from: https://stillmyrevolution.org/.

63. Clare E. Brilliant imperfection: grappling with cure. Durham: Duke
University Press; 2017.

64. Devaney J. My leaky body. Fredricton: Goose Lane Editions; 2012.

65. da Silva Gorman R [Internet]. Toronto: R da Silva Gorman; [cited 2018
Dec 29]. Revolutionary forms. Available from: http://www
.revolutionaryforms.org.

66. Peers D, Eales L. G.I.M.P. bootcamp [Internet]. [place unknown]: KingCrip Productions; 2008 [cited 2018 Dec 29]. Video: 8 min. Available from: https://vimeo.com/58160733?embedded=true&source=vi deo_title&owner=13589983.

67. Mingus M. Leaving Evidence [blog on the Internet]. [place unknown]: Mia Mingus; 2016 [cited 2018 Dec 29]. Available from: https://leavinge vidence.wordpress.com.

68. monoceros m [Internet]. [place unknown]: melannie monoceros [Internet]; [cited 2018 Dec 29]. Available from: http://melanniemonoceros .com

69. Piepzna-Samarasinha LL. Care work: dreaming disability justice. Vancouver: Arsenal Pulp Press; 2018.

15 LGBTQ Newcomers in Canada

MEGO NERSES, NICHOLAS HERSH,
AND CAROL GELLER

Introduction

Many LGBTQ newcomers have endured various forms of homophobia and transphobia perpetuated by their family members, communities, religious and medical institutions, and state authorities in their countries of nationality. Consequently, many arrive in Canada suffering from serious physical and mental health conditions for which accessing proper services may be a challenge. Barriers to appropriate health services include systemic cultural and language barriers, stigma surrounding their sexuality or gender identity, cross-cultural communication barriers with health care providers, and the burden of preparing cases for refugee protection.

This chapter focuses on the intersection between health, LGBTQ identities, and refugee-status determination in Canada. Our aim is to provide clinicians and other health allies with a broad foundational understanding of the unique health challenges for LGBTQ newcomers to improve their practices in working with this population.

Between 2013 and 2015, approximately 12 per cent of refugee claims in Canada were based on sexual orientation, representing a significant caseload for the Refugee Protection Division (RPD) of the Immigration and Refugee Board (IRB), which reviews these claims.[1] Moreover, the number of claims based on sexual orientation in 2015 rose to 1286 compared to a yearly average of 1132 claims in the preceding four years.[2] LGBTQ individuals may also arrive in Canada through other immigration channels such as on international student visas, as economic immigrants, or as resettlement as refugees from outside Canada. Although they may not experience the burdens of applying for refugee protection inside Canada, they often share similar needs for health care services as refugee claimants. Therefore, there are valid reasons to examine common health concerns for LGBTQ newcomers, as well as the role of health care professionals in supporting LGBTQ individuals navigating Canada's asylum system.

This chapter is divided into five parts. Part 1 is intended to describe the common experiences of LGBTQ individuals in their countries of origin and post arrival in Canada. Part 2 explains the legal and evidentiary requirements for refugee protection as they relate to claims based on sexual orientation and gender identity expressions. We focus particularly on the scope and importance of evidence tied to LGBTQ individuals' physical and mental health in their refugee claims. In Part 3, we turn to the physical and mental health challenges experienced by LGBTQ newcomers, particularly refugee claimants. Part 4 of this chapter highlights the important roles of health care professionals in service delivery and provides recommendations for ensuring effective care for LGBTQ newcomers. Finally, we conclude this chapter in Part 5 by recommending future research and directions.

For the purpose of this chapter, *LGBTQ* is used to describe individuals whose sexual orientation or gender identity expressions are at odds with societal expectations. We recognize this acronym is limited and problematic. It conjures different interpretations and may not sufficiently represent all unconventional identities and expressions, including sexual and gender minority refugee claimants. It is noteworthy that we did not include the 2S for *Two-Spirit* in the acronym for our chapter. Given that the term is used by some North American Indigenous communities to describe their identities, it is unlikely to be represented in refugee and newcomer communities.

The information reflected in this chapter is drawn from our professional experiences in an urban centre. We acknowledge that LGBTQ newcomers have varying experiences based on available health resources and geographical location in Canada.

Part 1: Experiences before and after Migration

Common Experiences in Countries of Nationality

LGBTQ newcomers experience various pre-migration struggles. In their countries of nationality, their sexual orientation or gender identity expressions are often considered against social, religious, and state laws.[3,4] Consequently, some may have been subjected to imprisonment, floggings, lashings, torture, and other forms of cruel and inhumane treatments for their unconventional sexualities and gender identities.[4] Even if homophobic and transphobic laws are not enforced, they create an environment in which state and non-state actors, such as families and communities, are enabled to cause harm to LGBTQ individuals.[5] Hence, LGBTQ newcomers may never feel safe in their countries of nationality.

In some countries in the Middle East, Africa, and South-East Asia, expressing unconventional sexual or gender identities is treated as being abnormal, demonic, or diseased.[4] For instance, individuals from these regions report being accused of having "the white disease" – a disease caused by white individuals.[3] They may experience cultural rituals to drain them of the "gay" disease.[4] These rituals include witch-hunting practices, forced consumption of blood or urine for cleansing fulfilments, and public humiliations such as corrective rape.[4] In 2013, Shidlo and Ahola described corrective rape as:

> Rape of a person because of their perceived sexual or gender orientation; the intended consequence of the rape, as seen by the perpetrator, is to "correct" their orientation – to turn them heterosexual or to make them act more in conformity with gender stereotypes.[6]

Many LGBTQ newcomers report feeling a strong sense of shame and dishonour ascribed to their families because of their sexual orientation or gender identity expressions.[4] Consequently, they report being rejected and disowned by family members who want to maintain their reputation in their communities.[4] Rejection may result in homelessness or emotional, physical, or sexual abuse at the hands of family members. In some instances, individuals who support rather than punish their LGBTQ family members may also face violence and societal disapproval, compounding the pressure for LGBTQ individuals to conceal their sexual or gender identities.[4]

For LGBTQ individuals who are threatened or face violence, escape becomes their only chance of survival.[4] They flee their homes and seek refuge in countries with stronger reputations for LGBTQ protections such as Canada, the United States, and western European countries.[4] Unless they hold valid travel documents and visas, LGBTQ individuals may turn to smugglers to facilitate their travel, which is costly and dangerous.[4] Fleeing their countries comes with a high emotional price, as they may be leaving behind their families, jobs, and partners.[4] Many people who turn to smugglers for assistance may not end up reaching a safe country as planned.[4] Some are sent back to their countries of nationality or are threatened by the smugglers if they refuse to act or perform sexual favours.[4]

Post-migration Acculturation: Reflection and Experiences

Commonly, immigrants and refugees, including LGBTQ individuals, are expected to acculturate into their new society after arrival.[7,8] The concept of acculturation has been studied extensively in psychological literature.[9–13] For example, Berry described two intersecting dimensions that comprise acculturation: cultural maintenance and cultural adaptation. Berry explained that individuals retain their cultural practices (maintenance) or choose to integrate with other ethnic groups in the host country (adaptation).[14] Additionally, he suggested that there are four possible outcomes resulting from the intersection of these two dimensions: *integration, assimilation, separation,* and *marginalization.* Individuals who *integrate* preserve their own cultural values and simultaneously learn new values of the host country. Individuals who *assimilate* adapt their own values and norms to fit with the host country but no longer maintain their own cultural norms. Contrarily, individuals who *separate* avoid social groups in the host country to maintain their own values and traditions. Finally, individuals who *marginalize* themselves reject both their cultural values and norms and those of the host country. Associated research has suggested that integration yields the best psychological outcomes while marginalization has been seen as having negative impacts on an individuals' psychological well-being.[14]

Unlike Berry's model, recent literature proposes that acculturation be conceptualized as a complex, multidimensional process.[15,16] This process is influenced by individuals' cultural values, knowledge, identity, family, neighbourhood, and community,[17] along with other contextual factors such as cognitive appraisals, and physical and symbolic meaning of the world.[18]

It is understood that similarly to other newcomers to Canada, LGBTQ refugee claimants usually enter mainstream Canadian society by acquiring a new language, adopting dominant social values and traditions, and learning to navigate Canadian systems, such as housing, employment, medical care, and education.[4] However, data on acculturation processes specific to LGBTQ refugee claimants are scant. For example, little is known regarding the extent to which pre-migration psychological trauma (such as torture, slavery, human trafficking, and corrective rape) hinder or advance the acculturation process of LGBTQ refugee claimants.

Unlike other newcomers, LGBTQ newcomers face additional challenges as they begin to acculturate into the Canadian LGBTQ communities, which espouse values and beliefs related to relationships and sexuality that often conflict with those in their former environment.[19,20] Dating and sexual scripts – the where, how, when, and what of sexual contact – are unique to each country and context.[4] For example, some report feelings of confusion about meeting potential partners online given that dating opportunities are arranged differently in their countries of origin.[3] They report that in their home countries, they may have only learned of and embraced being LGBTQ in a private context such as covert pubs, hotel rooms, or private residences where dating is arranged by fellow members of the LGBTQ community. For some, dating apps are considered unsafe in their countries of origin because of the potential for blackmail or the risk of being outed or otherwise harmed by homophobic/transphobic individuals.[3] Consequently, some still struggle to trust dating apps. Partners in mixed-orientation relationships with or without children will face different relationship negotiations, dynamics, and dating challenges.[21,22]

Another example of confusion commonly expressed concerns gay pride events.[4] While these are commonplace in Canada, some newcomers are apprehensive about attending them because they fear being recognized by someone in their ethnocultural community, thus potentially putting their lives or those of loved ones in their countries of origin at risk. At the same time, some newcomers who have participated in pride parades have reported feeling liberated of shame and guilt.

LGBTQ newcomers often have to adjust their expectations and create new sex scripts that fit their individual and cultural needs, as well as their understanding of sexuality and gender identity.[4] Most LGBTQ newcomers report feeling pressured to adhere to unfamiliar scripts, not only to fit into the gay community but also to prove their credibility as LGBTQ to refugee status decision makers.[23] From our experiences, LGBTQ newcomers eventually adjust and integrate newly acquired values into their lives.[4]

Part 2: Canadian Refugee Law and Clinical Reports

Refugee Protection Process

Applications for refugee protection in Canada are handled by the RPD, a section of the IRB. Individuals may submit their paperwork to claim protection either at a Canadian border entry point or at a local Immigration, Refugees, and Citizenship Canada (IRCC) office. Claimants are entitled to hire legal counsel at their own expense to prepare their cases. Eligible individuals may also apply for provincial legal aid certificates to cover the fees for legal representation.

Claimants eventually testify at a hearing, which takes place in an IRB office in Ottawa, Montreal, Toronto, Calgary, or Vancouver.[24] Generally, the adjudicator, known as a board member, begins the hearing by reviewing the documentation, asking the claimants to swear to tell the truth, and then questioning the claimants on their fears of returning to their countries of nationality. Then, counsel has an opportunity to question the claimants to clarify testimony or highlight particular experiences germane to the claim. Any witnesses are then brought into the hearing room to testify. Finally, counsel provides submissions to the IRB on why the claimants meet the requirements for refugee protection in Canada. Claimants are entitled to professional interpretation during the hearing. RPD hearings are not open to the public.[24]

Following the hearing, the IRB member determines whether claimants are Convention refugees. A convention refugee is defined as:

> A person who is outside of his or her country of nationality or habitual residence; who has a well-founded fear of persecution for reasons of race, religion, nationality, political opinion, or membership in a particular social group; and who is unable or unwilling to seek state protection in his or her country of nationality or habitual residence.[25]

Rejected claimants receive notice by mail of the RPD's decision and their right to file an appeal to the Refugee Appeals Division (RAD) of the IRB pending certain conditions. Claimants must file appeal notices with the RAD within 15 days of receiving the RPD's decision and then have another 15 days to provide written arguments. They may also include evidence if it is new or could not have reasonably been provided to the RPD. The RAD has the statutory authority to uphold the determination of the RPD, set the RPD's determination aside and substitute its own, or refer the matter back to the RPD for redetermination.[25] RAD board members are required to render their decisions with written reasons within 90 days or as soon as feasible after 90 days.[26] The overall grant rate of appeals involving sexual orientation is approximately 27.6 per cent.[1] Beyond an appeal, a claimant may submit an application to the Federal Court to judicially review the RPD's or RAD's decision.

Assessing the Credibility of Claims

While there is a presumption that claimants' statements are truthful unless there is a valid reason to doubt their truthfulness, claimants are required to provide sufficient credible evidence to establish their membership in a particular social group – in other words, that they are

LGBTQ. Adjudicators must judge whether this onus has been met by virtue of a claimant's testimony, witnesses, and documentary evidence such as affidavits or police and medical reports. Decision makers also refer to country of origin information on the social and legal realities of LGBTQ refugees before making credibility assessments.

The Scope and Purpose of Medical and Mental Health Reports

While members of the RPD and RAD have expertise in determining credibility, decisions on claimants' physical and mental health go beyond their scope of knowledge. Therefore, clinical reports often serve as crucial pieces of documentary evidence in refugee status determination proceedings.

First, reports provide the IRB with insight on the state of claimants' mental health and how it may impact their ability to recount their stories within the hearing process. Members are entitled to draw negative inferences from a claimant's demeanour, inconsistencies, omissions, and insufficiently spontaneous responses, all of which may be linked to issues of mental health.[27] The absence of a clinical report identifying mental health issues that may impact claimants' ability to accurately recollect and articulate relevant memories to their case may result in adverse credibility determinations.

Second, psychological and psychiatric reports may serve to bolster the grounds for procedural accommodations in accordance with *Chairperson Guideline 8: Procedures With Respect to Vulnerable Persons Appearing Before the IRB* (*Chairperson Guideline*) to allow claimants designated as vulnerable to meaningfully participate in their hearings.[28] Examples of accommodations include allowing the vulnerable person to provide evidence by videoconference or other means, allowing a support person to participate in a hearing, creating a more informal setting for a hearing, varying the order of questioning, and providing a panel and interpreter of a particular gender.[26] Though the IRB may not require expert evidence on the vulnerability of a claimant, it may consider whether such evidence could have reasonably been obtained to determine the applicability of the *Chairperson Guideline*.[28]

Third, reports may support other criteria for protection, such as explaining claimants' delays in applying for refugee protection because of their mental health. Generally, a delay in claiming refugee protection may raise doubts about a claimant's subjective fear, a required criterion to qualify as a Convention refugee. Reports may also explain the psychological impact on claimants if they were to return to their countries of nationality.

Finally, medical reports are also useful pieces of evidence to corroborate the testimony of LGBTQ refugee claimants, especially when they have reported experiences of physical abuse and violence in their countries of origin but do not have medical records produced at the time of the incidents. Claimants with visible bodily injuries such as scars and lacerations might consider submitting a report from a medical professional stating such injuries are consistent with the claimants' alleged experiences. While claimants are responsible for testifying on how they sustained injuries, the IRB cannot reject medical reports solely because they do not confirm that the only cause of those injuries is that alleged by the claimants.[29-31]

Recommendations for Writing Clinical Reports

Health professionals may consider the following recommendations to ensure their reports are given substantial weight before board members. While these recommendations reflect considerations gleaned from the jurisprudence and the *Chairperson Guideline*, each report should consider the claimant's unique circumstances and may require tailoring on a case-by-case basis.

First, medical and mental health professionals have more credibility when they indicate their qualifications, for example, by explaining them in the report or including their curriculum vitae or a copy of their licence to practise in their profession. Providing credentials helps to demonstrate they are qualified to provide expert evidence on a claimant's physical and mental state and are authorized to provide a clinical opinion by their professional regulatory body.

Second, clinical assessments are stronger if they are linked to the claimant's capacity to recount their stories during their RPD or RAD hearing.[29] A clinical diagnosis based solely on the claimant's version of events may prove problematic in determining credibility as opposed to being interpreted through a clinical lens. Thus, a nuanced distinction is required between a claimant's version of experiences and the health professional's personal observations of the claimant when articulating those experiences, such as their demeanour, eye contact, and emotional state. For example, clinicians can include their clinical impressions, mental health status exam (MHSE), and other observations in the report to make this distinction.

Next, health professionals are cautioned to not reach findings within the IRB's purview of expertise.[29] Conclusions of a claimant's merits for refugee protection, particularly the veracity of the claimant's allegations of abuse or persecution, may be perceived as an attempt to usurp the member's role, in turn diminishing the weight assigned to the report.[29] To illustrate, in a 2014 RAD decision, the IRB found that the psychologist attempted to influence the outcome of the case because his report:

> Explains the Appellant's delay in claiming [for reasons unrelated to his mental health], makes repeated appeals for him to be given status in Canada, and concludes that any evidentiary inconsistencies should not be considered as credibility problems.[29]

No weight was accorded to the psychological report in determining the claimant's credibility.[29]

Finally, reports should indicate how much time the health professional has spent with the claimant and confirm they have sufficient information based on that amount of time to reach their clinical impressions or else reports may be accorded little weight.[31] It is helpful to indicate whether claimants require follow-up care and if they have done so. A claimant's failure to pursue treatment may result in a rejection of the clinical report.[29] Beyond the suggestions proposed in this section, health professionals may consider furthering their skills and knowledge and receive supervision in assessing mental health and writing clinical reports in the context of immigration. It is likewise recommended that health professionals gain knowledge of legal and ethical implications for writing these reports.

Part 3: Physical and Mental Health of LGBTQ Newcomers

This section highlights physical and mental health experiences common to LGBTQ newcomers, particularly refugee claimants.

Physical Health

Generally, newcomers have unique, culturally bound understanding and terminology to describe their health, including their symptoms, self-care, and overall approach to achieving and maintaining their health. Moreover, before and during migration, newcomers often have limited access to health care services and, upon arrival in Canada, are unfamiliar with the availability and the importance of preventive care and chronic disease management. Generally, their pre-migration experience is based solely on accessing physical health care for acute health concerns. The concept of primary as opposed to specialist care is also new for many newcomers in our practice.

Certain health conditions, including infectious diseases such as chronic hepatitis B, genetic conditions such as sickle cell anemia and thalassemia, and chronic illnesses such as diabetes, are more prevalent in the newcomer population. The statutorily required immigration medical exam (IME) and diagnostic testing consist only of a chest X-ray, urinalysis, syphilis serology, and HIV testing for those older than 15 years of age.

In our practices, many newcomers do not have records or recollection of the vaccines they received before arriving in Canada. It is important to review whether a follow-up immunization schedule should be implemented depending on their country of nationality and transit countries.

Having access to resources on prevention and screening recommendations for newcomers, including lab work, recommended immunizations, and Mantoux testing is invaluable. The Canadian Collaboration for Immigrant and Refugee Health's website is an example that provides an evidence-based preventative care checklist for new Canadians, immigrants, and refugees.[32] Pottie et al. also provide evidence-based clinical guidelines for immigrants and refugees in Canada.[33]

Preventive health care is an important concept to explain to patients, including its context in the Canadian health care system, as it is often unfamiliar. It is important to implement age-appropriate screening, such as PAP tests, mammograms, screening for colon cancer, and tests for diabetes and high blood pressure. Finally, health care for newcomers involves identifying and managing acute and chronic illnesses. Common health issues include poor oral health and unmet contraceptive needs.

Mental Health

Newcomers' mental health issues can be affected by the degree of adversity they experienced before, during, and after resettlement.[4] Mental health may also be perceived differently based on newcomers' cultural background and social values.[34] Many LGBTQ newcomers feel disinclined to disclose their symptoms to mental health professionals because of fears of stigmatization or ostracism within their ethnocultural communities.[4,34] Others may have a fear of being judged and misunderstood by mental health professionals. An individual's mental health may also have multiple and contextual ramifications. For example, in Middle Eastern cultures, an identified family member with a mental illness is considered injurious to the reputation of the family.[35-37] Individuals report that their families are seen as unhealthy, that the mental health condition is felt to be contagious, and that women in the family will have fewer opportunities to get married.

Initially, the occurrence of anxiety and depression in newcomers and refugees is lower than the general population[38] but increases to a similar prevalence over time. Newcomers and refugees who have had exposure to violence often have higher rates of symptoms related to the traumatic events including post-traumatic stress disorder (PTSD), somatic symptoms, and chronic pain. Some guidelines recommend against routine screening for exposure to trauma, given that pushing for disclosure might cause harm.[33] On the other hand, undiagnosed and untreated trauma-related symptoms can have profoundly negative effects on individuals' psychological well-being and can impede the recovery process.[39]

We recommend that health providers mitigate the potential harms of screening for trauma and PTSD by embracing trauma-informed screening steps to safely explore and understand past trauma histories and their impact on patients. Health professionals should consider screening for PTSD symptoms only after a solid therapeutic rapport has been established, and they ensure that patients have healthy coping skills and access to appropriate supports. Similarly, routine screening for depression is not recommended unless appropriate supports are available for those who screen positive.[33]

Clinicians must also be alert to signs and symptoms of adjustment stress and various forms of abuse, including domestic and child abuse, as some LGBTQ newcomers may have experienced threats, violence, and abuse from their family members.[4] It is important to be mindful that underlying mental health issues can often present with unexplained somatic complaints or sleep issues.[33]

LGBTQ newcomers, particularly refugee claimants, can struggle with emotional stress because of the humiliation, violence, and abuse they endured before leaving their countries.[4] Many individuals who faced torture exhibit trauma symptoms, such as flashbacks, depression, nightmares, and isolation.[4] Others who have experienced sexual violence have reported experiencing dyspareunia, vaginismus, or challenges involving sexual desire.[4]

Systemically, LGBTQ newcomers, notably those from African, Caribbean, and Black (ACB) communities, face multiple forms of oppression such as racism, discrimination, Islamophobia, refugee-phobia, homophobia, transphobia, and sexism.[3,4,40] Additionally, ACB communities often face HIV-related stigma.[41] LGBTQ newcomers may also confront additional stressors and difficulties, beyond those of other newcomers, in accessing proper housing, food, income, medical care, and employment because of discrimination or fear of discrimination.[4,40] As outlined in the minority stress model, experiences of oppression and stigma have a negative impact on mental well-being and increase the risks of mental and physical health issues.[42]

Not all LGBTQ refugees categorically face mental health challenges because of past experiences of abuse or violence. In fact, some LGBTQ refugees exhibit strengths, skills, and resilience in the face of adversities they experienced in their lives before, during, and after migration.[4] Therefore, it is fundamentally important that health care professionals approach their patients individually without making assumptions about their migration and mental health experiences.

Challenges in Accessing Health Care Insurance

In Canada, certain categories of newcomers, including refugee claimants, receive their health care insurance through the Interim Federal Health Program (IFHP), funded by IRCC. IFHP provides limited health care coverage for refugee claimants until they are accepted as refugees, in which case the IFHP coverage expires after 90 days. In the case of refused refugee claimants, their IFHP coverage lasts until they are removed from Canada or obtain permanent resident status through a different immigration channel.

It is now relatively straightforward for health care providers (i.e., physicians, therapists, and nurses who are registered with their respective provincial or territorial regulatory bodies or colleges) to become IFHP providers. Providers are required to register with Medavie Blue Cross, the administrator of the program on behalf of IRCC, to be reimbursed for services. Information about the coverage for health care services, including prescriptions and supplemental coverage for hearing aids, mobility aids, and so on, can be found on the Medavie Blue Cross website. However, a separate system of payment from the provincial or territorial health plans may prove to be a barrier for some to provide care. Furthermore, some providers report lengthy delays in reimbursement.

Access to mental health services covered through IFHP is crucial for LGBTQ refugees; however, the process of receiving services through IFHP is not without its challenges.[43] For example, hormone replacement therapy and gender-affirming surgeries are not covered by the IFHP for trans refugees.[44]

There are specific conditions for IFHP coverage for psychotherapy or counselling. To obtain coverage, mental health professionals must submit to Medavie Blue Cross (1) a referral and mental health diagnosis by a medical doctor or a nurse practitioner and (2) a mental health assessment report. After these documents are submitted, the wait time for approval is typically one to two weeks. Following approval, mental health professionals are expected to call Medavie Blue Cross on every occasion before meeting with their patient to confirm their eligibility for services. Claims submitted online through Medavie Blue Cross's portal may have a faster turnaround time than those submitted by fax or mail.

While awaiting approval to provide mental health services under IFHP, health service providers have ethical decisions to make regarding the care of their patients. Providers may need to decide whether to initiate care before the approval of coverage. Clinicians should consider assessing the severity and seriousness of the mental health concerns, as well as the level of functioning of their patients to assist in decision making. In certain cases, immediate treatment should be provided. For example, patients who are at higher risk of self-harm or suicide, or who are exhibiting severe symptoms should receive services immediately.

Overall, easier and faster access to health services approved by Medavie Blue Cross under the IFHP would have a positive impact on the health of LGBTQ refugee claimants.

Part 4: Enhancing the Roles of Health and Mental Health Providers

Physicians and mental health professionals have both clinical and ethical roles to perform while working with LGBTQ newcomers.[4] They must be culturally competent and have adequate training and education to work with this vulnerable population.[4] Thus, they require extra training in the areas related to the intersection of sexuality, gender identity, culture, and refugee mental health.[3] Unfortunately, health professions' training and continuing education courses specific to the needs of the LGBTQ newcomer population are not widely available.[4]

Additionally, health professionals play a pivotal role in assisting LGBTQ newcomers with systems navigation, including appropriate referrals to settlement support services such as housing, medical care, and employment. Settlement organizations can also assist with accessing many post-migration services, including language classes, school, housing, job training, and employment searches.

In light of the barriers to publicly funded counselling services specific to LGBTQ newcomers, health professionals may consider advocating for access to time-sensitive services that are trauma and refugee informed.[4] In an effort to address this step, they can educate community partners about systemic barriers that have negative impacts on the wellness of LGBTQ newcomers.[4] Subsequently, they can work in coalition with other partners, such as professional associations, universities, and community centres to educate municipal and provincial funders about the lack of resources available to support this population.[4] Health care providers can empower their patients to voice their concerns about the lack of services offered to them by various social service agencies in Canada.

Health care providers can improve their practices by orienting LGBTQ newcomers to the Canadian health care system, including confidentiality and navigating appointment-based systems. From our experiences, many patients have difficulty completing health care-related tasks, such as undergoing diagnostic tests or filling prescriptions.

Accurate assessment of a patient requires clear communication. This is particularly challenging because of the difficulty of interacting with and assessing complex issues of someone with different cultural norms and who does not speak English or French. Systematic reviews have found that the use of professional interpreters improves communication and increases the disclosure of psychological and physical symptoms compared to recruiting volunteers such as family, friends, and staff.[38] However, providers should be wary that some LGBTQ newcomers may feel uncomfortable speaking in front of professional interpreters who share the same cultural identity. Systematic reviews have found the use of professional interpreters as compared to volunteers improves communication and increases the disclosure of psychological symptoms and delivery of psychological services.[38] Unfortunately, the cost of hiring a professional interpreter is also commonly a prohibitive barrier. IFHP partially covers interpretation services upon request.

Health care professionals must be able to provide culturally competent care to their patients. Culturally competent health care "provides care to patients with diverse values, beliefs and behaviors including tailoring delivery to meet patients' social, cultural and linguistic needs."[45] Without a cross-cultural perspective in the practice of health care, providers might offend or compromise medical and mental health care by limiting communication. Finally, health care professionals and organizations should consider basing their practice on anti-racism, social justice, trauma-informed care and refugee-informed perspectives.[4] Otherwise, they risk providing care that may be harmful to patients.

Part 5: Conclusion

This chapter suggests that LGBTQ newcomers, specifically refugee claimants, experience a wide variety of health-related challenges before and during migration, and following their arrival in Canada.

Individuals often hide their LGBTQ identities for fear of violent and discriminatory repercussions from their families and ethnocultural communities. They may also suffer from shame and stigma surrounding their sexual or gender identities, worsening their health status. Moreover, LGBTQ newcomers may struggle to receive adequate health care once in Canada because of previous experiences of discrimination in a medical context, a culturally different understanding of health care, language barriers, and administrative barriers.

Based on our research and professional experiences, we advocate for a deeper understanding of the unique health care needs of LGBTQ newcomers and call on further collaboration between legal counsel and health professionals to better ensure access to justice for LGBTQ refugee claimants before the RPD members. We hope that with further research on the topics touched on in this chapter, health care tailored to LGBTQ refugee claimants will improve across Canada.

References

1. Rehaag S. Sexual orientation in Canada's revised refugee determination system: an empirical snapshot. Can J Women Law. 2017;29(2):259–89.
2. Robertson DC. Why is Canada only now accepting more LGBT asylum claims? Xtra [Internet]. 2017 Feb 2 [cited 2018 Jan 21]. Available from: https://www.dailyxtra.com/why-is-canada-only-now-accepting -more-lgbt-asylum-claims-72932.
3. Nerses M, Kleinplatz PJ, Moser C. Group therapy with international LGBTQ+ clients at the intersection of multiple minority status. Psychol Sex Rev. 2015;6(1):99–109.
4. Nerses M, Kleinplatz PJ. Seeking safety: Context, trauma, resilience. Unpublished manuscript. 2018. Available from: https://www .megonerses.com.
5. UN High Commissioner for Refugees. Guidelines on international protection No. 9: Claims to refugee status based on sexual orientation and/or gender identity within the context of article 1A(2) of the 1951 convention and/or its 1967 protocol relating to the status of refugees. Geneva, Switzerland: UNHCR; 2012. Available from: https://www .refworld.org/pdfid/50348afc2.pdf.
6. Shidlo A, Ahola J. Mental health challenges of LGBT forced migrants. Forced Migr Rev. 2013;1(42):9.
7. Hamberger A. Immigrant integration; Acculturation and social integration. J Ident Migr Stud. 2009;3(2):2–21.
8. Nwangwu JT. Nigerian immigrants in the United States: Race, identity and acculturation. Int Bull Mission Res. 2012;36(4):221.

9. Gibson MA. Immigrant adaptation and patterns of acculturation. Hum Development. 2001;44:19–23.

10. Rogler LH, Malgady RG, Costantino G, Blumenthal R. What do culturally sensitive mental health services mean? The case of Hispanics. Am Psychol. 1987 Jun;42(6):565–70.

11. Berry JW. Acculturation as varieties of adaptation. In: Padilla A, editor. Acculturation: theory, models and findings. Boulder: Westview; 1980. p. 9–25.

12. Berry JW. Stress perspectives on acculturation. In: Sam DL, Berry JW, editors. The Cambridge handbook of acculturation psychology. UK: Cambridge University Press; 2006. p. 43–57.

13. Tadmor CT, Tetlock PE, Peng K. Acculturation strategies and integrative complexity: the cognitive implications of biculturalism. J Cross Cult Psychol. 2009;40(1):105–39.

14. Berry JW. Immigration, acculturation, and adaptation. Appl Psychol. 1997;46(1):5–34.

15. Miller MJ. A bilinear multidimensional measurement model of Asian American acculturation and enculturation: implications for counseling interventions. J Couns Psychol. 2007;54(2):118–31.

16. Yoon E, Langrehr K, Ong LZ. Content analysis of acculturation research in counseling and counseling psychology: a 22-year review. J Couns Psychol. 2011 Jan;58(1):83–96.

17. Yoon E, Chang CT, Kim S, Clawson A, Cleary SE, Hansen M, et al. A meta-analysis of acculturation/enculturation and mental health. J Couns Psychol. 2013 Jan;60(1):15–30.

18. Chirkov V. Critical psychology of acculturation: what do we study and how do we study it, when we investigate acculturation? Int J Intercult Relat. 2009;33(2):94–105.

19. Cox N, Vanden Berghe W, Dewaele A, Vincke J. Acculturation strategies and mental health in gay, lesbian, and bisexual youth. J Youth Adolesc. 2010 Oct;39(10):1199–210.

20. Carpenter LM. From girls into women: scripts for sexuality and romance in seventeen magazine, 1974–1994. J Sex Res. 1998;35(2):158–68.

21. Buxton AP. A family matter: when a spouse comes out as gay, lesbian, or bisexual. J GLBT Fam Stud. 2005 Mar 31;1(2):49–70.

22. Jordal CE. "Making it work": a grounded theory of how mixed orientation married couples commit, sexually identify, and gender themselves [dissertation]. [Blacksburg (VA)]: Virginia Tech; 2011. Available from https://vtechworks.lib.vt.edu/bitstream/handle /10919/27664/Jordal_CE_D_2011.pdf.

23. Hersh N. Challenges to assessing same-sex relationships under refugee law in Canada. McGill Law J. 2015;60(3):527–71.

24. Immigration and Refugee Board of Canada [Internet]. Ottawa: Government of Canada; 2018 [cited 27 January 2018]. Claimant's guide. Available from: https://www.irb-cisr.gc.ca/en/refugee-claims/Pages /ClaDemGuide.aspx#_Toc340245806.

25. Immigration and Refugee Protection Act, SC 2001, c 27.

26. Immigration and Refugee Protection Regulations, SOR/2002-227.

27. Immigration and Refugee Board of Canada [Internet]. Ottawa: Government of Canada; 2020 Dec [cited 2021 Oct 3]. Available from: https://irb.gc.ca/en/legal-policy/legal-concepts/Pages/Credib.aspx.

28. Immigration and Refugee Board of Canada [Internet]. Ottawa: Government of Canada; 2006 Dec 15 [amended 2012 Dec 15; cited 2018 Jan 27]. Chairperson guideline 8: Procedures with respect to vulnerable persons appearing before the IRB. Available from: https://irb.gc.ca/en /legal-policy/policies/Pages/GuideDir08.aspx.

29. X (Re), 2014 CanLII 95779 (CA IRB). Available from: https://canlii.ca/t/gl1hs.

30. Murji v Canada (Minister of Citizenship and Immigration), 2004 FC 148 (CanLII). Available from: https://canlii.ca/t/1gd6x.

31. X (Re), 2015 CanLII 52119 (CA IRB). Available from: https://canlii.ca/t /gkrwq.

32. Warmington R, Miller K, Pottie K [Internet]. Ottawa: Canadian Collaboration for Immigrant and Refugee Health and University of Ottawa; 2012 [cited 2021 Oct 18]. Evidence-based preventive care checklist for new immigrants and refugees. Available from: http://www.ccirhken .ca/ccirh/checklist_website/index.html.

33. Pottie K, Greenaway C, Feightner J, Welch V, Swinkels H, Rashid M, et al.; coauthors of the Canadian Collaboration for Immigrant and Refugee Health. Evidence-based clinical guidelines for immigrants and refugees. CMAJ. 2011 Sep;183(12):E824–925.

34. Marsella AJ, White GM. Introduction: cultural conceptions in mental health research and practice. In: Marsella AJ, White GM, editors. Cultural conceptions of mental health and therapy. Culture, illness and healing. Volume 4. London: Springer, Dordrecht; 1982. p.3–8.

35. Kleinman A. Anthropology and psychiatry: The role of culture in cross-cultural research on illness. Br J Psychiatry. 1987 Oct;151(4):447–54.

36. Abdullah T, Brown TL. Mental illness stigma and ethnocultural beliefs, values, and norms: an integrative review. Clin Psychol Rev. 2011 Aug;31(6):934–48.

37. Corrigan PW, Miller FE. Shame, blame, and contamination: a review of the impact of mental illness stigma on family members. J Ment Health. 2004;13(6):537–48.

38. Kirmayer LJ, Narasiah L, Munoz M, Rashid M, Ryder AG, Guzder J, et al.; Canadian Collaboration for Immigrant and Refugee Health (CCIRH).

Common mental health problems in immigrants and refugees: general approach in primary care. CMAJ. 2011 Sep;183(12):E959–67.

39. Center for Substance Abuse Treatment (US). Trauma-informed care in behavioral health services. Rockville (MD): Substance Abuse and Mental Health Services Administration (US); 2014. Report No.: (SMA) 14-4816. PMID: 24901203.

40. Logie CH, Lacombe-Duncan A, Lee-Foon N, Ryan S, Ramsay H. "It's for us – newcomers, LGBTQ persons, and HIV-positive persons. You feel free to be": a qualitative study exploring social support group participation among African and Caribbean lesbian, gay, bisexual and transgender newcomers and refugees in Toronto, Canada. BMC Int Health Hum Rights. 2016 Jul;16(1):18.

41. Kerr J, Burton K, Tharao W, Greenspan N, Calzavara L, Browne O, et al. Examining HIV-related stigma among African, Caribbean, and Black church congregants from the Black PRAISE study in Ontario, Canada. AIDS Care. 2021 Dec;33(12):1636–41.

42. Meyer IH. Prejudice, social stress, and mental health in lesbian, gay and bisexual populations: conceptual issues and research evidence. Psychol Bull. 2003 Sep;129(5):674–97.

43. McKeary M, Newbold B. Barriers to care: the challenges for Canadian refugees and their health care providers. J Refug Stud. 2010;23(4):523–45.

44. Jacob T. Embodied migrations: Mapping trans and gender non-conforming refugee narratives in Canada's refugee regime. Montreal: McGill University; 2020.

45. Betancourt JR, Green AR, Carrillo JE. Cultural competence in health care: emerging frameworks and practical approaches [Internet]. New York: Commonwealth Fund, Quality of Care for Underserved Populations; 2002 [cited 2021 Oct 18]]. Available from: http://www.cmwf.org/usr_doc/betancourt_culturalcompetence_576.pdf.

Glossary

AFAB/AMAB: an acronym denoting individuals who were assigned female at birth and assigned male at birth, respectively.

bisexual: a binary term denoting a person who is attracted to both men and women. Bisexual identities are not homogeneous – each person may be attracted in differing degrees to men and women over time and within changing contexts. Some people who identify as bisexual may also be attracted to non-binary individuals; however, many with a spectrum of attractions prefer the more inclusive term *pansexual*. Although bisexual attractions are not limited to one gender, do not presume non-monogamy.

butch: A form of gender expression. A masculine-identified person of any gender identity.

cis: Having a non-transgender identity (may also sometimes see *cis-sexual* or *cisgender*). It is preferable to use *cis* than to use terms such as *biological, genetic,* or *real*.

cissexism: The ideas and actions resulting from the belief that cis identities or bodies are more "real" or "valid" than trans ones. This is distinct from *transphobia* (which denotes hatred and fear towards trans persons).

coming out: The process of disclosing to others one's sexual orientation or gender identity that would not otherwise be known. This process

Adapted from Guidelines for Gender-Affirming Primary Care for Trans and Non-binary Patients. 4th ed., Toronto, ON: Rainbow Health Ontario, a program of Sherbourne Health; 2019 and Homophobia, heterosexism and AIDS: Creating a more effective response to AIDS. Ottawa, ON: Canadian AIDS Society; 1991.

may occur over a short, intense time, or it may be a gradual process wherein a person initially takes into confidence only a close friend. Coming out is a highly individualized process, governed by one's own comfort level and internal and external influences.

differences of sexual differentiation (DSDs): A term used to describe the various conditions experienced by those who are intersex. Used in this text in place of the more common but pathologizing term *disorders of sexual differentiation*. Persons with a DSD may be cis or trans, depending on how their gender identity relates to the one assigned to them at birth.

femme: A form of gender expression. A feminine-identified person of any gender identity.

FTM: An older term to describe transmasculine individuals. It has fallen out of favour because of its binary nature; it also conflates sex and gender identity and forever identifies the assignment that one is transitioning away from.

gay: A man (or masculine-spectrum individual) whose primary interest, sexually and intimately, is with his own gender. Although the term is often used when referring to both homosexual men and women, some women feel that this is similar to using masculine pronouns as inclusive terms and that *gay* does not satisfactorily establish their identity as distinct from men.

gender: Behavioural, cultural, or psychological traits commonly associated with one sex. Unlike sex, which is biologically determined, gender is considered to be a social construct.

gender expression: The social expression of gender. Often described as being on a spectrum between masculine and feminine. Often related to, but sometimes distinct from, gender identity.

gender identity: A person's internal self-awareness of being a boy/man, girl/woman, something in between, or something other altogether.

genderqueer: A person whose gender identity does not align with binary gender categories such as "man/woman" or "boy/girl." Genderqueer persons often identify as having an intermediary gender.

heterosexism: The promotion and perpetuation of the superiority of heterosexuality and the assumption that everyone is heterosexual. Heterosexism awards privileges to the dominant group while denying non-heterosexuals access to similar rights and privileges (legal, financial, and social). Examples of heterosexism in practice include the assumption that a person's partner is of the other sex or the denial of survivor benefits to a lesbian because she was not a legal "spouse" of the deceased.

homophobia: An irrational fear of, aversion to, or discrimination against homosexuality or homosexuals, which can be expressed through social ostracism, religious and legal interdiction, and verbal, physical, and sexual violence.

homosexual: An outmoded term used historically for diagnostic purposes, meaning attracted to persons of the same sex. It is preferable to use *gay* or *lesbian* or to use the term by which a person self-identifies.

internalized homophobia: Internalized fear or shame of and for one's own sexuality. Such feelings are often evoked by external messages that one's innate way of being is disgusting, sick, or unnatural, and may be expressed by feelings that this is true of one's self.

intersex: The state of being born with genitalia that is difficult to label as male or female or developing secondary sex characteristics of indeterminate sex or a combination of features of both sexes. Some intersex people are also trans, but intersex is not considered a subset of transgender, nor transgender a subset of intersex.

lesbian: A woman (or feminine-spectrum individual) whose primary interest, sexually and intimately, is with her own sex.

LG, LGB, LGBQ, 2SLGBQ: Acronyms that may be used (for example, in research) when describing only those who identify as lesbian, gay, +/– bisexual, +/– queer, +/– Two-Spirit, and not those who are trans or non-binary.

MSM: An acronym denoting men who have sex with men; it is used to capture the broad range of men who engage in sexual activity with other men irrespective of their sexual identity.

MTF: An old term to describe transfeminine individuals. It has fallen out of favour because of its binary nature; it also conflates sex and gender identity and forever identifies the assignment that one is transitioning away from.

non-binary: An umbrella term for anyone who does not identify with static, binary gender identities. Includes persons who may identify as having an intermediary gender (e.g., genderqueer), as being multiple genders, as having a constantly shifting gender, or as not having a gender altogether.

pansexual: A person who is attracted to others regardless of their biological sex, gender expression, or gender identity. Considered by some to be more inclusive than the term *bisexual*, as it more explicitly includes those who do not identify with binary categories of sex and gender. As with those who identify as bisexual, do not presume non-monogamy.

queer: A previously derogatory term for gays and lesbians now re-appropriated by sexual- and gender-minority people. It is more popular than terms such as *gay* or *lesbian* with younger generations because of the binary nature of these terms. Because of its historical derogatory use, some (particularly older adults) may continue to experience this word as offensive.

sex: Describes one's genotype and phenotype. Often determined by genital configuration at birth. Referred to in terms of *male, female,* or *intersex*. Often erroneously conflated with gender identity.

sexual identity: A chosen mode of self-presentation, based on social identity, sexual behaviour, or both. A person may choose to publicly identify using a term that does not strictly conform to their sexual behaviour (e.g., a man who identifies as heterosexual may engage in sex with other men, or a bisexual woman may be intimate only with women). How one identifies one's self is a personal choice.

sexual orientation: Refers to the group(s) of persons that someone may desire intimate emotional or sexual relationships with. This term is preferred over *sexual preference*, which implies that one's desires are a matter of choice rather than an inherent part of one's nature. Examples of sexual orientations include straight, queer, lesbian, gay, bisexual, pansexual, and asexual. Everyone, cis or trans, has a sexual orientation.

trans/transgender: An umbrella term for people who are not cis, includes persons who are (or identify as) non-binary as well as trans men and trans women.

transition: The sum total of changes involved in moving from living as one gender to another. Typically a stage in a trans person's life. May include social transition (e.g., name and pronoun change) or medical transition (e.g., hormones and surgery).

transphobia: An irrational fear of, aversion to, or discrimination against trans persons, which can be expressed through social ostracism, religious and legal interdiction, and verbal, physical, and sexual violence.

transsexual: Describes persons who undergo medical transition (typically including surgical interventions) and social transition to align the gender they live and present as with their internal gender identity.

trans man/transgender man/transmasculine: Umbrella terms to describe all persons assigned female at birth who transition to live as boys/men or somewhere on the masculine spectrum.

trans woman/transgender woman/transfeminine: Umbrella terms to describe all persons assigned male at birth who transition to live as girls/women or somewhere on the feminine spectrum.

Two-Spirit: An umbrella term describing the diversity of gender and sexual identities present in traditional belief systems held by North American First Nations persons.

WSW: An acronym denoting women who have sex with women; a term used to capture the broad range of women who engage in sexual activity with other women, irrespective of how they identify their sexual orientation.

Contributors

Ian Armstrong is a family physician practising at Maple Leaf Medical Clinic and Hassle Free sexual health clinic. After completing his residency in family medicine at McMaster University, he completed additional postgraduate training in HIV primary care and 2SLGBTQ health at the University of Toronto. They are also involved with the Trans Women HIV Research Initiative, with a focus on gender-affirming hormone therapy in the context of antiretroviral therapy.

Amy Bourns (she/her) – since completing the first 2SLGBTQ Enhanced Skills Residency Program with the Department of Family and Community Medicine at the University of Toronto in 2011, Amy Bourns has practised comprehensive primary care as part of the LGBT2SQ team at Sherbourne Health in Toronto, Ontario. Over the past decade, Amy has spear-headed multiple initiatives aimed at expanding the capacity of health care providers in caring for 2SLGBTQ patients, including authorship of Sherbourne Health's *Guidelines for Gender-affirming Primary Care with Trans and Non-binary* Patients and the adapted interactive online *Trans Primary Care Guide*. Amy takes an avid interest in medical education, having served as the inaugural faculty lead for 2SLGBTQ Health at the University of Toronto Temerty Faculty of Medicine and currently acting as the university's program director for the 2SLGBTQ Enhanced Skills Residency Program, offering family medicine residency graduates the opportunity to develop expertise and foster leadership in 2SLGBTQ health. Amy is a queer, cisgender, white settler descended from English and Irish immigrants, raised on the traditional lands of many Indigenous peoples, including the Mississaugas of the Credit, the Anishinaabe, the Haudenosaunee, and the Wendat, in the Greater Toronto Area. Amy currently resides in Toronto with her partner and daughter.

Alexandre Coutin (he/him, they/them) is a senior resident physician in emergency medicine at the University of Ottawa. Dr. Coutin completed their MD at the University of Toronto, where their passion for justice precipitated an interest in the care of sex- and gender-minority communities. They have been involved in numerous medical education initiatives to better train providers to care for the 2SLGBTQ community, thereby reducing medical violence. This includes educational tools now used internationally for clinical skills teaching, among others. They continue to bring a strong focus on advocacy in their role as senior editor with the EMOttawa Digital Scholarship and Knowledge Dissemination Program. They are an executive member of the Canadian Association of Emergency Physicians (CAEP) 2SLGBTQIA+ National Committee and have additional interests in health care worker wellness, addictions medicine, sexual health, public health, and point-of-care ultrasound. Dr. Coutin's work has been featured in *Resuscitation*, the *Canadian Journal of Medical Education*, and the *Canadian Journal of Emergency Medicine*, and at numerous national and international conferences, with the hope of creating a safer space for queer and trans patients within the health sphere. Dr. Coutin is a queer, white settler of French ancestry raised in the traditional and unceded land of the Kanien'kehà:ka in Montreal, Quebec.

Christopher (Kit) Fairgrieve is a physician. He completed his residency in family medicine at McMaster University and a clinical fellowship in addiction medicine at the University of British Columbia. He is currently a staff physician in the addiction medicine programs at St. Michael's Hospital in Toronto and St. Joseph's Healthcare Hamilton. He is an assistant professor in the Department of Family and Community Medicine at the University of Toronto and an assistant clinical professor (adjunct) in the Department of Family Medicine at McMaster University. Dr. Fairgrieve has also completed an addiction research fellowship with the BC Centre on Substance Use and the Research Addiction Medicine Scholars (RAMS) program at Boston Medical Centre. His primary research interests are in addiction medicine, specifically the use of managed alcohol programs in hospital. He has contributed to work published in *Substance Abuse, Journal of Addiction Medicine, Harm Reduction Journal, Medical Clinics of North America*, and the *Cochrane Database of Systemic Reviews*. Dr. Fairgrieve is a queer, cisgender, white settler of Scottish and English ancestry raised in the traditional territory of the Huron-Wendat, the Seneca, and the Mississaugas of the Credit First Nation in Toronto, Ontario.

Jacqueline Gahagan, PhD, is a medical sociologist, associate vice president of research, and professor of gender and women studies at Mount Saint Vincent University in Halifax, Nova Scotia, Canada. Jacquie has published widely in the areas of equity in access to health services among 2SLGBT populations, sex- and gender-based analysis in health promotion and public health, and has co-edited the book *Sex- and Gender-Based Analysis in Public Health* (2021), published by Springer.

Carol Geller is a family doctor who has been practising at Centretown Community Health Centre in Ottawa, Ontario, since 1999. She has a special interest in working with inner-city populations, and her practice has a large proportion of people new to Canada and those who are struggling with mental health and addiction problems. She is the co-founder of a clinic for those new to Canada that has been in existence since 2007, serving mostly refugee claimants and providing health care customized to their unique needs.

Jordan Goodridge is a lecturer with the Temerty Faculty of Medicine at the University of Toronto and is a family physician working at Sherbourne Health, where he has a focused practice in 2SLGBTQ+ health. He received his MD from Queen's University in Kingston, Ontario, completed his family medicine training at McMaster University in Hamilton, and did an Enhanced Skills year in HIV primary care through the University of Toronto. He has a strong interest in medical education and currently teaches in the undergraduate medicine program at the University of Toronto, in addition to teaching elective medical students and residents at Sherbourne Health. He is a faculty member of the Department of Family and Community Medicine and stays involved with the postgraduate family medicine residency program, delivering lectures in HIV primary care and sexual health as part of their academic half-day curriculum. He leads seminars in transgender health through Rainbow Health Ontario and the Centre for Addiction and Mental Health, geared towards health care providers in various stages of training.

Zongwe Binesikwe (Sounding Thunderbird Woman) Crystal Hardy (they/she) is a Two-Spirit Anishinaabe nurse practitioner. Zongwe is a PhD candidate in nursing at Queen's University, with a focus on cultural humility in action using Indigenous autoethnography to explore spiritual self-reflection and using expressive arts to address compassion fatigue.

Elizabeth Harrison is a registered nurse working to make health care accessible to systemically excluded and impoverished people. Elizabeth currently works on the Street Clinical Outreach for Unsheltered Torontonians team. Their practice is informed by their lived experience as a cancer survivor and survivor of suicide loss. Elizabeth is a white settler who works in Toronto, the traditional territory of many nations including the Mississaugas of the Credit, Anishnaabek, Chippewa, Haudenosaunee, and Wendat peoples and is now home to many First Nations, Inuit, and Métis peoples, and is covered by Treaty 13 with the Mississaugas of the Credit.

Nicholas Hersh (he/him) is an immigration and refugee lawyer at Community Legal Services of Ottawa and professor of the Refugee Sponsorship Support Program course at the University of Ottawa Faculty of Law. He has worked extensively in refugee private sponsorship since 2010 with Capital Rainbow Refuge, a community group committed to providing a safe haven for refugees with diverse sexual orientation, gender identity, gender expression, and sex characteristics (SOGIESC). Nicholas has published in peer-reviewed journals on credibility and evidentiary challenges facing LGBTQ claimants in refugee law, as well as a chapter on improving United Nations High Commissioner for Refugees protection services for LGBTQ refugees. In 2017 and 2018, he delivered professional development trainings to the Immigration and Refugee Board's adjudicators, registrar staff, and research directorate on the SOGIESC Guideline. In July 2021, he released the Queer Refugee Hearings Program Toolkit, an innovative and interactive tool to assist counsel representing SOGIESC refugee claimants.

Emily Hughes is an internal medicine resident physician at the University of Toronto and chief medical resident at Women's College Hospital (2022–2023). Dr. Hughes completed her MD at the University of Toronto. She is interested broadly in equity and leadership. In July 2017, she wrote *The Medical Post's* cover series of stories on gender equity in medicine. She credits her time volunteering at The 519 Space for Change in Toronto for inspiring her to pursue actionable change in health care settings such that healthcare providers are better equipped to be allies to members of 2SLGBTQ communities. Dr. Hughes is a cisgender, white settler of British ancestry raised on Treaty 7 territory in Calgary, Alberta.

Elise Jackson (she/her) is an internal medicine resident at the University of British Columbia and chief medical resident at Vancouver

General Hospital (2021–2022). She completed her undergraduate studies at McGill University and her MD at the University of Toronto. Dr. Jackson has a longstanding interest in social justice and throughout her training has been active in curriculum development focused on increasing content related to equity and anti-oppression in medical training, at both the undergraduate and the postgraduate level. Dr. Jackson is a cisgender, white settler of British ancestry, raised on the traditional territories of the Beothuk in St. John's, Newfoundland and Labrador, and the Guringai in Sydney, Australia, and is now living on the stolen and unceded territory of the Coast Salish Peoples, including the xwm kw y m (Musqueam), Skwxwú7mesh (Squamish), Stó:lō, and Səl̓ílwətaʔ/Selilwitulh (Tsleil-Waututh) Nations.

Edward Kucharski (he/him) is a practising family physician at the Southeast Toronto Family Health Team and chief medical officer for Casey House Hospital. Throughout his career, Ed has focused on the health inequities of communities that face barriers to care. He has taught about 2SLGBTQ primary care at various medical schools, centres and conferences. Ed was also a regional primary care lead (Toronto Central Local Health Integration Network, South) for Cancer Care Ontario and the Toronto Central Regional Cancer Program. In 2013, Ed was the recipient of both the Association of Family Health Team's Bright Lights Award – Improving the Health of the 5% and the University of Toronto's Department of Family and Community Medicine Excellence in Community Teaching Award. In 2015, Ed was recognized by The Change Foundation as one of Ontario's 20 Faces of Change for innovative, and patient-centred initiatives to improve cancer screening in 2SLGBTQ, newcomer, and homeless populations. Ed holds his doctorate in medicine from the University of Ottawa and completed his residency in family medicine at the University of Toronto. Ed is a gay, cisgender, white settler descended from English, Polish, Scottish, and Ukrainian immigrants, raised on the traditional lands of many indigenous peoples, including the Mississaugas of the Credit, the Anishinaabe, the Haudenosaunee, and the Wendat, in the Greater Toronto Area.

Laura MacDonald is a registered nurse who currently works in primary care at Regent Park Community Health Centre. She previously worked in attendant care and has a keen interest in adaptive design. She has been actively involved in the design and provision of low-barrier health care in Toronto's downtown east, with particular focus on harm reduction services and provision of low-barrier health care for people who use drugs. She is a white settler who grew up on the traditional lands of the Mi'kmaq people in Halifax, Nova Scotia, and currently lives on the traditional lands of many Indigenous peoples, including the Anishinabek Nation, the Haudenosaunee Confederacy, the Huron-Wendat, and the Métis, in Toronto, Ontario.

Catherine Maser (she/her) is a nurse practitioner in the Division of Adolescent Medicine at the Hospital for Sick Children, Toronto, where she has been the team lead (and a founding member) of the Transgender Youth Clinic since its opening in 2013 and the co-lead for the adolescent medicine consultation service. Cathy has over 35 years of experience working with children, youth, and their caregivers, and her clinical focus is with youth with chronic illness, substance misuse, sexual health, gender identity, and minor mood disorders. Cathy is actively involved in partnerships within the adolescent and transgender care communities and often provides education to schools, parents, health care providers, and community agencies on adolescent brain development, mental health, substance use, and gender-diverse identities. Cathy has academic and professional teaching credentials, having been on faculty at the Lawrence S Bloomberg Faculty of Nursing, University of Toronto for 12 years in both the undergraduate and the graduate programs.

Christopher McIntosh (BSc, MSc, MD, FRCPC, DFAPA) is an associate professor of psychiatry at the University of Toronto and editor-in-chief of *The Journal of Gay and Lesbian Mental Health*, one of the longest-running academic journals for LGBTQ+ mental health now in its 32nd year of publication. He is on the executive board of AGLP: The Association of LGBTQ+ Psychiatrists and is a senior fellow of the Group for the Advancement of Psychiatry. He is the past clinic head of the Adult Gender Identity Clinic at the Centre for Addiction and Mental Health.

Mego Nerses (he/him) is a clinical consultant and trauma-informed registered psychotherapist based in Ottawa, Ontario. He provides psychotherapy in English, Arabic, and Armenian. He integrates social justice perspectives into his psychotherapy practice. Specifically, he specializes in the trauma, sexuality, and mental health of LGBTQI+ refugees and asylum seekers. Mego has extensive experience working with LGBTQI+ refugees and asylum seekers in Canada. He was awarded the 2017 Humanitarian Award by the Canadian Counselling and Psychotherapy Association in recognition of his contributions to LGBTQI+ refugees and asylum seekers in Canada. Mego provides online courses, workshops, and consultations on trauma and mental health issues affecting LGBTQI+ refugees at the national and international level. His website is www.megonerses.com.

Quang Nguyen (he/him) is a clinical lecturer in the Department of Family and Community Medicine at the University of Toronto. Dr. Nguyen completed his MD degree at the University of Western Ontario and his post-doctoral medical training at the University of Toronto. Dr. Nguyen holds a dual MPH/MBA degree from Johns Hopkins University and has a strong commitment to health equity through community engagement and patient advocacy. As a family physician at Sherbourne Health, Dr. Nguyen specializes in 2SLGBTQ primary care, with a focus on HIV and gay men's health. Through his lived experience, Dr. Nguyen provides culturally competent and compassionate care to patients who face multiple barriers to health care access, including those who are homeless and underhoused, refugees and immigrants, racialized sexual and gender minorities, and people living with HIV/AIDS. As an educator, Dr. Nguyen enjoys teaching and preparing medical trainees to become future 2SLGBTQ allies and advocates in family medicine.

Carrie Schram is a family physician with a fellowship in women's health and a master of public health. Dr. Schram is an assistant professor at the University of Toronto in the Department of Family and Community Medicine and the medical director and medical chief of the Natural Conception Program at Hannam Fertility Centre in Toronto, Ontario. For over 10 years, Dr. Schram has been practising low-intervention fertility and low-risk obstetrics, within which she supports 2SLGBTQ families as they journey through these life events. Dr. Schram is an advocate for de-medicalized fertility care and honouring diverse populations and family types.

Lisa Smith (she/her) is a registered nurse who works at Toronto Public Health as a health promotion specialist on the Child Care Infection Prevention and Control team. She completed her BScN at Nipissing University in the Scholar Practitioner Program where she specialized in public health nursing. She holds a BA in English Literature and Religious Studies from Concordia University. Over the last several years, Lisa has worked as a counsellor on the Sexual Health Info Line Ontario (SHILO), in the needle exchange at The Works, and as a breast/chest feeding peer support worker. Before working in health care Lisa was a hairdresser and a musician. She is a queer, cisgender, white settler descended from British, Irish, German, Dutch, Spanish, and French immigrants. She grew up on the traditional territories of the Omàmìwininìwag and Anishinabewaki in Western Quebec. She currently lives in Toronto with her partner, their children, and their senior cats Vlad and Farrah.

Laura Stratton (she/her) is a lecturer in the Department of Family and Community Medicine at the University of Toronto. Dr. Stratton completed her medical degree at the University of Toronto and her family medicine residency at Women's College Hospital in Toronto, Ontario. After her family medicine training, she pursued an Enhanced Skills program at the University of Toronto in 2SLGBTQ+ health. Dr. Stratton currently provides comprehensive primary care to patients at Women's College Family Practice and virtual trans and gender diverse care to patients throughout Ontario at the Connect Clinic. She is actively involved in teaching 2SLGBTQ+ care to medical students and residents. Dr. Stratton is a queer, cisgender, white settler of English and Polish ancestry raised in the traditional territory of the Mississaugas of the Credit First Nation in Milton, Ontario. She currently lives in Toronto with her wife.

Sydney Tam is a queer, trans, Asian, settler, woman, family physician, and emergency room doctor. She has been in practice for over 30 years in Canada and the United States and has seen and overseen many changes in the care of 2SLGBTQ+ adolescents and adults over the decades. She is a lecturer at the University of Toronto Department of Family and Community Medicine. Teaching 2SLGBTQ+ competent care and anti-oppressive care to medical students and residents is an intrinsic part of her teaching practice. She has a special interest in anti-oppression, equity, diversity, and inclusion in medicine, and the intersections of the history of medicine and diverse populations. She has been a guest on multiple national television programs, most notably the *Oprah Winfrey Show*, and has received multiple practice quality awards, including the Gay and Lesbian Medical Association Provider of the Year award. Dr. Tam has multiple interests outside of medicine: she has various credits in music and filmmaking and is a passionate photographer and athlete. She lives with her partner and three grown children just outside Toronto, Canada.

Ashley Vandermorris (she/her) is a staff paediatrician in the Division of Adolescent Medicine at the Hospital for Sick Children (Sick-Kids) and a member of the SickKids Centre for Global Child Health. Dr. Vandermorris completed her undergraduate degree at Yale University;

her medical degree at Harvard Medical School; a residency in paediatrics and fellowships in adolescent medicine and global child health at SickKids; and an MSc in health policy, management, and evaluation at the University of Toronto. As an adolescent medicine physician, Dr. Vandermorris is committed to championing the ideals of accessibility, advocacy, equity, justice, and collaboration as the fundamental tenets that will enable improved health outcomes for youth. Dr. Vandermorris works in the Transgender Youth Clinic and the Young Families programs within the Division of Adolescent Medicine, where her clinical focus is on collaborating with youth navigating the intersections of structural and social determinants of health to achieve healthy developmental trajectories. Her research program emphasizes participatory methods and working with intersectoral, multidisciplinary teams to examine adolescent-responsive, rights-based approaches to transforming health systems to promote improved health outcomes for youth, in both the local and the global context.

A.J. Withers is a white settler who lives and works in Tkaronto/Toronto, the traditional territories of the Anishinabek, Chippewa, Haudenosaunee, and Wendat. They are adjunct faculty of critical disability studies at York University. They completed their PhD at the York University School of Social Work, and they centre social justice and an intersectional lens in all of their work. Their primary research interests are disability studies, homelessness, social movements, and social interventions. They are the author of *Fight to Win: Inside Poor People's Organizing* (Fernwood, 2021), *A Violent History of Benevolence: Interlocking Oppression in the Moral Economies of Social Working* (University of Toronto Press, 2019) with Chris Chapman, and *Disability Politics and Theory* (Fernwood, 2012). Their work has also appeared in *The Canadian Review of Social Policy* and multiple scholarly anthologies, and they have written journalistic pieces, including in *Everyday Feminism, Now Magazine, and Al Jazeera*. Dr. Withers is also a long-time social justice and disability justice activist, drawing on their lived experiences of being poor, disabled, queer, and trans/non-binary.

Index

Milton Keynes UK
Ingram Content Group UK Ltd.
UKHW011550150324
439587UK00025B/341